ESSENTIALS OF PERIODONTOLOGY AND PERIODONTICS

ESSENTIALS OF PERIODONTOLOGY AND PERIODONTICS

TORQUIL MACPHEE
BDS, FDSRCSE, DRD
Senior Lecturer in Oral Medicine and Pathology, University of Edinburgh
Head of the Department of Periodontology, Edinburgh Dental Hospital
Consultant in charge of the Edinburgh School of Oral Hygiene
Honorary Consultant Dental Surgeon to the Lothian Area Health Board

AND

GEOFFREY COWLEY
BDS, DDS
Professor of Preventive Dentistry, University of Dundee
Head of the Department of Periodontology and Community Dentistry,
Dundee Dental Hospital
Honorary Consultant Dental Surgeon, Tayside Health Board

THIRD EDITION

BLACKWELL SCIENTIFIC PUBLICATIONS
OXFORD   LONDON   EDINBURGH
BOSTON   MELBOURNE

© 1969, 1975, 1981 by
Blackwell Scientific Publications
Editorial Offices:
Osney Mead, Oxford OX2 0EL
8 John Street, London WC1N 2ES
9 Forrest Road, Edinburgh EH1 2QH
52 Beacon Street, Boston,
    Massachusetts 02108, USA
214 Berkeley Street, Carlton
    Victoria 3053, Australia

First Edition 1969
Reprinted 1972
Second Edition 1975
Japanese Edition 1979
Third Edition 1981

Printed and bound in Great Britain by
William Clowes (Beccles) Limited,
Beccles and London

DISTRIBUTORS

USA
    Blackwell Mosby Book Distributors
    11830 Westline Industrial Drive
    St Louis, Missouri 63141

Canada
    Blackwell Mosby Book Distributors
    120 Melford Drive, Scarborough
    Ontario, M1B 2X4

Australia
    Blackwell Scientific Book
    Distributors
    214 Berkeley Street, Carlton
    Victoria 3053

ISBN 0 632 00533 5

Contents

Foreword

This is a book which I think you will enjoy. It has all the attractions of a good book, well written, well illustrated and well worth reading. By its title it claims to contain the essentials of the subject but it seems to me that it contains much more than the bare essentials and very little, if anything, has been omitted. It is therefore a sound book for undergraduate and postgraduate students to use. It will be ideal for general practitioners seeking to get an up to date view of this important part of modern dental practice. The book I find is conveniently divided into two sections, from chapter eight to the end there is a full coverage of the clinical aspects and the preceding chapters deal with the basic pathology and the applied aspect of the biological sciences. The busy practitioner will probably first want to read onwards from chapter eight to get the authors' views on clinical practice and treatment. This he can do and he will find what is advocated has been thoroughly tried out but he should not ignore the first seven chapters. Let him settle in a comfortable chair and read these early chapters, he will find them rewarding. Sir William Osler said 'as your pathology so your treatment' this is still applicable to our practice to-day for we cannot adequately treat disease if we do not understand it. But to-day we have to prefix a phrase to this old aphorism and it is 'as your biology so your pathology' for modern biological sciences contribute so much to our understanding of disease that the scientific background to modern pathology has to be stated and this is one of the commendable features of this book.

This is the first text book produced by the members of staff of the Periodontal Department of the School of Dental Surgery, University of Edinburgh and for that reason it is very welcome. If the achievements of the department are anything to go by, the book will have much success.

JOHN BOYES

Preface

Conservative periodontics are the fashion of the times. There is increasing disenchantment with traditional diagnostic criteria such as plaque and gingival indices which do not distinguish between 'contained' and 'progressive' periodontitis and do not reflect active tissue destruction in the submarginal tissues. Periodontitis is a subgingival plaque associated disease and there is a refreshing growing acceptance that oral hygiene procedures have little effect on the ecology of subgingival plaque in crevices over 2.5 mm or on the progression of periodontitis. Good oral hygiene while eminently desirable may only serve to mask the presence of progressive disease.

There is presently no clear answer to these problems. Each chapter has been updated in the areas where apparently relevant information has emerged. The aetiology of periodontitis has been redeveloped as three chapters. The possibility that gingivitis and periodontitis are a series of sequential infections and the possible role of diagnostic bacteriology in assessment of treatment need are considered. This theme is further developed throughout the chapters on treatment planning and patient treatment.

While in sympathy with the present vogue for conservative periodontics the danger with enthusiasts is that they persisistently attempt to discredit all but the particular enthusiasm of the time. There is presently a reduced role for surgery and occlusal therapy in control of periodontitis but the need for knowledge and understanding of these techniques still exists. It is only the judgement of when to use them which has altered and it may be that there will be increased frequency of use under slightly different conditions within the forseeable future.

The diagnostic and treatment programmes described are in use in either or both of our clinics and represent a balanced approach on the basis of information presently available.

We thank Mrs Linda Lyall, Mrs Jan Chapman and Miss Anne Taylor for help in preparing the revised manuscript, and also Mr Ian Goddard for the new photographs.

T.M. *I take the view and always have done that if you cannot say what you have to say in twenty minutes you should go away and write a book about it.*
Lord Brabazon
Reported in the Press. June 1955.

G.C. *If a man will begin with certainties, he shall end in doubts; but if he will be content to begin with doubts he shall end in certainties.*
Francis Bacon,
The Advancement of Learning, I, v. 8.

Preface to First Edition

Something more than 40 per cent of teeth are extracted following caries, something less than 40 per cent following periodontal disease, and something more than 10 per cent for more bizarre reasons. The pattern of dental practice in Britain does not parallel the realities of tooth mortality and reorientation of the dental profession towards devoting a greater percentage of effort to control of periodontal disease is inevitable.

This book is about nonspecific periodontitis and its treatment. Periodontology is a rapidly developing science, and the practice of periodontics is to some extent still confused by the not inconsiderable mythology of the past. The object is to review the present state of knowledge of periodontology as we understand it and to relate this to a programme of patient treatment. The reference system shows the source of the information presented, and distinguishes mythology from what may be regarded as more responsible views.

The function of this book is to create an understanding of concepts and attitudes to the subject rather than didactic repetition of minutiae of techniques which are matters of personal preference, best learned at the chairside. For example, we have included a small section on technique of scaling largely to underline the need for a systematic and disciplined approach using suitable instruments. The particular system which is used, and the choice of instruments, are matters for the individual within the limitations of the general principles which are illustrated. Good technique automatically follows a clear understanding of the general principles underlying the procedure that the operator plans to carry out.

The book is intended to present a logical sequence of information on which to base a programme of patient treatment. Each chapter, however, is designed to be largely complete in itself, and intelligible without necessarily having read those preceding. The first chapters review the scientific aspect of the subject primarily for the convenience of present day undergraduate and postgraduate students. The clinical chapters are designed for the convenience of any student or dentist, and the system of treatment planning is that presently used by the Scottish Dental Estimates Board as a basis for estimates for periodontal treatment in the National Health Service.

We are indebted to the previous Heads of the Department of Periodontology in the Edinburgh Dental School, Dr J.W. Galloway and Professor G.S. Beagrie with whom we have worked during our years as students and as members of the staff and to Professors John Boyes and John Mansbridge for their constant encouragement. We have received much valuable advice and guidance during preparation of the manuscript from our self-chosen readers, Professor W.D. McHugh of the Chair of Dental Health, University of Dundee, Mr A.J.W. McKendrick, Senior Lecturer in the Department of Periodontology, University of Dundee, and Docent Jan Egelberg of the School of Dentistry, Malmö, Sweden. It must be made clear, however, that responsibility for the views expressed in this book lies entirely with us, and that the readers are in no way committed.

We thank Miss Mary Benstead, sometime Medical Artist in the Edinburgh Dental School for the drawings so signed; Mr Alex. Hunter, M.B.E. Chief Technician in the Edinburgh Dental School, Mr Robert Renton and Mr Ian Goddard for the quality of many of the photographs taken over the years: Mrs Jean Carus, Miss Edna Miller, Mrs C. Weir and other Secretaries who have assisted in preparation of the manuscript: Miss Anne Taylor for her assistance with the index.

T.M.   *As a rule disease as it stalks through*
        the land cannot keep pace with the
        incurable vice of scribbling about it.
        John Mayou de Rachitide, 1668

G.C.   *Oh that one would hear me! behold, my desire is,*
        that the Almighty would answer me and
        that mine adversary had written a book.
        Job 31:35

Preface to Second Edition

The format of this book remains similar to that of the first edition. Each chapter has been updated in the areas where it seemed that significant information had emerged during the six years since the original manuscript was prepared, and a short review of the epidemiology of gingivitis and periodontitis forms an additional chapter.

Laboratory studies have now confirmed the significance of immunologic mechanisms in periodontitis and what was to some extent 'crystal ball gazing' at the time of the first edition is now a reality to be appreciated at least to some degree by all undergraduates, post-graduates and practitioners of all fields of dentistry. The chapter on aetiology of periodontitis has been extended by some 30,000 words on the ecology of plaque, the basic principles of immunology, the host response to plaque and the mechanisms of tissue destruction in periodontitis.

We thank Miss Jenny Mitchell, sometime medical artist in the Edinburgh Dental School, for the drawings additional to those present in the first edition; Mr Alex Hunter, M.B.E. Chief Technician in the Edinburgh Dental School and Mr Ian Goddard for the photographs: Miss Anne Brennan, Miss Mary Ferguson and Mrs C. Weir for the preparation of the manuscript and Miss Anne Taylor for her assistance with the reference system.

T.M.   *'Obscurus fio'*
        It is when I am struggling to be brief that I become unintelligible.
        Horace. Ars Poetica v 25

G.C.   *'Sero in periculis est consilium quaerere'*
        'It is too late to seek advice after you have run into danger.'
        Publilius Syrus. Sententiae No. 684 c43 BC

CHAPTER 1

The periodontium

The supporting apparatus of the teeth, as defined by the term periodontium, consists of bone, cementum, periodontal membrane, and the investing sheath of the gingivae and oral mucosa. The adult tooth protrudes into the mouth through a cuff of mucous membrane closely adapted to the tooth surface, which acts as a seal between the environment of the clinical crown of the tooth, the mouth, and the environment of the root of the tooth, the epithelial and connective tissue elements of the supporting tissues (fig. 1.1). In the young adult, where the epithelial cuff is related entirely to enamel, an epithelial structure in origin, the mouth can be considered to be covered by a continuous epithelial sheath. With advancing age, the cuff

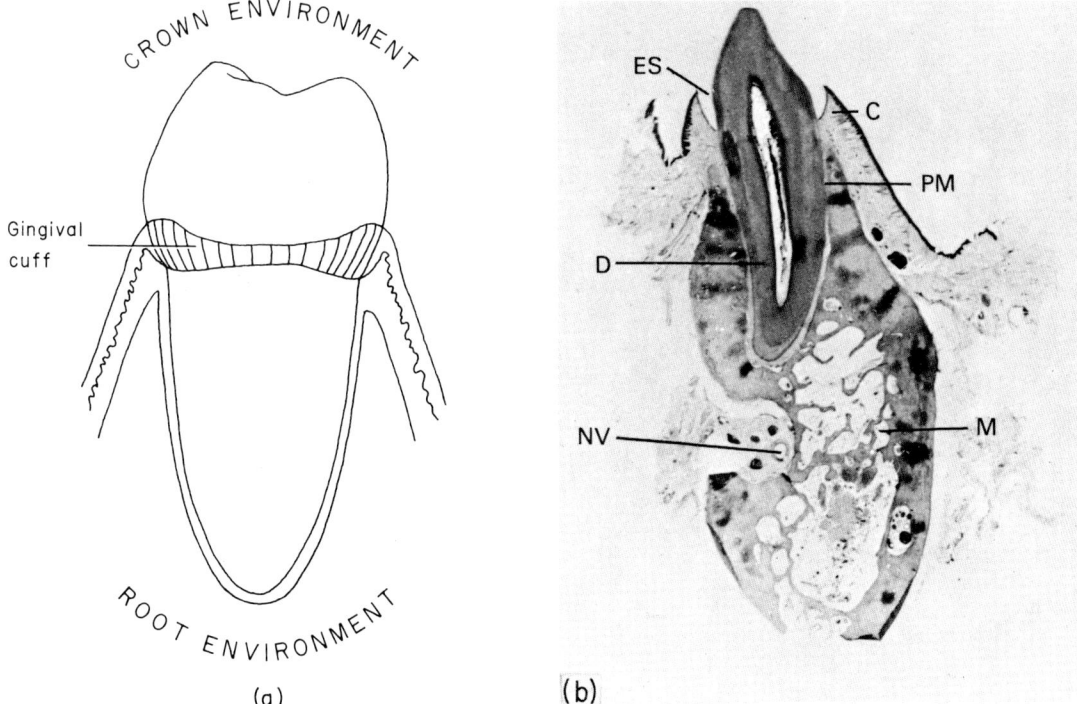

FIG. 1.1 (a) The tooth protrudes into the mouth through a cuff of mucous membrane which acts as a seal between the environment of the crown and the environment of the root. (b) Decalcified buccolingual section of a dog mandibular premolar; C, cuff; D, dentine of root; ES, enamel space; M, mandible; NV, inferior dental nerves and vessels; PM, periodontal membrane.

may become related to cementum, which is mesenchymal in origin, and the unique situation is established where the overall epithelial covering of the body is breached by the tooth. The connective tissues around the root of the tooth are at risk to the hazards of the external environment, probably to a greater degree than in any other area of the body.

BONE

Alveolar bone differs in no way from bone elsewhere in the body, with the exception of its dependence on the presence of the teeth. It is a transient tissue whose principal function is the support of teeth, and following their loss it is gradually resorbed. The bone lining the socket adjacent to the roots of the teeth is dense 'bundle' bone, called the lamina dura, into which collagen bundles of the periodontium are inserted; they are described as Sharpey's fibres (fig. 1.2a). The thin bundle bone of the lamina

dura is pierced by many small holes (Volkman canals) which act as channels for the vessels and nerves of the periodontium (fig. 1.3a). It is continuous with the buccal and lingual cortical plates at the crest of the ridge (fig. 1.3b). The bone between the external cortical plates and the cribriform lamina dura is of the cancellous type. Bone is a highly adaptable tissue, and there is a continuous process of resorption and remodelling in progress. The position and shape of the alveolar crestal bone depends upon the degree of eruption, angulation and position of the related teeth [1].

CEMENTUM

Cementum is a hard, calcified connective tissue arranged in layers around the root of the tooth [2 & 3], into which the Sharpey's fibres are inserted (fig. 1.4a). The cementum of the cervical two-thirds of the root is a thin, acellular, laminated tissue laid down by cementoblasts, which do not become embedded in the tissue during the

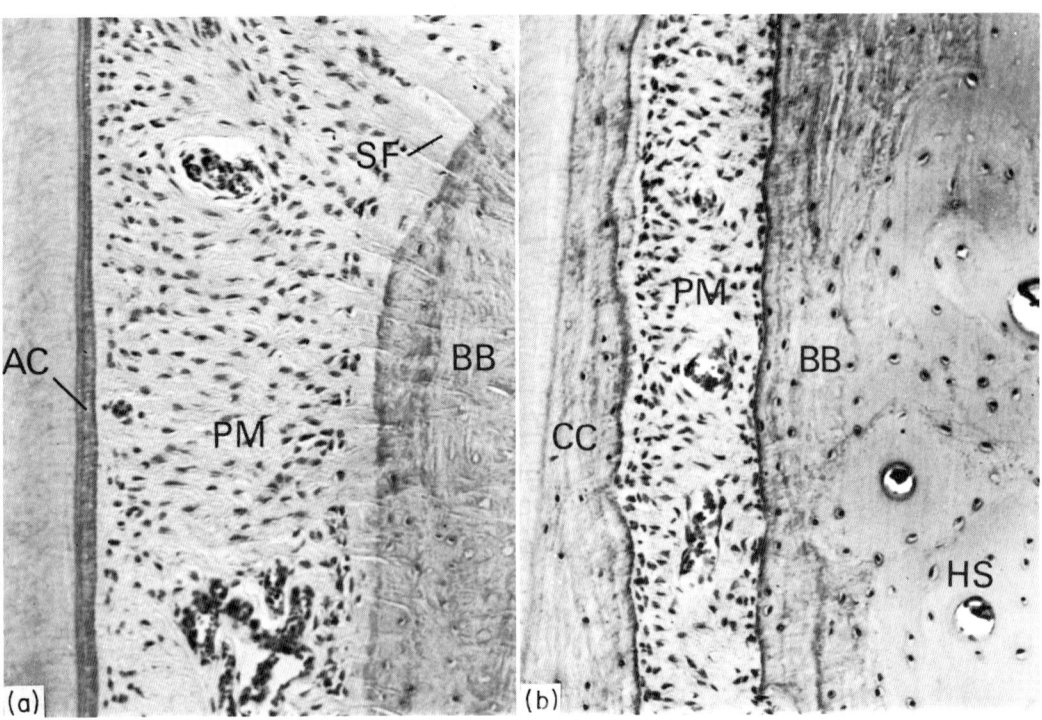

FIG. 1.2. Buccolingual sections through root of tooth, periodontal membrane and alveolar bone; (a) cervical area and (b) apical third of root. AC, acellular cementum; BB, bundle bone of lamina dura; CC, cellular cementum; HS, haversian systems; PM, periodontal membrane; SF, Sharpey's fibres.

apposition of further layers (figs. 1.2a & 1.4b). The cementum of the apical one-third of the root is cellular in character and is broadly comparable to bone in its general structure (fig. 1.2b). Cementum formation is probably a continuous process throughout life [4 & 5], the rate of formation being partly governed by the degree of function of the tooth. It does not, however, have the capacity for resorption and remodelling possessed by bone.

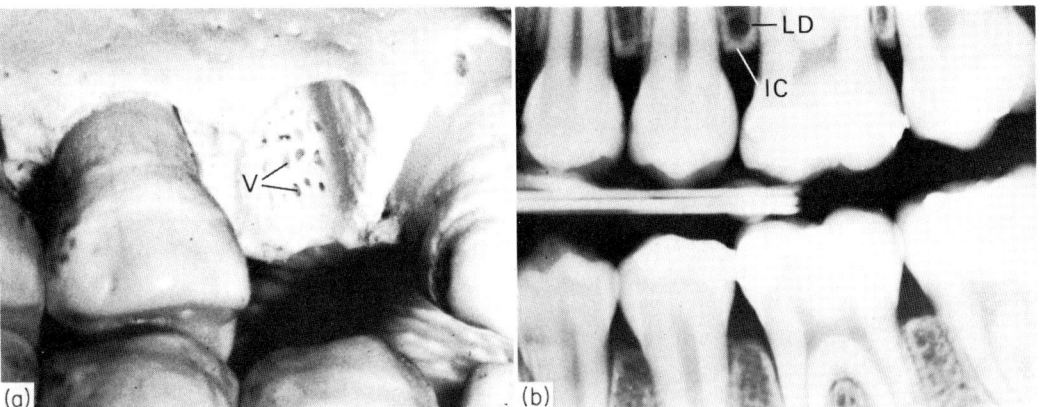

FIG. 1.3. (a) Skull socket. cribriform plate: V. Volkman canals. (b) Bitewing normal bone. The lamina dura (LD) of adjacent sockets appears to be continuous across the interdental crests (IC). Courtesy of Mr A. R. Bradshaw.

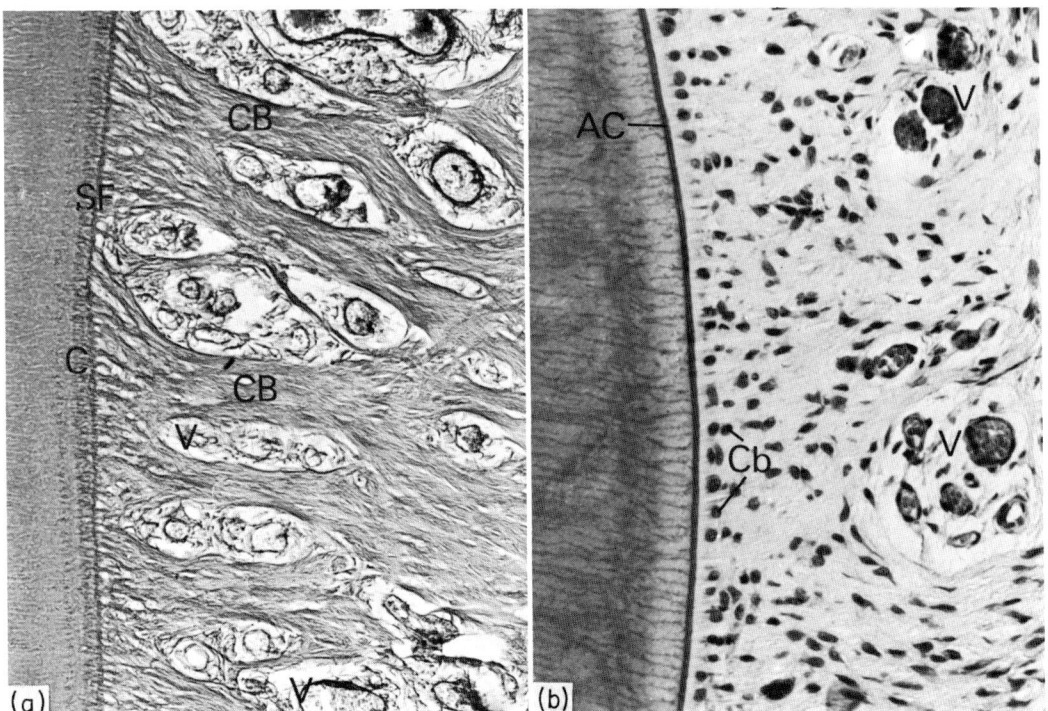

FIG. 1.4. Periodontal membrane. (a) Longitudinal section, silver impregnation; CB, collagen bundles; V, vessels; C, cementum; SF, Sharpey's fibres inserted into cementum. (b) Transverse section, haematoxylin and eosin; Cb, cementoblasts; AC, acellular cementum; V, vessels.

PERIODONTAL MEMBRANE

Periodontal membrane consists essentially of groups of collagenous connective tissue fibres that are formed by fibroblasts. Between these bundles run vessels, lymphatics and nerves, embraced in a loose connective tissue stroma (fig. 1.4a). This stroma is further penetrated by a network pattern of epithelial cells, the cell rests of Malassez, which is established following disintegration of Hertwig's sheath (the cervical loop) (fig. 1.5). Fullmer and Lillie [6] have described the presence of another fibre, the oxytalan fibre, in the periodontal membrane, but as yet its function and significance remains unknown. The width of the periodontal membrane of a tooth in normal function is about 0·25 mm.

PERIODONTIUM

Development

Before the onset of tooth eruption, the outer wall of the tooth follicle is in contact with, but not attached to, the bone of the crypt. When eruption commences, the fibres in the area of the amelocemental junction become attached to the rim of the alveolar bone which forms the opening of the crypt. As root formation proceeds, Hertwig's sheath (the cervical loop), which separates the connective tissues of the follicle from the root of the tooth, disintegrates over the first formed portion of the root becoming a network instead of a continuous layer, the epithelial cell rests of Malassez (fig. 1.5a & b). The innermost fibres of the follicle come into contact with the den-

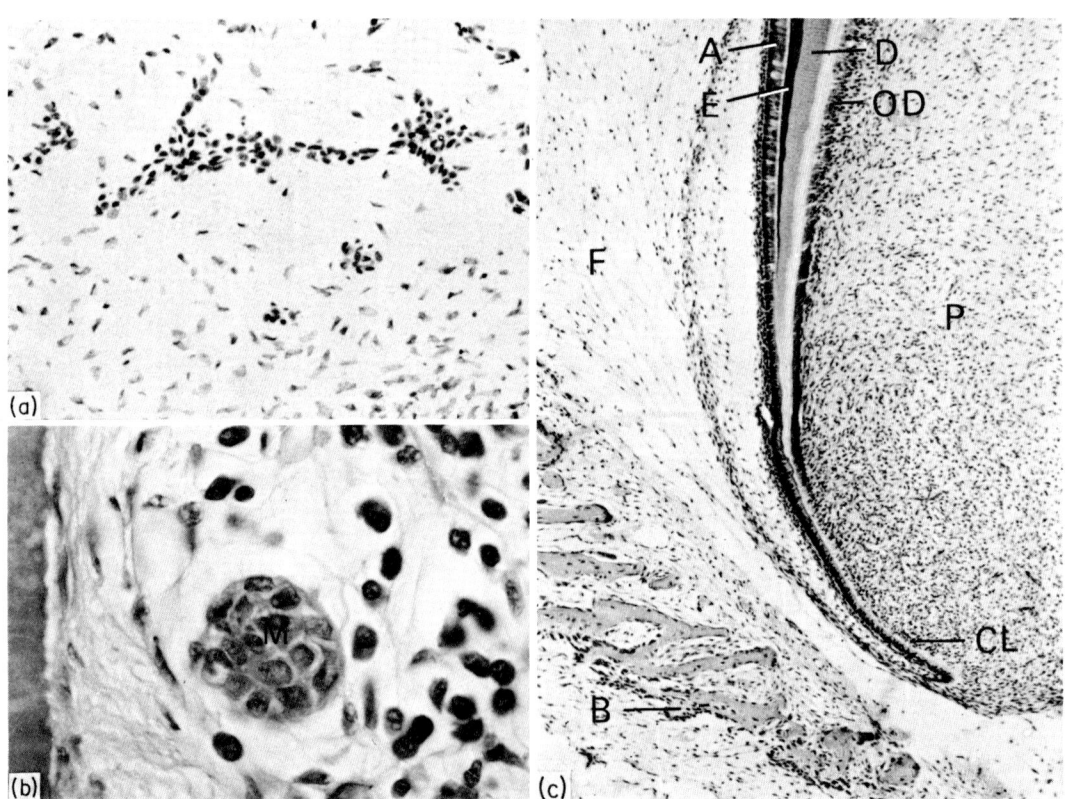

FIG. 1.5. (a) The network pattern of epithelial cell rests of Malassez which becomes established in the connective tissue stroma following disintegration of Hertwig's sheath (the cervical loop, fig. 1.5). (b) Epithelial cell rest of Malassez (M), high power. (c) Developing tooth in crypt; CL, cervical loop; P, pulp; F, follicle; B, bone crypt; D, dentine; OD, odontoblasts; E, enamel; A, ameloblasts.

tine, and by deposition of cementum, become attached to the root at the same time as the outermost fibres of the follicle are becoming attached to the wall of the developing socket. In this way the follicle, which is for the greater part of its development free of attachment to bone, becomes the periodontal membrane.

The principal bundles of fibres in the periodontal membrane are frequently described as:

(1) the alveolar crestal fibres, a condensation of fibre bundles which run from the cervical area of the root to the crest of the alveolar bone;

(2) the horizontal fibres, which run at right angles to the tooth and to the alveolar bone;

(3) the oblique fibres, which run in an apical direction from alveolar bone to cementum.

There is some question as to what extent such discrete groups of collagen fibres exist *in vivo*, since the histological appearance is partly governed by the process of tissue fixation and subsequent procedures involved in the preparation of tissue for microscopy.

The collagen fibres of the periodontal membrane show a moderately high rate of amino acid turnover [7], particularly on the alveolar bone side [8], and the tissue as a whole is capable of a high degree of functional adaption (chap. 12).

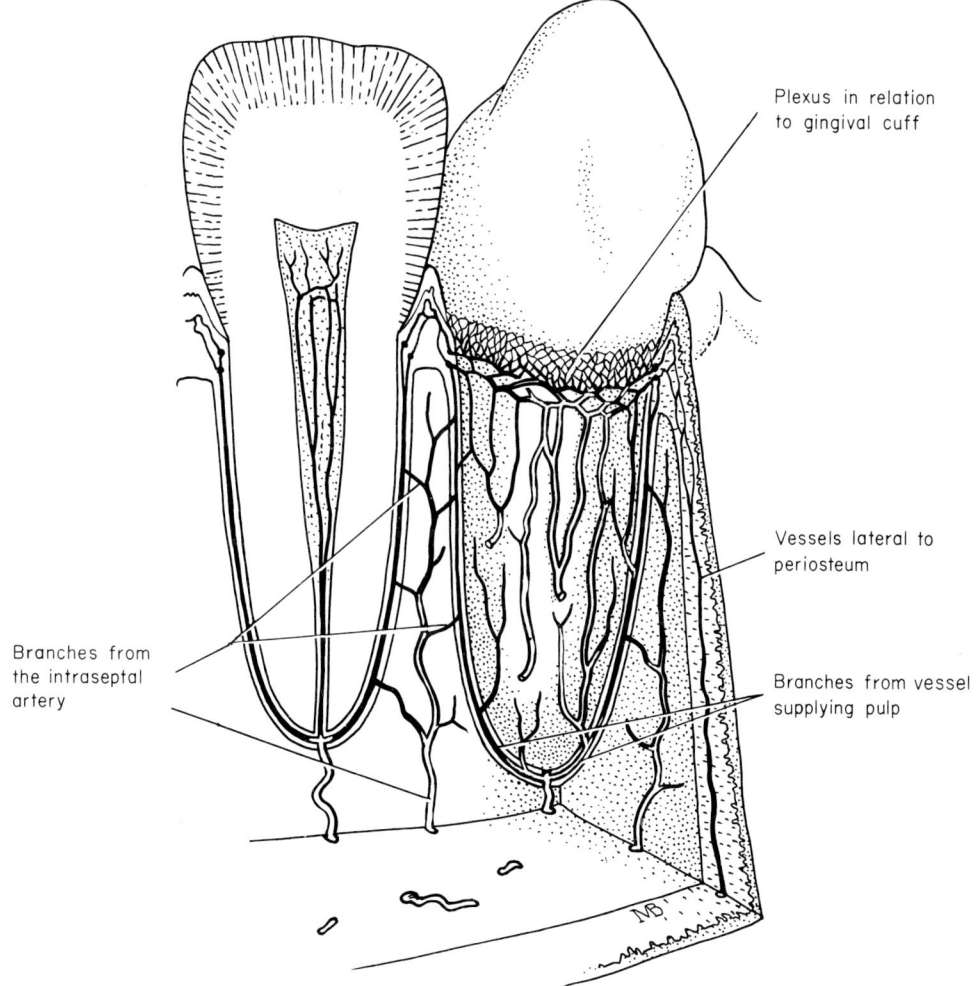

Plexus in relation to gingival cuff

Vessels lateral to periosteum

Branches from the intraseptal artery

Branches from vessel supplying pulp

FIG. 1.6. Blood supply to periodontium. Three sources: (a) branches from apical vessels, which form a network between the root and alveolar bone, (b) branches from intraseptal vessels, (c) branches from vessels lateral to the periosteum.

Blood supply

The blood supply to the periodontium is delivered from three sources [9, 10 & 11] (fig. 1.6):

(1) apical vessels which give off branches to the periodontal membrane before supplying the pulp;

(2) branches from the intraseptal arteries which penetrate the lamina dura at all levels and form an anastomosis between the periodontal vessels of apical origin and the vessels of the Haversian system of the alveolar bone;

(3) branches lying lateral to the periosteum supplying the gingival tissue and oral mucous membrane which anastomose with the vessels of the periodontal membrane forming a well-defined vascular plexus above the marginal ligament (figs 1.6 & 1.7a & b). The marginal ligament is formed by collagen fibres in the region between the amelocemental junction and the crest of the alveolar bone, and it thus lies immediately deep to the gingival cuff (see fig. 1.16).

The entire vascular system is such that the root of the tooth is in a fluid environment, where the fluid in the vessels of gingivae and periodontium is in continuity with the vascular reservoir in bone [12]. Shift of fluid in the system may contribute to the ability of the tooth to withstand stress in normal and abnormal function. The lymphatic system probably has a similar distribution to the blood vessels, although an adequate description is not present in the dental literature. It may also contribute to the fluid buffer system of the root.

Nerve supply

PERIODONTAL MEMBRANE

The nerve supply to the periodontal membrane is derived from two sources [13]. One group of fibres arises from the dental nerve as it passes through the alveolar plate prior to entering the apical foramen of the tooth. This group runs cervically and gives off branches which form a network within the membrane. The second main source of fibres is branches from the intra-alveolar nerve, which ascend through the bone toward the alveolar crest. The lateral nerves pass through the cribriform plate of the socket to end in the periodontal membrane. The branches terminate as a fine aborization within the periodontal membrane [14].

GINGIVAL INNERVATION

The terminal branches of the nerve supplying the periodontal membrane also supply the interdental area of the gingivae, whilst branches from the buccal, lingual, and palatal nerves supply the free and attached gingivae. The filaments penetrate the submucosa where further branching occurs; most of the nerves terminate as a fine network at the dermoepidermal junction. Intra-

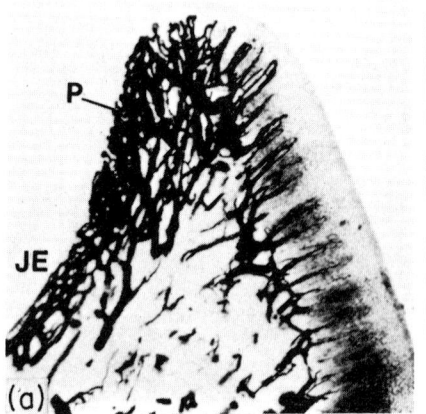
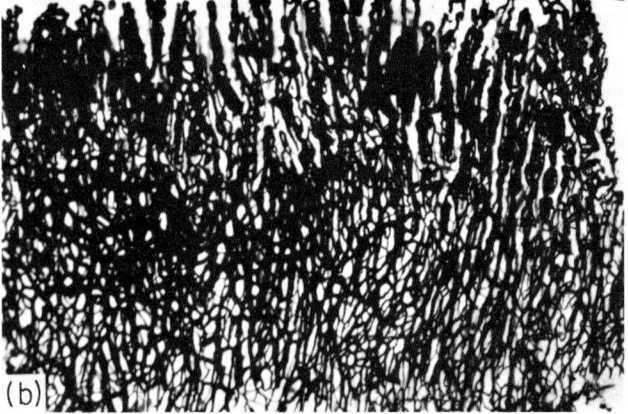

FIG. 1.7. India ink perfusion of chronically inflamed marginal gingivae of dog to show blood vessels. (a) Buccolingual section showing vascular plexus (P) deep to junctional epithelium (JE) and superficial to the marginal ligament (fig. 1.13). (b) Mesiodistal section showing the extreme complexity of the vascular plexus underlying the junctional epithelium. Courtesy of Dr J. Egelberg and the *Journal of Periodontal Research.*

epithelial nerves have been demonstrated to course from the dermal papillae towards the surface of the epithelium, ending in a small bulb-like structure [15]. Although many filaments throughout the gingivae appear to have no specialized ending, both Meissner and Krause corpuscles have been described [16].

THE INVESTING SHEATH

The mucosal covering of the attachment apparatus can be divided into several parts, the free gingivae, the attached gingivae and the reflected mucosa (fig. 1.8a & b), which develop from the oral mucous membrane, and the epithelium of the gingival cuff, which at the time of eruption is at least in part enamel organ epithelium in origin [17] (fig. 1.8c & d).

Gingivae

The gingivae is that mucous membrane which extends from the cervical region of the tooth to the alveolar mucosa. A potential space, the gingival sulcus, is formed where the marginal gingivae lies against the tooth.

In health the gingivae is coral pink in colour although this may vary to some extent with the amount of pigment present. The tissue is usually firm in consistency, and closely adapted to the

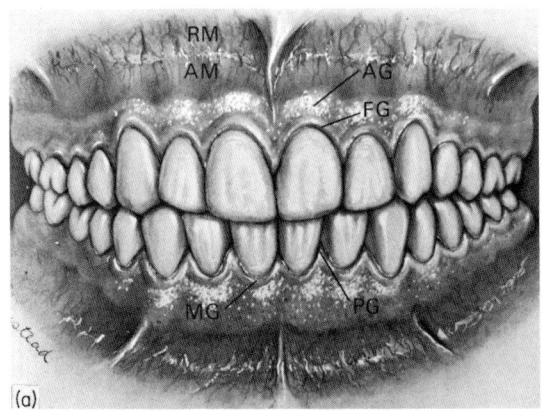

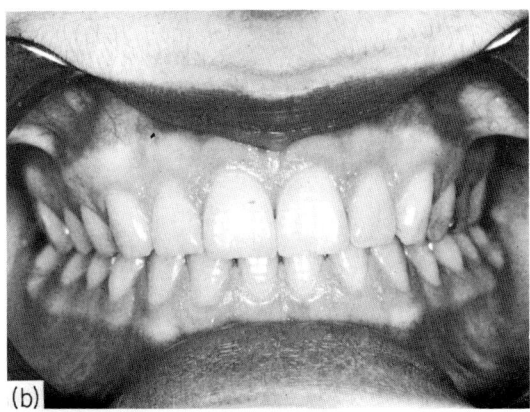

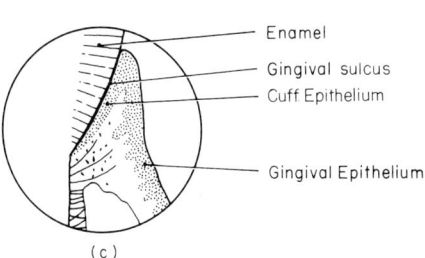

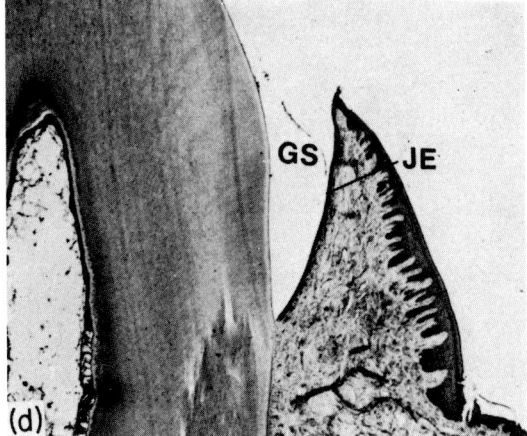

FIG. 1.8. The normal mouth. (a) FG, free gingivae; AG, attached gingivae; AM, alveolar mucosa; RM, reflected mucosa; PG, papillary gingivae; MG, marginal gingivae; drawing by courtesy of Dr A.R. McGregor. (b) Clinical photograph of a normal mouth. (c) Diagram of the dento-gingival junction. (d) Photomicrograph of a gingival cuff; GS, gingival sulcus; JE, junctional epithelium.

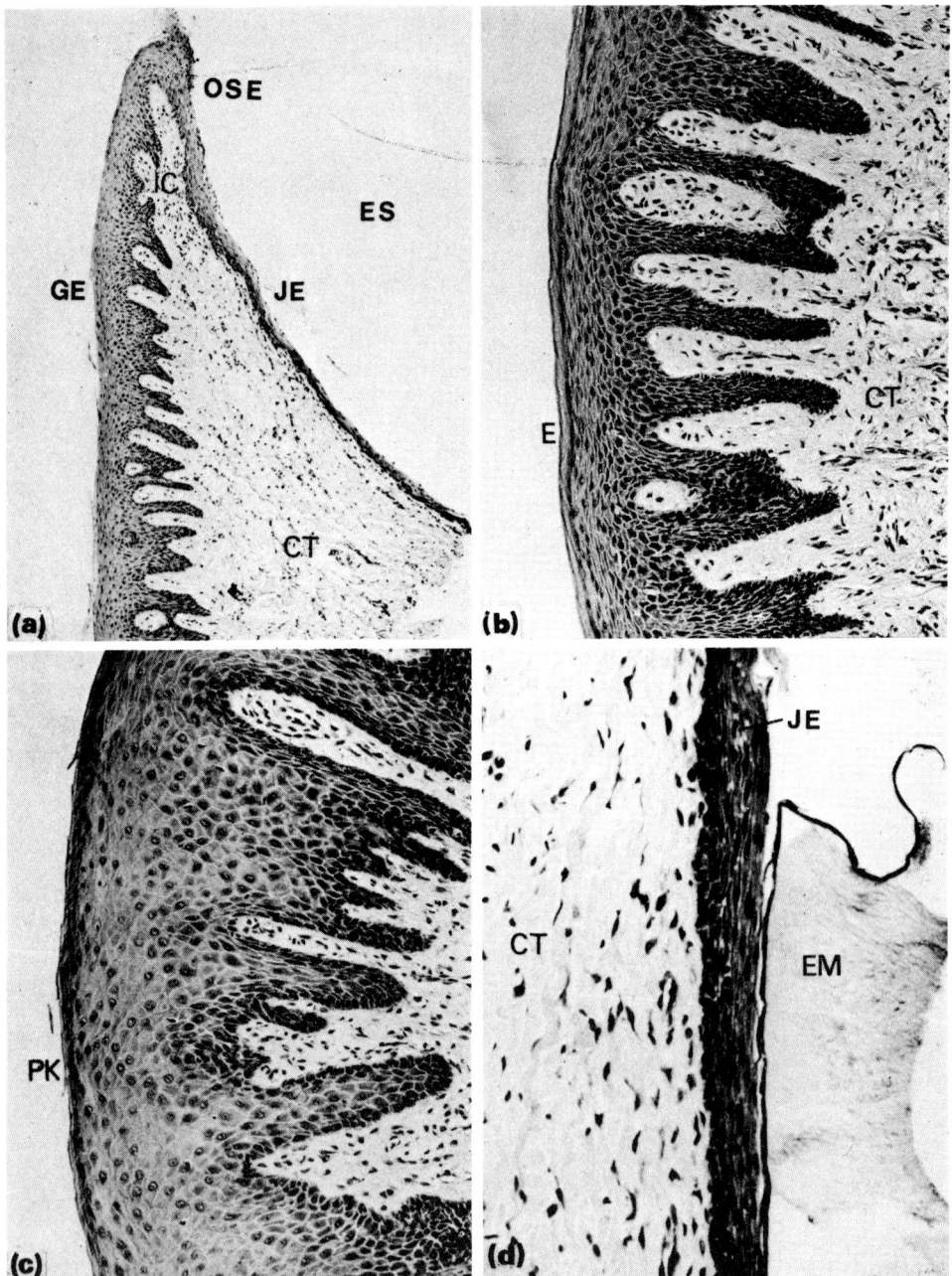

FIG. 1.9. (a) Buccolingual section through clinically healthy gingival cuff; JE, junctional epithelium; CT, connective tissue; ES, enamel space; GE, gingival epithelium; IC, inflammatory cells, present even in clinically healthy gingiva; OSE, oral sulcular epithelium. (b) Section of gingival epithelium with underlying connective tissue (CT); epithelium (E) shows keratinization (orthokeratinization). (c) Section of gingival epithelium showing parakeratinization (PK), i.e. presence of nuclei in keratinized layer. (d) High power of healthy junctional epithelium (JE) which is non-keratinized. Note the close relationship to the enamel matrix (EM) and the absence of inflammatory cells in the connective tissue (CT).

tooth at the cervical margin (fig. 1.8a & b). Histologically, the gingivae consist of a corium of connective tissue covered by stratified squamous epithelium (fig. 1.9a). On the labial and lingual aspects the gingival epithelium is usually keratinized (fig. 1.9b) or parakeratinized (fig. 1.9c), whilst the junctional epithelium is nonkeratinized (fig. 1.9d). The gingival tissues are held in close contact with the teeth by collagen bundles, which run from the papillary layer of the dermis to cementum and alveolar bone. Interposed between these fibre bundles are the cells, vessels, nerves, and ground substances of the connective tissue. Even in clinically healthy tissues a few mononuclear inflammatory cells can usually be observed in the gingival tissues (fig. 1.9a).

FREE GINGIVAE

The gingival tissue adjacent to the crown of the tooth is normally detached to a depth of 0·5 mm giving rise to the gingival sulcus and is termed the free gingivae. For descriptive purposes this is sub-divided into the marginal gingivae, situated labially and lingually, and the papillary gingivae, which is interdental in position (fig. 1.8a & b).

ATTACHED GINGIVAE

The attached gingivae extends from the apical margin of the free gingivae to the line of reflection of the oral mucosa from the alveolar process to the lips and cheeks. It has a stippled appearance due to well-developed collagen bundles that course at right angles to the bone, binding the mucosa down as firmly united mucoperiosteum (fig. 1.8a and b).

ALVEOLAR MUCOSA

The alveolar mucosa (fig. 1.8a and b) is loosely attached to the underlying periosteum in the region of the line of reflection and is increasingly separated from the underlying bone by a loose connective tissue stroma. Histologically, there is a gradual change from attached gingivae to alveolar mucosa (fig. 1.10). The most prominent change occurs at the epithelium connective tissue junction where the epithelial ridges become progressively shorter. The epithelium is nonkeratinized and an increase in the proportion of elastic fibres occurs in the underlying connective tissue.

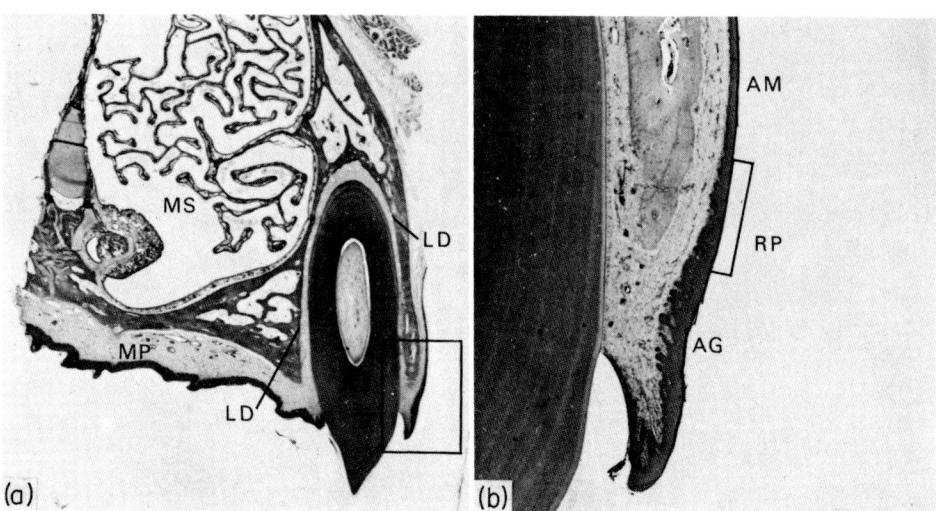

FIG. 1.10. Buccopalatal section of canine of cat. (a) Maxillary air sinus (MS), mucous membrane of palate (MP), lamina dura of socket (LD). (b) Higher power of area indicated in fig. 1.10a. A progressive shortening of the epithelial ridges (rete pegs, RP) occurs with the transition of tissue from attached gingiva (AG) to alveolar mucosa (AM).

Dentogingival junction

Immediately prior to the eruption of a tooth there is hyperplasia and downgrowth of the oral epithelium immediately overlying the crown. These cells come into association with the pro-liferating epithelial cells of the enamel organ of the erupting tooth. The tooth erupts through a mass of epithelial cells of mixed origin (fig. 1.11a), and there are few clear indications as to which cells originate from which source. In the early stages of eruption the crown is enclosed in a deep cuff of gingivae which is detached from the tooth to the level of any remaining enamel epithelium [18] (fig. 1.11b). When the tooth has fully erupted, however, the detached part of the cuff has been reduced to the 0·5–1 mm which constitutes the free gingivae (fig. 1.11c). At this stage the tooth has attained a functional position in the occlusion, and two-thirds to three-quarters of the enamel surface is exposed in the mouth; the remaining enamel is related to the junctional

epithelium. The accepted normal relation-ship for the fully erupted tooth is that the base of the junctional epithelium is in the region of the amelocemental junction. According to Gottlieb's theory of continuous eruption, from this stage there is a rootward shift of the cuff in the process of passive eruption, so that the cuff becomes re-lated to the cementum [19]. On the other hand Cohen believes that when the connection of the gingival fibres to the cementum is destroyed, and the junctional epithelium is permitted to occupy the cementum, disease is always present [20]. Cohen has stated: 'Contrary to previous clinic-ally oriented concepts of this phase of eruption representing a normal passive stage, it must be emphasized that pathologic changes must have occurred before the epithelium migrates onto the root surface.'

The latter view has been supported by a num-ber of studies including one of a group of Canadian Eskimos [21]. No macroscopic in-crease in distance from the amelocemental junc-

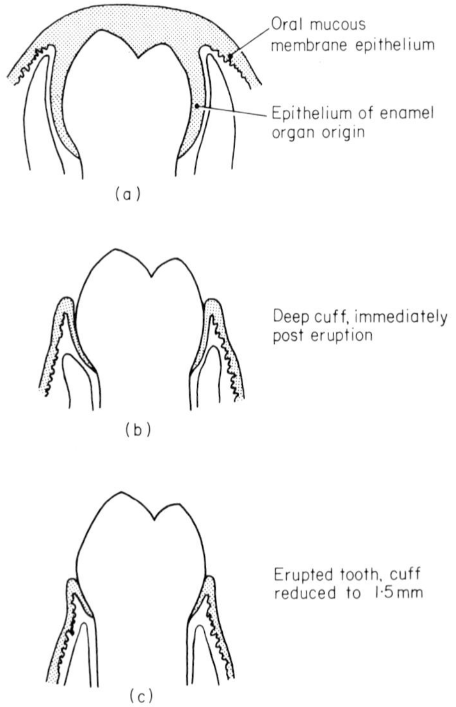

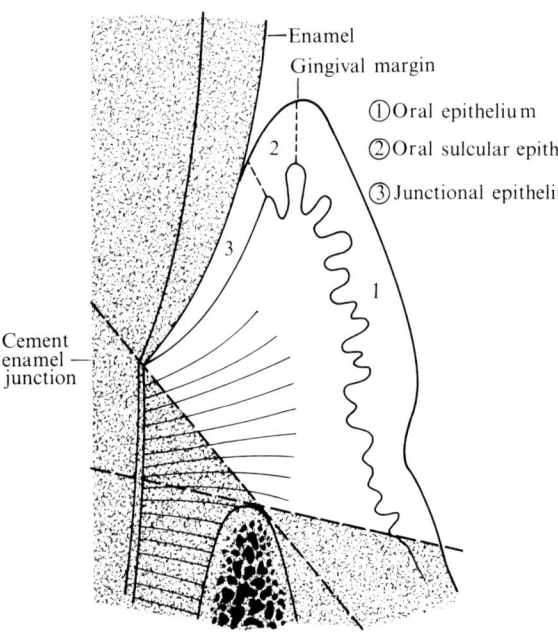

FIG. 1.11. Eruption of tooth and development of the dentogingival junction.

Oral mucous membrane epithelium

Epithelium of enamel organ origin

(a)

Deep cuff, immediately post eruption

(b)

Erupted tooth, cuff reduced to 1·5mm

(c)

Enamel
Gingival margin
①Oral epithelium
②Oral sulcular epithel
③Junctional epitheliur

2

3

1

Cement enamel junction

FIG. 1.12. Diagrammatic view of a labio-lingual section of gingiva. The gingival epithelium consists of oral epithelium, oral sulcular epithelium and junc-tional epithelium. After Listgarten M. (1972) Normal development, structure, physiology and repair of gingival epithelium. *Oral Sci. Rev.* **1**, 3.

tion to the alveolar crest occurred, even in the presence of complete loss of the crown by attrition.

For the sake of clarity it is convenient to adopt the terminology proposed by Schroeder and Listgarten [22]. The gingiva comprises that portion of the oral mucosa surrounding the teeth which is limited coronally by the gingival margin and apically by the mucogingival junction externally, and the supracrestal collagen fibres internally. Gingival epithelium lines the gingival surface on the vestibular as well as the tooth side. The gingival epithelium (fig. 1.12) may be considered to consist of:

(1) *Oral epithelium:* This includes the epithelium which extends from the mucogingival junction to the gingival margin (i.e. the imaginary line passing through the most coronal points of the gingiva).

(2) *Sulcular epithelium:* This is the epithelium which lines the gingival sulcus (i.e. the shallow groove surrounding each tooth which is limited coronally by the sulcular orifice and apically by the free surface of the junctional epithelium. It consists of a coronal portion, the oral sulcular epithelium which morphologically resembles the oral epithelium and an apical part which is formed by the coronal surface of the junctional epithelium).

(3) *Junctional epithelium:* This is the epithelium which joins the internal (toothside) surface of the gingiva to the tooth. The actual junction of this epithelium to the tooth surface represents the epithelial attachment. The most coronal extension of the junctional epithelium, which lines the bottom of the gingival sulcus, is its free surface (i.e. the surface from which cell desquamation takes place). As defined by this terminology cuff epithelium consists of two morphologically distinct areas, the oral sulcular epithelium and the junctional epithelium.

Junctional and sulcular epithelium constitute the gingival cuff epithelium. There is evidence [23 & 24] that shortening of the ameloblasts after deposition of the enamel matrix is not a sign of cellular degeneration, but rather the reflection of a change in function of these cells from a secretory to a resorptive role. Concomitant with this change of function of the ameloblasts, an attachment apparatus appears between the ameloblasts and the enamel that consists of a basement lamina and hemidesmosomes which has been described as the primary epithelial attachment [22 & 25].

Prior to tooth eruption, the reduced enamel epithelium consists of an internal layer of reduced ameloblasts and several layers of epithelial cells external to the ameloblasts which are derived from odontogenic epithelium, probably from the stratum intermedium in particular. As the crown of the erupting tooth approaches the overlying oral epithelium, the reduced ameloblasts over the unerupted part of the crown undergo further intracellular re-organization, resulting in their transformation into squamous cells indistinguishable from those of oral epithelium (fig. 1.11a) [22 & 26]. During this transformation the cells remain attached to the enamel by hemidesmosomes and the internal basement lamina. While it is widely accepted that these cells lose the ability to divide at the time of their differentiation into ameloblasts, the external cells of the reduced enamel epithelium are not similarly affected [27 & 28]. Consequently, as a result of cell turnover, the external cells of the reduced enamel epithelium eventually displace the transformed ameloblasts to take their place as the innermost epithelial cell layer. The external cells of the reduced enamel epithelium thus give rise to an epithelium with a relatively high turnover rate [29], which replaces the relatively inactive reduced enamel epithelium as the epithelium uniting what is now the gingival connective tissue to the enamel surface. The epithelium in which the ameloblasts can no longer be identified is now called the junctional epithelium. Its attachment to the tooth surface via hemidesmosomes and a basement lamina forms the secondary epithelial attachment (fig. 1.14).

Although the origin of the junctional epithelium from the external cells of the reduced enamel epithelium has been widely accepted it has also been suggested that junctional epithelium may be derived from the oral epithelium [30 & 17]. It seems likely that at the time of fusion between oral and reduced enamel epithelium, the oral epithelium contributes to the formation of the coronal portion of the junctional epithelium, the reduced enamel epithelium giving rise to the remaining portion. As these epithelia become joined it may no longer be possible to attribute the origin of a particular cell in the coronal portion of the junctional epithelium to one epithelium or the other, particularly after several renewals of the cell population have taken place. It is, however, possible to observe small areas of reduced enamel epithelium near the cervical margin of a fully erupted tooth for a certain length of time following tooth emergence into the oral cavity and it has been estimated that this epithelium might persist following eruption from one to two years in man [22]. Eventually, however, the epithelial attachment is entirely mediated by junctional epithelium and it should be noted that it is clearly possible for oral epithelium alone to reconstitute an entirely new junctional epithelium following gingival surgery.

Oral epithelium

The oral epithelium of the gingiva, which extends from the mucogingival junction to the gingival margin, is a stratified squamous epithelium showing all the histological characteristics of skin except for the absence of stratum lucidum and a less well developed stratum granulosum (fig. 1.9). The underside of this epithelium in man is characterized by ridges of varying depth and thickness, that intersect in a variety of patterns and which in some cases run more or less parallel to one another and to the margins of the gingiva [31]. The characteristic stippling of healthy human gingiva, observed clinically, appears to be due to depressions in the epithelial surface, which are associated with intersecting epithelial ridges on the under surface of the epithelium [31]. Oral epithelium is capable of completing the process of keratinization, although para-keratinization is frequently seen in specimens of healthy tissue. In contrast, junctional epithelium is a thin stratified squamous epithelium, approximately 15–30 cells thick in the vicinity of the sulcus, which never keratinizes in man. The thickness of the epithelium tapers to a single cell at its most apical extension and throughout its length there are nucleated cells apparent at its enamel surface. The epithelial-connective tissue junction is generally straight and there are

no epithelial ridges comparable to those in oral epithelium. The intercellular spaces of junctional epithelium are much more prominent than those of oral epithelium and account for almost one fifth of the tissue volume [32]. Varying numbers of leucocytes may be seen within these intercellular spaces, the number increasing in proximity to the gingival sulcus. In terms of its relationship to the tooth the junctional epithelium may be described as a wedge having three surfaces, (1) an internal surface facing the tooth, (2) an external surface facing the gingival connective tissue and (3) a coronal surface which forms the bottom of the gingival sulcus. Thus, the most apical part of the sulcular epithelium consists of the coronal portion of the junctional epithelium which it resembles histologically. In the more coronal portion of the sulcus, the oral sulcular epithelium is stratified in a manner similar to that of oral epithelium, but the superficial cells do not achieve the same degree of keratinization as do oral epithelial cells. The intercellular spaces are narrow and seldom contain leucocytes. The junctional epithelial cells facing the tooth surface are characterized by hemidesmosomes lining the cell membrane adjacent to the tooth and a basement lamina which links the epithelium to the underlying tooth surface or dental cuticle [22]. Junctional epithelium may be united to a variety of surfaces including enamel, fibrillar or afibrillar cementum or dentine [22 & 33]. In all cases this union is morphologically similar and is characterized by the presence of hemidesmosomes and basement lamina (fig. 1.14). Schroeder [34] has estimated that in the vicinity of the gingival sulcus leucocytes may occupy from 2–64 per cent of the relative volume of the junctional epithelium. The degree of this leucocytic infiltrate seems to be unrelated to the degree of clinical inflammation or the relative volume of the inflamed connective tissue.

Histological versus clinical sulcus [35]

At a histological level the gingival sulcus is a shallow furrow approximately 0·5 mm in depth, whose base is formed by the junctional epithelium (fig. 1.13a). Due to its structural weakness, junctional epithelium is readily disrupted, either by the introduction of foreign objects such as metal, plastic or paper strips or periodontal probes, or by attempts at separating the gingiva from the tooth surface. This disruption usually occurs within the epithelium rather than at the dentoepithelial junction (fig. 1.13b), The depth of the clinical gingival sulcus may be defined as

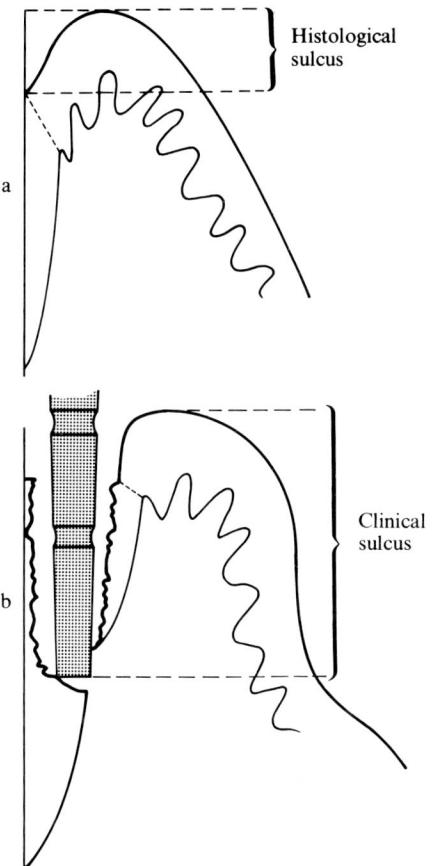

FIG. 1.13. Diagrammatic views of the histological and the clinical sulcus. (a) The histological sulcus is best observed in block sections of tooth and undisturbed gingiva. Its depth is the distance between two lines drawn perpendicular to the tooth surface which intersect the free surface of the junctional epithelium and the margin of the gingiva. (b) The clinical sulcus is the depth to which a foreign object, such as a periodontal probe, will penetrate past the gingival margin. Because of varying degrees of tissue disruption, the clinical sulcus depth will generally exceed the histological depth. After Listgarten M. (1972). Normal development. structure, physiology and repair of gingival epithelium. *Oral Sci. Rev.* **1**, 3.

the depth past the gingival margin to which a periodontal probe will penetrate when introduced with light pressure [35]. Thus, the histological and clinical sulcus depths are different entities which should not be confused with each other.

In the embrasure region the gingival tissues rise to two peaks, the buccal and lingual papillae. There is continuity of epithelium joining these peaks through the embrasure below the contact point, along the line of a concavity between the peaks described by Cohen as the interdental col [36] (fig. 1.15). Immediately following eruption, the epithelium of this region is of the thin non-keratinizing type, developmentally related to the enamel organ. These cells are gradually replaced by cells of oral mucous membrane origin, which proliferate through the embrasure following eruption of the tooth. It has been suggested that failure of oral mucous membrane to become established in this region, before the thin post-eruptive epithelium is breached by factors from the mouth, is an initiating cause of periodontal disease [30 & 37].

ADAPTATION OF THE CUFF TO THE TOOTH

The seal between the crown environment and the root environment is dependent on the continuity of the epithelial sheath as a whole and particularly on the degree of adaptation of the gingival cuff to the tooth (fig. 1.14).

Factors which may influence the relationship of the cuff epithelium to the tooth are:

(1) The products of the superficial cells of the cuff epithelium may contribute to a cuticle on the tooth surface, to which the cells themselves adhere. The factors concerned with the stickiness of cells and adhesion of epithelium to enamel have been reviewed by Schultz-Haudt *et al.* [34 & 38].

(2) The condition of the gel structure of the surrounding gingival connective tissue is governed partly by the central factors controlling local tissue metabolism and partly by the constantly changing crown environment (see chap. 7). Simple pressure is sufficient to produce a gel–sol change and an altered permeability of the connective tissue [39].

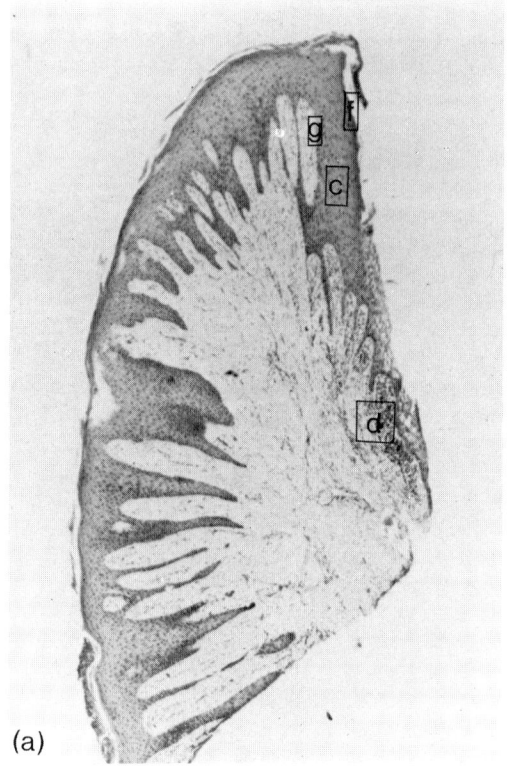

(a)

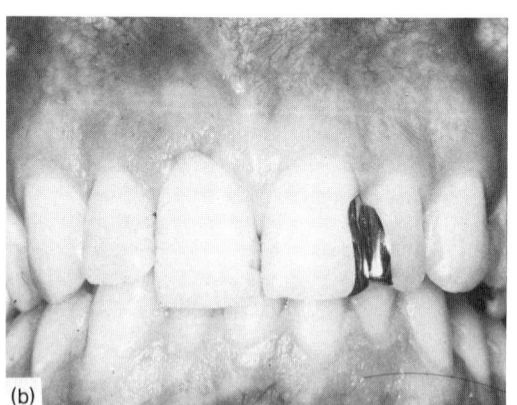

(b)

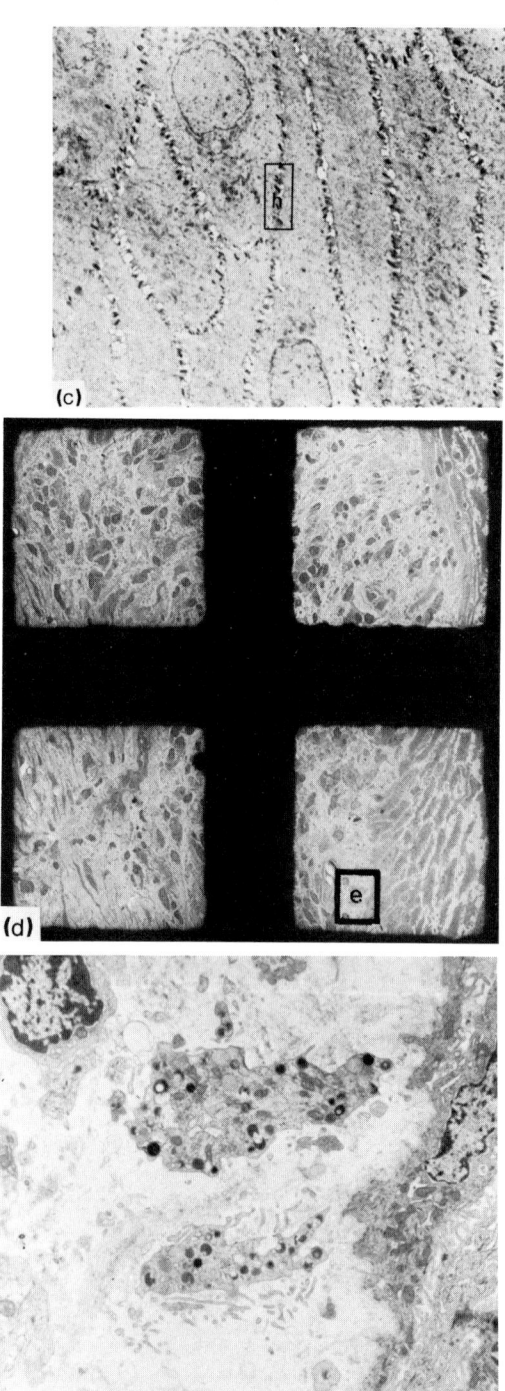

(c)

(d)

(e)

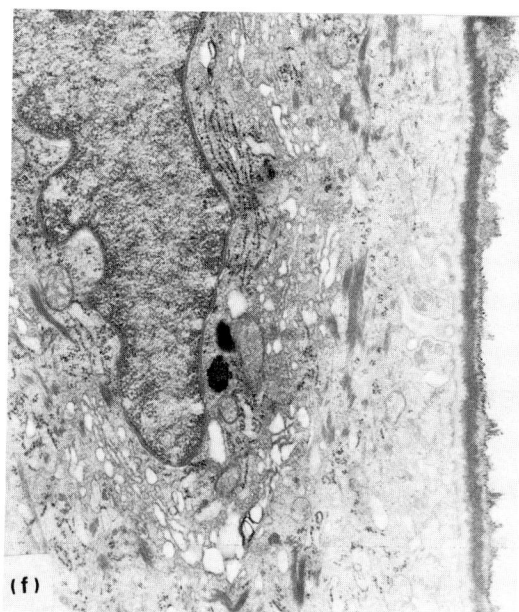

(f)

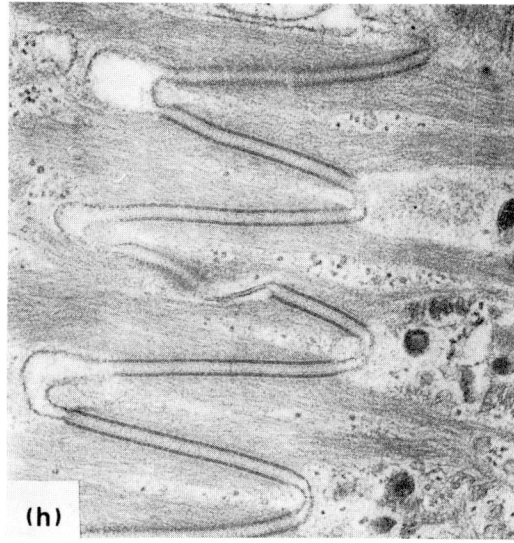

(h)

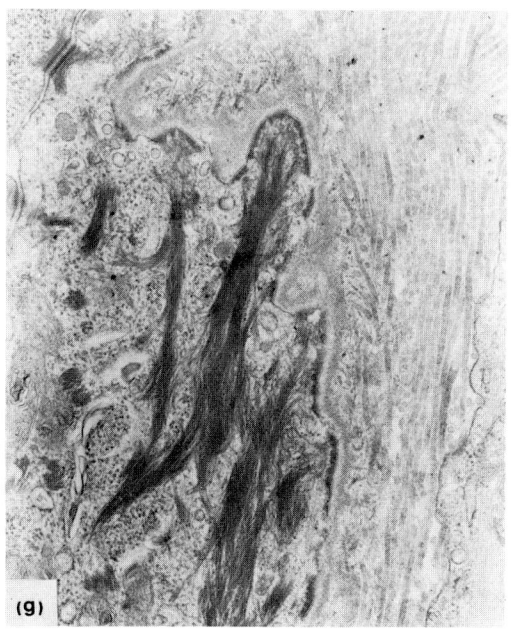

(g)

FIG. 1.14. (a) Orientation photomicrograph, bucco-lingual section through clinically healthy gingiva from 1⌋ shown in (b); healing margin one week post-operatively can be seen. (c) Low power E.M. photo-micrograph showing inter-epithelial cell zone and junctional epithelial cells from area ⎺c⎽. (d) E.M. grid with low power view showing mixed inflammatory cells underlying junctional epithelium. (e) High power of two macrophages in connective tissue immediately below junctional epithelium. (f) Epithelial cell with basal lamina in contact with enamel crystals on right. (g) Epithelial cell with tonofibrils attached to hemi-desmosomes lying immediately below lamina densa; collagen can be seen at the right. (h) High power of zone beneath two epithelial cells showing several desmosomes, with attached tonofibrils. Note the com-plexity of the so-called inter-cellular zone.
zone between two epithelial cells showing several plexity of the so-called inter-cellular zone. Photo-micrographs (f), (g) and (h) are courtesy of Prof. H. E. Schroeder.

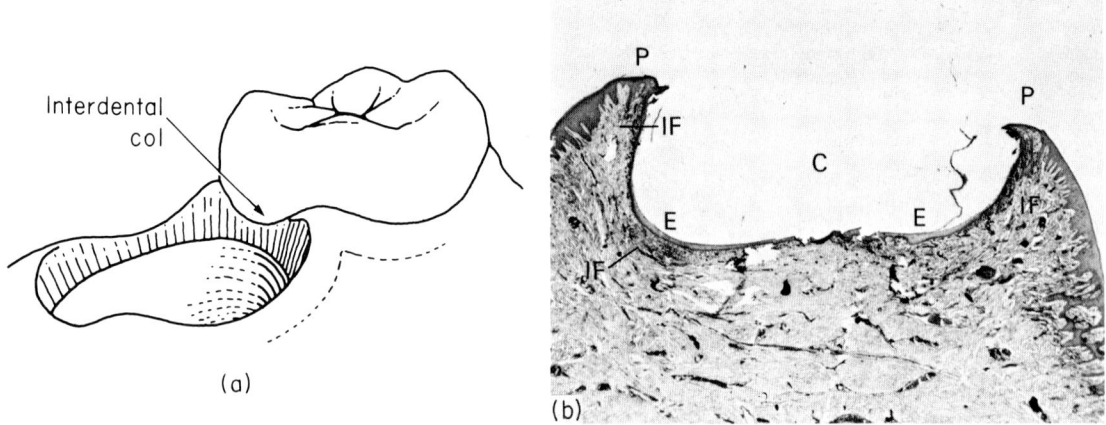

FIG. 1.15. Interdental col. The histological section (buccolingual) shows continuity of epithelium (E) through the col (C) which joins the interdental papillae (P). Some scattered foci of chronic inflammatory cells are present (IF).

(3) Connective tissue is a dynamic structure, and there is constant exchange of soluble collagen between the bundles and the ground substance. The degree of condensation into fibres is variable, and it is governed by a wide range of factors such as the degree of function of the teeth, or the presence of tissue intoxicating factors such as hydantoin drugs (see chap. 13).

Marginal ligament

The ligament consists of a well defined condensation of collagen fibres which circumscribes the teeth [40]. For practical purposes it may be visualized as a figure-of-eight weave of collagen bundles having a highly specialized arrangement in the region of the embrasure (fig. 1.16a).

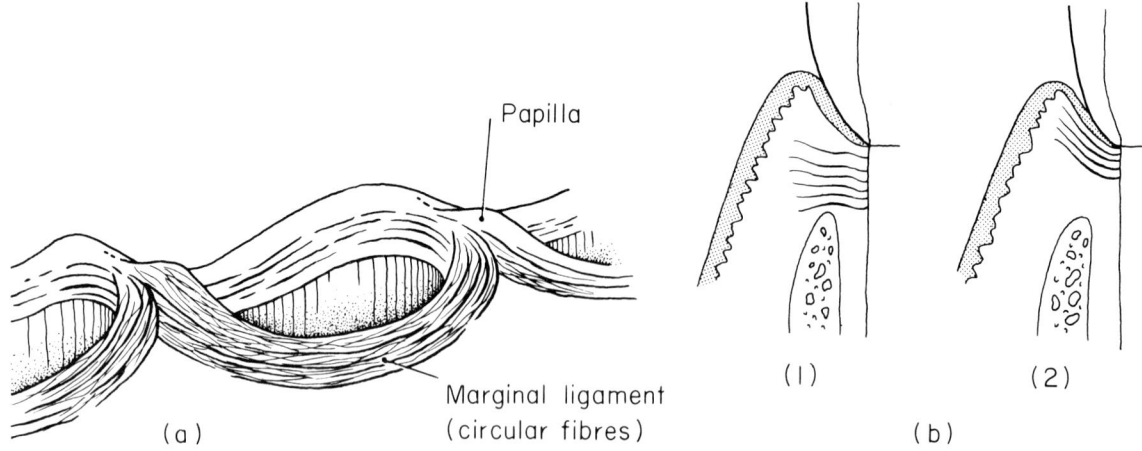

FIG. 1.16. (a) Diagram of the marginal ligament. (b) Principal groups of fibres which play a part in maintaining the close relationship of the gingival cuff to the tooth and alveolar crest; (1) and (2) dentogingival fibres; (3) free gingival fibres, binding gingiva to alveolar crest; (4) circular fibres of marginal ligament; (5) transeptal fibres; (6) dentoperiosteal fibres; modified from J. Erausquin, Buenos Aires.

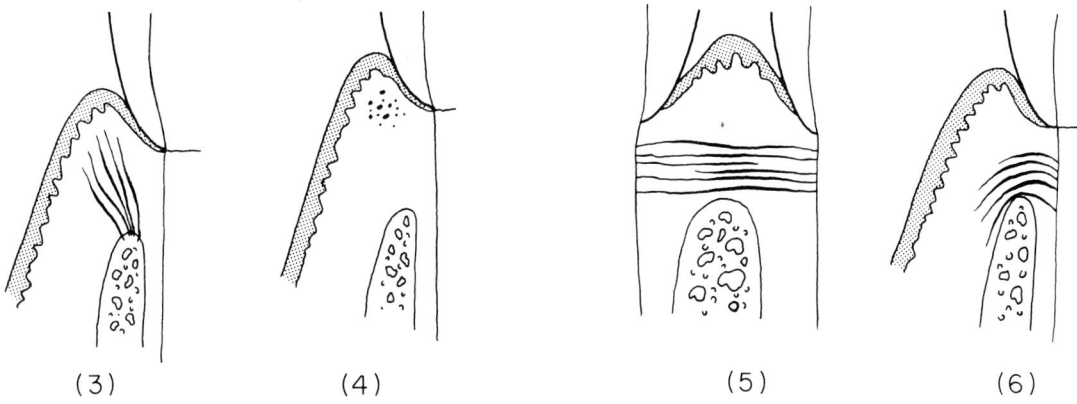

(3)   (4)   (5)   (6)

FIG. 1.16(b) *continued*

In this region five groups of fibres have been said to contribute to maintaining the relationship of the epithelial cuff to the tooth (fig. 1.16b). These are dentogingival fibres which attach the gingival tissue to cementum; free gingival fibres which attach gingival tissue to bone; circular fibres which circumscribe the tooth; transeptal fibres which cross the embrasure from tooth to tooth coronal to the alveolar crest; dentoperiosteal fibres which course from the cementum to the periosteum of the alveolar crest.

Disruption of this anatomical arrangement of the connective tissues, and loss of continuity of the buccal and lingual papillae through the embrasure, are the first major clinical signs of an established periodonitis (41) (fig. 1.17).

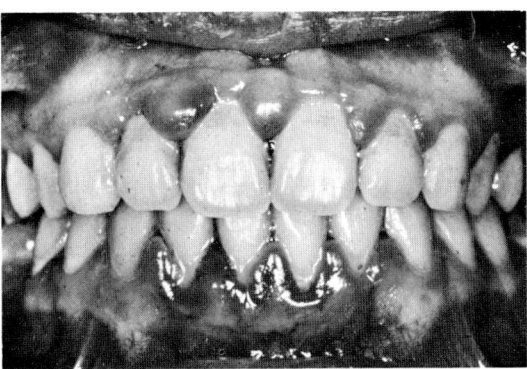

FIG. 1.17. Clinical photograph showing disruption of the collagen structure of the marginal ligament and loss of continuity of the buccal and lingual papillae through the embrasure.

REFERENCES

[1] RITCHEY B. & ORBAN B. (1953) Crests of the interdental alveolar septa. *J. Periodont.* **24**, 75–87.

[2] KERR D.A. (1961) The cementum: its role in periodontal health and disease. *J. Periodont.* **32**, 183–189.

[3] SELVIG K.A. (1965) The fine structure of human cementum. *Acta odont. scand.* **23**, 423–441.

[4] RAMFJORD S.P. & ASH M.M. (1971) *Occlusion*, 2nd Edition. Philadelphia: Saunders.

[5] GUSTAFSON A.G. & PERSSON P. (1957) The relationship between the direction of Sharpey's fibres and the deposition of cementum. *Odont. T.* **65**, 457–463.

[6] FULLMER H.M. & LILLIE R.D. (1958) The oxytalan fiber: a previously undescribed connective tissue fiber. *J. Histochem. Cytochem.* **6**, 425–430.

[7] CARNEIRO J. & FAVA DE MORAES F. (1965) Radioautographic visualization of collagen metabolism in the periodontal tissues of the mouse. *Arch. oral Biol.* **10**, 833–848.

[8] STALLARD R.E. (1963) The utilization of H^3 proline by the connective tissue elements of the periodontium. *Periodontics* **1**, 185–188.

[9] KELLER G.J. & COHEN D.W. (1955) India ink perfusions of the vascular plexus of oral tissues. *Oral Surg.* **8**, 539–542.

[10] KINDLOVA M. & MATENA V. (1962) Blood vessels of the rat molar. *J. dent. Res.* **41**, 650–660.

[11] CARRANZA F.A., ITOIZ M.E., CABRINI R.L. & DOTTO C.A. (1966) A study of periodontal vascularization in different laboratory animals. *J. periodont. Res.* **1**, 120–128.

[12] CASTELLI W.A. & DEMPSTER W.T. (1965) The periodontal vasculature and its responses to experimental pressures. *J. Amer. dent. Ass.* **70**, 890–905.

[13] JERGE C.R. (1965) Comments on the innervation of the teeth. *Dent. Clin. N. Amer.* March, 117–127.

[14] BERNICK S. (1957) Innervation of teeth and periodon-

tium after enzymatic removal of collagenous elements. *Oral Surg.* **10**, 323–332.

[15] TOLMAN D.E., WINKELMAN R.K. & GIBILISCO J.A. (1965) Nerve endings in gingival tissue. *J. dent. Res.* **44**, 657–663.

[16] GAIRNS F.W. & AITCHISON J. (1950) A preliminary study of the multiplicity of nerve endings in the human gum. *Dent. practit. dent. Rec.* **70**, 180–194.

[17] McHUGH W.D. (1961) The development of the gingival epithelium in the monkey. *Dent. practit. dent. Rec.* **11**, 314–324.

[18] WAERHAUG J. (1952) The gingival pocket. *Odont. T.* **60**, Suppl. 1.

[19] GOTTLIEB B. & ORBAN B. (1938) *Biology and Pathology of the Tooth and its Supporting Mechanism.* New York: Macmillan.

[20] COHEN D.W. (1965) Pathology of periodontal disease, in *Oral Pathology*, Ed. Tiecke R. W. New York: McGraw-Hill.

[21] WILLIAMS C.H.M. (1943) Investigation concerning the dentition of the Eskimos of Canada's Eastern Arctic. *J. Periodont.* **14**, 34–37.

[22] SCHROEDER H.E. & LISTGARTEN M.A. (1971) Fine structure of the developing epithelial attachment of human teeth, in *Monographs in Developmental Biology*, Ed. Wolsky A. Basel: S. Karger.

[23] KALLENBACH E. (1970) Fine structure of rat incisor enamel organ during late pigmentation and regression stages. *J. Ultrastruct. Res.* **30**, 38–63.

[24] REITH E.J. (1970) The stages of amelogenesis as observed in molar teeth of young rats. *J. Ultrastruct. Res.* **30**, 111–151.

[25] GRANT D.A., STERN I.B. & EVERETT F.G. (1968) *Orban's Periodontics*, 3rd Edition, p. 32–33, St. Louis: C.V. Mosby Co.

[26] PROVENZA D.V. & SISCA R.F. (1970) Fine structure features of monkey (Macaca mulatta) reduced enamel epithelium. *J. Periodont.* **41**, 313–319.

[27] SKOUGAARD M.R. & BEAGRIE G.S. (1962) The renewal of gingival epithelium in marmosets (Callithrix Jacchus)

as determined through autoradiography with thymidine-H^3. *Acta odont. scand.* **20**, 467–484.

[28] GLAVIND L. & ZANDER H.A. (1970) Dynamics of dental epithelium during tooth eruption. *J. dent. Res.* **49**, 549–555.

[29] SKOUGAARD M.R. (1965) *Cell Population Kinetics of the Gingival Epithelium.* Copenhagen: Internat. Sci. Publ.

[30] COHEN B. (1959) Morphologic factors in the pathogenesis of periodontal disease. *Brit. dent. J.* **107**, 31–39.

[31] KARRING T. & LOE H. (1970) The three-dimensional concept of the epithelium-connective tissue boundary of gingiva. *Acta odont. scand.* **28**, 917–933.

[32] SCHROEDER H.E. & MUNZEL-PEDRAZZOLI S. (1970) Morphometric analysis comparing junctional and oral epithelium of normal human gingiva. *Helv. Odont. Acta.* **14**, 53–66.

[33] LISTGARTEN M.A. (1972) Ultrastructure of the dentogingival junction after gingivectomy. *J. periodont. Res.* **7**, 151–160.

[34] SCHROEDER H.E. (1970) Quantitative parameters of early human gingival inflammation. *Arch. oral Biol.* **15**, 383–400.

[35] NEIDERS M.E. (1972) Contact phenomena of epithelial cells. *Oral Science Reviews* **1**, 69–101.

[36] COHEN B. (1959) Pathology of the interdental tissues. *Dent. practit. dent. Rec.* **9**, 167–173.

[37] FISH W. (1961) Etiology and prevention of periodontal breakdown. *Dent. Progr.* **1**, 234–247.

[38] SCHULTZ-HAUDT S.D., WAERHAUG J., FROM S.H. & ATTRAMADAL A. (1963) On the nature of contact between the gingival epithelium and the tooth enamel surface. *Periodontics* **1**, 103–108.

[39] GERSH I. & CATCHPOLE H.R. (1960) The nature of ground substance of connective tissue. *Perspect. Biol. Med.* **3**, 282–319.

[40] ARNIM S.S. & HAGERMAN D.A. (1953) The connective tissue fibers of the marginal gingiva. *J. Amer. dent. Ass.* **47**, 271–281.

[41] MELCHER A.H. (1962) The pathogenesis of chronic gingivitis: The spread of the inflammatory process. *Dent. practit. dent. Rec.* **13**, 2–7.

CHAPTER 2

The environment of the tooth

HOMEOSTASIS

Homeostasis may be defined as the tendency of an organism or tissue to maintain its integrity in face of a changing environment. The stability and integrity of the periodontal tissues are influenced by the everchanging balance between conditions in the mouth which constitute the environment of the crown and the local tissue environment of the root (fig. 2.1). The balance is such that change in one environment is likely to be reflected by change in the other.

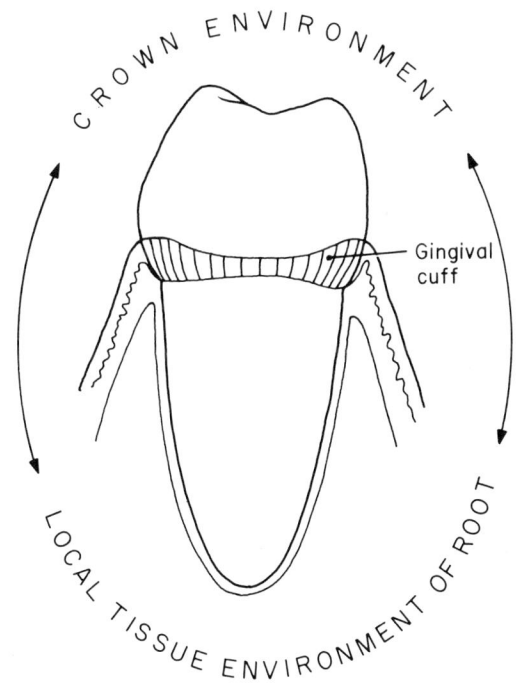

FIG. 2.1. Homeostasis.

The environment of the crown

The oral cavity is host to one of the densest and most varied of known microbial populations [1]. The literature records that at least twenty-eight species of microorganisms have been isolated from the mouth. The salivary microbial count has been variously reported to be between 43×10^6 and 5500×10^6 per ml of saliva [2]. The number of organisms in deposits on teeth such as bacterial plaque is even higher, and has been stated to be of the order of $1 \cdot 7 \times 10^{11}$ microorganisms per gramme wet weight of plaque [3]. This latter figure corresponds to that obtained in an equivalent weight of packed cells from a centrifuged broth culture of streptococci. Conditions in the mouth are therefore influenced greatly by this parasitic population. The mouth should be regarded as a dynamic biological system, not only in terms of a population of many different groups of microorganisms in balance with each other, but also in terms of an overall commensal population which is in balance with the host [4].

Infectious disease may be defined as the impairment of function which an organism suffers through the activities of some other organism that lives within or upon it [4]. The concepts of health and disease are difficult to define, as one is usually explained in terms of the other. Thus health may be defined as an absence of disease. According to Topley and Wilson the basis of all harmful effects of bacterial infection is 'quite certainly chemical' [5].

Parasitism is a universal phenomenon in biology. Only a small percentage of the obligatory parasites, harboured by every form of higher life, is involved in the causation of disease. The fact that parasitism is universal, whereas frank disease is relatively infrequent, indicates that, in general, host–parasite relationships tend towards equilibrium.

Microbial interactions are important in determining the outcome of an attempt by a microbe to establish itself in an area where there is a stable resident flora. These interactions may take the form of indifference (commensalism), antagonism (antibiosis), mutual benefit (symbiosis) or cooperation (synergism). Not all host–parasite interactions are detrimental to the host. The normal flora of the intestinal tract produces vitamin K and also some of the vitamin B complex. The benefit derived by the host from a commensal parasitic population is, however, relatively small.

The microbial population in the sulcus area is large and varied, and as yet large scale comprehensive studies to compare the flora in health and disease are only beginning to emerge.

The findings from some small scale investigations have suggested that whilst quantitatively there is an increase in bacteria with the onset of gingivitis there appears to be relatively little qualitative change [3 & 6]. It has been reported that when a small group of dental students ceased cleaning their teeth an increase in bacterial plaque was noted, followed by clinically evident gingivitis [7]. Study of the bacterial population in these subjects, however, showed both quantitative and qualitative changes with the onset of inflammation. It was reported that smears taken from the cervical region of clean teeth showed a sparse flora, consisting almost entirely of gram positive cocci and rods. After 2 days of plaque accumulation, in addition to an increase in the numbers of these microorganisms, about 30 per cent of the total number was gram negative cocci and rods. During the next few days fusobacteria and filaments appeared (up to 7 per cent) and by 7–9 days the flora was supplemented with spirilla and spirochaetes (2 per cent). Following reinstitution of oral hygiene the numbers and types of microorganisms reverted to those found at the onset of the study. It was also noted that the gingival inflammation resolved 1 day after plaque removal [7]. Present evidence suggests that there may be clearly detectable differences in the relative proportions of microorganisms in bacterial samples from healthy and diseased sites. It has been suggested that in areas of health the proportion of coccoid cells may be more than three times as high as in areas of disease and may account for more than three-quarters of the microbial population in a healthy sulcus [8]. (See chapter 4.)

The indigenous microbial population of the mouth tends to maintain its balance as a whole and resists invasion of its territories by exogenous organisms which it attempts to suppress [9, 10 & 11]. It follows that exogenous infections of the mouth are relatively infrequent and breakdown of the system is most commonly expressed as an endogenous infection [12 & 13], where one or more groups of the commensal population have become relatively increased.

MECHANICAL IRRITATION

Superimposed on this bacterial factor will be some degree of mechanical trauma during mastication and normal function, with the added possibility of further irritation from the edges of carious cavities, overhanging fillings or poorly fitting crowns. Food impaction may occur where there are inadequate contact points between the teeth, and a variable degree of inflammation is frequently found in association with orthodontic appliances or prostheses.

The local tissue environment of the root

The local tissue environment of the root is governed by the nutritional, endocrine and enzymatic factors responsible for epithelial and connective tissue metabolism throughout the body as a whole. Any failure of biochemical control of tissue metabolism may be reflected as a decreased capacity of the tissues to maintain their health in relation to the commensal population of the mouth (chap. 5).

DYNAMIC BALANCE

The balance between the two environments is such that the periodontium cannot be considered within strict limits as inflamed or not inflamed.

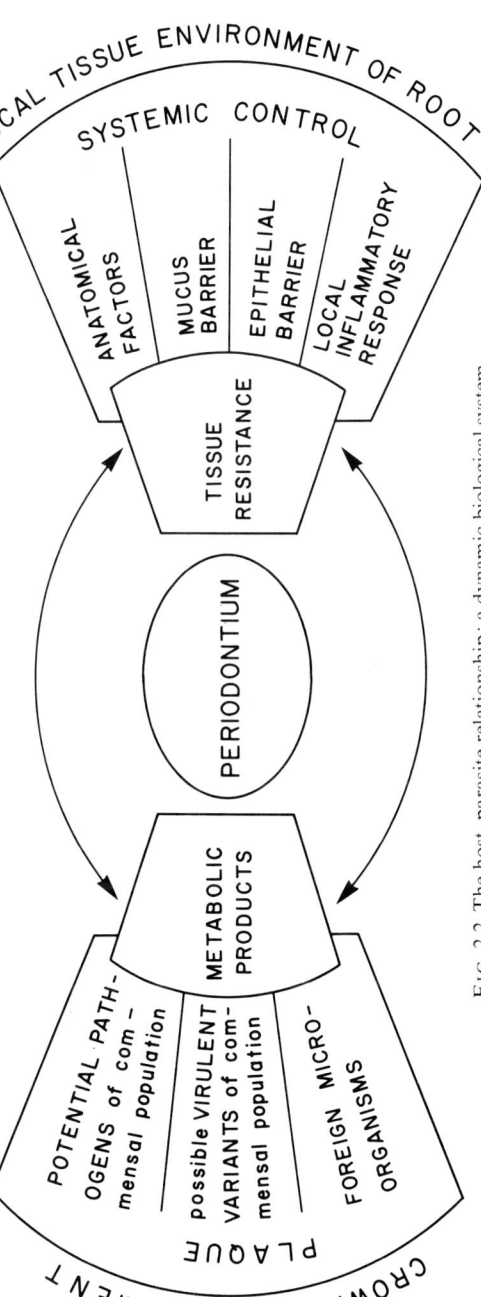

FIG. 2.2 The host–parasite relationship; a dynamic biological system.

CROWN ENVIRONMENT

Conditions in the mouth are influenced by the commensal population. The number of organisms in deposits on teeth is of the order of 1.7×10^{11} micro-organisms per g wet weight of plaque. Tissue damage results from the high concentration of metabolic products from the commensal organisms of plaque which overcomes the host resistance. There is, at present, no evidence of virulent variants of the commensal population arising as mutants. A commensal population tends to suppress foreign microorganisms introduced into its habitat.

TISSUE RESISTANCE

Host tissue resistance to the metabolic products of the commensal population of the mouth can be considered as a series of four barriers; breach of one or more of which is evidenced by disease.

Anatomical factors

Functional anatomical relationships of the tissues in the mouth are designed for effective comminution of food and clearance of food debris from the oral cavity. Plaque accumulates where functional tissue relationships are poor (stagnation areas) and causes disease.

Mucus barrier

Saliva is the direct environment of the commensal population of the mouth. It contains enzymes and antibodies which control growth of the commensal population, and an essential feature of saliva is rapid transportation of material to the oesophagus. The clearance time of saliva from the mouth is of the order of 30 min. Saliva trapped in a stagnation area may contribute to the substrate of plaque.

Epithelial barrier

The crowns of the teeth protrude into the mouth through a continuous epithelial sheath consisting of gingival and cuff epithelium. Plaque products may cause a 'biochemical lesion', or frank ulceration, of the thin epithelium of the embrasure which is the area of maximum risk, and cause disease.

The local inflammatory response

The balance of the dynamic system of the mouth is such that there is frequent low grade inflammation of gingivae as a result of irritants from the crown environment. In the presence of an adequate inflammatory response such inflammation is transient and resolves when the irritant is removed from the sulcus. The adequacy of the inflammatory response is reduced in presence of severe debilitating disease, such as diabetes or leukemia.

There is frequently a minimal threshold of inflammation of the connective tissues in relation to the tooth, demonstrable at least in histological terms [14]. Disturbance of the balance of the biological system (fig. 2.2) may occur as a result of either increase in intensity of local irritants in the mouth or decrease in the capacity of gingival tissue to maintain its health in relation to these irritants. This disturbance will be reflected as an increase in the level of nonspecific inflammation which is present. The increased level of non-specific inflammation may be considered as the general 'environmental expression' of any imbalance of the host–parasite system of the mouth. This form of expression remains similar for a wide range of different causative factors. Factors causing imbalance generally do not give rise to clinically distinct entities.

Dental plaque

Dental plaque consists of microorganisms embedded in a mass of protein and carbohydrate which is partly endogenous in origin, being derived from saliva and the products of tissue metabolism and catabolism, and partly exogenous in origin, being derived from the diet. Plaque is initially populated by gram positive rods and cocci, gram negative rods and cocci, fusobacteria, spirilla, spirochaetes, and subsequently by gram positive and negative filamentous forms, predominantly actinomyces and leptotrichia [7, 15, 16, 17 & 18]. Histological survey of gingival connective tissue has shown that the presence of organisms within inflamed tissue is a relatively rare finding [19]. As a result of quantitative and qualitative changes, the commensal population may become pathogenic due to the high concentration of bacterial metabolites which accumulates adjacent to the gingival sulcus. This population has little capacity to survive out of its own environment and is not ordinarily pathogenic. That the potential for pathogenicity exists is shown by

(1) subacute bacterial endocarditis related to *Streptococcus viridans*,

(2) bronchiectasis and postural lung abscesses related to dental infection [20],

(3) bite wound infections,

(4) gangrenous stomatitis (cancrum oris, noma).

There is considerable weight of evidence that periodontitis is a direct result of the reaction of the periodontal tissues to the metabolic products of the high concentration of microorganisms in dental plaque. There is no evidence that virulent variants of the commensal population, arising as a result of mutation, produce the tissue response, and exogenous infections of the mouth are rare.

Tissue resistance

The resistance of the periodontal tissues to irritation from the crown environment may be visualized as a series of barriers, the breach of one or more of which is evidenced by disease.

THE ANATOMICAL BARRIER

The health of individual tissues of the mouth is dependent on good functional anatomical relationships of the masticatory apparatus as a whole. The teeth, the supporting bone of the maxilla and mandible, the temporomandibular joint, the masticatory muscles and the investing sheath of the oral mucosa act as a single functional unit within which the individual tissues are mutually interdependent (fig. 2.3). Changes in one component of the unit are reflected in the other tissues. If teeth are lost, the remaining teeth are free to move through the supporting bone (fig. 2.4c). This change in position of the teeth may result in a change in pattern of movement of the joint or change in the functional relationship of the gingival tissues to the teeth. The functional efficiency of the masticatory apparatus as a whole is thereby reduced.

The teeth are set in catenary arches; each tooth meeting its neighbour in a narrow zone of contact below which there is epithelial continuity from buccal to lingual. The teeth of each arch meet along the plane of occlusion which curves upwards, backwards and outwards. The lips and cheeks lie close against the buccal and labial surfaces of the teeth, and the tongue lies against the lingual and palatal surfaces. Movement of these tissues during mastication and speech has a cleansing action by virtue of this functional contact against the teeth.

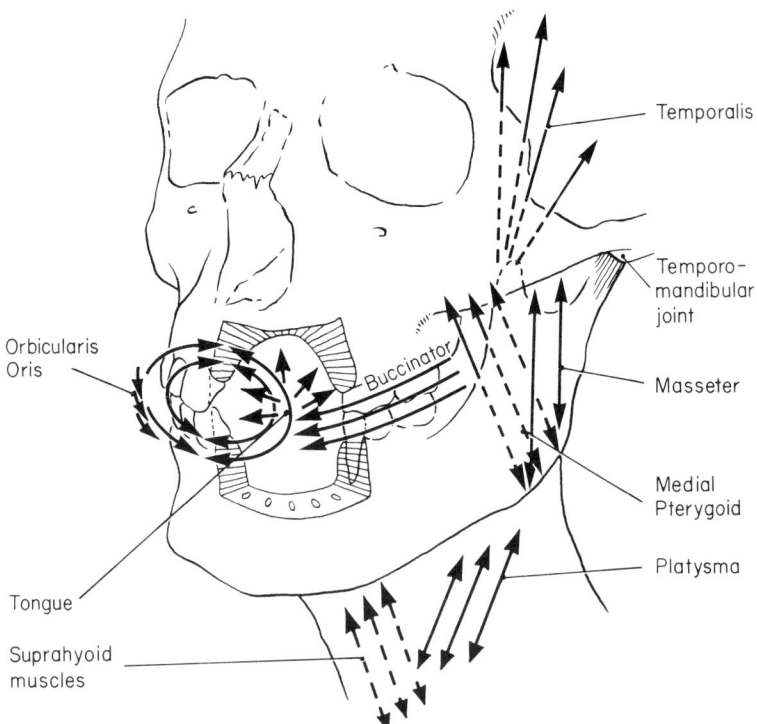

Temporalis

Temporo-
mandibular
joint

Masseter

Medial
Pterygoid

Platysma

Orbicularis
Oris

Buccinator

Tongue

Suprahyoid
muscles

FIG. 2.3. The mouth is a functional unit. The teeth, the supporting bone of maxilla and mandible, the temporo-mandibular joint, the masticatory muscles and the investing sheath of the oral mucosa act as a single functional unit within which the individual tissues are mutually interdependent.

The teeth themselves have a shape which deflects food from the junction of soft tissue and tooth and may thereby protect the gingival margins from damage during mastication (fig. 2.4).

The buccal surface of incisor teeth is convex, so that during incision food is deflected clear of the gingival margin (fig. 2.4). The interstitial surface is convex so that each tooth meets its neighbour in a narrow zone of contact to prevent food being forced down between the teeth, which would affect the continuity of the soft tissues through the embrasure. With interproximal wear, the area of contact increases (fig. 2.5), and it has been estimated that the anteroposterior length of the dental arch decreases 1 cm by the time middle age has been reached [21 & 22].

The posterior teeth follow the same principle, the primary function of cusps and fissures being mastication; and the equally important secondary function is the deflection of food along defined paths over the buccal and lingual convexities, clear of the junction of the soft tissues with the tooth.

In ideal terms, where functional anatomical relationships are good, the mouth should be largely self-cleansing of food but not of bacterial plaque [11 & 23]. Tooth shape, tooth position and the occlusal pattern assume an added significance in the mouth of the patient with periodontal disease, and the basis of treatment lies in the creation of acceptable functional anatomical relationships. Casual extraction, and restorative procedures undertaken without respect to functional anatomical form, tend to exaggerate an existing periodontitis.

THE MUCUS BARRIER

The mucous membrane of the mouth is covered

by a layer of saliva which acts as a primary barrier to the spread of infection and constitutes the environment of the commensal population throughout the mouth as a whole.

Saliva

Saliva is a colourless, odourless fluid of varying viscosity secreted by three paired major glands, the parotid, submandibular and sublingual

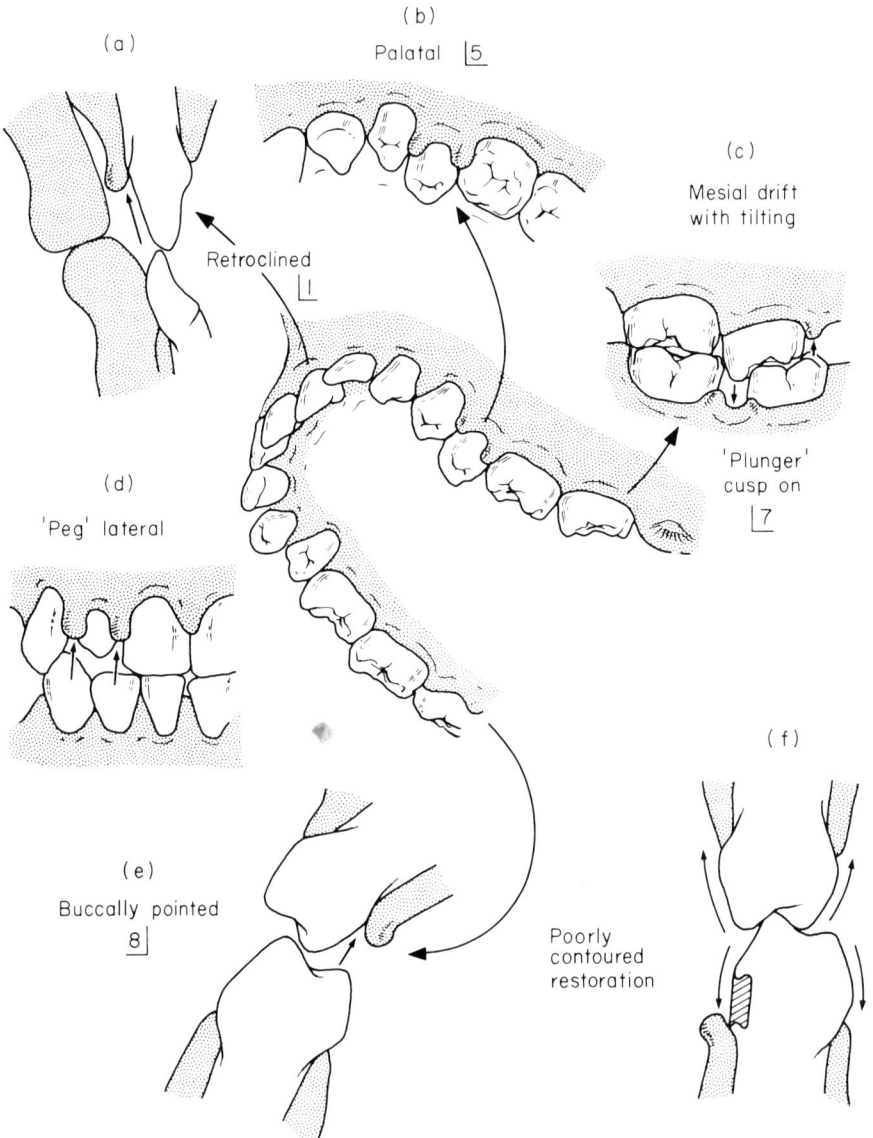

FIG. 2.4. (a) Retroclined maxillary incisor causing food impaction in the buccal sulcus. (b) Gingival inflammation in stagnation area caused by palatally displaced ⊥². (c) Plunger cusp relationship resulting from mesial drift and tilting of ⫤⅞ following removal of ⫤⁷. (d) Inflammation associated with lack of contact area protection of embrasure due to malformed lateral incisor. (e) Palatal food packing due to tilting of ⅞⊢. (f) Food packing due to poorly designed restoration which does not follow contour of tooth.

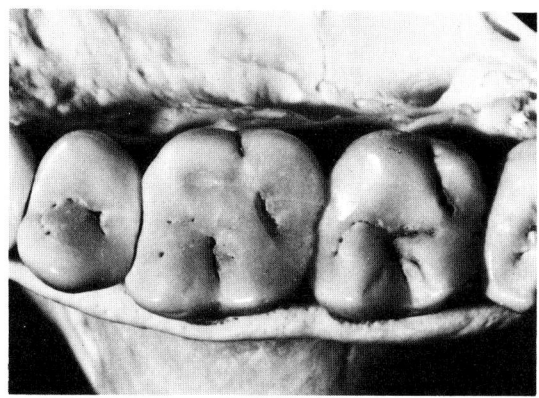

FIG. 2.5. An occlusal view of maxillary posterior teeth in the dried skull showing proximal wear resulting in a broader contact area and shortening of the antero-posterior length of the arch.

glands, and by a large number of small accessory glands distributed throughout the oral mucous membranes [24].

The total volume of saliva secreted each day is probably in the region of 800–1000 ml although a figure of 500 ml per day has been reported for two patients with oesophageal fistulae [25].

The secretions of the various glands differ in composition, and great variation is found in the composition of saliva among individuals and in the same individuals at different times. Glandular secretion is under the control of the sympathetic and parasympathetic nervous systems [26]. No hormone has yet been isolated which controls the rate of salivary flow, although ACTH has been shown to influence the sodium but not the potassium levels [27]. There is evidence, however, of a close relationship between the activity of salivary glands and the endocrine system [28].

Mixed saliva has a specific gravity of between 1·00 and 1·01 which increases with the rate of flow. Saliva has an average pH of 6·7 which varies considerably with the rate of flow [29]. Although proteins afford the main buffering capacity in plaque, bicarbonates are the most important buffers in saliva.

Saliva is supersaturated with regard to calcium and phosphorus [30]. Other inorganic constituents include potassium, sodium, thiocyanate, chloride and carbonates.

Microorganisms, epithelial cells, leucocytes and food debris are found in saliva once the glandular secretion has reached the mouth and give rise to its opalescent appearance. The organic component comprises plasma protein, enzymes (table 4.2), urea, amino acids, phospholipids, citrates, vitamins, mucin and sialic acid.

A number of functions have been attributed to saliva, apart from its function of initiating the breakdown of some carbohydrates. These include lubrication, facilitating chewing and swallowing, and speech; it has antibacterial properties and forms one of the barriers to the penetration of bacteria into host tissue.

The mucus sheath acts as a barrier to dissemination of infection in three essential ways.

(1) Its capacity as a lyophilic sol enables it to absorb water. The fixed water in the mucus does not wet the underlying epithelium and so reduces the permeability of epithelium to bacterial toxins [31].

(2) Its antibody and lysozyme content contributes to the control of the commensal bacterial population of the mouth [32].

(3) The sheath is not static. It was shown by Bloomfield [33 & 34] that: 'Its essential feature is direct and rapid transportation of material towards the oesophagus'. Studies of the clearance of charcoal particles from the mouth have shown that mucus takes a direct and relatively constant course along specific routes towards the oesophagus, and in this way bacteria inoculated into the mouth do not spread widely. The clearance time is of the order of 30 min. This barrier breaks down when there is primary insufficiency of saliva as in Sjögrens syndrome, or more commonly where functional anatomical relationships are such that a stagnation area exists. Breakdown products of mucus trapped in a stagnation area contribute to the substrate of dental plaque. Mouthbreathing caused by incomplete lip seal or inadequate nasal airway results in drying of the gingiva in the upper anterior region leading frequently to breach of the mucous barrier and gingival hyperplasia [35].

THE EPITHELIAL BARRIER

The ability of an epithelial surface to resist

penetration of bacterial toxins is related to the thickness of the epithelium, the degree of keratinization and the rate of turnover of the cell population. The oral mucosa is keratinized to varying degrees throughout the mouth, to some extent in proportion to the degree of functional stimulation in each area. This tissue has a well developed capacity to respond to irritation by hyperplasia and downgrowth of the basal layers, and frequently to return to a normal histological appearance after the irritant has been removed. The degree of chronic irritation is maximal in the region of the gingival sulcus since plaque is constantly present in that area. The nonkeratinized, thin, sulcular epithelium is easily damaged and is a less effective barrier to penetration of the connective tissues by bacterial products than is the oral mucosa in other areas of the mouth. While it may be fragile and permeable, however, it is also uniquely equipped to deal with the repeated injuries to which it is subjected as a result of its location between the gingival connective tissue and the tooth [36]. The structural characteristics of this region suggest that the floor of the sulcus, formed by the most superficial layers of the junctional epithelium is the most permeable portion. It is readily disrupted by the introduction of foreign objects, such as metal or plastic strips or periodontal probes. This disruption generally occurs within the epithelium rather than at the tooth-epithelial junction and may be facilitated by the presence of large numbers of leucocytes in the junctional epithelium [37]. The permeability of the dento-gingival junction has been studied with respect to both the passage of irritant material from the mouth into the gingival connective tissues and the outward passage of an inflammatory exudate across the epithelium into the sulcus, which this stimulus may provoke. It is now widely accepted that junctional epithelium represents no real barrier to penetration of biologically active material from plaque. Experiments by Egelberg [38] have shown that at least small molecules can penetrate through intact epithelium and Fine [39] has reported that carbon particles 1–3 μm in diameter pass through junctional and sulcular epithelium in normal human gingiva into the underlying connective tissues. Tolo [40]

used tritiated albumen to show that a protein with a molecular weight of 68,000 would easily penetrate the intracellular spaces of junctional epithelium, but not as readily the underlying connective tissues. McDougall [41] has stated that horse-radish peroxidase fails to penetrate through keratinized epithelium of rat gingiva, but rapidly enters the intercellular spaces of the non-keratinized junctional epithelium, reaching the most apical cells of the junctional epithelium after as little as 10 min. It was further reported that application of the enzyme resulted in enlargement of the intercellular spaces and stimulation of polymorphonuclear leucocyte emigration. A number of reports have suggested that certain enzymes may have the capacity to increase the permeability of junctional epithelium by enlarging the intercellular spaces [42, 43, 44 & 45]. The increased numbers of leucocytes which occupy enlarged intercellular spaces of inflamed junctional epithelium may be a response to chemotactic factors originating from the mouth. While some of these chemotactic factors may originate from dental plaque [46 & 47], it has been shown that leucocytes can also be attracted to this site in germfree animals [48, 49 & 50], possibly as a result of chemotactic factors which are not dependent on the presence of live bacteria. While some work has suggested that demonstrable ulceration of sulcular or junctional epithelium is a necessary precursor to antigen penetration [51], micro-ulceration of such epithelia is likely to be a frequently occurring event. The majority of studies suggest that antigenic substances will penetrate from the sulcus into the underlying connective tissues [52 & 53]. The formation of specific antibodies in gingival connective tissues following sensitization of animals by antigens penetrating via the gingival sulcus has also been demonstrated [54].

Junctional epithelium acts as a two way filter in that these stimuli result in the outflow of gingival fluid into the sulcus region.

Since the investing sheath is subject to a degree of trauma in normal function, and plaque is ubiquitously present in sheltered areas of the mouth, the presence of exudate in the sulcus is a consistent finding in the inflamed mouth. All the evidence suggests that gingival fluid is a major factor in government of the ecology of the bacterial population of the sulcus [55] and of subgingival plaque in particular. Egelberg [56] underlined the importance of gingival fluid in the statement '. . . here the environment must be governed primarily by factors such as gingival fluid, desquamated epithelial cells, and emigrated white blood cells. The gingival fluid as a substrate for bacterial growth is different from saliva. The subgingival microbiota has to develop in co-existence with the crevicular leucocytes.'

Bacteria artificially introduced into healthy sulci are cleared by the inflammatory response within 24 hours [57] and do not seem to be able to remain below the gingival margin unless retained in the stroma of dental plaque.

The composition of gingival fluid is variable and consists of differing proportions of the humoral elements associated with the inflammatory response, and large numbers of leucocytes [58, 59 & 60].

Gingival fluid has been shown to contain:

(1) Amino acids [61 & 62].

(2) Plasma proteins such as albumin, $\alpha 1$, $\alpha 2$, β and γ globulins as revealed by immunoelectrophoresis [62].

(3) Electrolytes, i.e. sodium, potassium, calcium and phosphorous [58].

(4) A fibrinolytic system [63].

(5) Cellular material [64 & 65].

A correlation between pocket depth, inflammation and the amount of gingival fluid obtained has been demonstrated [66 & 67]. Other factors which have been shown to influence the amount of gingival fluid in both pathologically involved and healthy mouths are chewing [61], mechanical stimulation and gingival massage [68], circadian rhythms [69], hormonal changes [70] and enzymes [71].

LOCAL INFLAMMATORY RESPONSE

The final and perhaps the most significant barrier to penetration of the connective tissues by factors from the crown environment is the local inflammatory response. The balance of the biological system of the mouth is such that inflammation is usually chronic, and the cells characteristic of periodontitis are thus plasma cells and lymphocytes (fig. 2.6). Where acute inflammation exists, it most commonly arises as an exacerbation of a pre-existing chronic condition, and polymorphonuclear leucocytes are seen against a background of mononuclear cells.

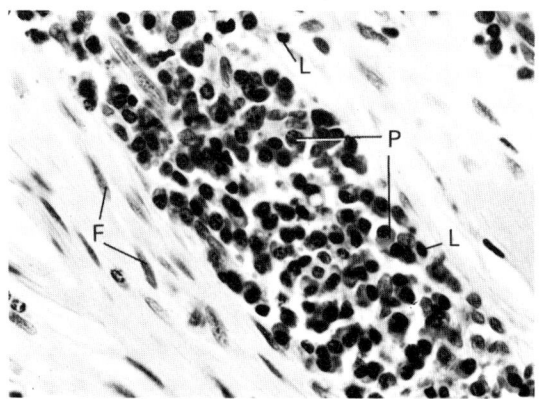

FIG. 2.6. Histological section showing an infiltrate of chronic inflammatory cells between bundles of collagen fibres; F, fibroblasts; L, lymphocytes; P, plasma cells.

Sections of gingival tissue frequently show inflammation of the connective tissues underlying the junction of junctional and sulcular epithelium, immediately adjacent to plaque adherent to the tooth surface.

The main factors in tissue resistance, which govern the balance between the mouth environment and the local tissue environment, are the integrity of anatomical form of the tissues, nutritional and endocrine control of local tissue metabolism, and the ability of the patient to produce an adequate inflammatory response (fig. 2.7).

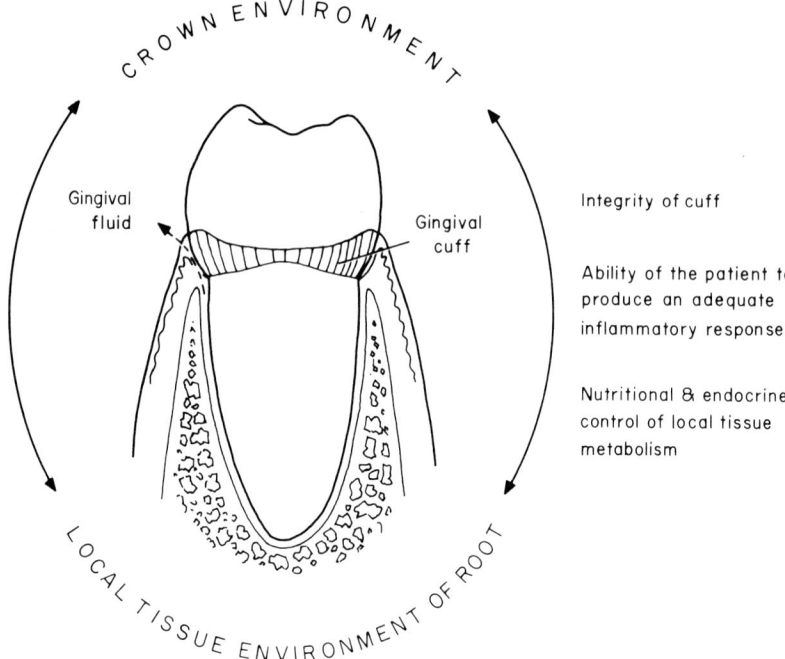

FIG. 2.7. The main factors in tissue resistance.

REFERENCES

[1] SCHERP H.W. & BURNETT G.W. (1956) Host–parasite interaction in relation to dental disease. *Norske Tannlaegeforen. Tid.* April, 25.

[2] STRÅLFORS A. (1950) Investigations into the bacterial chemistry of dental plaques. *Odont. T.* **58**, 155.

[3] SOCRANSKY S.S., GIBBONS R.J., DALE A.C., BORTNICK L., ROSENTHAL E. & MACDONALD J.B. (1963) The microbiota of the gingival crevice area of man: total microscopic and viable counts of specific organisms. *Arch. oral Biol.* **8**, 275.

[4] BURNETT G.W. & SCHERP H.W. (1966) *Oral Microbiology and Infectious Disease*, 2nd Edition. Baltimore: Williams and Wilkins.

[5] WILSON G.S. & MILES A.A. (1955) *Principles of Bacteriology and Immunity*, 4th Edition. London: Arnold.

[6] GIBBONS R.J., SOCRANSKY S.S., SAWYER S., KAPSIMALIS B. & MACDONALD J.B. (1963) Microbiota of the gingival crevice area of man. II, the predominant cultivable organisms. *Arch. oral Biol.* **8**, 281–289.

[7] THEILADE E., WRIGHT W.H., BORGLUM JENSEN S. & LÖE H. (1966) Experimental gingivitis in man. II. a longitudinal clinical and bacteriological investigation. *J. periodont. Res.* **1**, 1–13.

[8] LISTGARTEN M.A. & HELLDEN L. (1978) Relative distribution of bacteria at clinically healthy and periodontally diseased sites in humans. *J. Clin. Periodont.* **5**, 115, 132.

[9] BJÖRNSJÖ K.B. (1950) Studies on the antibacterial factors of human saliva. *Acta chem. scand.* **4**, 835–841.

[10] BURROWS W. (1959) *Textbook of Microbiology*, p. 283. Philadelphia: Saunders.

[11] ALEXANDER A.G., MORGENSTEIN S.I. & RIBBONS J.W. (1969) A study of the growth of plaque and the efficiency of self-cleansing mechanisms. *Dent. practit. dent. Rec.* **19**, 293–297.

[12] ROSEBURY T. (1952) The role of infection in periodontal disease. *Oral Surg.* **5**, 363–370.

[13] ROSEBURY T. (1961) Infection and inflammatory periodontal disease. *J. West Soc. Periodont.* **9**, 105.

[14] BERNIER J.L. (1950) Histologic changes of the gingival tissues in health and periodontal disease. A preliminary report. *Oral Surg.* **3**, 1194–1199.

[15] McDOUGALL W.A. (1963) Studies on the dental plaque. I. The histology of the dental plaque and its attachment. *Aust. dent. J.* **8**, 261–273.

[16] McDOUGALL W.A. (1963) Studies on the dental plaque.

II. The histology of the developing interproximal plaque. *Aust. dent. J.* **8**, 398–407.

[17] McDougall W.A. (1963) Studies on the dental plaque. III. The effect of saliva on salivary mucoids and its relationship to the regrowth of plaques. *Aust. dent. J.* **8**, 463–467.

[18] McDougall W.A. (1964) Studies on the dental plaque. IV. Levans and the dental plaque. *Aust. dent. J.* **9**, 1–5.

[19] Wertheimer F.W. (1964) A histologic study of microorganisms and human periodontal tissues. *J. Periodont.* **35**, 406–409.

[20] Fallon M. & Main D.M.G. (1963) Dental sepsis and lung infection. *Dent. practit. dent. Rec.* **13**, 281–284.

[21] Goldman H.M., Schluger S., Fox L. & Cohen D.W. (1964) *Periodontal Therapy*, 3rd Edition. Saint Louis: Mosby.

[22] Lammie G.A. & Posselt U. (1965) Progressive changes in the dentition of adults. *J. Periodont.* **36**, 443–454.

[23] Lindhe J. & Wicen P.O. (1969) The effect on the gingivae of chewing fibrous foods. *J. periodont. Res.* **4**, 193–201.

[24] Sreebny L.M. & Meyer J. (1964) *Salivary Glands and their Secretions*. Oxford: Pergamon.

[25] McKeown K.C. & Dunstone G.H. (1959) Some observations on salivary secretion and fluid absorption by mouth. *Brit. med. J.* **ii**, 670.

[26] Burgen A.S.V. & Emmelin N.G. (1961) *Physiology of the Salivary Glands*, Monographs of the Physiological Society, Number 8. London: Arnold.

[27] Dreizen S. *et al.* (1952) The effect of ACTH and cortisone on the sodium and potassium levels of human saliva. *J. dent. Res.* **31**, 271–280.

[28] Shafer W.G. & Muhler J.C. (1956) Some observations on the relationship between the salivary glands and the endocrine system. *J. Amer. Coll. Dent.* **23**, 193.

[29] Brawley R.E. (1935) Studies on the pH of normal resting saliva. *J. dent. Res.* **15**, 55–77.

[30] Rathje W. (1956) Oversaturation of saliva with hydroxyapatite. *J. dent. Res.* **35**, 245–248.

[31] Lammie G.A. (1966) *Dental Orthopaedics*. Oxford: Alden.

[32] Brandtzaeg P. (1966) Local factors of resistance in the gingival area. *J. Periodont. Res.* **1**, 19–42.

[33] Bloomfield A.L. (1921) Dissemination of bacteria in the upper air passages. I. The circulation of foreign particles in the mouth. *Amer. Rev. Tuberc.* **5**, 903–914.

[34] Bloomfield A.L. (1922) Dissemination of bacteria in the upper air passages. II. The circulation of bacteria in the mouth. *John Hopk. Hosp. Bull.* **33**, 145–139.

[35] Jacobson L. (1973) Mouthbreathing and gingivitis. *J. periodont. Res.* **8**, 269–277.

[36] Listgarten M.A. (1972) Normal development, structure, physiology and repair of gingival epithelium. *Oral Science Reviews* **1**, 3.

[37] Schroeder H.E. & Listgarten M.A. (1971) Fine structure of the developing epithelial attachment of human teeth, in *Monographs in Developmental Biology*. Ed. Wolsky A. Basel: S. Karger.

[38] Egelberg J. (1963) Diffusion of histamine into the gingival crevice and through the crevicular epithelium. *Acta odont. scand.* **21**, 271–282.

[39] Fine D.H. *et al.* (1969) The penetration of human gingival sulcular tissue by carbon particles. *Arch. oral Biol.* **14**, 1117–1119.

[40] Tolo K.J. (1971) A study of permeability of gingival pocket epithelium in guinea pigs and Norwegian pigs. *Arch. oral Biol.* **16**, 881–888.

[41] McDougall W.A. (1971) Penetration pathways of a topically applied foreign protein into rat gingiva. *J. periodont. Res.* **6**, 89–99.

[42] Schultz-Haudt S.D., Dewar M. & Bibby B.G. (1953) Effects of hyaluronidase on human gingival epithelium. *Science* **117**, 653.

[43] Thilander H. (1963) Effect of leucocyte enzyme activity on the structure of the gingival pocket epithelium in man. *Acta odont. scand.* **21**, 431–451.

[44] Murphy P.J. & Stallard R.E. (1968) An altered gingival attachment epithelium: a result of the enzyme hyaluronidase. *Periodontics* **6**, 105–108.

[45] Stallard R.E. & Awwa I.A. (1969) The effect of alterations in the external environment on the dento-gingival junction. *J. dent. Res.* **48**, 671–675.

[46] Schroeder H.E. (1970) Quantitative parameters of early human gingival inflammation. *Arch. oral Biol.* **15**, 383–400.

[47] Tempel T.R., Snyderman R., Jordan H.V. *et al.* (1970) Factors from saliva and oral bacteria, chemotactic for polymorphonuclear leucocytes: their possible role in gingival inflammation. *J. Periodont.* **41**, 71–80.

[48] Magnusson B. (1969) Mucosal changes in erupting molars in germfree rats. *J. Periodont. Res.* **4**, 181–188.

[49] Listgarten M.A. & Heneghan J.B. (1971) Chronic inflammation in the gingival tissue of germfree dogs. *Arch. oral Biol.* **16**, 1207–1213.

[50] Courant P.R. (1971) Electron microscopic observations on neutrofil infiltration of germfree gnotobiotic rat interdental gingiva. *57th Annual Meeting Amer. Acad. Periodont.* Chicago.

[51] Rizzo A.A. (1970) Histologic and immunologic evaluation of antigen penetration into oral tissues after topical application. *J. Periodont.* **41**, 210–213.

[52] Courant P.R. & Bader H. (1966) *Bacteroides melaninogenicus* and its products in the gingiva of man. *Periodontics* **4**, 131–136.

[53] Wittwer J.W., Toto P.D. & Dickler E.H. (1969) *Streptococcus mitis* antigens in inflamed gingiva. *J. Periodont.* **40**, 639–640.

[54] Ranney R.R. (1970) Specific antibody in gingiva and submandibular nodes of monkeys with allergic periodontal disease. *J. periodont. Res.* **5**, 1–7.

[55] Brill N. & Brönnestam R. (1960) Immuno-electrophoretic study of tissue fluids from gingival pockets. *Acta odont. scand.* **18**, 95–100.

[56] Egelberg J. (1970) A review of the development of dental plaque, in *Dental Plaque*. Ed. McHugh W.D. p. 13. Edinburgh: E & S Livingstone.

[57] Waerhaug J. & Steen E. (1952) Presence or absence of bacteria in gingival pockets and the reaction in healthy pockets to certain pure cultures. A bacteriological and histological investigation. *Odont. T.* **60**, 1–24.

[58] Krasse B. & Egelberg J. (1962) The relative propor-

tions of sodium, potassium and calcium in gingival pocket fluid. *Acta odont. scand.* **20**, 143–152.

[59] EGELBERG J. (1963) Cellular elements in gingival pocket fluid. *Acta odont. scand.* **21**, 283–287.

[60] CIMASONI G. (1974) The crevicular fluid. *Monographs in Oral Science.* Vol. 3. Ed. Myers H.M. Basel: S. Karger.

[61] BRILL N. (1959) Effect of chewing on flow of tissue fluid into human gingival pockets. *Acta odont. scand.* **17**, 277–284.

[62] MANN W.V. & STOFFER H.R. (1964) Identification of protein components in fluid from gingival pockets. *Periodontics* **2**, 263–266.

[63] GUSTAFFSSON G.T. & NILSSON I.M. (1961) Fibrinolytic activity in fluid from the gingival crevice. *Proc. Soc. exp. Biol. Med.* **106**, 277.

[64] LÖE H. (1961) Physiological aspects of the gingival pocket. An experimental study. *Acta odont. scand.* **19**, 387.

[65] ATTSTROM R. (1971) Studies on neutrophil poly-morphonuclear leucocytes at the dento-gingival junction in health and disease. *J. periodont. Res.* Suppl. 8.

[66] BRILL N. (1962) The gingival pocket fluid. Studies of its occurrence, composition and effect. *Acta odont. scand.* **20**, Suppl. 32.

[67] MANN W.V. (1963) The correlation of gingivitis, pocket depth and exudate from the gingival crevice. *J. Periodont.* **34**, 379.

[68] BRILL N. & KRASSE B. (1959) Effects of mechanical stimulation on flow of tissue fluid through the gingival pocket epithelium. *Acta odont. scand.* **17**, 115.

[69] BISSADA N.F., SCHAFFER E.M. & HAUS E. (1967) Circadian periodicity of human crevicular fluid flow. *J. Periodont.* **38**, 36.

[70] LINDHE J. & SONESSON B. (1966) The effect of sex hormones on inflammation. 1. The effect of progestorone. *J. periodont. Res.* **1**, 212.

[71] AWWA I. (1968) Interpretation of present epidemiological indices for periodontal disease. Master of Science and Dentistry Thesis. University of Minnesota.

CHAPTER 3

The pathology of periodontitis

Pathological change and deviation from the normal anatomical arrangement of the periodontal tissues is commonly associated with a variable degree of clinically evident inflammation (fig. 3.1). It is now generally agreed that the great majority of children and adults with periodontal disease suffer from a condition which is essentially inflammatory in nature. The inflammatory reaction in the periodontal tissues is not different from that of any other part of the body, and before considering periodontitis in particular the general features of inflammation should be reviewed.

INFLAMMATION

Burdon-Sanderson has stated that: 'the process of inflammation is the succession of changes which occur in a living tissue when it is injured, provided that the injury is not of such a degree as at once to destroy its structure and vitality' [1]. Menkin has put forward a narrower definition in which inflammation is: 'a complex, vascular, lymphatic, and local tissue reaction, elicited in higher animals by the presence of microorganisms, or of non-viable irritants' [2]. It should be stressed that the process is dynamic and not static.

Many forms of injury invoke an inflammatory response, but the host reaction remains essentially the same. The outcome of injury is conditioned by the severity and type of the irritant, the time period over which the injurious agent acts and the physiological state of the cells. Whereas an intense stimulus will elicit an acute reaction, characterized by increased vascular permeability and polymorph emigration, a stimulus of lower grade may evoke a more chronic type of reaction. Should the body not be able to remove the irritant, as in the case of bacterial plaque on teeth, a disease process develops in which there is a mixture of destruction, repair, and regeneration. This is called chronic inflammation, and such a mixture of tissue destruction and regeneration is a prime feature of chronic periodontitis. Walter and Israel have defined chronic inflammation as a process in which inflammatory destruction is proceeding at the same time as attempts at healing [3]. Whereas polymorphonuclear leucocytes are characteristic of the acute inflammatory response, mononuclear cells, principally macrophages and plasma cells, but including lymphocytes, are associated with chronic irritation of a minimal but persistent nature. Associated with the vascular and exudative changes in inflammation is alteration of the colloidal system of the ground substance of connective tissue (chap. 7). There is a tendency for the complex macromolecular ground substance to be disaggregated, with transformation from the gel to sol state, and subsequent alteration of the immediate environment of cells within the affected tissue.

The integrity of the cell, its continued existence and the maintenance of its specialized functions depend ultimately on the constant supply of energy and the stability of its immediate environment. Interference with energy supply may occur as a result of a variety of injuries, including the action of toxic substances. Such cellular changes may be reversible or irreversible.

A low grade of injury is usually associated with reversible change, but with increasing degrees of injury, cell death and autolysis may ensue [4].

Investigations of injured cells have given support to the view that a wide range of noxious substances may affect cell surface membranes and organelles. It is thought that the mechanism regulating ionic concentration within the cell

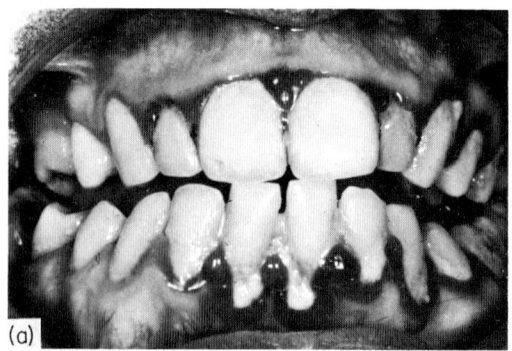

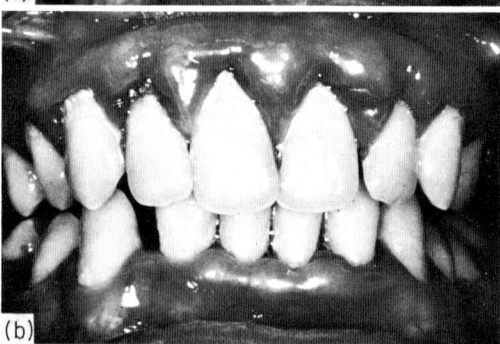

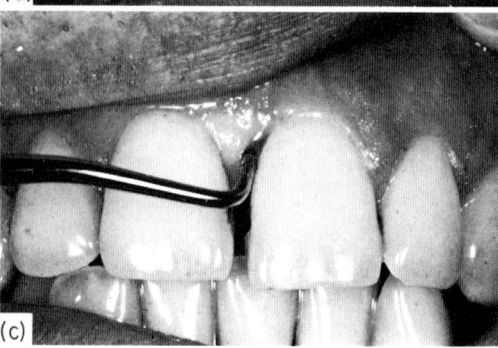

FIG. 3.1. (a) Chronic nonspecific inflammation principally of the marginal and papillary gingivae. (b) Chronic nonspecific inflammation associated with gingival enlargement showing obvious disorganization of the collagen structure of the marginal ligament and the presence of deep pockets. (c) Disorganization of the collagen structure of the marginal ligament and deep pocket formation associated with little clinically evident inflammation or distortion of gingival form.

is impeded. Sodium and water accumulate within the cell, which tends to become waterlogged. Although progressively the electrolytes can pass the cell membrane more freely, intracellular protein cannot escape. There is thus a tendency for the cell to become hypertonic with respect to its surroundings, and this may be increased if intracellular breakdown of protein follows. To counteract the hypertonicity, water passes into the cell. If the causal agent is removed during the early stages of this process, a return to normal may be possible, whilst progressive damage over a period of time may lead to cell death. The lipoprotein membrane of intracellular lysosomes appears to become ruptured, releasing the various hydrolytic enzymes which are associated with autolysis of cells.

The usual, although not inevitable, outcome of inflammation in connective tissue is the replacement of damaged tissue by newly formed tissue or, where regeneration is minimal, by fibrosis. Whether resolution immediately follows the exudative and cellular changes, or whether suppuration is interposed, depends on the nature of the irritant and the resulting tissue response.

Clinical features of gingivitis

Inflammation of the gingivae, gingivitis, is a widespread disease which affects approximately half the child and almost the total adult world populations [5]. Gingivitis usually starts at the tips of the interdental papillae and subsequently involves the gingival margins. It may be localized or generalized, and it frequently runs a protracted but progressive course with numerous exacerbations and remissions. The clinical features may vary, as they reflect the type and extent of inflammation present, which may be either acute or chronic. Any or all of the following signs may be noted (fig. 3.2).

(1) Discoloration of the gingival tissue from pink to bluish red occurs as a result of the increased degree of vascularization and stasis.

(2) The presence of pitting oedema is a result of extravasation of fluid and alteration in the state of aggregation of the connective tissue ground substance.

(3) Loss of stippling is a result of disaggrega-

tion and loss of attachment of the collagen bundles binding the attached gingivae to the underlying periosteum.

(4) Retraction of the gingivae is a result of disaggregation of the collagen bundles of the

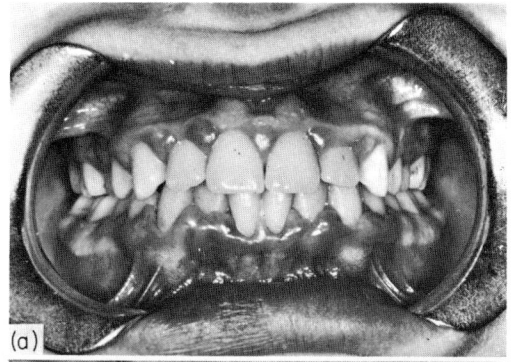

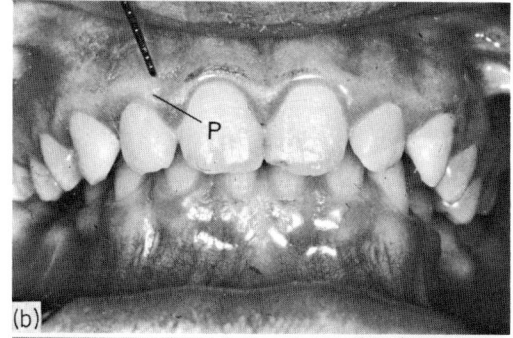

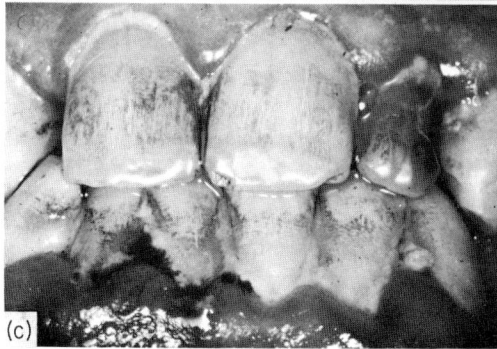

FIG. 3.2. (a) Discoloration of gingival tissue from pink to bluish red. The loss of stippling of attached gingivae and retraction of gingival tissue from the teeth is also shown. (b) Pitting oedema (P) following steady pressure with the rounded end of a periodontal probe. (c) Presence of gingival bleeding and a visible inflammatory exudate.

marginal ligament and loss of tissue tone.

(5) Bleeding, and the presence of a visible inflammatory exudate follows ulceration of the cuff epithelium. Ulceration may be defined as having occurred when there is a break in the continuity of an epithelial surface. Although previously there has been a tendency to use the term only when gross lesions were present, with advances in molecular biology and the concept of a biochemical lesion [6], the word is here used in the wider sense to include ultra structural and biochemical changes as well as those discernible at clinical or light microscopic levels.

The tissue changes of chronic periodontal disease may be expressed in one of three ways, or more commonly as a combination of these basic changes.

(1) Predominantly as oedema associated with disaggregation of the gel structure of connective tissue, and hyperplasia of the epithelial tissues, resulting in pocket formation (fig. 3.3a).

(2) Predominantly as hyperplasia of the connective tissues in relation to the tooth (fig. 3.3b). This may or may not be associated with hyperplasia of the epithelial tissues and pocket formation.

(3) Predominantly as recession and atrophy of the epithelial and connective tissue elements in relation to the tooth (fig. 3.3c & d).

Although acute gingivitis is only rarely found in mouths where chronic inflammation has not been present, it is a frequent finding superimposed on a pre-existing chronic condition. Ulceromembranous and acute coccal gingivitis are examples of this type of change and are discussed in chap. 9.

Microscopic features of inflammatory periodontal disease

CHANGES IN THE CUFF AND GINGIVAL EPITHELIA

The essential change of the early lesion is thinning and ultimate ulceration of the cuff epithelium, exposing the underlying connective tissue to irritating factors from the crown environment. As a result of this irritation there is hyperplasia of the cuff epithelium and of the gingival epithelium in an attempt to restore the continuity of the epithelial barrier (fig. 3.4). Such epithelium shows a varying degree of inflammatory change in terms of inter- and intracellular oedema, and neutrophils and other inflammatory cells may be evident between the epithelial cells. The superficial zone of the gingival epithelium also shows an increased tendency towards parakeratinization, probably due to an increased rate of cell turnover.

CHANGES IN THE CONNECTIVE TISSUE

The connective tissue is the seat of the inflammatory response. An inflammatory cell infiltrate is evident in the connective tissue subjacent to

the ulcerated areas of the cuff epithelium. Dilated and engorged capillaries are surrounded by the inflammatory infiltrate which varies in nature depending on the extent, and the acuteness or chronicity of the inflammation. In acute inflammation principally polymorphonuclear leucocytes are seen (fig. 3.5a), whereas in chronic inflammation mononuclear cells predominate (fig. 3.5b). The presence of inflammation of the connective tissues results in alteration of the degree of aggregation of the ground substance and disintegration of the collagen bundles of the periodontium, which lose their attachment to cementum or alveolar bone and which are gradually replaced by the chronic cellular infiltrate (fig. 3.6).

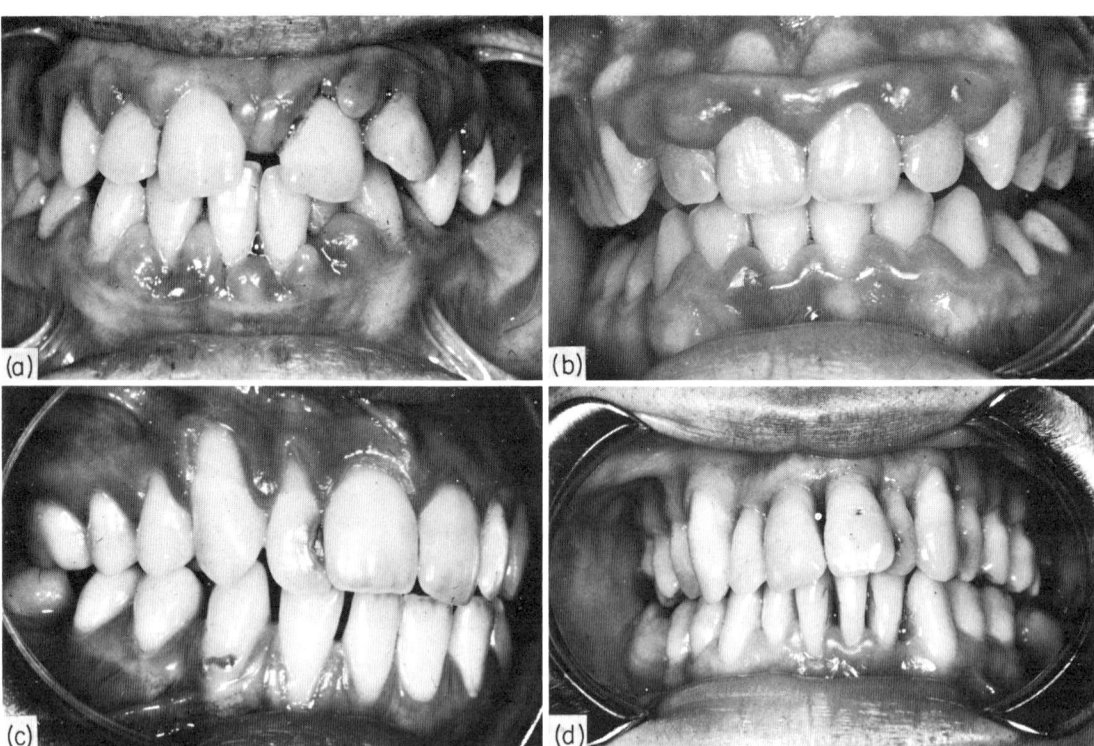

FIG. 3.3. Chronic nonspecific periodontitis may present as: (a) Predominantly inflammation and oedema associated with disaggregation of the gel structure of connective tissue and hyperplasia of the epithelial tissues resulting in pocket formation. (b) Predominantly hyperplasia of the connective tissues in relation to the tooth. This may or may not be associated with hyperplasia of the epithelial tissues and true pocket formation. (c) & (d) Recession and atrophy of both epithelial and connective tissue elements in relation to the tooth.

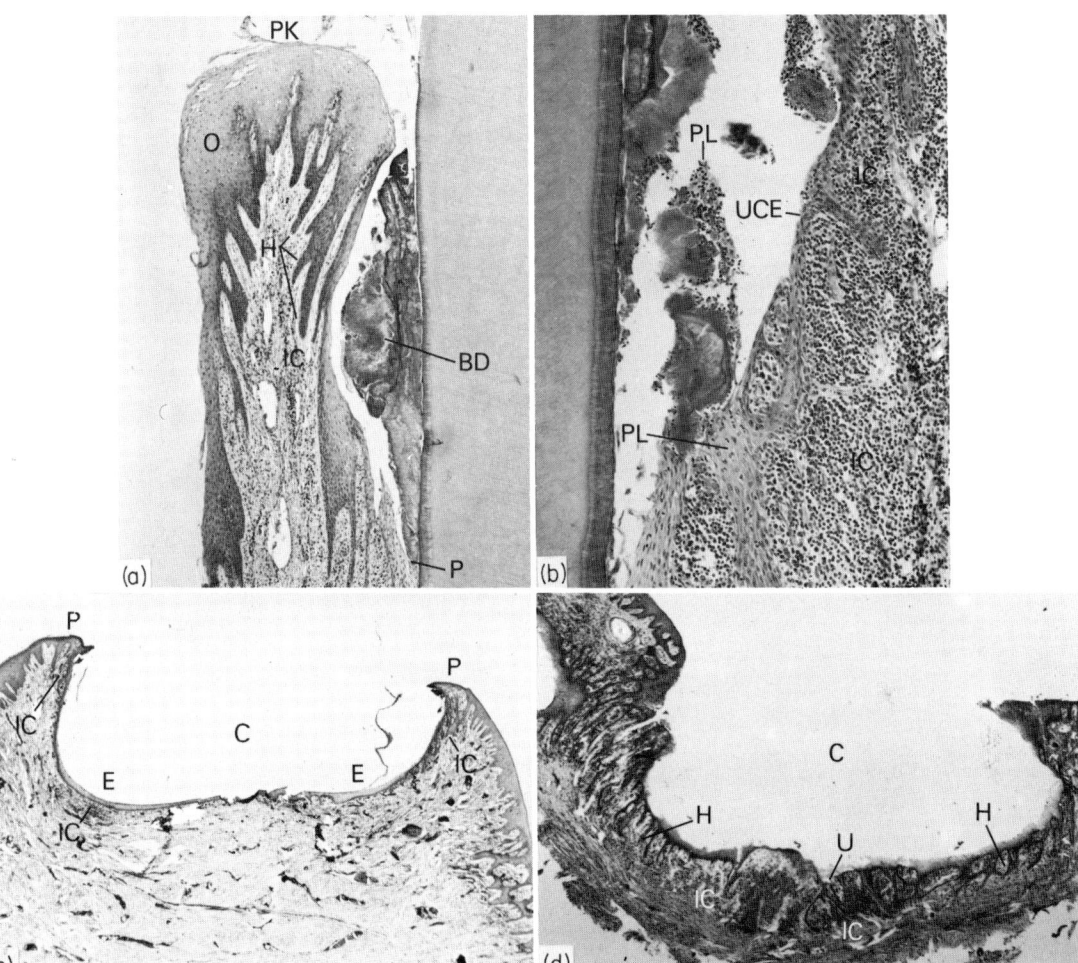

FIG. 3.4. Reaction of gingival tissues to irritation by bacterial deposits. (a) Pocket showing hyperplasia of cuff epithelium (H), parakeratosis (PK) and intracellular oedema (O). Chronic inflammatory cells (IC) are present in the connective tissue. Bacterial deposits (BD) are present, extending to the base of the pocket (P). (b) High power section of bacterial deposits in pocket with thinning and ulceration of cuff epithelium (UCE). A dense mononuclear inflammatory cell infiltrate (IC) is present in the gingival connective tissue, and polymorphonuclear leukocytes (PL) are present within the cuff epithelium and surrounding the bacterial deposits. (c) Low power buccolingual section through a clinically healthy col (C). There is no hyperplasia of the epithelium (E) joining the papillae (P), and only a few foci of inflammatory cells (IC) are present. (d) Low power buccolingual section through inflamed col (C). There is ulceration (U) and hyperplasia (H) of the epithelium lining the col, and a dense infiltrate of chronic inflammatory cells (IC) is present in the underlying connective tissue.

Progression of periodontitis

Whereas in some cases gingivitis remains localized to the marginal tissues for a considerable
period (gingivally contained lesion), in many
instances progression into the deeper structures
follows more rapidly. The clinical features become those of a gingivitis superimposed upon
involvement of the deeper tissues (non-gingivally
contained lesion). At this stage bone loss can be
detected both clinically and radiographically
(fig. 3.7), the teeth progressively become more
mobile, and the soft tissues become less well
adapted to the form of the underlying teeth and
bone.

Extension of the infiltrate into the deeper
tissues occurs with breakdown of the main fibre
bundles at the cervical margin, resorption of
alveolar bone and proliferation of the cuff
epithelium apical to the amelocemental junction.
When this stage of pocket formation has been
reached, the disease, now involving all the tissues
of the periodontium, is termed periodontitis
(fig. 3.8).

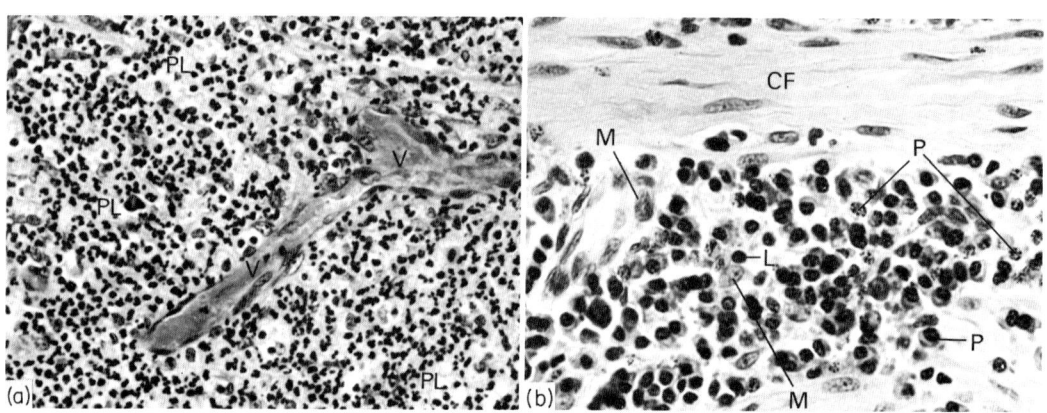

FIG. 3.5. (a) Dense infiltrate of polymorphonuclear leukocytes (PL) in acutely inflamed tissue. A vessel (V) is present
in the centre of the field. (b) Dense infiltrate of chronic inflammatory cells between collagen fibres (CF); L, lymphocyte;
M, macrophage; P, plasma cells with typical 'clock face' pattern of nuclear chromatin and eccentric nuclei.

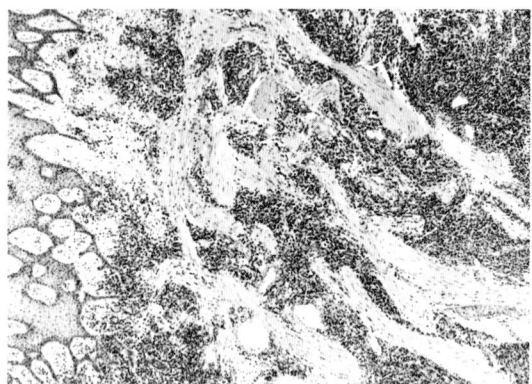

FIG. 3.6. Disintegration of collagen bundles and replacement with chronic cellular infiltrate.

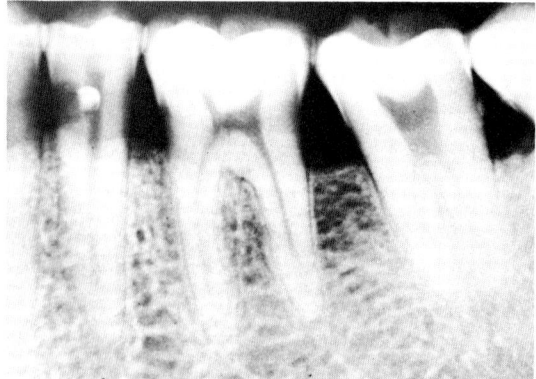

FIG. 3.7. Radiograph of mandibular posterior teeth
with early periodontitis. Resorption of the crests of
the interdental alveolar septa has occurred. Resorption is evenly distributed in all areas, and the pattern
of bone loss is horizontal.

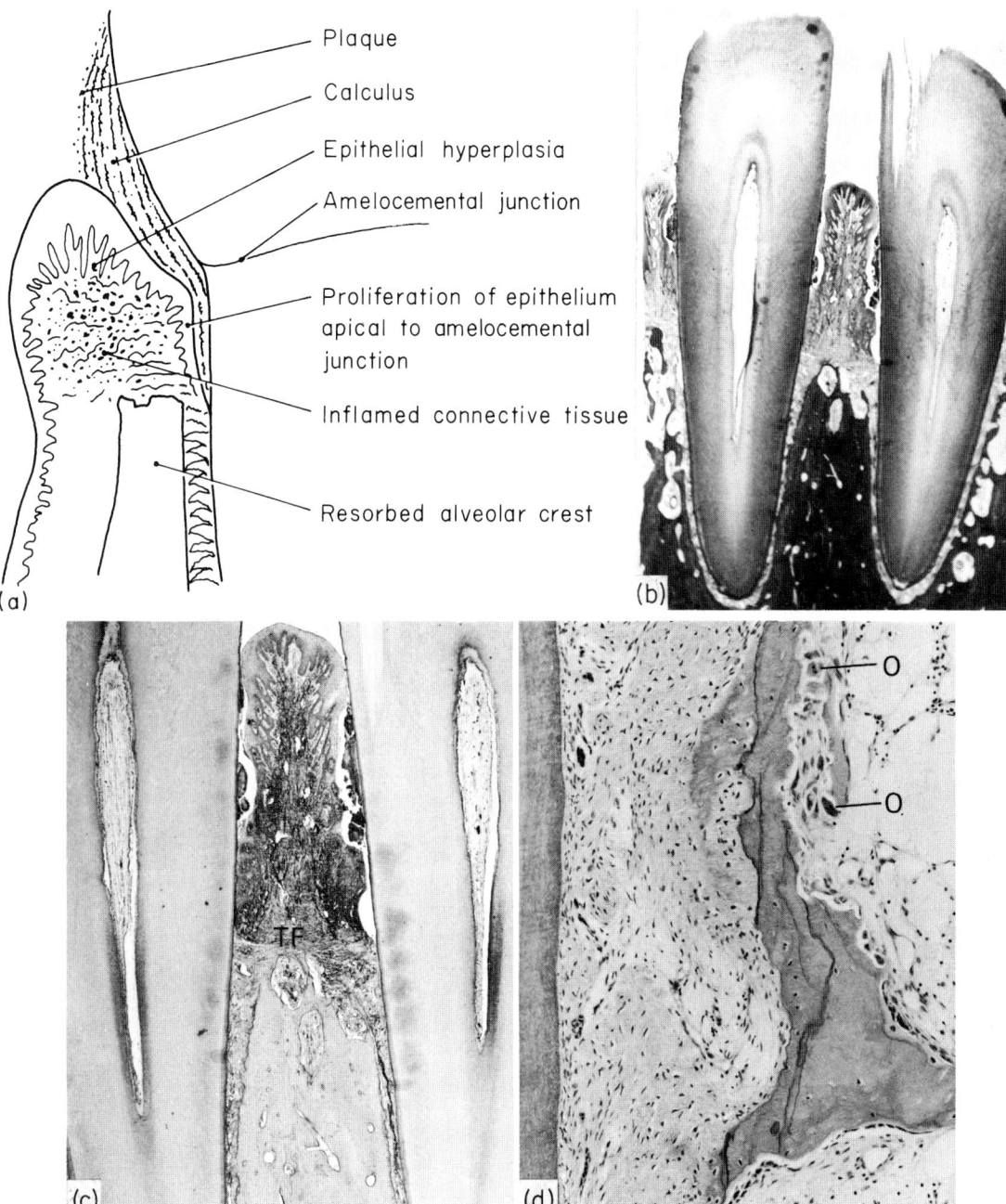

FIG. 3.8. (a) Diagram of established periodontitis (true pocket). Irritation from bacterial deposits has caused disaggregation of connective tissue, apical proliferation of epithelium onto cementum and resorption of the alveolar crest. While collagen bundles may reorganize during a subsequent phase of repair, reattachment of collagen bundles to tooth substance is prevented by proliferated epithelium which extends to the base of the pocket. (b) True pocket, mandibular incisors. (c) True pocket showing dense inflammatory cell infiltrate, disaggregation of transeptal fibres (TF) and resorption of alveolar crest. (d) High power section showing resorption of alveolar bone; O, osteoclasts.

As the balance between the virulence of the factors from the crown environment and the resistance of the tissues changes, there is an alternating pattern of tissue destruction and repair. In the phase of repair there is reorganization of the connective tissue structure and reformation of the collagen structure of the periodontal membrane. Such a tissue may be considered to be in a constant state of wound healing. The reformed collagenous tissue is prevented from becoming attached to the tooth surface by the apical proliferation of the cuff epithelium, and the overall result is rootward migration of the epithelial cuff and the most coronal point of attachment of the connective tissues to the root of the tooth. This sequence of events results in pocket formation (fig. 3.8). As the disease progresses there is resorption of the alveolar crest and replacement of bone by granulation tissue (fig. 3.8). This may be partly a result of the influence of toxic factors from the crown environment on bone metabolism. and partly a result of the loss of functional stimulation, which follows detachment of the collagen bundles from the alveolar crest. Over the long term the ultimate result of this progression is loss of the dentition (fig. 3.9).

Plaque and observable gingival inflammation are universal phenomena throughout the animal kingdom, but with the exception of humans and sheep, tooth loss prior to death as a result of chronic periodontitis is relatively rare [7]. It is well documented that both the prevalence and severity of periodontitis increase linearly with age [8], and while it has been assumed predominantly by epidemiologists, from cross sectional rather than longitudinal studies, and by clinicians that gingivitis inevitably progresses to destructive periodontitis, this assumption remains unproven and it appears that at least in some cases this progression does not occur [7, 9 & 10].

The present state of knowledge has been well summarized by Page and Schroeder [11].

'Chronic periodontitis, a common disease of microbial origin, is the major cause of tooth loss in adult humans. The disease serves as a convenient experimental model for analysis of many aspects of chronic inflammation. A considera-

tion of currently available data has permitted the formulation of a new concept of the pathogenesis of this disease . . .

The gingival tissues respond within two to four days to a beginning accumulation of microbial plaque with a classic acute vasculitis which we have termed the *initial lesion*. This response, which includes loss of perivascular collagen, is comparable to that elicited in most other tissues, subjected to acute injury and may be a consequence of the elaboration and release of chemotactic and antigenic substances by microbial plaque.

Within four to ten days, the *early lesion* develops. It is characterized by a dense infiltrate of lymphocytes and other mononuclear cells, pathologic alteration of fibroblasts, and continuing loss of connective tissue substance. The structural features of the early lesion are consistent with those expected in some forms of cellular hypersensitivity, and a mechanism of this kind may be important in the pathogenesis.

The early lesion is followed by the *established lesion* which develops within two to three weeks, and is distinguished by a predominance of plasma cells, in the absence of significant bone loss.

The established lesion, which is extremely widespread in humans and in animals, may remain stable for years or decades or it may become converted into a progressive destructive lesion.

Factors causing this conversion are not understood. In the advanced lesion, plasma cells continue to predominate although loss of the alveolar bone and periodontal ligament, and disruption of the tissue architecture with fibrosis are also important characteristics. The initial, early and established lesions are sequential stages in gingivitis and they, rather than the advanced lesion which is manifest clinically as periodontitis, make up the major portion of inflammatory gingival and periodontal disease in humans . . .'

The most common form of inflammatory disease of the periodontal tissues appears to begin during childhood or young adulthood in most individuals and to be associated with the presence of microbial plaque on the surfaces of the teeth [8].

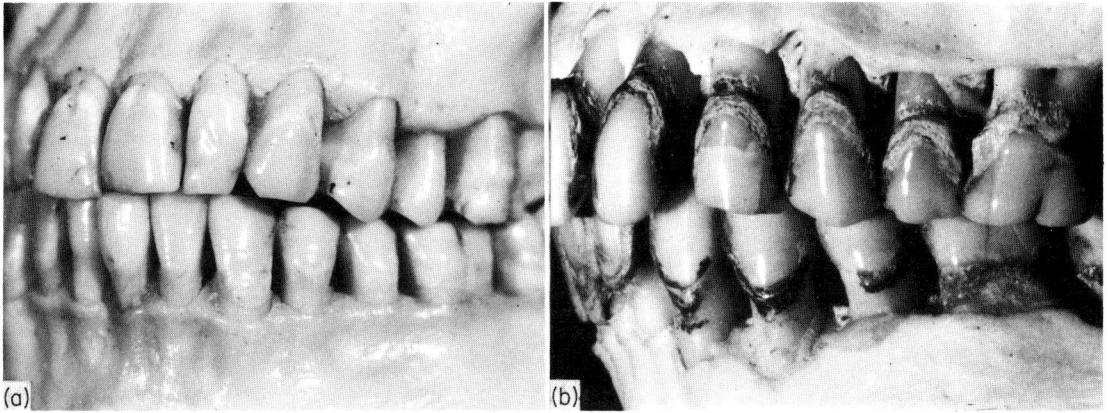

FIG. 3.9. The skull; (a) normal bone architecture; (b) heavy deposits on all teeth and extensive alveolar resorption.

While it is now widely accepted that observable gingival inflammation is common enough to be the norm in child and adult populations, several studies have reported evidence of destructive periodontitis in a significant proportion of the teenage population. For example, it has been shown that 31 per cent of 11–14 year olds show pockets in excess of 3 mm in some areas of the mouth [12]. Forty-six per cent of 15-year-olds had loss of attachment to 1 mm including 11 per cent with loss to 2 mm on at least one tooth [13]. On the basis of a standardized technique 51·5 per cent of 14-year-olds showed radiographic evidence of chronic periodontitis [14].

While localized bone resorption resulting in loss of support of teeth, particularly the first molars, has been demonstrated from the age of eight upwards [13 & 15], there is little evidence for the assumption that except in extremes those earliest affected in childhood are those whose teeth are earliest lost in adult life.

It has been proposed that an explanation for the extreme tissue destruction and immunological findings in juvenile periodontitis (see chap. 6) is that a selective defect in response to some Gram-negative organisms affects T. lymphocytes but that B. lymphocyte activity remains intact and is responsible for producing antibodies and MIF [16].

The time scale of progression of gingivitis to periodontitis is not linear. 'In many cases, the lesion remains confined indefinitely to the marginal and to the coronal portion of the inter-dental gingiva where it may exhibit clinical manifestations, or it may be observed as a mild, frequently transient gingivitis. On the other hand, in some individuals the lesion converts to a destructive periodontitis leading to complete disruption of the architecture of the gingival connective tissue with severe fibrosis, conversion of the junctional epithelium to pocket epithelium and loss of variable amounts of alveolar bone.

These tissue alterations underlie the pocket formation, tooth mobility, periodontal abscess formation and eventual tooth exfoliation which are characteristic of the advanced stages of peridontal disease . . .' [11].

Although the frequency of destructive lesions increases with increasing age, the prevalence of progressive disease in humans is probably far less than is commonly believed. While definitive observations have not yet been made, longitudinal studies on large groups of individuals by Lovdal et al. [17 & 18], and Suomi et al. [19] tend to support this view. In the Lovdal experiments, gingivitis was found to be almost universal although, in those groups of individuals still possessing 50 per cent or more of their teeth, only 10–15 per cent of the teeth exhibited inter-proximal pockets of 5 mm or more.

In the Suomi [19] experiments, several hundred individuals between the ages of 18 and 40 years were allocated by computer matching into an experimental group, which was examined and given frequent prophylaxis and intensive training in oral hygiene techniques, and a control group which was only examined. Adults who had received no instruction to change their usual pattern of oral hygiene showed an average apical migration of the attachment level of 0·10 mm per year over a three year period. In a similar group where the oral hygiene condition was kept at the highest possible level the mean loss of attachment was only 0·08 mm during the whole three year period [19]. The control group thus showed a loss of epithelial attachment at a rate more than three and a half times greater than the experimental group over the three years. It is notable however that over the three years the difference between the experimental and control does not appear to be clinically significant and after five years and ten months it was still not significant.

During another preventive programme where the experimental child group was subjected to professional tooth cleaning at fortnightly intervals for the first two years, the interval being extended to four weeks during the third year 'practically no new caries lesion was developed . . . and inflammation of the marginal gingiva almost entirely disappeared'. [20]

A further conclusion of the studies of Suomi and colleagues [19] was that 'the findings of this study indicate that it may not be reasonable to expect most individuals to maintain absolute oral cleanliness or to eliminate all traces of gingival inflammation from their mouths', a fact which has been well demonstrated in a number of populations.

It seems clear that gingival inflammation is, variably, progressively tissue destructive. At the present time there are no definitive criteria which distinguish progressively destructive inflammation from the stabilized 'contained' gingivitis.

It has been suggested that the key factor may be the proportion of lymphocytes to plasma cells in the inflammatory infiltrate of the connective tissues subjacent to the junctional epithelium. Where an inflammatory infiltrate was present in biopsies from relatively healthy sites

it was dominated by mononuclear cells with lymphocytes clearly predominating over plasma cells [21]. The biopsies from diseased sites were characterised by a markedly infiltrated connective tissue which sometimes involved most of the gingiva. Although the extent and pattern of distribution of the inflammatory infiltrate varied widely, the infiltrate consisted of a mixture of plasma cells and lymphocytes which was generally dominated by plasma cells. The ability of plasma cells from human gingiva to produce a wide range of potentially destructive hydrolytic enzymes has been reported by Cowley [22].

The non-infiltrated connective tissue contained well defined bundles of collagen fibres. At infiltrated sites the collagen bundles appeared to have been largely replaced by inflammatory cells. Diseased tissue often contained pale enlarged fibroblasts which resembled cells having undergone degenerative changes.

It may be that the proportion of lymphocytes to plasma cells in the infiltrated connective tissue subjacent to the junctional epithelium may be largely influenced by the presence of particular groups of organisms in subgingival plaque. Plasma cells may be produced in response to antigenic stimulation by certain members of the periodontal flora particularly from the Gram-negative groups. For example, a clear association seems to exist between the nature of the connective tissue infiltrate and the presence of spirochaetes in the bacterial sample of plaque. In one particular study [21] plasma cells tended to dominate in those tissues which were associated with a microbial flora containing 5 per cent or larger proportions of spirochaetes. Infiltrates dominated by lymphocytes tended to come from biopsies associated with microbial floras containing 5 per cent or fewer spirochaetes.

In the same study it was demonstrated that the inflammatory infiltrate of diseased sites was dominated by plasma cells which constituted close to 50 per cent of all cells present. Following treatment lymphoid cells accounted for approximately 50 per cent of the cells in the infiltrate with plasma cells present only occasionally. It may be that 'contained' gingivitis is associated with connective tissue infiltrates which are lymphoid cell dominated while destructive progressive periodontitis is associated with infiltrates which are plasma cell dominated. The key factor may be the anti-genic stimulus from particular groups of the subgingival plaque flora (see chap. 6).

REFERENCES

[1] BURDON-SANDERSON (1962) In *General Pathology*, 3rd Edition, p. 21. Ed. Florey H. London: Lloyd-Luke.

[2] MENKIN V. (1956) *Biochemical Mechanisms in Inflammation*, 2nd Edition. Springfield, Ill.: Thomas.

[3] WALTER J.B. & ISRAEL M.S. (1963) *General Pathology*. London: Churchill.

[4] MAJNO G., LA GUTTUTA M. & THOMPSON T.E. (1960 Cellular death and necrosis: Chemical, physical and morphological changes in rat liver. *Virchows. Arch. path. Anat.* **333**, 421–465.

[5] WORLD HEALTH ORGANISATION (1961) Report of an expert committee on dental health. No. 207.

[6] PETER SIR R. (1973) *Biochemical Lesions and Lethal Synthesis*. Oxford: Pergamon.

[7] PAGE R.C., SIMPSON D.M. & AMMONS W.F. (1975) Host tissue response in chronic inflammatory periodontal disease. 4. The periodontal and dental status of a group of aged apes. *J. Periodont.* **46**, 144.

[8] SCHERP H.W. (1964) Current concepts in periodontal disease research: epidemiological contributions. *J. Amer. Dent. Assoc.* **68**, 667.

[9] AMMONS W.F., SCHECTMAN L.R. & PAGE R.C. (1972) Host tissue response in chronic periodontal disease. The normal periodontium and clinical and anatomical manifestations of periodontal disease in the marmoset. *J. Periodont. Res.* 7, 131.

[10] SCHECTMAN L.R., AMMONS W.F., SIMPSON D.M. & PAGE R.C. (1972) Host tissue response in chronic periodontal disease. 2. Histologic features of the normal periodontium and histopathologic and ultrastructural manifestations of the disease in the marmoset. *J. Periodont. Res.* 7, 195.

[11] PAGE R.C. & SCHROEDER H.E. (1976) Pathogenesis of inflammatory periodontal disease. A summary of current work. *Lab. Invest.* **33**, 3,235.

[12] DOWNER M.C. (1970) Dental caries and periodontal disease in girls of different ethnic groups. A comparison in a London secondary school. *Brit. dent. J.* **128**, 379.

[13] LENNON M.A. & DAVIES R.M. (1975) A method of defining the level of periodontal treatment needs in a population of 15-year-old schoolchildren. *Community Dent. Oral Epidemiol.* **3**, 244.

[14] HULL P.S., HILLAM D.G. & BEALE J.F. (1975) A radiographic study of the prevalence of chronic periodontitis in 14-year-old English schoolchildren. *J. Clin. Periodont.* **2(4)**, 203.

[15] PARFITT G.J. (1967) Periodontal disease in children. *Clinical Paedodontics*. Philadelphia and London: Saunders.

[16] LEHNER T. (1975) Immunological aspects of dental caries and periodontal disease. *Brit. Med. Bulletin* **31**, 2.

[17] LOVDAL A., ARNO A., SCHEI O. & WAERHAUG J. (1961) Combined effect of sub-gingival scaling and controlled oral hygiene on the incidence of gingivitis. *Acta Odont. Scand.* **19**, 537–555.

[18] LOVDAL A., ARNO A. & WAERHAUG J. (1958) Incidence of clinical manifestations of periodontal disease in light of oral hygienic and calculus formation. *J. Amer. dent. Ass.* **56**, 21–33.

[19] SUOMI J.D., GREENE J.C. & VERMILION J.R. (1971) The effect of controlled oral hygiene procedures on the progression of periodontitis in adults; results after the third and final year. *J. Periodont.* **42**, 152.

[20] LINDHE J., AXELSSON P. & TOLLSKOG G. (1975) Effect of proper oral hygiene on gingivitis and dental caries in Swedish school children. *Commun. Dent. Oral Epidemiol.* **3(4)**, 150.

[21] LISTGARTEN M.A., LINDHE J. & HELLDEN L. (1978) Effect of tetracycline and/or scaling on human periodontal disease. *J. Clin. Periodont.* **5**, 246–271.

[22] COWLEY G.C. (1972) Enzyme activity in gingival immunocytes. *J. dent. Res.* **51**, 284–292.

CHAPTER 4

Plaque and calculus

It is inherent in the concept of the mouth as a balanced biological system that periodontitis is the result of a broad spectrum of interaction between the commensal population of the mouth and the tissues of the host. Failure of biochemical control of tissue metabolism is rarely the entire cause of periodontitis, but it may predispose the tissues to disease in the presence of factors in the crown environment which are of low pathogenicity. Local factors in the mouth may, of themselves, be of sufficient intensity to produce clinically evident disease, which would become exacerbated if the control of local tissue metabolism is impaired. At the present stage of knowledge there is insufficient data to define the role of bacteria in relation to

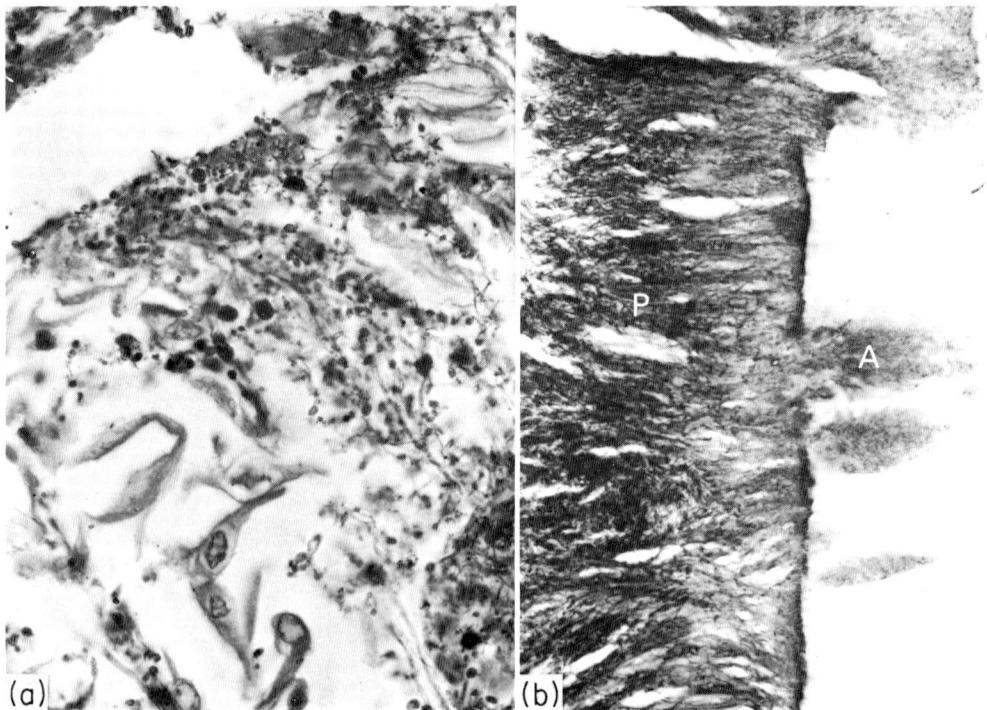

FIG. 4.1. (a) Outer plaque layers consisting of food debris, desquamated epithelial cells, microorganisms and leucocytes, with a poorly defined histological architecture. (b) Decalcified section of tooth with bacterial plaque (P). Highly organized palisade structure of filamentous organisms at right angles to tooth surface (A) indicates areas of plaque which have gained attachment in defects on the root surface.

the disease, and understanding of the control of tissue metabolism is limited. Periodontitis is, therefore, a complex disease involving a wide range of possible interactions between parasites and host tissues.

The key to the aetiology of periodontitis lies in the study of three main groups of factors [1]:

(1) the metabolic functions and products of the organisms in dental plaque;

(2) the local environmental factors which may enhance or inhibit the expression of bacterial pathogenicity;

(3) the central factors governing metabolism of host tissues which may condition the response to bacterial products.

DEPOSITS ON THE TOOTH SURFACE

Unless an immaculate oral hygiene regimen is carried out, deposits form on teeth. Although it has been suggested that all soft extraneous material adhering to the teeth should be called dental plaque [2], this term has been frequently reserved for the firmly adherent bacterial masses, which possess a recognizable histological architecture. A soft, amorphous, light-coloured deposit which consists of food debris, desquamated epithelial cells, microorganisms and leucocytes [3] which does not have the organized structure of dental plaque has been termed materia alba or sordes (fig. 4.1). These traditional terms are of limited value and all visible soft deposits on teeth should be regarded as plaque.

PLAQUE

The formation of dental plaque has been divided into two stages [4 & 5]:

(1) formation of an initial, nonbacterial plaque matrix, the acquired pellicle (secondary cuticle);

(2) the proliferation of microorganisms within the plaque matrix to give a well defined structure as in mature plaque (chap. 2).

CALCULUS

Calculus is a hard deposit formed by the mineralization of plaque. Both dental plaque and calculus may become stained, the colour probably depending on chromogenic microorganisms present in the deposit, and the presence of substances absorbed from tobacco, tea or coffee and various metals. Brown, black, green and orange extrinsic stains may occasionally be observed, and they must be distinguished from intrinsic discoloration such as that seen in fluorosis (fig. 4.2).

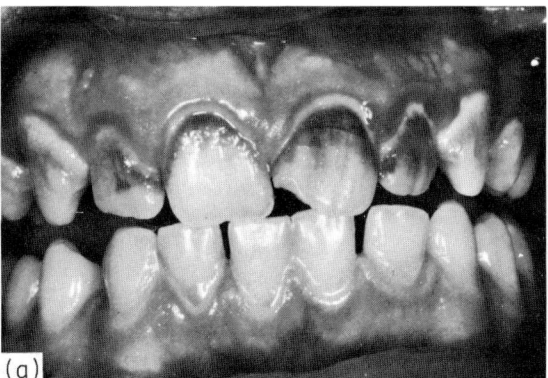 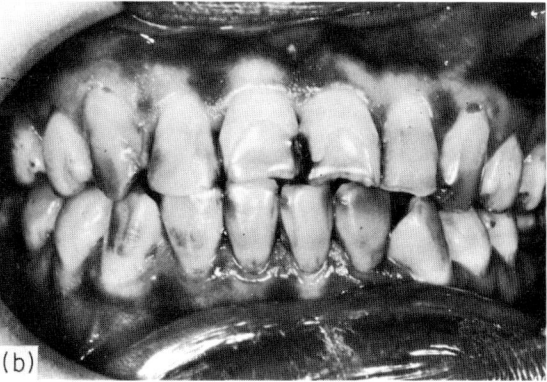

FIG. 4.2. (a) Extrinsic green stain associated with chromogenic bacteria. This is a superficial deposit on the enamel surface that can be removed by careful polishing of the teeth, viz., stain removed from mandibular incisors. (b) Intrinsic staining of enamel, endemic fluorosis, where the fundamental defect is in the outer part of the enamel rod. This alters the optical properties of enamel and therefore the appearance, and secondarily allows substances from the mouth to diffuse into the enamel and cause the brown pigmentation [6].

METABOLIC FUNCTIONS AND PRODUCTS
OF ORGANISMS IN DENTAL PLAQUE

The initial plaque matrix consists of an accumulation of protein and carbohydrate partly endogenous in origin, derived from saliva and the products of tissue metabolism and catabolism, and partly exogenous being derived from the diet (fig. 4.3). This acts as a substrate for higher concentrations of microorganisms than are found generally in other areas of the oral cavity. Microorganisms constitute at least 70 per cent of the bulk of plaque [7]. Each individual area of

the mouth has a particular physicochemical environment, and consequently its own microflora, dependent on the symbiotic relationships of the individual groups of organisms and the antibiotic and nutritional factors which the particular environment provides [1]. Bacterial metabolism is capable of changing the plaque environment by altering physicochemical conditions within the plaque and its immediate area. Metabolism of an essentially proteinaceous substrate with little available carbohydrate creates a relatively alkaline environment as a result of the decarboxylation and deamination

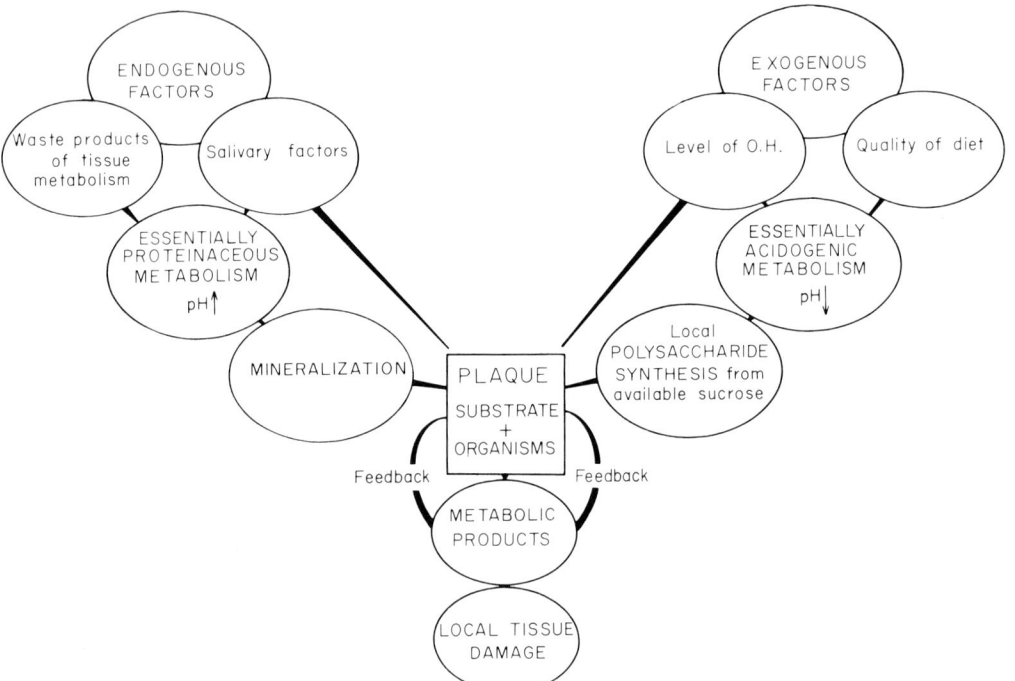

FIG. 4.3. Diagram of plaque metabolism. Plaque consists of substrate and organisms. The substrate is derived partly from endogenous sources, such as saliva and products of tissue metabolism and catabolism, and partly from exogenous sources, such as the diet.

Metabolism of an essentially proteinaceous substrate with little available carbohydrate creates a relatively alkaline environment. In the presence of an essentially proteinaceous metabolism the pH tends to rise and the plaque tends to mineralize.

Metabolism of a substrate with an appreciable proportion of fermentable carbohydrate creates an acidogenic plaque, and an acid environment, as a result of local accumulation of lactic acid. The pH tends to fall, there is a reduced tendency towards mineralization and large quantities of plaque may accumulate.

Plaque organisms metabolize a mixed substrate at any given time, but the substrate varies principally with the amount of fermentable carbohydrate present in the diet. Research has shown that a major factor in plaque growth is the quantity of available sucrose. Sucrose is used in the synthesis of intra- and extracellular polysaccharide by organisms. Such polysaccharide may subsequently contribute available carbohydrate to the substrate of plaque through a feedback mechanism. Plaque does not have to calcify sufficiently to produce a clinically obvious deposit to cause tissue damage. Tissue damage results from the production of toxic metabolic products by plaque organisms.

of amino acids following breakdown of protein chains. Metabolism of a substrate with an appreciable proportion of available fermentable carbohydrate creates an acidogenic plaque and an acid environment as a result of local accumulation of lactic acid. The pH of plaque may vary in the range of 4–8 according to the quantity of carbohydrate available at any given time and the buffering capacity of the proteins present.

Plaque has been described as the environmental membrane between saliva and tooth [8], and this concept is equally applicable to the relationship of saliva to the tissues of the dento-gingival junction. Conditions in the immediate area are governed by the presence or absence of plaque, the type of plaque which may be present and its metabolic functions at any given time. Plaque, therefore, creates its own environment which is constantly changing as a result of variation in physicochemical conditions, such as degree of function, rate of salivary flow and the exogenous contribution to the substrate from the diet (figs 4.4 & 4.5).

Conditions in the mouth are such that all surfaces are covered by a layer of mucoprotein which is apparently of salivary origin. It is generally accepted that this is the origin of the pellicle. The accumulation of such a pellicle on a tooth is partly governed by the degree of functional cleansing of the surface, and where this is inadequate, an amorphous thin mucoprotein layer is formed. Bacteria progressively colonize this pellicle from defects in the tooth surface and from saliva [4 & 5].

The addition of different sugars to a standardized protein–fat diet has shown, in man, that the amounts of plaque are considerably greater following the addition of sucrose, than following the addition of glucose or fructose [9]. It is clear that the accumulation of plaque is not directly related to the change in physicochemical conditions which follows metabolism of any available sugar, but it is at least governed partly by the particular sugar which is available as a bacterial nutrient. The evidence suggests that the rate of growth is maximal, in the presence of available sucrose, as a result of synthesis of intra- and extracellular polysaccharide by coccal organisms. Berman and Gibbons [10] have shown that plaque streptococci, diphtheroids, fusobacteria and bacteroides produce abundant amounts of iodine-staining intracellular polysaccharide, whereas veillonella, anaerobic streptococci, lactobacilli and *Vibrio sputorum* form little or none. The former group constitute about 80 per cent of the cultivable supragingival plaque flora and are responsible for most of the polysaccharide synthesis within plaque. Sucrose is the principal dietary sugar which serves as a substrate for the synthesis of these polysaccharides [9]. It has been shown that the plaque content of polysaccharide more than doubles after a 40 per cent sucrose rinse [11]. Plaque growth is thus related to the number of

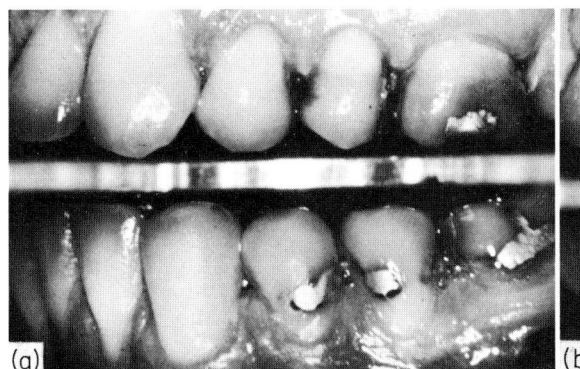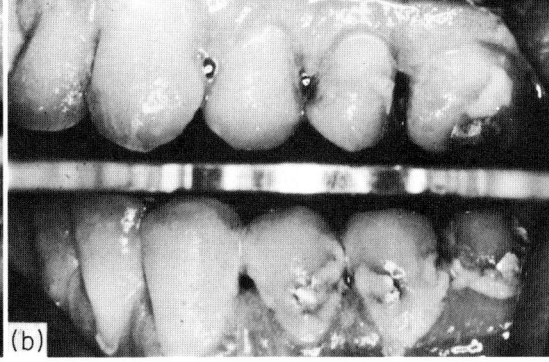

FIG. 4.4. (a) Degree of plaque accumulation in the absence of any oral hygiene care after one week on a basic carbohydrate free diet. (b) Degree of plaque accumulation in the absence of any oral hygiene care after one week on the basic diet supplemented with sucrose. Courtesy of Drs J. Carlsson, J. Egelberg and *Odont. Revy* (1965), **16**, 112–125.

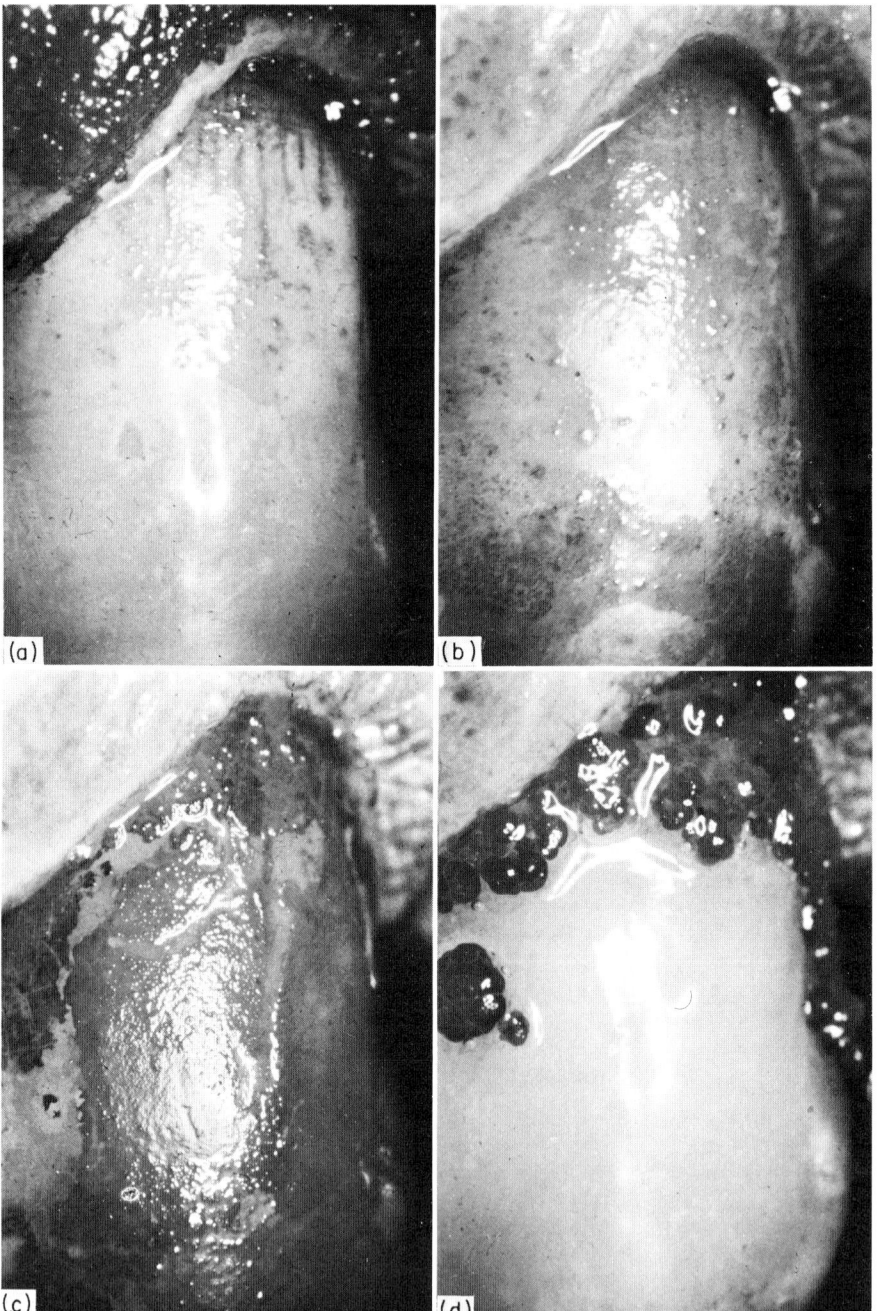

FIG. 4.5. (a) Disclosed tooth with one day's plaque accumulation on the basic diet supplemented with fructose. (b) Same tooth disclosed after three days plaque accumulation on basic diet supplemented with fructose. (c) Disclosed tooth after three days basic diet supplemented with glucose. (d) Disclosed tooth after three days basic diet supplemented by sucrose. Note accumulation at the cervical margin and resemblance to bacterial colonies. Courtesy of Drs J. Carlsson, J. Egelberg and *Odont. Revy* (1965), **16**, 112–125.

microorganisms and to the volume of extra-cellular polysaccharide synthesis by coccal organisms. It has been estimated that 95 per cent of polysaccharide of the plaque matrix is the polyglucan dextran and about 1 per cent levan [12 & 13].

Individual groups of organisms within plaque are probably mutually interdependent, and the metabolic products of one group may act as the substrate for another. Locally synthesized poly-saccharide may contribute to the general sub-strate available in plaque through a feedback mechanism in the absence of available carbo-hydrate from the diet (fig. 4.3).

Human plaque is the product of bacterial growth, mature plaque having a definite micro-scopic architecture (fig. 4.6a). It consists of a meshwork of filamentous and coccoidal organ-isms with a pallisade type organization at right angles to the tooth substance and closely ad-herent to the tooth surface. Plaque is a precursor of calculus, but the extent to which it calcifies to form clinically obvious calculus is variable and

is a function of the chemistry of its particular environment. Although there is a close relation-ship between the distribution of periodontal disease and calculus, it is apparent that perio-dontal disease is more common than calculus. There is much evidence that plaque may play a major role in the aetiology of periodontitis with-out calcifying sufficiently to form a clinically obvious deposit, and that mechanical irritation by the calcified deposits is not the major factor in the aetiology of periodontitis.

Dental plaque is part of the total body flora and is a normal finding in any mouth. The body flora does not generally cause disease but main-tains a commensal or symbiotic relationship with the host from which the host may obtain direct advantage, as from the synthesis of Vitamin K by gut organisms. The commensal microflora of the mouth is an important body defence mechanism which prevents foreign microorganisms becoming established whose presence would cause disease. Alteration or elimination of normal flora by antimicrobial

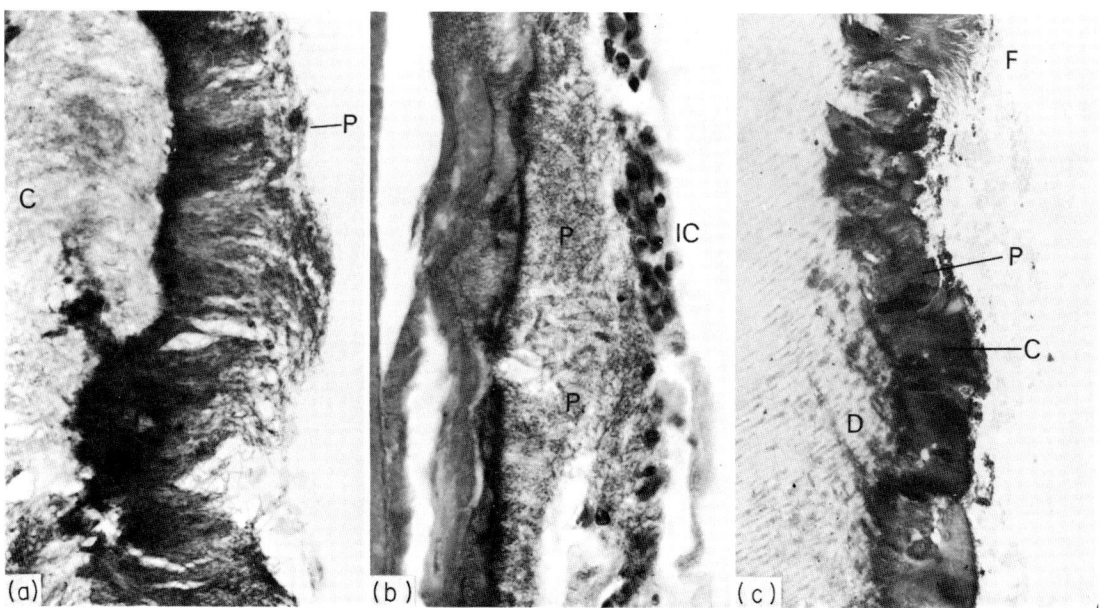

FIG. 4.6. (a) Pallisade arrangement of organisms in dental plaque (P) on the surface of a layer of calculus (C). There is a predominance of filamentous organisms in the plaque. (b) Microorganisms in dental plaque (P) where the pallisade type of organization is less well defined, compare with figs 4.6 (a) and (c). A layer of inflammatory cells (IC) is present on the surface of the plaque. (c) Layer of bacterial plaque (P) attached to carious dentine (D). The organisms are predominantly cocci (C) but filamentous forms are also present (F).

drugs or other means may result in the establishment of an altered secondary flora. This may be characterized by overgrowth of particular groups of the commensal population possibly to pathogenic levels, a change in environment which may allow establishment of foreign microorganisms, or both. As a general principle, such induced commensal shifts tend to result in disadvantage to the host.

The development of the oral microbiota

The mouth is sterile at birth, but is from that time continuously inoculated with large numbers of organisms which display a wide variety of metabolic requirement. Initially, it is colonized by those organisms which find the existing physicochemical, nutritional, and antibiotic factors conducive to their growth and retention. The metabolic activities of this initial bacterial population change the environment and influence the subsequent composition of the indigenous flora. This control may be positive or negative with respect to incoming organisms [14]. In positive control, one group of organisms provides favourable conditions for another by regulating the environment to a suitable Eh or pH, or by producing an adequate level of nutrients and essential growth factors by virtue of its metabolic functions. In negative control, the environment is altered so that conditions become unsuitable for other inoculated groups of organisms to survive and become established. Most oral organisms have fastidious growth requirements and different microorganisms tend to colonize different sites in the mouth. For example, the microbial composition of a dental plaque on a single tooth is unique to that site at that time. Removal of that plaque will be followed by the development of a new plaque with possibly a different qualitative, quantitative and spatial arrangement of the organisms [15]. Although all indigenous organisms can be found in almost any site in the mouth at one time or another, it is clear that many organisms have a 'primary ecologic niche' [16]. Quantitative differences in the types of microorganisms present can be demonstrated in samples from the gingival sulcus [17], dental plaque [18], the dorsum of the tongue [19], and

in saliva of different individuals [20]. For example, *S. salivarius* appears to reside principally on the tongue [21] while *S. mutans* appears to have a predilection for tooth surface in hamsters and in man [22 & 23]. *S. sanguis* also appears to reside primarily on the tooth surface [22], whereas spirochaetes and *Bacteroides melaninogenicus* are found in highest numbers in the gingival sulcus of man [24]. There is also considerable variability of the bacterial population within the same site in the same individual. Repeated culturing of the same site within an individual's mouth reveals that a marked variability exists in the microbial composition of that site at different times [25]. The microbial population of the mouth changes throughout life with the eruption of the teeth, the development of caries and periodontitis, the loss of teeth and the insertion of dentures.

From 6–10 hours following birth, there is a rapid increase in the number of detectable organisms and the bacterial composition for the first few days of life appears to be very variable [16]. However, *S. salivarius*, which normally resides on the tongue and which is not dependent on the presence of teeth for survival, has been found in 80 per cent of infants at approximately 1 day of age and has been shown to remain at a consistently high level thereafter [26]. At this stage, there appears to be a total absence of organisms such as spirochaetes whose 'primary ecologic niche' is the gingival sulcus but many other organisms, including some anaerobes, have been demonstrated to occur sporadically in the oral flora of the child of less than 1 year of age [27]. The infant mouth is continuously inoculated with microorganisms normally indigenous to the adult, and following eruption of the teeth, the proportions of the predominant cultivable organisms from the gingival sulcus area of the pre-school child appear to resemble generally those of the adult (Table 4.1) [28] with the exception that spirochaetes and *Bacteroides melaninogenicus* are not present in all children. The prevalence of *Bacteroides melaninogenicus* in children about 5 years of age ranges from 18–40 per cent, but by 13–16 years of age essentially all individuals appear to harbour this organism [29]. There is a gradually increasing incidence of organisms such as *S. mutans* with a predilection for attachment to the tooth surface [26], and spirochaetes also appear to increase in prevalence with increasing age, and are constantly present in the adult [30]. The microbial population varies with the presence of dental caries in the mouth. Retentive sites are created for organisms with little adhesive capability and dietary substrates for microorganisms are present in the carious tooth which may not be as available in other areas of the mouth. It is likely that similar changes in the gingival sulcus flora follow the presence of increased levels of gingival inflammation, and consequently of gingival exudate and the presence of pocket formation, but the obvious difficulties of sampling subgingival plaque make such changes difficult to define. Following complete loss of the teeth there is a marked reduction in the presence of spirochaetes, lactobacilli, certain yeasts, *S. mutans* and *S. sanguis* in the edentulous mouth [31, 32, 33 & 34].

DENTAL PLAQUE

The development of plaque

FORMATION OF THE ACQUIRED PELLICLE

Most studies of the successional changes in developing plaque have used polished or etched tooth surface in an adult mouth as a starting point. If a tooth surface is scaled and polished so that no plaque or pellicle is left, a deposit forms within 15–30 minutes which has been called the acquired pellicle. The formation of this pellicle has been confirmed by electron-microscopy. Lenz and Muhlemann [35] observed a pellicle-like layer covering the surface of etched enamel after 2 hours' exposure to the oral environment. The presence of an electron dense pellicle developing on the tooth surface, ranging in thickness from 0·05–0·4 mm, has been confirmed by a number of other studies [36, 37, 38, 39 & 40]. The main source of the acquired pellicle has generally been supposed to be saliva and its amino acid composition parallels fairly closely the acid precipitates of submaxillary or whole saliva mucin [41]. Based upon the presence of muramic acid, which is a specific bacterial cell wall component, Armstrong concluded that the pellicle protein is derived from the submandibular gland secretion and is associated with significant amounts of bacterial cell wall protein material [42].

Mucin precipitation from saliva which may contribute to the acquired pellicle and subsequently to the plaque matrix has been thought to be due to:

(1) Local production of acid by bacterial deposits on the teeth.

(2) The action of calcium ions.

(3) The alteration of salivary mucins by bacterial enzymes.

The basic structure of plaque may be a floc, which is a type of aggregate where cells and intercellular bridging proteins provide a porous structure through which fluid (saliva, gingival fluid or liquids from the diet) can diffuse [41]. The porosity and filtration rate of such a structure would depend upon the specific arrangement existing between the cells and the intercellular material [43] and the presence within the intercellular spaces of extracellular polysaccharide, synthesized by plaque microorganisms from dietary carbohydrate, particularly sucrose.

Until recently, the main source of the endogenous contribution to the substrate of plaque was considered to be precipitation of mucoids from saliva as a direct result of the fall in pH of the plaque environment which follows metabolism of fermentable carbohydrate of dietary origin [44]. Investigation has shown, however, that plaque accumulates in the mouths of dogs on a protein/fat carbohydrate free diet [45] and laboratory studies have shown that precipitation of mucoids from saliva as a direct result of physiochemical change does not take place above pH 3·5 [46], whereas pH 4 is estimated to be the lowest pH found in acidogenic plaque.

Experiment has suggested that calcium ions may induce matrix formation by enhancing mucin precipitation [47] and increase adsorption of mucins to glass and to hydroxyapatite [48]. The source of calcium ions in sufficient concentration to induce mucin precipitation may be saliva or gingival exudate and plaque when acidified releases calcium to its environment. There is good evidence of bacterial interactions with salivary constituents and it is clear that high molecular weight salivary proteins asso-

TABLE 4.1. Mean percentages of cultivable organisms in the adult oral cavity.

	Gingival crevice area	Dental plaque	Tongue	Saliva
Gram positive facultative cocci	28·8	28·2	44·8	46·2
Streptococci	27·1	27·9	38·3	41·0
S. salivarius	N.D.	N.D.	8·2	4·6
Enterococci	7·2		N.D.	1·3
Staphylococci	1·7	0·3	6·5	4·0
Gram-positive anaerobic cocci	7·4	12·6	4·2	13·0
Gram-negative facultative cocci	0·4	0·4	3·4	1·2
Gram-negative anaerobic cocci	10·7	6·4	16·0	15·9
Gram-positive facultative rods	15·3	23·8	13·0	11·8
Gram-positive anaerobic rods	20·2	18·4	8·2	4·8
Gram-negative facultative rods	1·2	N.D.	3·2	2·3
Gram-negative anaerobic rods	16·1	10·4	8·2	4·8
Fusobacterium	1·9	4·1	0·7	0·3
B. melaninogenicus	4·7	N.D.	0·2	N.D.
V. sputorum	3·8	1·3	2·2	2·1
other Bacteroides	5·6	4·8	5·1	2·4
Spirochaetes	1·0	N.D.	N.D.	N.D.

N.D. = not detected
From Socransky S.S. & Manganiello S.D. (1971) The oral microbiota of man from birth to senility. J. Periodont. **42**, 491.

ciated with the mucin fraction act as effective bacterial aggregating systems [49 & 50].

It has been suggested by Leach that neuraminidase, a bacterial enzyme which cleaves the terminal sialic acid residues from salivary mucins could cause mucin precipitation by this mechanism. Many oral bacteria produce neuraminidase [51 & 52] and it has been shown that plaque samples contained little or no sialic acid [53]. It has not been shown, however, that the sialic acid was removed from the mucins prior to their incorporation in dental plaque rather than after. In the subgingival region in particular, there is probably a further contribution to the acquired pellicle from the protein of gingival exudate and disintegrating tissue cells.

A cleaned tooth surface is rapidly recolonized by significant numbers of organisms by a process of selective adsorption [54 & 55]. Bjorn and Carlsson [54] studied the morphogenesis of dental plaque directly on the tooth surface by examining developing plaque with a stereomicroscope after staining with disclosing solution. The teeth were thoroughly cleaned and the patients asked to refrain from toothbrushing. The facial surfaces of the anterior teeth were

examined every day for a week. At the first inspection 24 hours after the surface was cleaned, a very weak affinity to fuchsin was regularly observed over a large area of the tooth. The material gradually filled up cracks in the tooth surface and later formed ridges protruding out over the surface of the teeth. Within 1–4 days, discrete small hemispherical intensely stained accumulations could be seen scattered over the tooth surface, especially along the gingival margin and in areas of tooth surface irregularity. These bacterial aggregates gradually increased in size and after a few days closely resembled bacterial colonies on an agar plate. The microcolonies gradually increased in size and eventually coalesced to form a continuous bacterial layer which grew in thickness until it became limited by abrasive forces.

Löe et al. [56] and Jensen et al. [57] studied the accumulation of plaque during a period of no oral hygiene, on the basis of microscopic study of impression preparations taken from the gingival margin. Following withdrawal of all oral hygiene measures from twelve human subjects, it was possible to recognize three distinct phases in this new bacterial colonization of the gingival margin. The first phase started immediately after the beginning of the experiment and was characterized by a massive increase of the coccal flora. Large numbers of desquamated epithelial cells completely overgrown with cocci, and large mats of cocci probably loosened from the underlying epithelial tissue were dominant. At the same time, small accumulations of leucocytes were observed along the gingival margin.

The second phase of bacterial proliferation usually started 2–4 days after tooth cleaning had been abolished. It was characterized by the presence of filamentous forms and slender rods, although cocci were still present in fairly large numbers. According to morphological criteria, the filamentous bacteria were predominantly leptotrichia and fusobacteria which were found in varying numbers. Leucocyte accumulations increased in number.

While the transition from the first to the second phase of bacterial colonization was rather easily observed, the transition from second to third phase was more gradual and somewhat difficult to time. The bacterial flora in this last stage was primarily characterized by the appearance of vibrios and spirochaetes. Cocci, rods and filamentous organisms were still present. On the average, the transition from second to third phase took place 6–10 days after tooth cleaning had ceased. Leucocyte accumulations were usually very heavy during this phase which persisted for varying intervals of time until clinical gingivitis was diagnosed. The time required to develop clinical gingivitis varied considerably amongst the twelve subjects. Some had gingivitis after 10 days, but the majority of the subjects required from 15–21 days for clinically evident gingivitis to develop. Smears taken at the beginning of the experiment showed that the bacterial population in the very small amounts of plaque which could be collected at that stage was dominated by Gram-positive cocci and short rods. These organisms accounted for 90–100 per cent of the total organisms counted in nine out of the twelve subjects. By the time clinical gingivitis had developed, the composition of the gingival flora had altered radically. In all the subjects Gram-positive cocci and short rods now only

accounted for 45–60 per cent of the micro-organisms in the plaque along the buccal gingiva. The distribution of other bacteria constituting the remaining 40–55 per cent of the flora were as follows:

Gram-negative cocci and short rods 22 per cent (range 11–31 per cent)
Gram-positive filaments 10 per cent (range 5–16 per cent)
Fusobacteria 10 per cent (range 4–15 per cent)
Vibrios 6 per cent (range 1–12 per cent)
Spirochaetes 1 per cent (range 0–2 per cent)

The originally predominating flora of Gram-positive cocci and short rods was reduced to 50–70 per cent of the total flora during the first 4–7 days of plaque formation and remained fairly constant at 45–60 per cent throughout the rest of the experimental period. A number of studies have confirmed that population shifts may occur as plaque ages, such that streptococci predominate in young plaques while with increasing age, filamentous organisms and Gram-negative bacteria increase in proportion [25, 58 & 59]. Plaques are therefore heterogeneous with a variable microbial population and a variable potential to elicit disease. Differences in biochemical activity exist from plaque to plaque and even within different regions of the same plaque.

Traditionally, it has been implied that bacteria become incorporated in plaque in a random, non-specific fashion but this theory does not account for the bacterial specificity involved in plaque formation or the cohesive nature of formed dental plaque. It has been suggested that two types of bacterial interactions are necessary for the formation of dental plaque [60]. Organisms must first adhere to the surface of the acquired pellicle and secondly there must be adhesive interactions occurring between bacteria, mediated by components of the plaque matrix to permit the organisms to accumulate and to impart cohesive properties. These adhesive interactions require a chemical or physical interaction between constituents present on the bacterial cell surface, and components of the acquired pellicle or the plaque matrix. Plaque formation on a clean tooth surface is initiated by rapid and selective adsorption of bacteria from saliva to the acquired enamel pellicle. Subsequent to their adsorption, bacteria must accumulate. It appears that in this latter phase two general classes of polymer are essential. Some bacteria synthesize extracellular polymers which bind their cells together (intraspecies binding), while other organisms may interact with salivary constituents which serve as the binding material. The cell surface components of bacteria vary widely from species to species and organisms may be expected to have a variable capacity to interact with and adhere to constituents of the enamel pellicle. Similarly, chemical analysis has shown that the matrix of pooled plaque consists of an array of both bacterial and salivary constituents which may react with cell surfaces as binding agents for different groups of organisms.

THE INITIAL PHASE OF PLAQUE DEVELOPMENT

Experiment has shown that a clean tooth surface is rapidly recolonized. After 1 hour up to 10^6 viable bacteria can be recovered per mm^2 of tooth surface. Bacteria show a variable capacity to adsorb to human enamel powder *in vitro* or to teeth *in vivo* and it would appear that there is selective adsorption of bacteria to the surface of the acquired enamel pellicle [60, 61 & 62]. If enamel powder is exposed to saliva *in vitro* to form a film of selectively adsorbed salivary constituents mimicking the natural enamel pellicle, the adsorption of some bacterial species is enhanced while that of other organisms is either unaffected or reduced. Adsorption of strains of *S. sanguis* and *S. mitis* is increased whereas adsorption *S. salivarius* or *S. mutans* tends to be unaffected or reduced [61 & 63]. Organisms such as *S. sanguis* and *S. mitis* are adsorbed from saliva to a much greater extent than are species such as *S. salivarius* or veillonella [64 & 65]. This explains why higher proportions of *S. sanguis* and *S. mitis* are recovered from early plaque than of *S. salivarius* or veillonella, even though the latter organisms are present in higher proportions in saliva. The relative adherence of bacteria to teeth and to all epithelial surfaces has been found to correlate with their proportions present naturally in these sites. It appears

that the composition of the flora which initially colonizes a clean, non-retentive tooth surface is almost entirely determined by the innate capacity of the organisms to become firmly attached, and by their numbers available for adsorption. Once the initial population has been acquired, population shifts caused by differences in microbial growth rates may occur relatively quickly. Plaque growth is further governed by the ability of bacterial cells to adhere one to the other.

BACTERIAL COHESIVE INTERACTIONS MEDIATED BY EXTRACELLULAR BACTERIAL POLYMERS

S. mutans forms adherent microbial deposits on the walls of culture vessels when provided with sucrose [66 & 67], and forms large bacterial plaques in experimental animals fed diets containing sucrose [66 & 68]. This organism has been shown to synthesize extracellular polysaccharides consisting of glucans and fructans specifically from sucrose but not from other common sugars [66, 69 & 70]. It has been suggested that since this organism metabolizes other sugars such as glucose for energy as readily as sucrose, its apparent dependence on sucrose for colonization may be related to developing a capacity for attachment. There is direct evidence for the involvement of some glucans in the adhesive interactions of *S. mutans*. Glucose grown cells of *S. mutans* form homogeneous cell suspensions but the addition of sucrose or only a few molecules of high molecular weight dextran per streptococcal cell causes rapid bacterial aggregation [71 & 72]. Such dextran-induced aggregation occurs with high molecular weight glucans of the dextran type but not with polysaccharides such as starch or levan [71]. Specific glucan molecules appear to bind directly to receptor sites on the surface of *S. mutans* cells linking the organisms together. The ability to aggregate in this way with dextran is a unique property of this organism. Other types of plaque bacteria, including strains of *S. sanguis* which also synthesize glucans from sucrose, do not possess this characteristic. Dextran-induced aggregation is thus specific to a particular species of organism and is not a universal mechanism for binding plaque bacteria on the surfaces of teeth, which accounts for the failure of dextranase preparations to remove all human plaque [73, 74 & 75]. Clearly, plaque bacteria use a variety of adhesion mechanisms to become established. *A. viscosus* and *A. naeslundii* form plaque deposits *in vitro* in experimental animals and are capable of synthesizing constituents which enable them to form cohesive bacterial masses [76, 77 & 78]. These organisms form surface constituents which impart cohesive properties and while the nature of these surface polymers remains undefined it is clear that glucans and fructans are not involved. *S. mutans* and actinomyces represent examples of bacteria which synthesize polymers which bind similar cells together, intra-species binding. Surface polymers of one bacterial species can also bind to those of a dissimilar organism, interspecies binding. For example, it has been reported that veillonella species unable to adhere to hard surfaces *in vitro* have the capacity to attach to preformed plaques formed by *A. viscosus* [79]. As plaque matures, filamentous organisms and Gram-negative bacteria increase in proportion, a change which has been attributed to the in-

creased growth rate of these organisms relative to streptococci due to changing conditions within maturing plaque. Electron microscope studies have shown that large numbers of filamentous bacteria are frequently found to radiate out from the surface of plaque apparently freely exposed, associated with little or no surrounding matrix material [80]. These filamentous bacteria form an enormous surface area of a specific nature with which bacteria capable of interacting with these surfaces would have a greater opportunity to attach and accumulate in a developing plaque (fig. 4.7). It has been suggested that such interbacterial interactions could account for some of the population shifts observed during plaque developments [60].

Plaque contains many organisms which do not appear to synthesize or interact with bacterial extracellular polymers. Organisms such as *S. sanguis* and *S. mitis* which are unable to form plaque-like deposits *in vitro* are present in human plaque in significant proportions which suggests such organisms may have the capacity to react with other substances in the plaque environment such as components of saliva or

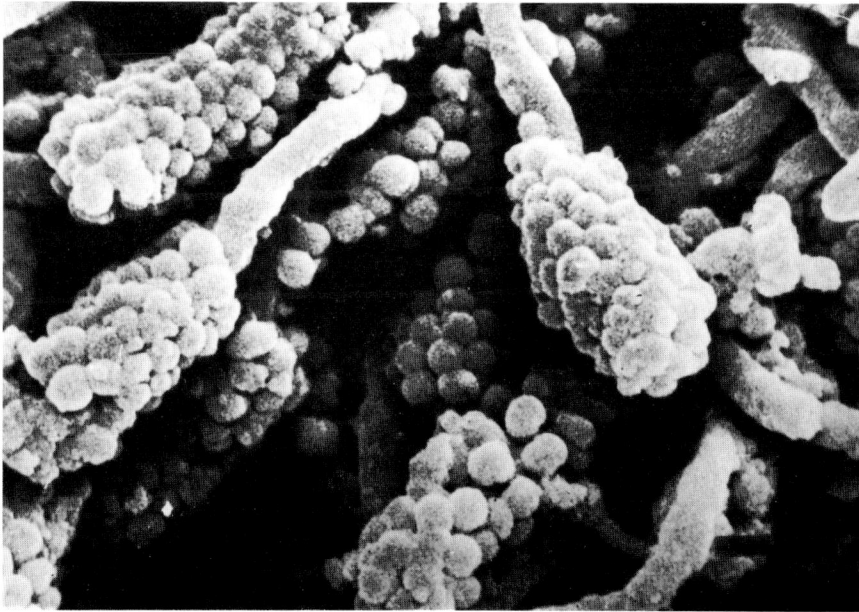

FIG. 4.7. Scanning electron photomicrograph of human dental plaque showing coccal forms attached to filamentous bacteria to form 'corn on the cob' structures. Photograph provided by Dr C.A. Saxton, Unilever Research Laboratory, 455, London Road, Isleworth, Middlesex.

gingival fluid. Strains of *S. mitis* and *S. sanguis* have been found to aggregate when incubated with either whole clarified saliva or with parotid and submaxillary secretions [49, 50 & 63]. Saliva contains a number of bacterial aggregating systems. Samples from some individuals possess secretory antibody with agglutinating activity [81 & 82], and high molecular weight constituents from the mucin fraction also act as effective bacterial aggregating systems [83]. Experiment suggests that separate mucinous polymers are involved in the aggregation of *S. sanguis* and *S. mitis* [84], and that calcium ions are required in both cases, since the addition of EDTA inhibits aggregation. Calcium ions appear to be involved in a number of mechanisms which contribute to plaque matrix formation and to imparting cohesive properties to plaque, and have been shown to increase the adsorption of mucins to glass and to hydroxyapatite [47 & 78]. Past theories of plaque formation have implied that salivary polymers were present in the plaque matrix as the result of precipitation. It is now clear that at least some salivary constituents can bind directly to surface components of certain types of prominent plaque bacteria and thereby become incorporated into the plaque [50]. Pooled plaque has been shown to contain significant quantities of IgA [85] and in some cases serum albumin [60]. Both IgA and albumin are effective bacterial aggregating systems and their presence in plaque is probably due to their capacity to bind directly to bacteria. While such mechanisms give cohesion to supragingival plaque, saliva does not penetrate the gingival sulcus. Components of gingival fluid may play an analogous role in lending cohesion to subgingival plaque.

MICROBIAL FEATURES OF PLAQUE
RELATED TO HEALTH AND DISEASE

Present evidence suggests that different forms of peridontal disease may have specific microbial aetiologies. The widely held view that the composition of dental plaque is reasonably consistent from individual to individual and from site to site is no longer valid. There are clear differences in the microbial composition of plaque associated with a healthy sulcus and that associated with gingivitis, early periodontitis and advanced periodontitis.

In health (fig. 4.8), the flora associated with the sulcus is scanty and located almost entirely supragingivally on the tooth surface. Microbial cell accumulations are 1–20 cells in thickness, and are mainly Gram-positive coccal forms. Organisms commonly found in such sites in adults include *S. mitis*, *S. sanguis*, *Staphylococcus epidermis*, *Rothia dentocariosa*, *Actinomyces viscosus*, *Actinomyces naeslundii*, and occasionally species of *Neisseria* and *Veillonella* [86].

The bacteriological criteria for a healthy sulcus appear to be scanty microflora consisting of approximately 85 per cent Gram-positive organisms usually of the actinomyces and streptococcus species [87]. In the early stages of gingivitis the actinomyces group of organisms tends to be the dominant genus associated with supragingival plaque, frequently comprising 50 per cent or more of isolates. In longstanding gingivitis approximately 25 per cent of the microbiota may be Gram-negative, including species of *Veillonella*, campylobacter and *Fusobacteria*. The Gram-negative cells appear to be located primarily on the surface of the plaque, in subgingival sites [88].

A 'contained' gingivitis is thus associated with a marked quantitative increase of the microflora and up to a three-fold increase in the proportion of Gram-negative organisms in comparison to that found in the healthy sulcus.

Plaque associated with gingivitis and early periodontitis is complex and heterogeneous and at least a portion appears to be firmly attached to tooth surface. In contrast, microbiologic examination of plaque in the apical parts of deep periodontal pockets in adults has revealed a predominance of Gram-negative anaerobic rods. The advanced periodontitis microbiota is characterised by the presence of large numbers of asaccharolytic microorganisms, including *Fusobacterium nucleatum*, *Bacteroides melaninogenicus*, *Eikenella corrodens*, *Bacteroides corrodens*, *Bacteroides capillosus* and anaerobic vibrios. Such organisms have been shown to comprise up to 75 per cent of the isolates from such sites in the mouth [89].

Studies of the microbial composition of

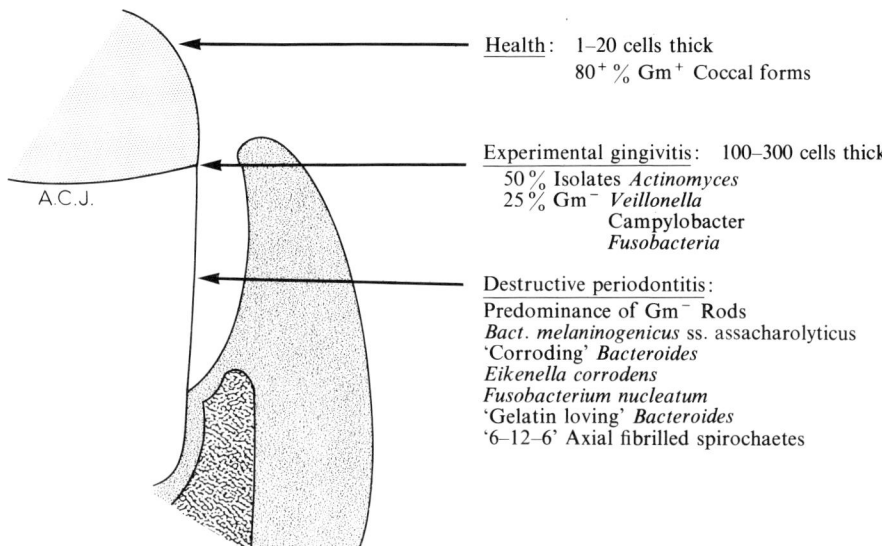

Health: 1–20 cells thick
         80⁺% Gm⁺ Coccal forms

Experimental gingivitis: 100–300 cells thick
     50% Isolates *Actinomyces*
     25% Gm⁻ *Veillonella*
              Campylobacter
              Fusobacteria

Destructive periodontitis:
Predominance of Gm⁻ Rods
Bact. melaninogenicus ss. assacharolyticus
'Corroding' *Bacteroides*
Eikenella corrodens
Fusobacterium nucleatum
'Gelatin loving' *Bacteroides*
'6–12–6' Axial fibrilled spirochaetes

A.C.J.

FIG. 4.8. Bacterial populations in health and disease.

pockets in juvenile periodontitis patients revealed the presence of a sparse microbiota which was dominated by Gram-negative capnophilic and anaerobic rods [90 & 91]. One of the organisms most frequently isolated and isolated in the highest numbers was a Gram-negative fusiform shaped rod which would glide on agar surfaces. The characteristics of this organism are consistent with the species *Bacteroides ochraceus*. The juvenile periodontitis microbiota appears to be characterised by saccharolytic microorganisms of five distinct groups, now classified under the new genus capnocytophaga [92]. It is now clear that this group of organisms can also be isolated with a much lower frequency from healthy sites in patients without juvenile periodontitis.

Structural studies of *in situ* plaque associated with destructive periodontitis in adults revealed a more complex picture than that observed in juvenile periodontitis. Plaque is usually more abundant and often consists in part of a zone of primarily Gram-positive organisms which are apparently firmly attached to the surface. Between this zone and the pocket epithelium, one finds a zone of loosely packed Gram-negative organisms and spirochaetes. This loose

zone extends to the apical portion of the pocket [93].

It has been proposed that it is possible to develop a diagnostic and therapeutic regimen for patients on the basis of monitoring the percentage of bacteria present in scrapings obtained from tooth surface as assessed by either dark ground illumination or phase contrast microscopy [94, 95 & 96]. On this basis it might become possible to decide the presence or absence of active disease, the prognosis or outcome of therapy, and the frequency of recall visits which an individual patient may require (see chap. 12).

Chemical control of plaque accumulation

In some individuals established gingivitis may stabilise and remain quiescent without leading to further destruction of the periodontium for many years, while in others it is rapidly progressive to destructive periodontal disease. Present evidence suggests that progression of periodontal disease is episodic rather than linear with periods of exacerbation and remission over the long term. It may be that periods of active disease can be associated with the presence or absence in plaque of particular groups of mouth organism as previously defined. There is growing interest in the possibility of chemotherapeutic control of the microbial populations of dental plaque. This subject has been well reviewed by Loesche [97]. The 'non specific' plaque hypothesis proposes that if periodontal diseases are non-specific microbial infections, then all species in plaque will have to be suppressed continually throughout the individual's life to achieve control. Chemotherapeutic agents would have to be chosen which were broad spectrum in activity, would not select resistant forms and have no additional biological side effects. The ubiquitous occurrence of gingivitis and widespread presence of its associated organisms suggest that less specificity may exist in gingivitis and the early stages of periodontitis and that the degree of bacterial specificity associated with tissue damage may increase as the disease progresses. The demonstration of distinct microbial populations in healthy sites and sites with different forms of periodontal disease, the differences in pathogenic potential of different human pocket isolates, and the efficacy of therapy which suppresses some but not all members of the periodontal microbiota all suggest the likelihood that different levels of periodontal disease have specific microbial aetiologies.

While it is possible that a single microbial species may be responsible for all destructive disease, such a possibility appears unlikely. The probability is that infectious diseases of the periodontium can be initiated by any of a number of pathogens. Socransky [86] has suggested that perhaps six to twelve microbial species may be responsible for the majority of destructive periodontal disease, and additional forms may be responsible for destructive disease in a small percentage of the population. On this basis chemotherapy of plaque might come to have a valuable role in prevention and treatment of active periodontal disease (see chap. 12).

Chemical control of dental plaque may involve prevention of plaque formation, removal or dispersion of existing plaque, inhibition of calcification of existing plaques, or alteration of the pathogenicity of plaque. It has been suggested that formation and retention of bacterial plaque on teeth might theoretically be interfered with at various stages of development [98].

(1) Microorganisms responsible for plaque formation may be eliminated or reduced in number.

(2) The formation of bacterial and salivary products which constitute the intermicrobial substance in plaque may be inhibited.

(3) Established plaques may be dissolved.

(4) Calcification of plaque may be counteracted.

(5) Colonization of bacteria on the tooth surface may be inhibited.

(6) The pathogenicity of plaque may be reduced by interference with the metabolism of the plaque bacteria.

A number of broad spectrum antibacterial compounds have been used to inhibit plaque formation. Cetylpyridinium chloride, benzalkonium chloride and chlorhexidine salts have been shown to have the capacity to inhibit plaque formation *in vivo* [99–106].

Daily mouth rinses with 0·2 per cent aqueous solutions of chlorhexidine reduce the number of bacteria in saliva by 95 per cent in the course of a few days. After about 15 days there was a slight increase in the number of bacteria and a new equilibrium was established at a level of 85–90 per cent reduction, which was maintained over a 40 day experimental period [104].

Various broad spectrum antibiotics have been shown to have inhibitory effects on both caries and periodontitis [107–112], but the use of broad spectrum antibiotics in this preventive role is limited by the danger of developing resistant strains of organisms and sensitivity reactions.

Vancomycin, which is active against Gram-positive bacteria, including streptococci, staphylococci and pneumococci, and spiramycin which has a similar spectrum of activity to erythromycin and penicillin, have been shown to reduce plaque formation and control dental caries and periodontitis [113–116].

Erythromycin has been shown to cause a mean decrease of 35 per cent in the amount of plaque in humans following 7 days administration as a liquid suspension of 250 mg dissolved in a small volume of water rinsed through the teeth and swallowed four times a day. The drug caused a marked rise in the percentage of erythromycin resistant organisms. Spirochaetes, which were initially present in all subjects, virtually disappeared for 5–18 weeks after antibiotic administration [117].

In other studies only temporary effects on plaque formation have been obtained with vancomycin and polymyxin B which is active against Gram-negative bacteria [112 & 118]. Both vancomycin and spiramycin have been shown to be effective plaque inhibitors in hamsters [119].

Actinabolin has been shown to have *in vitro* inhibitory activity against cariogenic streptococcal strains and mixed microbial cultures obtained from dental plaque of human subjects. This antibiotic is relatively non-toxic, is not appreciably absorbed when administered orally and has limited use in other fields of medicine [120].

The fact that a limited spectrum of noncariogenic oral Gram-positive bacteria appeared to show some sensitivity to actinabolin, and that yeasts and Gram-negative bacteria were found to be insensitive to inhibition by this antibiotic, suggest that undesirable microbial population shifts following long term administration might outweigh any advantage gained over the short term. This is the general problem of attempts to control commensal microbial populations by chemical means.

A macrolide antibiotic CC10232 obtained from the fermentation of a strain of *Streptomyces caelestis* NRRL2821, with strong antibacterial activity against a variety of Gram-positive microorganisms has been shown to inhibit plaque and calculus formation and to prevent gingivitis [121 & 122].

In common with actinabolin this drug has no other reported medical use and is not significantly absorbed either orally or systemically. It has been subjected to extensive pharmacological and toxicological evaluations and has been demonstrated to be relatively non-toxic [122].

It has been reported that CC10232 causes substantial reductions in formation of human dental plaque of the order of 70–77 per cent at a variety of concentrations and clinical test conditions [115]. The same report suggested that a mouth rinse containing 0·01 per cent CC10232 provided an approximately 75 per cent reduction

in dental calculus formation during a 12 week human clinical study. A further study showed a statistically significant 57 per cent reduction in plaque formation after 6 months and a significant 33 per cent reduction of calculus formation after 9 months following use of a 0·01 per cent CC10232 mouth rinse. While this antibiotic does not readily inhibit Gram-negative bacteria, yeasts and moulds, no adverse manifestations followed the use of a 0·01 per cent mouth rinse for a period of 9 months [122].

Attempts to interfere with the oral bacterial flora by use of vaccines have not been encouraging. Guggenheim *et al.* [123] superinfected rats with a strain of streptococcus mutans. A vaccine against this bacteria effected no reduction in plaque formation or caries incidence. Studies by Genco and Evans [124] have shown that antibodies against one strain of plaque forming *Streptococcus mutans* effectively inhibit plaque formed by this particular strain, whereas plaque formed by other cariogenic mutans strains was not affected. This demonstrates the high degree of specificity of antibodies to components of the oral microbiota which appears to be general. While there has been some success in producing caries reduction in experimental animals by use of vaccines, the mechanisms involved are incompletely understood. Since culture of organisms such as spirochaetes associated with periodontal disease is difficult in comparison, control of periodontal disease by these means seems unlikely in the immediate future [125].

INTERFERENCE WITH THE FORMATION OF BACTERIAL AND SALIVARY PRODUCTS

Streptococcal strains such as *S. mutans* and *S. sanguis* have been regarded as mainly responsible for plaque formation by virtue of their ability to produce extracellular polysaccharides [126–130].

These branched dextrans are thought to be necessary for the maintenance of the structural integrity of plaque, and to act as an energy store when the supply of simple sugars and levans is exhausted. They may be further used by bacteria as a means of concentrating ions or other essential nutrients [131].

Experiment has shown that amine fluorides can reduce the plaque forming capacity of three strains of *S. mutans* whereas inorganic fluorides showed no plaque inhibition. Kepner and Berman [132] demonstrated that cariogenic streptococci exposed to benzalkonium chloride and sodium lauryl sulphate did not form capsules which suggested interference with their production of extracellular polysaccharides. A vaccine against the dextran sucrases produced by a strain of *S. mutans* has been tested in rats in an attempt to interfere with extracellular polysaccharide synthesis but no effect on plaque formation or caries incidence was detected [133]. It has been shown that the synthesis of dextrans in plaque can be inhibited by adding dextranase to a polysaccharide synthesizing system and plaque is readily dissolved by crude dextranases *in vitro* [134 & 135]. Plaque inhibition, caries retardation and prevention of periodontitis in animals have been obtained using dextranases [136, 137 & 138].

Dextranases have not, however, proved to be effective plaque inhibitors in human studies, perhaps because the maximum activity of some dextranases is at a relatively low pH (3·5–5·5) [133 & 139] and because of the heterogeneity of the polyglucans and the presence of small amounts of levan in the plaque matrix.

INTERFERENCE WITH MICROBIAL COLONIZATION ON THE TOOTH SURFACE

Plaque formed on silicate fillings has been shown to differ chemically from plaque formed on other dental restorations and on tooth surfaces [140]. *In vivo*, plaque and calculus form at different rates on teeth and on Mylar strips when exposed to chlorhexidine [141]. Turesky *et al.* [142] have shown that inhibition of artificial plaque by chemical agents is dependent on the surface used for plaque growth. The observations suggest that interference with the nature of the tooth surface might influence the process of plaque formation. Complete plaque inhibition has been reported when 0·2 per cent aqueous solutions of chlorhexidine digluconate have been used as mouth rinses [103 & 104]. Gjermo, Baastad and Rolla [105] compared the *in vivo* and *in vitro* plaque inhibiting ability of

eleven antimicrobial agents against salivary bacteria. Chlorhexidine gluconate and acetate proved to be most effective *in vivo*, while other agents such as cetyl-pyridinium chloride and dequalinium chloride, equally or more effective *in vitro* against salivary bacteria, exhibited no effect *in vivo*. It was concluded since there was no direct correlation between the *in vivo* and *in vitro* effects that 'factors other than the general antibacterial activity are presumably important'. The antimicrobial action of chlorhexidine is exerted against a wide range of bacteria with Gram-negative species being generally less sensitive than Gram-positive types. It has been proposed [143 & 144] that the primary action of chlorhexidine is adsorption on to the bacterial cell surface. This adsorption is followed by a disruption of the cytoplasmic membrane, but further events depend on the concentration of chlorhexidine present. Low concentrations allow leakage of cytoplasmic components while higher concentrations coagulate the cytoplasmic components and are thus more rapidly bactericidal. Schroeder [145] reported the effect of thrice daily mouth rinses with chlorhexidine diacetate (Hibitane) on supragingival dental plaque in ten human subjects over a 3 day period and found a 73 per cent inhibition of deposit formation (by dry deposit weight) at 0·1 per cent concentration, 40 per cent at 0·05 per cent and 30 per cent reduction at 0·025 per cent. Following the use of the human experimental model system originally developed by Löe, Theilade and Jensen [56], it was concluded that in individuals who rinse with 10 ml of 0·2 per cent chlorhexidine gluconate for 1 minute in the morning and at night plaque will not form and no gingivitis will develop [103]. In a follow-up experiment by Löe [104] it was confirmed that two daily mouth rinses with 0·2 per cent chlorhexidine does effectively prevent plaque formation, as does one daily topical application of 2 per cent chlorhexidine. While chlorhexidine has a general antimicrobial effect in the mouth in that repeated rinses with it can reduce the salivary bacterial flora by 85–95 per cent [146], it has been shown that there is an additional tooth surface antimicrobial effect in that chlorhexidine gluconate has an affinity for hydroxyapatite and acidic salivary proteins and adsorbs to tooth surfaces *in vitro* [147]. A study of the retention of chlorhexidine in the mouth [148] reported that antibacterial properties were retained by saliva for 2 hours following a 0·2 per cent chlorhexidine rinse. Results of antibacterial activity and adsorption tests with chlorhexidine led to the conclusion that 'substances usually found on tooth surfaces—hydroxyapatite, pellicle, bacterial polysaccharide and streptococci all bind chlorhexidine *in vitro*'. In a long term human evaluation of chlorhexidine, Flotra *et al.* [149] studied the effects of a 0·1 per cent or 0·2 per cent chlorhexidine (gluconate and acetate) rinse and a placebo when used as a twice-daily mouth-wash in fifty young volunteer soldiers over a 4-month period. The subjects continued their ordinary oral hygiene procedures. Over the initial 8-week period the plaque index showed a 66 per cent reduction and the gingival index a 24 per cent reduction. Following a thorough scaling and an additional 9-week period, the respective reductions in the plaque and gingival indices were 84 per cent and 43 per cent.

Chlorhexidine has been shown to prevent the development of gingivitis and resolve experimentally induced gingival inflammation *in vivo* [103 & 150]. It has, however, only a limited effect on the bacterial population of pathological pockets and has brought about only slight improvement of gingival condition when subgingival plaque and calculus are present [106].

While chlorhexidine in the concentrations used for plaque inhibition is of low toxicity, there have been a number of reports of complaints of bitter taste and interference with taste sensation for some time after application. Discoloration and staining of teeth, fillings and tongues have been seen in human and animal studies [103, 104, 105, 145 & 151]. Animal experiment, however, confirms the relatively low toxicity of chlorhexidine [152].

Studies were done of the effect of topically applied chlorhexidine gluconate on chronically inflamed gingiva in three beagle dogs and healing of standardized gingival wounds in two other beagles over a 42-day period. It was concluded that in dogs it was possible to resolve chronic gingivitis and establish and maintain a plaque and gingivitis free dentition through the use of 2 per cent chlorhexidine topically applied once each day. It was further concluded that the chlorhexidine solution had no detrimental effect on the healing of open gingival wounds. Studies by Hirst *et al.* [153] suggested that chlorhexidine solution had a beneficial effect on gingival tissue when compared to either mechanical cleansing or application of saline solutions. Lindhe *et al.* [154] studied the effect of local application of 2·2 mmol (approximately 0·2 per cent chlorhexidine gluconate) on the oral mucosa of the hamster. When applied onto intact or dekeratinized cheek pouch epithelium no reaction was produced in the underlying connective tissue. However, the test solution caused rapid vascular disturbances (reduced flow, microthrombi formation, stasis etc.) when applied to exposed connective tissue. These observations indicate that chlorhexidine does not penetrate undamaged oral epithelium. Furthermore, it was found that the influence of extended chlorhexidine treatment (12 weeks) on epithelialized tissue is insignificant. By excluding substances known to neutralize chlorhexidine (phosphates, sulphates) from dentifrices it has been possible to retain its plaque inhibiting capacity [155].

Significant plaque inhibition was shown in a 2-month study on chlorhexidine-containing dentifrices [156]. No discoloured tongues and no lesions of the oral mucosa were detected. Teeth and silicate fillings however were frequently stained. Since the 'technical skill, time, effort and perseverance' required to continually maintain a high standard of oral cleanliness exceeds the ability of the average human being [157], a means of chemical plaque control to replace or supplant mechanical oral hygiene procedures would be valuable.

While the results of short-term evaluation of chlorhexidine are encouraging much more information is required on the long term effect on oral mucous membrane, on the ecological shifts induced in the oral flora and the effects of swallowed chlorhexidine on the gastrointestinal tract. Studies in dogs have demonstrated that resistant strains of *Proteus*, *Citrobacter* and *Klebsiella* may occur after 6 months of application of 0·2 per cent chlorhexidine, twice daily, to teeth [158].

The proposition [159] that the human oral

microflora has no essential physiologic function requires re-evaluation. Plaque is a normal part of the body flora which in general constitutes an important body defence mechanism. Chronic periodontitis appears to be a function of the metabolic activities of plaque rather than of its presence or absence and it may be that a modification of the diet or the plaque without the use of antiseptics, antibiotics or other agents, which are likely to produce cures worse than the disease, is the desirable approach to microbial population control. Stralfors [160] has reported 100 per cent disinfection of human dental plaque applying the antibacterial compound chloramine-T as a powder directly on the teeth with cap splints. Newly formed plaque is readily dissolved by frequent mouth rinses with 0·2 per cent chlorhexidine digluconate [103]. Inhibition of calcification of plaque seems to be possible by chemicals such as proteolytic enzymes, urea, vitamin C, but the results of trials are inconsistent and the value in prevention of disease is questionable.

DENTAL CALCULUS

Calculus forms as a result of the mineralization of plaque and is classified according to its position on the tooth in relation to the gingival margin. Mineralization of plaque may occur intracellularly and extracellularly in response to bacterial metabolism. There are two patterns of bacterial calcification [161]. In one, mineralization begins within the microorganism and progresses outward, whereas in the other, mineralization begins at the outer surface and progresses inward. The high levels of calcium and phosphorus in young plaque suggest that these elements may function as reservoirs to protect the enamel surface during periods of exposure to carbohydrate and low pH levels.

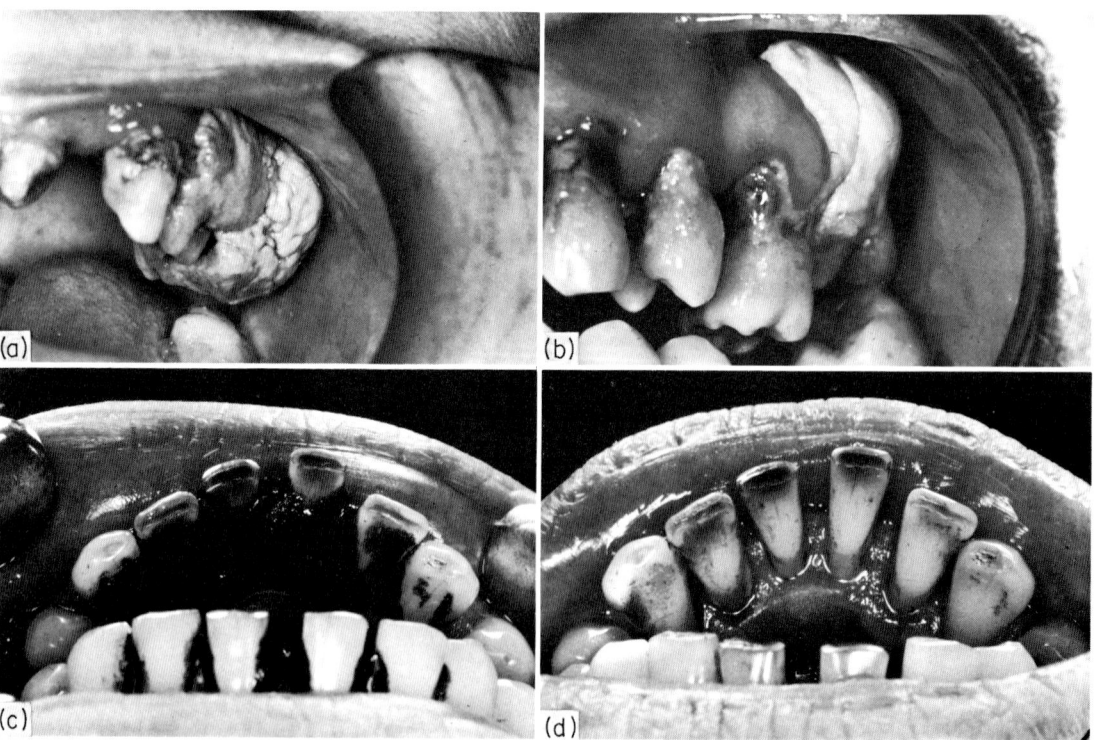

FIG. 4.9. (a) and (b) Gross supragingival calculus on the buccal surface of maxillary molars opposite Stensen's duct. (c) Gross deposits of heavily stained supragingival calculus, lingual to the mandibular incisors. (d) Following initial scaling.

SUPRAGINGIVAL CALCULUS

Supragingival calculus forms coronal to the gingival margin. It ranges in colour from white to yellow, but it may become stained by tobacco, tea or coffee. It is of hard, clay like consistency, easily detachable from the tooth with a scaler.

Such deposits occur most frequently, and in the greatest quantity, on the buccal surface of maxillary molars opposite Stenson's duct and on the lingual surface of lower incisors in relation to the submandibular and sublingual ducts (fig. 4.9). X-ray diffraction has shown that four major types of crystalline calcium phosphates

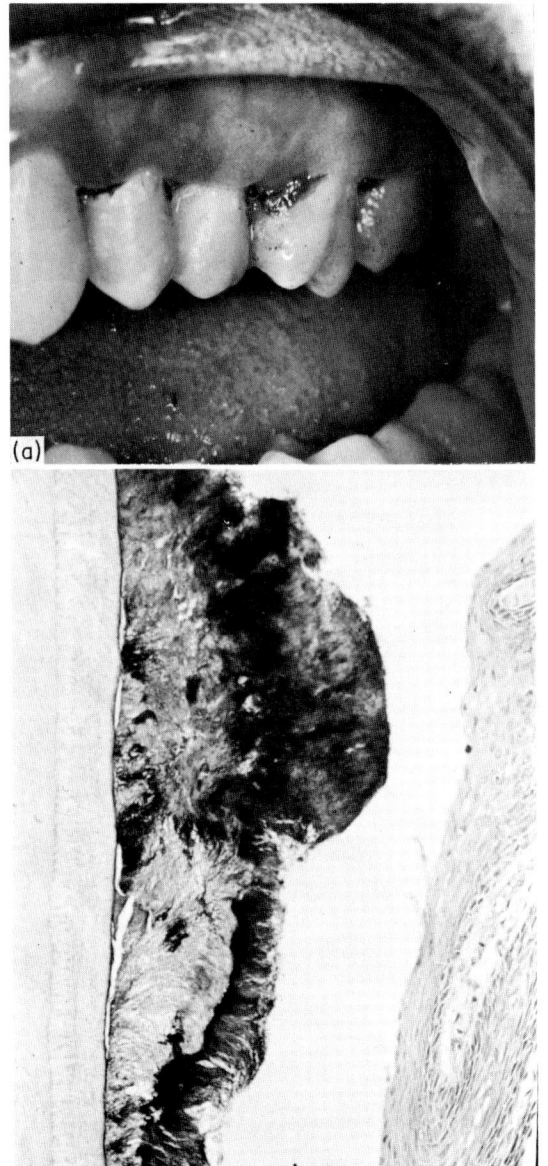

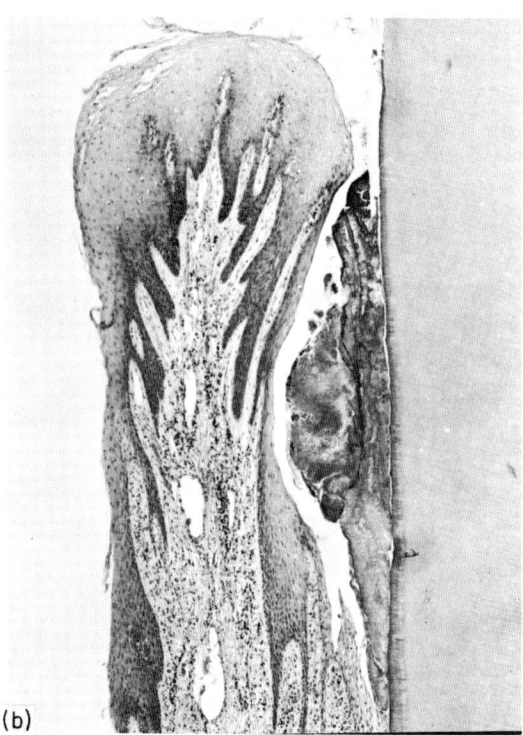

FIG. 4.10. Subgingival calculus. (a) A dense dark deposit firmly attached to tooth. Frequently not visible unless the gingivae are deflected by an air syringe or probe. (b) Photomicrograph, subgingival calculus and plaque which has caused hyperplasia of gingival epithelium, thinning and hyperplasia of crevicular epithelium and pocket formation. (c) High power subgingival calculus and plaque. Deep layers adjacent to tooth are highly calcified. Plaque on the surface of calcified layers has a pallisade structure of filamentous organisms.

may be present in supragingival calculus. These are brushite, whitlockite, octacalcium phosphate and hydroxyapatite [162].

This forms below the crest of the marginal gingiva and is not detectable on oral examination without the benefit of an air syringe or Cross type of calculus probe (fig. 4.10). It is usually dense, dark brown or green–black in colour, and very firmly attached to the tooth. Supragingival and subgingival deposits may occur separately, or together, in the same mouth, and they are sometimes referred to as salivary and serumal calculus respectively. The term serumal calculus was coined on the assumption that this type of calculus is at least partly derived from exudate of serum into the sulcus. Exudate from the sulcus may mediate the composition of subgingival calculus, which is relatively isolated from direct contact with saliva [163].

The structure of calculus

Calculus consists of an inorganic and organic fraction, the inorganic fraction being in the range of 70–90 per cent according to the degree of calcification (fig. 4.11). At least two-thirds of the inorganic component is crystalline, principally hydroxyapatite, but at least four other crystalline salts with a different Ca/P ratio have been demonstrated [164 & 165].

The organic component of calculus consists of mucopolysaccharide ground substance derived from saliva, desquamated epithelial cells, leucocytes, food debris and various types of bacteria and fungi. The predominant filamentous organisms, which form the stroma in which calcification takes place, belong to the families of actinomyces and leptothrix. In vitro investigation of the role of such organisms in calcification has shown that viability of the organisms is not a prerequisite for calcification to occur [166]. It has been suggested that specific carbohydrate–protein complexes derived from many sources may determine the potential of tissues to calcify. Further evidence that the presence of organisms is not essential to the mechanisms of calcification is indicated by the fact that calculus deposits are

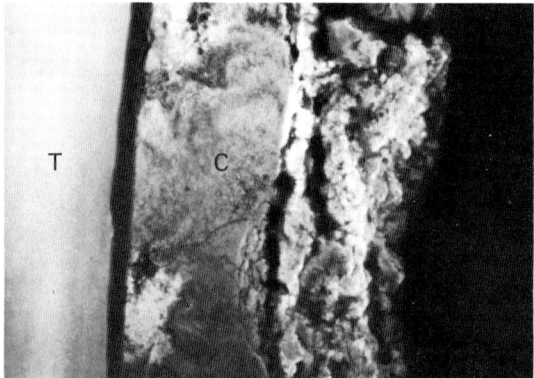

FIG. 4.11. Microradiograph of undecalcified section of calculus (C) on tooth (T). The superficial layers are incremental and progressively less mineralized towards the surface.

known to occur in germ free rodents [167 & 168]. It has been shown that the frequency of deposition of calculus is roughly the same in conventional and germ free rodents, and that the structure and composition of such deposits does not suggest a different mode of deposition under germ free conditions.

Administration of broad spectrum antibiotics to produce a major change in the oral flora of conventional animals does not significantly affect the rate of deposition of calculus, although topical applications of penicillin have been shown to reduce plaque formation on rat molars [169]. It has been concluded from such evidence that there is more than one calcifying mechanism, and that a calculus forming mechanism exists operating under sterile conditions compared to that underlying deposition in the presence of organisms.

It is probable that calculus formation occurs as a result of alteration of physicochemical conditions brought about by a wide range of factors where plaque is present; both the metabolic functions of the plaque and its mucoprotein composition are of importance in the process of calcification. Factors which have been considered of importance in relation to such physicochemical changes are well described by Jenkins [47].

Theories of calculus formation

CARBON DIOXIDE LOSS

In the past it has been considered that carbon dioxide loss caused precipitation of calcium as a direct result of rise in pH. Recent evidence suggests that carbon dioxide may have a specific effect in keeping calcium phosphate in solution, probably through formation of a complex ion. It has been shown that carbonic anhydrase may favour calculus formation *in vitro*, and that a high carbon dioxide tension reduces the tendency to calcification. The production of carbonic anhydrase by the plaque microbiota provides a logical explanation for variation in carbon dioxide tension.

THE FORMATION OF AMMONIA

The formation of ammonia from urea may produce local alkalinity as a result of catabolism of saliva in areas of reduced rate of flow or as a result of the production of ammonia by the organisms of plaque. No direct relationship between ammonia production and plaque formation has yet been demonstrated.

THE PHOSPHATASE THEORY

This theory was based on the observation that phosphatase from the gingival tissues is capable of releasing phosphate ions from organic phosphates in saliva *in vitro*. Many workers failed to confirm the action of this mechanism, and it was concluded that the concentrations of phosphatase in saliva were too low. The concentration of phosphates, and of acid and alkaline phosphatase in plaque, are sufficiently high to have revived interest in this as a possible mechanism.

PROTEIN PRECIPITATION

The protein molecules of saliva react on contact with a tooth surface, to become precipitated on the surface as an insoluble pellicle. The release of protein bound calcium as a result of this mechanism may be a factor in calculus formation.

THE SEEDING THEORY

The filamentous organism, diphtheroids, veillonella and some streptococci of plaque have the capacity to form intracellular crystals of apatite [170–173], and a protein can be extracted from some organisms, which mineralizes if placed in a calcifying solution. In a guest editorial in the *Journal of Calcified Tissue Research*, Ennever and Creamer have drawn attention to the need for further study of the mechanisms whereby bacteria calcify [174]. As early as 1925 Bulleid reported that leptothrix have a precipitating action: 'due to some inherent property of the organism' [175]. This microorganism has since been identified as *Bacterionema matruchotii*, a member of the Actinomycetales.

As plaque matures, there is an increase in the number of organisms, and the evidence suggests that some constituent of the organisms may act as a seeding substance, which results in the crystallization of calcium phosphate probably from saliva. Experiments with plaque on celluloid strips have shown that pretreatment of the strips with 10 per cent formalin does not significantly affect the ability of the strip to calcify when placed in a calcifying solution. The facts that viability of the organisms is not a determining factor and that calcification occurs in germ free rats, suggest that a variety of mucoproteins may also have the capacity to act as seeding agents.

REFERENCES

[1] BURNETT G.W. & SCHERP H.W. (1966) *Oral Microbiology and Infectious Disease*, 2nd Edition. Baltimore: Williams and Wilkins.

[2] STEPHAN R.M. (1953) Dental plaque in relation to the etiology of caries. *Int. dent. J.* **4**, 180–195.

[3] TURESKY S., RENSTRUP G. & GLICKMAN I. (1961) Histologic and histochemical observations regarding early calculus formation in children and adults. *J. Periodont.* **32**, 7–14.

[4] McDOUGALL W.A. (1963) Studies on the dental plaque. I. The histology of the dental plaque and its attachment. *Aust. dent. J.* **8**, 261–273.

[5] McDOUGALL W.A. (1963) Studies on the dental plaque. II. The histology of the developing interproximal plaque. *Aust. dent. J.* **8**, 398–407.

[6] JENKINS G.N. (1966) *The Physiology of the Mouth*, 3rd Edition. Oxford: Blackwell Scientific Publications.

[7] WINKLER K.C. & BACKER DIRKS O. (1958) The mechanism of the dental plaque. *Int. dent. J.* **8**, 561–585.

[8] KLEINBERG I. & JENKINS G.N. (1964) The pH of dental plaques in the different areas of the mouth before and after meals and their relationship to the pH and rate of flow of resting saliva. *Arch. oral Biol.* **9**, 493–516.

[9] CARLSSON J. & EGELBERG J. (1965) Effect of diet on early plaque formation in man. *Odont. Revy* **16**, 112–125.

[10] BERMAN K.S. & GIBBONS R.J. (1966) Iodophilic polysaccharide synthesis by human and rodent oral bacteria. *Arch. oral Biol.* **11**, 533.

[11] McDOUGALL W.A. (1964) Studies on the dental plaque. IV. Levans and the dental plaque. *Aust. dent. J.* **9**, 1–5.

[12] WOOD J.M. (1967) The amount, distribution and metabolism of soluble polysaccharides in human dental plaque. *Arch. oral Biol.* **12**, 849.

[13] McDOUGALL W.A. (1964) Studies on the dental plaque. (4) Levans and the dental plaque. *Aust. dent. J.* **9**, 1.

[14] HOBSON P.N. (1969) Growth of mixed cultures and their biological control, in *Microbial Growth*, p. 43. Eds. Meadow P. & Pirt S.J. Cambridge: Cambridge University Press.

[15] POOLE D.F.G. & NEWMAN H.N. (1971) Dental plaque and oral health. *Nature* **234**, 329.

[16] SOCRANSKY S.S. & MANGANIELLO S.D. (1971) The oral microbiota of man from birth to senility. *J. Periodont.* **42**, 485.

[17] GIBBONS R.J., SOCRANSKY S.S., SAWYERS S., KAPSIMALIS B. & MACDONALD J.B. (1963) The microbiota of the gingival crevice area of man. II. The predominant cultivable organisms. *Arch. Oral Biol.* **8**, 281.

[18] GIBBONS R.J., SOCRANSKY S.S., DE ARAUJO W.C. & VAN HOUTE J. (1964) Studies of the cultivable microbiota of dental plaque. *Arch. Oral Biol.* **9**, 365.

[19] GORDON D.F. & GIBBONS R.J. (1966) Studies of the predominant cultivable organisms from the human tongue. *Arch. Oral Biol.* **11**, 627.

[20] GORDON D.F. & JONG B.B. (1968) Indigenous flora from human saliva. *Appl. Microbiol.* **16**, 428.

[21] KRASSE B. (1954) The proportional distribution of *streptococcus salivarius* and other streptococci in various parts of the mouth. *Odont. Revy.* **5**, 203.

[22] CARLSSON J. (1967) Presence of various types of nonhaemolytic streptococci in dental plaque and in other sites in the oral cavity in man. *Odont. Revy.* **18**, 55.

[23] KRASSE B. & EDWARDSSON S. (1966) The proportional distribution of caries inducing streptococci in various parts of the oral cavity of hamsters. *Arch. Oral Biol.* **11**, 1137.

[24] GIBBONS R.J., KAPSIMALIS B. & SOCRANSKY S.S. (1964) The source of salivary bacteria. *Arch. Oral Biol.* **9**, 101.

[25] RITZ H.L. (1967) Microbial population shifts in developing human dental plaque. *Arch. Oral Biol.* **12**, 1561.

[26] ZINNER D.D. & JABLON J.M. (1969) Cariogenic streptococci in infants. *Arch. Oral Biol.* **14**, 1429.

[27] McCARTHY C., SNEIDER M.L. & PARKER R.B. (1965) The indigenous oral flora of man. I. The new born to the one year old infant. *Arch. Oral Biol.* **10**, 65.

[28] DE ARAUJO W.C. & MACDONALD J.B. (1964) Gingival crevice microbiota of pre-school children. *Arch. Oral Biol.* **9**, 227.

[29] KELSTRUP J. (1966) The incidence of *Bacteroides melaninogenicus* in human gingival sulci and its prevalence in the oral cavity at different ages. *Periodontics* **4**, 14.

[30] SOCRANSKY S.S., GIBBONS R.J., DALE A.C. & BORTNIK L. (1963) The microbiota of the gingival crevice area of man. I. Total microscopic and viable counts and counts of specific organisms. *Arch. Oral Biol.* **8**, 275.

[31] CARLSSON J., SODERHOLM G. & ALMSFELDT I. (1969) Prevalence of *Streptococcus sanguis* and *Streptococcus mutans* in the mouth of persons wearing full dentures. *Arch. Oral Biol.* **14**, 243.

[32] LILIENTHAL B. (1950) Studies of the flora of the mouth. III. Yeast-like organisms: Some observations on their incidence in the mouth. *Aust. J. Ex. Biol. Sci.* **28**, 279.

[33] SHKLAIR I.L. & MAZZARELLA M.A. (1961) Effects of full-mouth extraction on oral microbiota. *D. Progress.* **1**, 275.

[34] ROSENTHAL S.L. & GOOTZEIT E.H. (1942) The incidence of *Bacteroides fusiformis* and spirochetes in the edentulous mouth. *J. Dent. Res.* **21**, 373.

[35] LENZ H. & MUHLEMANN H.R. (1963) Repair of etched enamel exposed to the oral environment. *Helv. Odont. Acta.* **7**, 47.

[36] THEILADE J. (1964) Electron microscope study of calculus attachment to smooth surfaces. *Acta Odont. Scand.* **22**, 379.

[37] MECKEL A.H. (1965) The formation and properties of organic films on teeth. *Arch. Oral Biol.* **10**, 585.

[38] FRANK R.M. & BRENDEL A. (1966) Ultrastructure of the approximal dental plaque and the underlying normal and carious enamel. *Arch. Oral Biol.* **2**, 883.

[39] LEACH S.A. & SAXTON C.A. (1966) An electron microscopic study of the acquired pellicle and plaque formed on the enamel of human incisors. *Arch. Oral Biol.* **11**, 1081.

[40] ARMSTRONG W.G. (1968) Origin and nature of the acquired pellicle. *Proc. Roy. Soc. Med.* **61**, 923.

[41] KLEINBERG I. (1970) Biochemistry of the dental plaque. *Advances Oral Biol.* **4**, 43.

[42] ARMSTRONG W.G. (1967) The composition of organic films formed on human teeth. *Caries Res.* **1**, 89.

[43] HEALEY T.W. & LA MER V.K. (1964) The energetics of flocculation and redispersion by polymers. *J. Colloid. Sci.* **19**, 323.

[44] KIRK E.C. (1910) A consideration of the question of

susceptibility and immunity to dental caries. *Dent. Cosmos* **52**, 729–737.

[45] CARLSSON J. & EGELBERG J. (1965) Local effect of diet on plaque formation and development of gingivitis in dogs. II. Effect of high carbohydrate versus high protein–fat diets. *Odont. Revy* **16**, 42–49.

[46] DAWES C. (1964) Is acid precipitation of salivary proteins a factor in plaque formation? *Arch. oral Biol.* **9**, 375–376.

[47] JENKINS G.N. (1968) The mode of formation of dental plaque. *Caries Res.* **2**, 130.

[48] McGAUGHEY C. & STOWELL E.C. (1966) Plaque formation by purified salivary mucin in vitro: Effects of incubation, calcium and phosphate. *Nature* **209**, 897.

[49] GIBBONS R.J. & SPINELL B.M. (1970) Salivary induced aggregation of plaque bacteria, in *Dental Plaque*, p. 207. Ed. McHugh W.D. Edinburgh: E. & S. Livingstone.

[50] HAY D.I., GIBBONS R.J. & SPINELL B.M. (1971) Characteristics of some high molecular weight constituents with bacterial aggregating activity from whole saliva and dental plaque. *Caries Res.* **6**, 111.

[51] LEACH S.A. & HAYS M.L. (1967) Isolation in pure culture of human oral organisms capable of producing neuraminidase. *Nature* **216**, 599.

[52] PINTER J.K., HAYASHI J.A. & BAHN A.N. (1969) Carbohydrate hydrolases of oral streptococci. *Arch. Oral Biol.* **14**, 735.

[53] LEACH S.A. (1963) Release and breakdown of sialic acid from human salivary mucin and its role in the formation of dental plaque. *Nature* **199**, 486.

[54] BJÖRN H. & CARLSSON J. (1964) Observations on a dental plaque morphogenesis. *Odont. Revy.* **15**, 23.

[55] SAXTON C.A. (1971) Scanning electron microscope study of bacterial colonization of the tooth surface, in *Tooth Enamel*, II, p. 218. Eds. Fearnhead R.W. & Stack M.V. Bristol: Wright.

[56] LÖE H., THEILADE E. & JENSEN S.B. (1965) Experimental gingivitis in man. *J. Periodont.* **36**, 177.

[57] JENSEN S.B., LÖE H., SCHIOTT C.R. & THEILADE E. (1968) Experimental gingivitis in man. IV. Vancomycin induced changes in bacterial plaque composition as related to development of gingival inflammation. *J. Periodont. Res.* **3**, 284.

[58] THEILADE E. & THEILADE J. (1970) Bacteriological and ultrastructural studies of developing dental plaque, in *Dental Plaque*, p. 27. Ed. McHugh, W.D. Edinburgh: E. & S. Livingstone.

[59] CARLSSON J. & EGELBERG J. (1965) Effect of diet on early plaque formation in man. *Odont. Revy.* **16**, 112.

[60] GIBBONS R.J. & VAN HOUTE J. (1973) On the formation of dental plaques. *J. Periodont.* **44**, 347.

[61] VAN HOUTE J., GIBBONS R.J. & BANGHART S.B. (1970) Adherence as a determinant of the presence of *Streptococcus salivarius* and *Streptococcus sanguis* on the tooth surface. *Arch. Oral Biol.* **15**, 1025.

[62] LILJEMARK W.F. & GIBBONS R.J. (1972) The proportional distribution and relative adherence of *Streptococcus miteor (mitis)* on various surfaces in the human oral cavity. *Infect. and Immun.* **6**, 852.

[63] HILLMAN J.D., VAN HOUTE J. & GIBBONS R.J. (1970) Sorption of bacteria to human enamel powder. *Arch. Oral Biol.* **15**, 899.

[64] LILJEMARK W.F. & GIBBONS R.J. (1971) Ability of *Veillonella* and *Neisseria* species to attach to oral surfaces and their proportions present indigenously. *Infect. and Immun.* **4**, 264.

[65] VAN HOUTE J., GIBBONS R.J. & PULKKINEN A.J. (1971) Adherence as an ecological determinant for streptococci in the human mouth. *Arch. Oral Biol.* **16**, 1131.

[66] GIBBONS R.J., BERMAN K.S., KNOETTNER P & KAPSIMALIS B. (1966) Dental caries and alveolar bone loss in gnotobiotic rats infected with capsule forming streptococci of human origin. *Arch. Oral Biol.* **11**, 549.

[67] McCABE R.M., KEYES P.H. & HOWELL A. Jr. (1967) An in vitro method of assessing the plaque forming ability of oral bacteria. *Arch. Oral Biol.* **12**, 1653.

[68] KEYES P.H. (1968) Research in dental caries. *J.A.D.A.* **76**, 1357.

[69] GIBBONS R.J. & BANGHART S.B. (1967) Synthesis of extracellular dextran by cariogenic bacteria and its presence in human dental plaque. *Arch. Oral Biol.* **12**, 11–23.

[70] GIBBONS R.J. & NYGAARD M. (1970) Synthesis of insoluble dextran and its significance in the formation of gelatinous deposits by plaque-forming streptococci. *Arch. Oral Biol.* **13**, 1249.

[71] GIBBONS R.J. & FITZGERALD R.J. (1969) Dextran-induced agglutination of *Streptococcus mutans*, and its potential role in the formation of microbial dental plaques. *J. Bacteriol.* **98**, 341.

[72] GUGGENHEIM B. & SCHROEDER H.E. (1967) Biochemical and morphological aspects of extracellular polysaccharides produced by cariogenic streptococci. *Helv. Odont. Acta.* **11**, 131.

[73] CALDWELL R.C., SANDHAM H.J., MANN W.C. Jr., FINN S.B. & FORMICOLA A.J. (1971) The effect of dextranase mouthwash on dental plaque in young adults and children. *J. am. dent. ass.* **82**, 124.

[74] KEYES P.H., HICKS M.A., GOLDMAN B.M., McCABE R.M. & FITZGERALD R.J. (1971) Dispersion of dextranous bacterial plaques on human teeth with dextranase. *J. am. dent. ass.* **82**, 136.

[75] LOBENE R.R. (1971) A clinical study of the effect of dextranase on human dental plaque. *J. am. dent. ass.* **82**, 132.

[76] JORDAN H.V. & HAMMOND B.F. (1972) Filamentous bacteria isolated from human root surface caries. *Arch. Oral Biol.* **17**, 1333.

[77] JORDAN H.V., KEYES P.H. & BELLACK S. (1972) Periodontal lesions in hamsters and gnotobiotic rats injected with actinomyces of human origin. *J. Periodont. Res.* **7**, 21.

[78] SOCRANSKY S.S., HUBERSAK C. & PROPAS D. (1970) Induction of periodontal destruction in gnotobiotic rats by a human oral strain of *Actinomyces naeslundii*. *Arch. Oral Biol.* **15**, 993.

[79] BLADEN H., HAGEAGE G., POLLOCK F. & HARR R. (1970) Plaque formation *in vitro* on wires by Gram-negative oral microorganisms (Veillonella). *Arch. Oral Biol.* **15**, 127.

[80] BOYDE A. & LESTER K.S. (1968) A method of preparing bacterial plaque lining carious cavities for examination by scanning electron microscopy. *Arch. Oral Biol.* **13**, 1413.

[81] SIRISINHA S. (1970) Reactions of human salivary immunoglobulins with indigenous bacteria. *Arch. Oral Biol.* **15**, 551.

[82] WILLIAMS R.C. & GIBBONS R.J. (1972) Inhibition of bacterial adherence by secretory immunoglobulin A: A mechanism of antigen disposal. *Science* **177**, 697.

[83] GIBBONS R.J. & NYGAARD M. (1970) Interbacterial aggregation of plaque bacteria. *Arch. Oral Biol.* **15**, 1397.

[84] KASHKET S. & DONALDSON C.G. (1972) Saliva-induced aggregation of oral streptococci. *J. Bacteriol.* **112**, 1127.

[85] TAUBMAN M.A. (1972) Immunoglobulins of plaque. *I.A.D.R. Abstr.* 881.

[86] SOCRANSKY S.S. (1977) Microbiology of periodontal disease—present status and future considerations. *J. Periodont.* **48**, 9, 497.

[87] SLOTS J. *et al.* (1978) Microbiota of gingivitis in man. *Scand. J. Dent. Res.* **86**, 174–181.

[88] LISTGARTEN M.A. (1976) Structure of the microbial flora associated with periodontal disease and health in man. A light and electron microscopic study. *J. Periodont.* **47**, 1.

[89] SLOTS J. (1977) The predominant cultivable microflora of advanced periodontitis. *Scand. J. Dent. Res.* **85**, 114–121.

[90] SLOTS J. (1976) The predominant cultivable organisms in juvenile periodontitis. *Scand. J. Dent. Res.* **84**, 1.

[91] NEWMAN N.G. & SOCRANSKY S.S. (1977) Predominant cultivable microbiota in periodontosis. *J. Periodont. Res.* **12**, 120.

[92] SAVITT E.D., SOCRANSKY S.S. *et al.* (1975) Characterisation of fusiform organisms isolated from periodontosis. *J. Dent. Res.* **54**, 208.

[93] LISTGARTEN M.A., MAYO H.E. *et al.* (1975) Development of dental plaque on epoxy resin crowns in man. A light and electron microscopic study. *J. Periodont.* **46**, 10.

[94] KEYES P.H., WRIGHT W.E. & HOWARD S.A. (1978) The use of phase contrast microscopy and chemotherapy in the diagnosis and treatment of periodontal lesions. An initial report (1). *Quintessence International* **1**, 1.

[95] KEYES P.H., WRIGHT W.E. & HOWARD S.A. (1978) The use of phase contrast microscopy and chemotherapy in the diagnosis and treatment of periodontal lesions. An initial report (2). *Quintessence International* **2**, 7.

[96] LISTGARTEN M.A. & HELLDEN L. (1978) Relative distribution of bacteria at clinically healthy and periodontally diseased sites in humans. *J. Clin. Periodont.* **5**, 115–132.

[97] LOESCHE W.J. (1976) Chemotherapy of dental plaque infections. *Oral Sci. Reviews* **9**, 65.

[98] GJERMO PER (1972) Chemical cleaning of teeth, in *Oral Hygiene*, p. 64. Ed. Fransden Asger. Munksgaard.

[99] RENGLI H. (1966) Zanhbeloge und gingivale entzyngdung unter dem einfluss eines antibakteriellen mundspülmittels. Thesis. Zurich: Schippert, K. & Co.

[100] SCHROEDER H.E. (1969) *Formation and Inhibition of Dental Calculus*. Stuttgart: Hans Huber, 129–160.

[101] VOLPE A.R., KUPCZAK L.J. & BRANT J.H. (1969) Antimicrobial control of bacterial plaque and calculus and the effects of these agents on oral flora. *J. Dent. Res.* **48**, 832.

[102] LÖE H. (1969) Present day status and direction for future research on the etiology and prevention of periodontal disease. *J. Periodont.* **40**, 678.

[103] LÖE H. & SCHIOTT R.C. (1970) The effect of suppression of the oral microflora upon the development of dental plaque and gingivitis, in *Dental Plaque*, p. 274. Ed. McHugh W.D. Edinburgh: E. & S. Livingstone.

[104] LÖE H. & SCHIOTT R.C. (1970) The effect of mouth rinses and topical application of chlorhexidine on the development of dental plaque and gingivitis in man. *J. Periodont. Res.* **5**, 79.

[105] GJERMO P., BAASTAD K.L. & RØLLA G. (1970) The plaque inhibiting activity of 11 antibacterial compounds. *J. Periodont. Res.* **5**, 102.

[106] FLØTRA L. (1970) The effect of chlorhexidine mouthwashes. Thesis: Universitetforlaget, Oslo.

[107] HILL T.J. & KNIESNER A.H. (1949) Penicillin dentifrice and dental caries experience in children. *J. Dent. Res.* **28**, 263.

[108] HILL T.J.; SIMS J. & NEWMAN M. (1953) The effect of penicillin dentifrice on the control of dental caries. *J. Dent. Res.* **32**, 448.

[109] LUNIN M. & MANDEL I.D. (1955) Clinical evaluation of penicillin dentifrice. *J. Amer. Dent. Ass.* **51**, 696.

[110] SHIERE F.R. (1957) The effectiveness of tyrothricin dentifrice in the control of dental caries. *J. Dent. Res.* **36**, 237.

[111] HANDLEMAN S.R., MILLS J.R. & HOWES R.R. (1966) Caries incidence in subjects receiving long-term antibiotic therapy. *J. Oral Ther.* **2**, 338.

[112] LÖE H., THEILADE E., JENSEN S.B. & SCHIØTT R.C. (1967) Experimental gingivitis in man. III. The influence of antibiotics on gingival plaque development. *J. Periodont. Res.* **2**, 282.

[113] MITCHELL D.F. & HOLMES L.A. (1965) Topical antibiotic control of dentogingival plaque. *J. Periodont.* **36**, 202.

[114] MITCHELL D.F., HOLMES L.A., MARTIN P.W. & SAKURAI E. (1967) Topical antibiotic maintenance of oral health. *J. Oral Ther.* **4**, 83.

[115] VOLPE A.R., KUPCZAK L.J., BRANT J.H. *et al.* (1969) Antimicrobial control of bacterial plaque and calculus and the effects of these agents on the oral flora. *J. Dent. Res.* **48**, 832.

[116] COLLINS J.F. (1970) Effect of vancomycin on plaque after periodontal surgery. *J. Dent. Res.* **49**, 1478.

[117] LOBENE R., BRION M. & SCORANSKY S.S. (1969) Effect of erythromycin on dental plaque and plaque-forming micro-organisms of man. *J. Periodont.* **40**, 287.

[118] JENSEN S.B., LÖE H., SCHIØTT R.C., THEILADE E. & MIKKELSEN L. (1967) The effect of vancomycin and

polymyxin B on experimental gingivitis in man. *J. Periodont. Res.* **2**, 242.

[119] KEYES P.H., ROWBERRY S.A., ENGLANDER H.R. & FITZGERALD R.J. (1966) Bio-assays for medicaments for the control of dentobacterial plaque, dental caries and periodontal lesions in Syrian hamsters. *J. Oral Ther. Pharmacol.* **3**, 157.

[120] HUNT D.E., SANDHAM H.J. & CALDWELL R.C. (1970) *In vitro* antibiotic sensitivity of oral microorganisms to actinobolin. *J. Dent. Res.* **49**, No. 1, 137.

[121] STALLARD R.E., VOLPE A.R., ORBAN J.B. & KING W.J. (1969) The effect of an antimicrobial mouth rinse on dental plaque calculus and gingivitis. *J. Periodont.* **40**, 683.

[122] VOLPE A.R., SCHULMAN S.M., GOLDMAN H.M., KING W.J. & KUPCZAK L.J. (1970) The long term effect of an antimicrobial formulation on dental calculus formation. *J. Periodont.* **41**, 463.

[123] GUGGENHEIM B., MUHLEMAN M.H.R., REGOLATI B. & SCHMID R. (1970) The effect of immunization against streptococci or glucosyl transferases on plaque formation and dental caries in rats, in *Dental Plaque.* Ed. McHugh W.D. Edinburgh: E. & S. Livingstone.

[124] GENCO R.J. & EVANS R.T. (1971) Studies of plaque inhibition by antibodies to *Streptococcus mutans. I.A.D.R.* **49**, Gen. Meet. Chicago. Abstract No. **786**, 249.

[125] GENCO R.J. (1976) Immunological aspects of dental caries. *Journal of Dental Research* **55**, Special Issue C, C1–C230.

[126] GIBBONS R.J. & BANGHART S.B. (1967) Synthesis of extracellular dextran by cariogenic bacteria and its presence in human dental plaque. *Arch. Oral Biol.* **12**, 11–24.

[127] GUGGENHEIM B. & SCHROEDER H.E. (1967) Biochemical and morphological aspects of extracellular polysaccharides produced by cariogenic streptococci. *Helv. Odont. Acta* **11**, 131.

[128] FITZGERALD R.J. & JORDAN H.V. (1968) Polysaccharide producing bacteria and dental caries, in *The Art and Science of Dental Caries Research.* Ed. Harris S.R. New York: Academic Press.

[129] FITZGERALD R.J. (1968) Plaque microbiology and caries. *Ala. J. Med. Sci.* **5**, 239.

[130] GIBBONS R.J. & NIGAARD M. (1968) Synthesis of insoluble dextran and its significance in the formation of gelatinous deposits by plaque forming streptococci. *Arch. Oral Biol.* **13**, 1249.

[131] BOWEN W.H. (1971) The effects of calcium, magnesium, and manganese on dextran production by a cariogenic streptococcus. *Arch. Oral Biol.* **16**, 115.

[132] KEPNER G.R. & BERMAN K.S. (1971) Effect of cationic and anionic detergents upon capsule formation in oral streptococci. *I.A.D.R.* 49th General Meeting, Chicago, Abstract **56**, 66.

[133] GUGGENHEIM B. (1970) Enzymatic hydrolysis and structure of water insoluble glucan, produced by glucosyl transferases from a strain of *Streptococcus mutans. Helv. Odont. Acta* **14**, 89 Suppl. 5.

[134] FITZGERALD R.J., SPINELL D.M. & STOUDT T.H.

(1968) Enzymatic removal of artificial plaques. *Arch. Oral Biol.* **13**, 125.

[135] BOWEN W.H. (1969) Effects of dextranase on cariogenic and non-cariogenic dextrans. *Brit. Dent. J.* **124**, 347.

[136] FITZGERALD R.J., KEYES P.H., STOUDT T.H. & SPINELL D.M. (1968) The effects of a dextranase preparation on dental caries in hamsters. *J. Amer. Dent. Ass.* **76**, 301.

[137] BLOCK P.L., DOOLEY C.L. & HOWE E.E. (1969) The retardation of spontaneous periodontal disease and the prevention of caries in hamsters with dextranase. *J. Periodont.* **40**, 105.

[138] GUGGENHEIM B., KÖNIG K., MUHLEMAN H.R. & REGOLATI B. (1969) The effect of dextranase on caries in rats harbouring an indigenous cariogenic flora. *Arch. Oral Biol.* **14**, 555.

[139] BAASTAD K.L. & RØLLA G. (1970) Purification and properties of dextranase from penicillium funiculosum. *Scand. J. Dent. Res.* **78**, 452.

[140] NORMAN R.D., VIRMANI R., SWARTZ M.L. & PHILLIPS R.W. (1971) The effects of restorative materials on plaque composition. *I.A.D.R.* 49th Gen. Meet. Chicago. Abstract No. 162, p. 95.

[141] CANCRO L.P., CURRY J. *et al.* (1971) Effects of chlorhexidine gluconate. *I.A.D.R.* General Meeting, Chicago. March Abstr. **1847**, 81.

[142] TURESKY S., CLICKMAN I. & SANDBERG R. (1971) Chemical inhibition of *in vitro* plaque formation. *I.A.D.R.* 49th Gen. Meet. Chicago. Abstract No. 143, p. 88.

[143] HUGO W.B. & LONGWORTH A.R. (1964) Some aspects of the mode of action of chlorhexidine. *J. Pharm. Pharmacol.* **16**, 655.

[144] HUGO W.B. & LONGWORTH A.R. (1966) The effect of chlorhexidine on the electrophoretic mobility, cytoplasmic constituents, dehydrogenase activity and cell walls of *Escherichia coli* and *Staphylococcus aureus. J. Pharm. Pharmacol.* **18**, 569.

[145] SCHROEDER H.E. (1969) *Formation and Inhibition of Dental Calculus,* p. 147. Berne: Hans Huber.

[146] **SCHIOTT C.R., LÖE H., JENSEN S.B., KILIAN M., DAVIES R.M. & GLAVIND L. (1970) The effect of chlorhexidine mouth rinses on the human oral flora. *J. Periodont. Res.* 5, 84.**

[147] ROLLA G., LÖE H. & SCHIOTT C.R. (1970) The affinity of chlorhexidine for hydroxyapatite and salivary mucins. *J. Periodont. Res.* **5**, 90.

[148] ROLLA G., LÖE H. & SCHIOTT C.R. (1971) Retention of chlorhexidine in the human oral cavity. *Arch. Oral Biol.* **16**, 1109.

[149] FLOTRA L., GJERMO P., ROLLA G. & WAERHAUG J. (1972) A four-month study of the effects of chlorhexidine mouth washes on fifty soldiers. *Scand. J. Dent. Res.* **80**, 10.

[150] SYMPOSIUM (1976) Hibitane in the mouth. *Journal of Clinical Periodontology* **4**, 1–147.

[151] FLOTRA L., GJERMO P., ROLLA G. & WAERHAUG J. (1971) Side effects of chlorhexidine mouth washes. *Scand. J. Dent. Res.* **79**, 119.

[152] LINDHE J., HAMP S.E., LÖE H. & SCHIOTT C.R. (1970)

Influence of topical application of chlorhexidine on chronic gingivitis and gingival would healing in dogs. *Scand. J. Dent. Res.* **78**, 471.

[153] HIRST R.C., EGELBERG J., HORNBUCKLE G.C., OLIVER R.C. & RATHDUN E. (1972) Microscopic evaluation of topically applied chlorhexidine gluconate on gingival wound healing in dogs. Masters thesis. Loma linda University.

[154] LINDHE J., HEYDEN G., SVANBERG G., LÖE H. & SCHIOTT C.R. (1970) Effect of local application of chlorhexidine on the oral mucosa of the hamster. *J. Periodont. Res.* **5**, 177.

[155] GJERMO P. & ROLLA G. (1970) Plaque inhibition by antibacterial dentifrices. *Scand. J. Dent. Res.* **78**, 464.

[156] GJERMO P. & ROLLA G. (1971) The plaque inhibiting effect of chlorhexidine-containing dentifrices. *Scand. J. Dent. Res.* **79**, 126.

[157] LÖE H. (1970) A review of the prevention and control of plaque, in *Dental Plaque*, p. 259. Ed. McHugh W.D. Edinburgh: E. & S. Livingstone.

[158] HAMP S.E., LINDHE J. & LÖE H. (1973) Long-term effect of chlorhexidine on developing gingivitis in the Beagle dog. *J. Periodont. Res.* **2**, 63.

[159] LÖE H. (1969) Present day status and direction for future research on the aetiology and prevention of periodontal disease. *J. Periodont.* **40**, 678.

[160] STRALFORS A. (1962) Disinfection of dental plaques in man, in *Caries symposium*, p. 154. Zurich. Eds. Muhleman H.R. & Konig G. Berne: Hans Huber.

[161] RIZZO A.A., SCOTT D.B. & BLADEN H.A. (1963) Calcification of oral bacteria. *Ann. N.Y. Acad. Sci.* **109**, 14.

[162] SAXTON C.A. (1968) Identification of octocalcium phosphate in human dental calculus by electron diffraction. *Arch. Oral Biol.* **13**, 243.

[163] WAERHAUG J. (1955) Source of mineral salts in subgingival calculus. *J. dent. Res.* **34**, 563–568.

[164] JENSEN A.T. & DANO M. (1954) Crystallography of dental calculus and the precipitation of certain calcium phosphates. *J. dent. Res.* **33**, 741–750.

[165] JENSEN A.T. & ROWLES S.L. (1957) Magnesium whitlockite, a major constituent of dental calculus. *Acta odont. scand.* **15**, 121–139.

[166] WASSERMAN B.H., MANDEL I.D. & LEVY B.M. (1958) In vitro calcification of dental calculus. *J. Periodont.* **29**, 144–147.

[167] BAER P.N. & NEWTON W.L. (1959) The occurrence of periodontal disease in germ-free mice. *J. dent. Res.* **38**, 1238.

[168] GUSTAFSSON B.E. & KRASSE B. (1962) Dental calculus in germ free rats. *Acta odont. scand.* **20**, 135–142.

[169] KÖNIG K.G. & MÜHLEMANN H.R. (1959) Alterations in rat gingivae due to plaque accumulations. *Helv. odont. Acta* **3**, 44–48.

[170] ZANDER H.A., HAZEN S.P. & SCOTT D.B. (1960) Mineralization of dental calculus. *Proc. Soc. exp. Biol. (N.Y.)* **103**, 257–260.

[171] GONZALES H.A. & SOGNNAES R.F. (1960) Electron microscopy of dental calculus. *Science* **131**, 156–158.

[172] RIZZO A.A., MARTIN G.R., SCOTT D.B. & MERGENHAGEN S.S. (1962) Mineralization of bacteria. *Science* **135**, 439–441.

[173] RIZZO A.A., SCOTT D.B. & BLADEN H.A. (1963) Calcification of oral bacteria. *Ann. N.Y. Acad. Sci.* **109**, 14–22.

[174] ENNEVER J. & CREAMER H. (1967) Microbiologic calcification: Bone mineral and bacteria. *Calc. Tiss. Res.* **1**, 87–93.

[175] BULLEID A. (1925) An experimental study of *leptothrix buccalis. Brit. dent. J.* **46**, 289–300.

CHAPTER 5

Host–parasite interactions

THE RANGE OF REACTION

In view of the wide variety of microorganisms which normally inhabit the body, but which are rarely implicated as primary agents of disease, it is evident that ability to cause disease depends upon factors other than the maintenance of a life cycle in or on the hosts' tissues. Disease can be caused by:

(1) the resident host flora, when relationships, either among the microorganisms or between the host and its indigenous flora, are disturbed;

(2) by organisms implicated as specific aetiological agents in a recognized disease process.

The variations in severity and course of a disease depend not only on the various noxious products associated with the parasite but also on host factors.

In most cases, some mode of entry is required for an organism to produce disease. An exception to this rule is *Clostridium botulinum*, which causes disease following the absorption of its toxic products through the gut wall. In chronic gingivitis, bacterial plaque situated at the gingival margin acts as a reservoir for microorganisms which thus remain in close contact with the gingival tissue. Opinion has been divided as to whether microorganisms actually multiply in the gingival tissues, but it is now accepted that even the clinically healthy sulcus contains bacteria [1 & 2]. Fish, Wertheimer and others have expressed the view that in gingivitis, bacteria produce damage without invading the tissues [3, 4 & 5], whilst Beckwith *et al.*, Box and, more recently, Haberman have claimed that bacteria can be demonstrated in diseased gingival tissues [6–9]. This difference of opinion is probably a reflection of the fact that staining and identification of microorganisms in tissue sections is hampered by lack of specific stains. In general there is no reliable evidence of organisms in healthy or chronically inflamed gingival tissues even when viewed under the electron microscope.

There is a difference between the ability and the potential of organisms to cause disease. Many experimental studies, where microorganisms are introduced directly into host tissues, measure only microbial potential. Attempts to produce periodontal disease experimentally have measured only microbial potential, as in the fusospirochaetal type of infection investigated by MacDonald, Gibbons and Socransky [10]. Although in experimental fusospirochaetal infections of guinea pigs, the flora remains strikingly similar to that of human periodontal disease [10], an abscess is produced only after animal inoculation, and this does not provide any evidence that the organisms can gain entry to the tissues unaided. It is important to distinguish this approach, which only measures microbial potential, from that in which the actual capacity to initiate disease is measured.

Site of entry is also important, and as species susceptibility to particular microorganisms varies immensely, it is hazardous to apply results gained from studies in one species to disease in a different species.

Other factors governing initiation of disease are as follows:

(1) A suitable biochemical environment in or on the host is necessary.

(2) The pathogen must have the ability to survive in the altered host environment which its

presence occasions. The ensuing inflammatory reaction increases glycolysis; an increase in lactic acid occurs; the oxygen tension is reduced and the pH falls [11].

These conditions are bactericidal for many strains of bacteria, which may account for the absence of organisms in inflamed gingival tissue, but the pathogenic strains may multiply even in these circumstances.

The range of possible reactions between metabolic products of organisms in plaque and the epithelial and connective tissues is wide. There is as yet little evidence to suggest that one particular reaction or type of reaction is responsible for the prevalence of periodontal disease.

The virulence factors of the organisms in dental plaque may be considered as:

(1) factors interfering with the metabolism of host cells.

(2) factors directly toxic to host tissues.

(3) indirect toxic factors, mediated by altered sensitivity of host tissues.

Factors interfering with metabolism of host cells

In experimental animals, injection with rat virus and polyoma virus causes replacement of alveolar bone by granulation tissue, with subsequent apical migration of the cuff epithelium [12 & 13]. There is no evidence to suggest that viruses are causal agents in the initiation or progression of periodontitis in man.

Factors directly toxic to host tissues

EXOTOXINS

Reproduction of all the essential features of tetanus, diphtheria and botulism, by cell free filtrates of their respective causal organisms, and the relatively low toxicity of these bacterial cells themselves, points to the existence of an exotoxin. It is, however, in relatively few diseases that the pathological manifestations are due to such specific soluble poisons.

Typical exotoxins are either secreted by or are readily separated from the cell. They are usually lethal in extremely minute quantities. e.g. diphtheria toxin contains about 10000 guinea

pig LD_{50} per mg, whilst tetanus toxin contains several million LD_{50} per mg. Their action is neutralized by specific antitoxin. The LD_{50} is the amount of toxin required to kill 50 per cent of animals in a group, all given the same amount of toxin. Exotoxins are readily inactivated by heat, and when treated with formaldehyde they are converted into 'toxoids', which retain the power to stimulate specific antitoxins in man.

Substances other than exotoxins diffuse out from the living cell and sometimes have been classed with exotoxins. As these do not have similar properties and are usually enzymic in nature, e.g. streptococcal hyaluronidase, they will be considered under the heading of lytic enzymes.

There is no evidence to implicate exotoxins in the initiation or subsequent progression of periodontitis, nor have they been isolated from the oral microflora.

ENDOTOXINS

Endotoxins are complex macromolecules sometimes described as protein–lipopolysaccharide complexes, which are commonly found in the cell walls of Gram-negative organisms. The lipopolysaccharide fraction has been widely held to be responsible for the action of endotoxins, which are considered to be integral parts of bacterial cell walls, and which only cause tissue damage following their release by autolysis of the cell [14]. Many of their properties are the converse of those of the classical exotoxins. Endotoxins are relatively heat stable; their pharmacological effects are nonspecific; they do not differ from organism to organism and tend to be confined to the area of bacterial multiplication. The potency of endotoxins is relatively low, and although they appear to stimulate antibody formation, their action is not neutralized by such antibody.

The main effects of endotoxins are stereotyped, although various preparations may differ in potency. Their effects include:

(1) profound vasomotor disturbances terminating in shock;

(2) metabolic disturbances consisting of hyperglycaemia, followed by hypoglycaemia, and a build up of lactic acid in blood and tissues;

(3) high fever, sometimes followed by hypothermia;

(4) polymorphonuclear leucopenia followed by leucocytosis;

(5) production of haemorrhagic necrosis;

(6) with frequent sublethal doses, the appearance of resistance against the same or other endotoxins [15].

These substances are also characterized by their ability to provoke, in suitably prepared animals, the local and general Schwartzman reactions [15].

The local Schwartzman reaction may be produced in the rabbit by giving a preparing injection of endotoxin in the skin and, after a period of 18–24 hours, a provoking injection of endotoxin by vein. Within a few hours of the provoking dose, a localized haemorrhagic necrosis occurs at the prepared skin site.

The general Schwartzman reaction is produced by giving both preparing and provoking doses intravenously. The most characteristic lesion is bilateral cortical necrosis of the kidney. In both Schwartzman reactions heparin exerts an inhibitory effect, and the presence of polymorphonuclear leucocytes appears to be essential. Lesions similar to those of the local Schwartzman reaction are seen in typhoid fever, which is caused by a Gram-negative bacillus; the mechanism of the reaction, however, remains obscure [16].

The occurrence of endotoxins in human saliva has been reported [17], and the ability of endotoxins from oral *Veillonella* to cause mucosal necrosis has been described [18].

Lipopolysaccharide endotoxins have been isolated from *Borrelia vincentii, Borrelia buccalis*, small oral *treponemes, Fusobacteria, Bacteroides melaninogenicus, Selenomas sputigena* and *Veillonella* [19].

The dermal inflammatory response in rabbits to the inoculation of viable bacteria can be modified by prior intravenous injection of endotoxin [20]. In this investigation, endotoxin from oral *Veillonella* was injected from 1 hour to 2 days prior to subcutaneous inoculation with bacteria, and the subsequent inflammatory response observed macroscopically and microscopically.

It has been concluded from this type of experiment that endotoxins possess the potential to inhibit or to stimulate local cellular defence mechanisms, and they may modify host–parasite relationships in the periodontium.

The effect of endotoxins on mast cell integrity has been studied by Gustafsson and Cronberg who concluded that mast cell alterations do not seem to be an essential or a primary effect of endotoxins [21]. Thus it would appear that histamine is not involved in the series of reactions which follow the intradermal injection of endotoxins.

Although there is evidence of endotoxin production by oral bacteria, and it has been shown that these endotoxins have the capacity to produce dermal necrosis, no direct evidence is available concerning the role of endotoxins in either the initiation or the progression of gingival inflammation.

Bazin and Délauney have shown that polysaccharides and lipopolysaccharides of bacterial origin are capable of competing with chondroitin sulphate in the precipitation of a complex from solutions of collagen [22]. This, therefore, raises the question whether such competition plays a part in the progression of periodontal breakdown by modifying connective tissue formation or turnover.

A macromolecular complex of C polysaccharide and a peptide, from Group A streptococci, which is capable of producing 'a multinodular, remittent and intermittent lesion of dermal connective tissue' after a single intradermal injection, has been reported [23 & 24]. The mechanism of tissue damage following the introduction of this complex is not understood, although the hypothesis has been put forward that the polysaccharide–peptide complex may alter the sol–gel state of essential components of connective tissue [23].

In a paper concerned with immunological aspects of the host reaction to endotoxins, Stetson has stated: 'Whether or not the primary biological activity of endotoxins hinges on their antigenicity, circulating antibodies play a role in modification of the host response to these agents' [25].

After half a century of research, it is still not clear whether endotoxins produce their effects by virtue of some intrinsic pharmacological activity, or whether the reactions are mediated by immunological or hypersensitivity phenomena.

It is possible that the similarity between endotoxin and hypersensitivity reactions merely represents a final common pathway of tissue reaction triggered in different ways but expressed in a similar manner [25].

Much remains to be clarified before a definite role in the initiation or progression of periodontal disease can be assigned to endotoxin from oral bacteria. The World Workship in Periodontics *concluded on the basis of review of the literature: 'While little evidence is yet available in this area, expanded investigations using more refined techniques may yield promising information'* [26].

ANTIPHAGOCYTIC FACTORS AND LYTIC ENZYMES

Bacteria possess certain mechanisms for resisting phagocytosis. Well differentiated capsules, polysaccharide in nature, probably constitute the outermost defence layer. In the case of pneumococci the presence of a capsule is associated with virulent organisms, rough mutants having no capsule are avirulent. These noncapsular mutants can, however, cause disease if leucopenia is produced. Some pathogenic bacteria do not have a definite capsule; cell wall components of some strains may serve a similar function. The 'M' protein of group A haemolytic streptococci and the K substance of group B meningococci are thought to have these properties. In the case of Gram-negative bacteria, a similar function may be attributed to the complex cell wall.

The lytic enzymes which break down host tissues may also help in the dissemination of bacteria and their products. Increasing attention has been given recently to the possible role of bacterial enzymes in the disruption of host tissues. These substances are soluble products of the bacterial cell, are thermolabile and show some specificity of action (table 5.1). Their action may be inhibited by specific antibody.

Such a formidable array of bacterial enzymes has been isolated that it is difficult to establish

TABLE 5.1. Bacterial enzymes.

Affecting protein	Collagenases, proteases, peptidases
Affecting fluid portion of blood	Coagulase, streptokinases
Affecting the cellular elements of blood	Lysins
Affecting component parts of cells	Streptodornase, lecithinase
Affecting ground substance of connective tissue	Hyaluronidase, β Glucuronidase Chondroitinase Chondrosulphatase Phenolsulphatase

their precise relationship to disease. A wide variety has been isolated from culture filtrates of gingival bacteria; collagenase, protease, beta glucuronidase, chondrosulphatase, phenolsulphatase, hyaluronidase and neuraminidase have all been identified [27–31]. At the present time, however, there is little direct evidence implicating any of these enzymes in the initiation of gingivitis [32 & 33].

As breakdown of collagen fibres occurs in periodontitis [34], the demonstration of collagenase production by cell suspensions of *Bacteroides melaninogenicus* [30] may be of importance. Gibbons and MacDonald have shown by hydroxyproline determinations that collagen in untreated rat tail tendon and human gingival tissue is degraded during incubation with cell suspensions of *Bacteroides melaninogenicus* [30]. It has been subsequently shown that an enzyme of apparently endogenous origin, which is capable of lysing a reconstituted collagen gel, is present in inflamed gingival tissue [35 & 36]. The role of this enzyme in periodontitis is as yet speculative.

Schultz-Haudt has shown that when crude gingival polysaccharide mixtures are incubated with broth supernatants of mixed gingival bacteria, no hyaluronic acid, or chondroitin sulphate A, can subsequently be detected by paper electrophoresis [37]. This suggests that enzymes produced by gingival bacteria can hydrolyse gingival polysaccharides *in vitro*, but it does not demonstrate that they necessarily have the same capacity *in vivo*.

According to Lisanti the salivary level of hyaluronidase in persons with periodontitis is higher than in individuals with clinically healthy gingivae [38]. It does not necessarily follow that such an increase is related to the cause rather than the result of periodontal disease.

The production of hyaluronidase by viridans streptococci from the human gingival sulcus has been reported [27], and the production of hyaluronidase by oral streptococci has been demonstrated [37]. It has been postulated by many workers that hyaluronidase, either by itself or in combination with other enzymes, might be responsible for the initial breach in host tissue integrity. Hyaluronidase is thought to attack the acid mucopolysaccharides that might be present in the intercellular spaces of human gingival epithelium [39], thus opening tracts and allowing other bacterial products access to gingival connective tissue. In a histo-chemical investigation concerning the substances present in the intercellular zone of human gingival epithelium, the presence of sulphated acid mucopolysaccharides was not confirmed [33].

It would appear that evidence is available to show that hyaluronidase is produced by members of the oral microflora, and that its substrate may be present in human gingival tissues. The important question remains as to whether the enzyme breaks down its substrate *in vivo*.

The relationship between hyaluronidase production and the transmission of fusospirochaetal type abscesses in the guinea pig has been investigated by MacDonald *et al.* [10]. The data suggests that although hyaluronidase production occurs in the complex mixed anaerobic infection of guinea pigs, it is neither essential nor necessarily contributory to the pathogenesis. Other workers have failed to demonstrate a difference in hyaluronidase levels in debris from normal and inflamed mouths [40].

It has been shown that the quantitative change in the oral flora which is associated with gingivitis and periodontitis is such that the concentration of organisms in deposits on the teeth is of the order of 2×10^{11} organisms per gramme wet weight of plaque; approximately the same concentration of organisms as a centrifuged pure culture of streptococci. There is evidence that there is increase in the bacterial enzymes of saliva as a result of this change (tables 5.1 & 5.2).

The carbohydrate–protein complexes of gingival epithelium and connective tissue may act as a substrate for such enzymes, which may contribute in this way to the progression of periodontitis. Alteration in the state of aggregation of the mucopolysaccharide pool in epithelium and connective tissue, brought about by hyaluronidases, mucolytic and proteolytic enzymes, may be a mechanism in periodontitis, but it is not necessarily a primary cause. Alteration in the balance of the biological system of the mouth following reduction in tissue resistance would produce the same result. Metabolism in the plaque environment is further complicated by the presence of enzymes secreted in saliva and those freed by autolysis of tissue cells (table 5.2). At the present time, deficiency of the enzyme catalase, resulting in the accumulation of hydrogen peroxide of bacterial origin in the tissues, is the only known example of a genetically determined biochemical lesion of tissue resistance which may give rise to a nonspecific periodontitis [41].

TABLE 5.2. Additional sources of enzymes; salivary glands and autolysis of cells.

Carbohydrases
    Maltase, invertase, β-glucuronidase, β-galactosidase, hyaluronidase, mucinase, amylase
Esterases
    Acid and alkaline phosphatase, hexose diphosphatase, lipase, pseudocholinesterase, chondrosulphatase, aryl-sulphatase
Transferring enzymes
    Catalase, phenyl-oxidase, succinic dehydrogenase, hexo-kinase
Proteolytic enzymes
    Proteinase, peptidase, collagenase
Other enzymes
    Carbonic anhydrase, pyrophosphatase, aldolase, urease

Indirect toxic factors mediated by altered sensitivity of host tissues

It has already been stated that the cells typical of chronic gingivitis, which are to some extent also present in clinically healthy gingivae, are cells frequently associated with immune mechanisms. Bacteria in the sulcus, and their products, provide a constant source of antigenic material in the area of the cuff epithelium, and there is mounting evidence that immune or allergic re-actions have a role at some stage in the patho-genesis of periodontitis.

As a high proportion of the adult population of the western world suffers to some degree from periodontal disease [42] it would seem that in-nate immunity, although it may well be opera-tive, cannot combat the cumulative effects of the dense microflora in the gingival sulcus. Although acquired immunity may have some beneficial effects in relation to periodontal disease, acquired hypersensitivity also appears to occur and could be associated with the initia-tion or progression of the disease. Burnett and Scherp have stated that in practically every in-fectious disease which has been adequately ex-plored, the host develops an allergy to some of the constituents or products of the causal agent [16].

ACQUIRED IMMUNITY

Following Jenner's utilization of cowpox vac-cination as a protection against smallpox, it was not until Pasteur's classical experiments with fowl cholera, rabies, and anthrax, that acquired immunity was placed on a firm footing as a pro-tective mechanism.

The basis of this phenomenon is the hosts' ability to 'recognize' foreign material and to pro-duce substances (antibodies) which will react against the foreign material (antigen).

Although in recent years the occurrence of autoimmune disease has become accepted, the general principle of 'horror autotoxicus' is still the basis for present concepts of antibody for-mation. It is assumed that an individual's own antigens have 'self' markers which are recog-nized by immunologically competent cells. According to Burnet's 'Clonal Selection' theory the ability of host tissues to recognize these 'self' markers is learned by contact of the antigen with immunologically competent cells during em-bryonic development [43]. Thus certain body products, e.g. thyroglobulin and spermatozoa, which do not come into contact with immuno-logically competent cells during early develop-ment, may under some circumstances sub-sequently cause antibody formation which may lead to disease. This concept is strengthened by

other phenomena, e.g. active acquired tolerance where viable foreign cells introduced into a very young animal are not rejected as they would be by a mature animal that had no previous contact with the foreign cells.

Although for a long time circulating anti-bodies were regarded as the most important fac-tors in the immune response, many other factors are involved in the development of both im-munity and hypersensitivity. Many of these fac-tors are associated with cells and may not be related to γ-globulins in plasma. This can be illustrated by the observation that should chil-dren having hypogammaglobulinaemia recover from a specific infectious disease, they are sub-sequently immune. This, clearly, cannot be mediated by the classical circulating antibodies, as in hypogammaglobulinaemia there are few, if any, demonstrable gamma globulins.

In man the cells associated with cellular im-munity are lymphocytes and macrophages. These cells play an important part in immunity to infection, and are of special interest as they are regularly found in gingival tissues.

It is well established that antibodies are not formed in any one particular organ. In general, organs containing reticuloendothelial cells form antibodies, although the actual site depends to some extent on the route of administration of the antigen. When an antigen is introduced locally, the antibody may be produced at the site of in-jection or in the lymph nodes draining the area. Experiments with fluorescent antibodies have suggested that plasma cells are intimately associated with antibody production [44 & 45]. The ultrastructure of plasma cells has been shown by electron microscopy to be consistent with that of cells synthesizing protein [46].

As lymphocytes are usually present in chronic inflammation and are prominent in the rejection of grafts their role in the production of antibody must be considered. It would appear that the lymphocyte has prior claim to be the immuno-logically competent cell [47].

THE HOST RESPONSE

Antibodies

Circulating antibodies acquired by a process of

passive transfer across the placenta from the mother are present in the sera of new-born babies. With that exception, antibodies are substances which appear in the serum or external secretions, e.g. saliva, of an animal in response to stimulation with specific antigen, and which are subsequently capable of combination with that particular antigen. The presence of antibodies in a serum is demonstrable by their ability to form antigen-antibody (Ag:Ab) complexes *in vitro* with their corresponding antigens. The form of antigen-antibody reaction which may take place is variable, but in general these reactions involve observable deposition of a precipitate, agglutination of cells, or consumption of complement. Antibodies are therefore frequently described as being predominantly precipitins, agglutinins or complement fixing antibodies.

The serum proteins can be separated electrophoretically into a number of components such as albumins, Alpha 1 (α) globulins, Beta (β) globulins and Gamma (γ) globulins (fig. 5.1). Immunoelectrophoresis is the technique of immunological identification of electrophoretically separated serum proteins by use of precipitating anti-sera against separated proteins, which results in the formation of precipitin bands where antigen-antibody complexes have been formed. At least thirty components of human sera have been detected by this technique. Antibody activity has been found predominantly in the slow moving γ-globulin fraction, and to some extent in the β-globulin region. Antibodies have also been isolated by using a centrifuge capable of very high speeds producing gravitational fields of the order of $1\,000\,000 \times g$.

Heavy molecules exposed to gravitational fields of this order are deposited more rapidly than lighter molecules, and the rate of sedimentation according to molecular weight (mol. wt.) is expressed as Svedberg (S) units. Most globulins have an S value of 7, a mol. wt. of the order of 150 000, and many antibodies are found in this fraction. A heavier globulin fraction with an S value of 19 and a mol. wt. of 900 000 has been shown to be present in serum and certain antibodies, particularly agglutinins against erythrocytes and bacterial somatic or '0' antigens, have been found in this 'macro-globulin' fraction. Immunoelectrophoretic analysis of the serum proteins has shown that each group is heterogeneous in that it consists of many different proteins all of approximately the same electrophoretic mobility, but all quite different in their antigenic and other chemical properties. The term 'immunoglobulin' includes all the globulins which have antibody activity, which are predominantly of the γ and β fraction and similar serum proteins which have no such activity, such as some myeloma proteins. The γ-globulins form a family of related proteins, each seen as an individual precipitin arc in the immunoelectrophoretic separation. Antibody to a specific antigen, however, may be found in any or all of the immunoglobulin fractions.

THE STRUCTURE OF IMMUNOGLOBULINS

Immunoglobulins are classed according to antigenic specificity, and the notation recommended in the 1964 and 1968 World Health Organization Memoranda is universally used. Two symbols have been used for 'immunoglobulin', Ig and

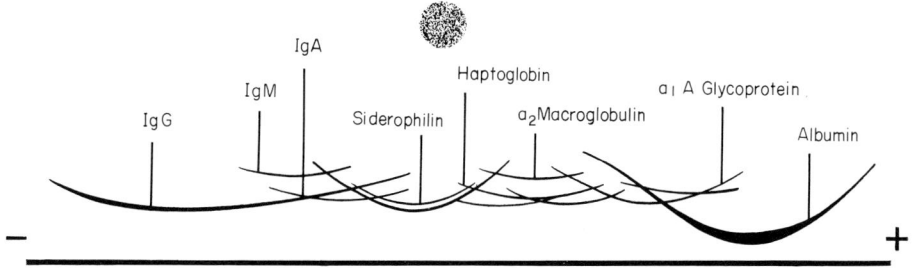

FIG. 5.1. Immunoelectrophoretic pattern of human serum.

Gamma. These symbols are accompanied by a capital letter indicating the antigenic class. In order of discovery, the class notation is as follows; IgG (for the major 7 S components), IgM (for the 19 S macro-gamma-globulin), IgA, IgD and IgE. Alternatively these are described as Gamma (γ) G, Gamma M, Gamma A, Gamma D and Gamma E. While the various immunoglobulins have a similar molecular structure, the various classes differ in electrophoretic mobility, molecular weight, sedimentation coefficient, concentration in serum, and carbohydrate content as shown in table 5.3.

The basic form of the immunoglobulin molecule is four polypeptide chains, two heavy (H) chains with a mol. wt. of 50 000–70 000 and two light (L) chains with molecular weight about 20 000, held together by three disulfide bonds (fig. 5.2).

The heavy chains of the various classes of immunoglobulin differ antigenically, being specific for each immunoglobulin, and at least five different kinds of heavy chains have been identified called Gamma (γ), Alpha (α), Mu (μ), Delta (δ) and Epsilon (ε). Two types of light chains called Kappa (κ) and Lambda (λ) have been identified by immunological methods. Normal human serum appears to have two to three times more immunoglobulin with light chains of type Kappa (κ) than of type Lambda (λ). Where possible, immunoglobulins are named according to their constituent chains. Thus, IgG describes an immunoglobulin which has a pair of

γ heavy chains, and IgA an immunoglobulin with a pair of α heavy chains. If, in addition, the identity of the light chains is known, then this information is conveyed in the name such that IgG K refers to an immunoglobulin with two heavy γ chains and two light κ chains.

The structure of the immunoglobulin molecule was defined by digestion with proteolytic enzymes such as papain and pepsin. Papain splits the peptide bonds between certain amino acids of IgG breaking the molecule into three large fragments (fig. 5.2). Whole γ-globulin has two combining sites for antigen, each molecule is capable of reacting with two antigen molecules and it is therefore known as divalent antibody. Two of the three fragments are able to act as a kind of univalent antibody, each combining with one molecule of antigen. Each therefore contains one of the two combining sites present on the whole immunoglobulin molecule. These fragments are called the Fab fractions (fig. 5.2). Binding of antigen to the immunoglobulin molecule occurs at a combining site formed by areas of the ends of the light and heavy chains which have a variable sequence of amino acids, and which have been described as the two arms of Fab. Since each immunoglobulin molecule has at least two antigen combining sites, the antigen-antibody reaction may result in precipitation or agglutination type of complexing. That part of the heavy chain which forms part of the Fab fraction is called the Fd piece. The other fragment of immunoglobulin produced by papain

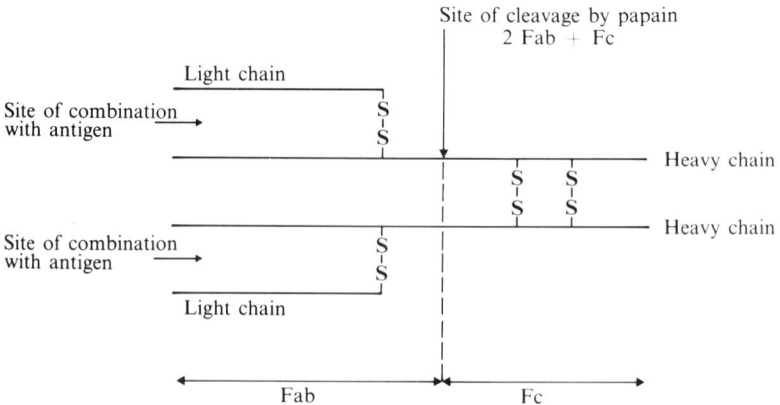

F IG. 5.2. Diagram of the four chain structure of IgG proposed by R.R. Porter.

digestion has no antibody activity and is called the Fc piece (Fragment capable of crystallization) because it has a tendency to crystallize in neutral salt solution. Antibody molecules are flexible and in combining with antigen the molecule can spring open on the disulphide bonds which join the two H chains, so that it takes up a shape of a Y with the Fab fragments as the two arms and the Fc fragment as the stem. In this way each combining site has room to react with a separate antigen molecule at some distance apart. Combination with antigen can pivot the arms of Fab to varying degrees, the pivot seeming to occur at the 'hinge' region near the site vulnerable to papain (figs. 5.2 & 5.3) and pepsin. The degree to which antibody molecules may open out in

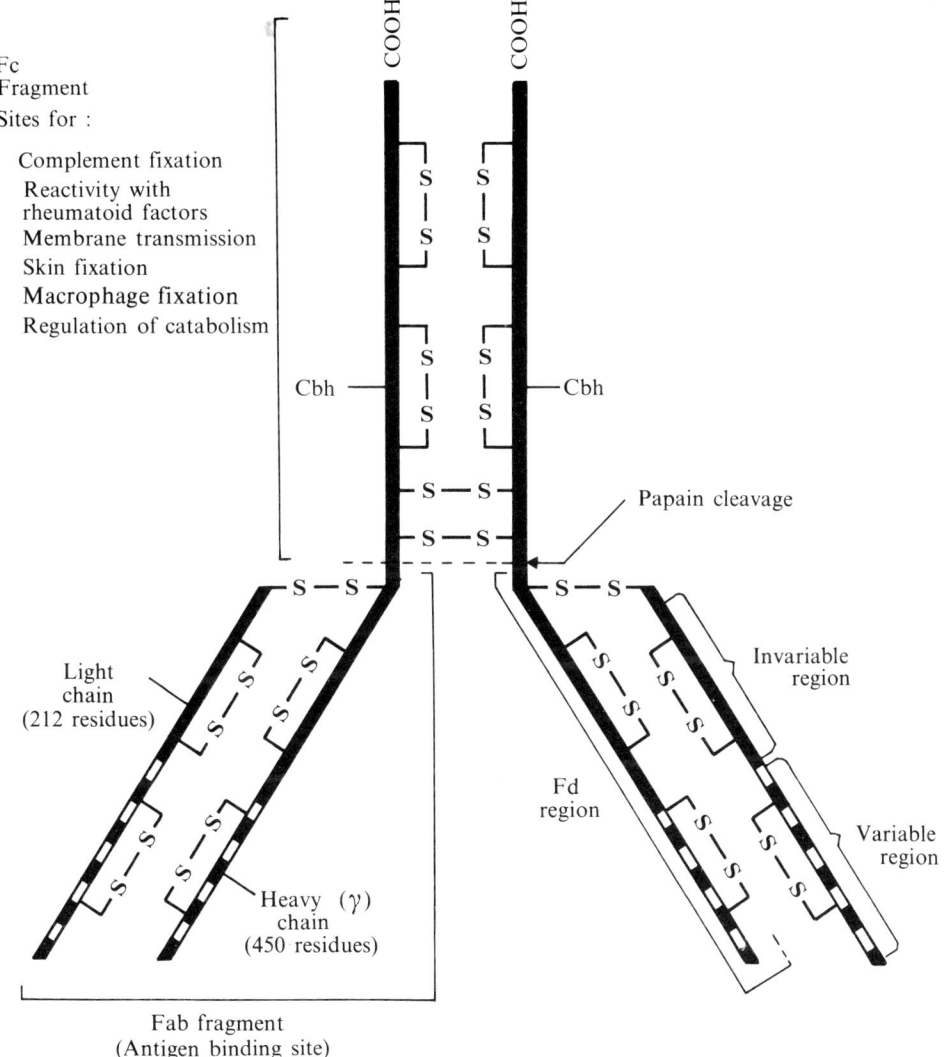

Fc
Fragment

Sites for :

Complement fixation
Reactivity with rheumatoid factors
Membrane transmission
Skin fixation
Macrophage fixation
Regulation of catabolism

Cbh

Papain cleavage

Light chain
(212 residues)

Invariable region

Fd region

Variable region

Heavy (γ) chain
(450 residues)

Fab fragment
(Antigen binding site)

FIG. 5.3. Diagrammatic representation of the four chain structure of IgG showing both inter- and intra-chain disulphide bridges. From Stanworth D.R. & Turner M.W. (1973) Immunochemical analysis of immunoglobulins and their subunits, in *Handbook of Experimental Immunochemistry*, 2nd Edition. Ed. Weir D.M. p. 10.3. Oxford: Blackwell Scientific Publications.

this way depends to some extent on the relative proportion of antigen to antibody. In a situation where the Fab fragments remain close together both combining sites may join with closely spaced determinants on the same antigen molecule.

The Fc fragment contains sites for complement fixation, reactivity with rheumatoid factors, membrane transmission, skin fixation, macrophage fixation and regulation of catabolism (fig. 5.3).

THE BIOLOGICAL PROPERTIES OF IMMUNOGLOBULINS

IgG is the most abundant of the serum immunoglobulins, and is distributed equally between the blood and the extravascular fluids where it has a major role in neutralizing bacterial toxins and binding to organisms to enhance their phagocytosis. The complexes of bacteria with IgG can adhere to phagocytic cells because these cells have specialized surface receptors for sites on the Fc piece of IgG. Only IgG antibodies coating target cells will sensitize them for extracellular cytotoxic killing by lymphoreticular cells. IgG molecules are probably particularly well adapted in structure to form macromolecular lattices with antigen and are therefore usually good precipitating antibodies.

IgM molecules are pentamers of the basic four chain immunoglobulin unit, linked together by disulfide bonds like a five-pointed star with antibody combining sites facing outwards. IgM molecules should therefore have a valency of 10, but have usually been found experimentally to have a valency of 5. This high valency gives IgM the advantage that a single antibody molecule can react with numerous closely spaced antigenic determinants on the surface of the cell or with several determinants on the surface of two contiguous cells. IgM is therefore extremely efficient in agglutinating or clumping red cells and bacteria. ABO blood group agglutinins, and antibodies against bacterial somatic antigens such as the O-antigens of Gram-negative bacteria are of the IgM type.

A primary antigenic stimulation via the parenteral route results in an initial synthesis of IgM antibodies, followed within a few days by the appearance of IgG antibodies. The formation of IgM antibodies lasts only a short time and ceases altogether after about 10 days, whereas the production of IgG antibodies may continue for many months. A secondary antigenic stimulation is followed by a rapid increase in the production of IgG antibodies with titres many times higher than occur in the primary antibody response. During the secondary response few or no IgM antibodies are formed. Repeated immunization may result in high titres of IgG antibodies which may persist for years providing a permanent defence mechanism. Macromolecular IgM is predominantly intravascular and functions as a quick acting short-lasting early defence mechanism.

IgA is less abundant than IgG in serum but is preferentially secreted into colostrum, milk, saliva, tears, nasal and bronchial fluid, the gastrointestinal secretion, bile, and urine. Most of the IgA in secretions is locally produced. IgA producing cells in the lamina propria in the region of exocrine glands produce IgA in a dimeric form of the usual immunoglobulin chain structure which sediments as an 11 S rather than a 7 S component (table 5.3). The IgA in these secretions is transported to the surface of the mucous membranes, after coupling to a special transport protein called 'secretory piece' which is probably synthesized by the glandular epithelial cells. Secretory IgA is therefore a dimer of two IgA molecules coupled to one molecule of secretory piece, the whole being particularly resistant to the action of proteolytic enzymes. IgA antibodies appear to have a special role in protection of conjunctiva, mouth and gastrointestinal tract and upper respiratory tract from infection. The IgA in the serum exists mainly as 7 S monomer, and originates from extra mucosal lymphoid tissues, such as spleen and lymph nodes.

The existence of IgD was recognized from the study of certain rare forms of myeloma. While its presence has been confirmed in variable but usually small concentrations in the plasma of normal persons, little is known about its biological properties and no specific antibody activity has yet been shown to be associated with this class of immunoglobulin.

IgE (reaginic antibody) is present in human serum only in trace amounts. Inhaled antigens

TABLE 5.3. Physicochemical, metabolic and biological properties of the five known classes of human immunoglobulins.

Class	Sedimentation coefficient	Molecular weight	Carbohydrate (%)	Type of heavy chain	Molecular weight of heavy chain†	Known subclasses	Mean serum concentration (mg/ml)‡ and range	Distribution (% intravascular)	Fractional catabolic rate (% intravascular pool/day)	Half-life (days)	Synthetic rate (mg/kg/day)	Complement fixation	Placental transmission	Skin sensitization Heterologous species	Skin sensitization Homologous species ||	Reactivity with rheumatoid factor	Antibody activity
IgG	7S	160 000	2·9	γ	53 000	4	13·23 (7·56–22·10)	45	6·7	23·0	33·0	+	+	+	?	+	Major anti-bacterial and anti-viral activity in serum. Antitoxins.
IgA Serum	7S(9, 11.13S)	170 000*	9·9	α1 α2	56 000 (±1700) 52 000 (±700)	2	1·6 (0·5–3·4)	42	25·0	5·8	24·0	0§	0	0	0	0	Several anti-bacterial and anti-viral activities.
Secretions	11S	385 000	11·7									0	0	0	0	0	Major anti-bacterial and anti-viral activity in secretions.
IgM	19S	900 000	11·8	μ	65 000 (±1800)	2	0·88 (0·2–2·8)	76	18·0	5·1	6·7	++	0	0	0	0	Anti-polysaccharide antibodies.
IgD	7S	184 000	12·0–14·0	δ	69 700	2	0·11 (<0·1–0·5)	75	37·0	2·8	0·4	0	0	0	?	?	Antibodies to penicillin, diphtheria toxoid and insulin detected. Major function unknown.
IgE	8S	188 100	11·6	ε	72 500 (±2400)	?	0·00033 (0·0001–0·0013)	51	89·0	2·3	0·02	0	0	0	++	?	Reaginic antibodies. Raised in helminthic infections.

* Monomeric type. † With carbohydrate moiety. ‡ Adult Caucasian population. §IgA is known to activate C3 proactivator and hence be capable of initiating C3–C0 consumption. || Guinea-pigs. N.B. Data from [10–15] have been included.

From Stanworth D.R. & Turner M.W. Immunochemical analysis of immunoglobulins and their subunits, in *Handbook of Experimental Immunology*. 1. Immunochemistry. 2nd Edition (1973). Ed. Weir D.M. p. 10.4. Oxford: Blackwell Scientific Publications Ltd.

such as pollens, and infections with helminths appear particularly to elicit reaginic antibody formation, but many other antigens have the same ability. IgE antibodies have a uniquely developed property of fixing themselves to body tissues and remaining so fixed. These antibodies cannot be detected in serum by conventional methods of serology as they do not appear to form precipitates with antigen, or to fix complement. The 'reaginic' antibodies of immediate hypersensitivity prominent in asthma, hay fever and drug and food allergies are of the IgE type. The antibodies have an affinity for cell surfaces possibly mediated by a cell attachment site on their Fc fragment. In man IgE sensitizes mast cells and leucocytes in this way and when the next encounter with appropriate antigen occurs, its specific combination with the cell bound IgE triggers histamine release from the cells. IgE antibodies are, for the most part, fixed on the surface of cells which may at some time be affected by the biological consequences of their specific reactions as antibodies, and this presumably explains

TABLE 5.4. Types of allergic response.

'Immediate' or dependent on circulating antibody

Anaphylaxis
    Result of quick release of pharmacologically active agents by antigen interacting with selected immunoglobulin forms of antibody fixed (sessile) on tissue cells, e.g. mast cells. Local and systemic.

Arthus reaction
    Local inflammatory response to formation of antigen-antibody complexes, especially within vessel walls. Slower in development than anaphylaxis. Evoked by different immunoglobulin forms of antibody than those concerned in anaphylaxis; especially by IgG and γ_2 antibodies which are complement-fixing.

Serum sickness
    Generalized result of a single introduction of a large amount of antigen, so that antigen is still in circulation when antibody is made and antigen-antibody complexes are formed in the presence of excess antigen. Manifestations mainly those of scattered Arthus reactions.

Lesions due to antibodies against cell or tissue antigens
    Auto-antibodies (or hetero-antibodies) can cause complement-mediated lysis of the target cells or excite inflammation by reacting with tissue antigen.

'Delayed' or cell-mediated hypersensitivity reactions
See page 87.

From White R G. & Timbury M.C. (1973). *Essentials of Immunology and Microbiology*, London: Pitman Medical.

the very low concentration of free IgE found in serum.

When an antigen provokes a response which is beneficial to the host, the term 'immune' is used but when harmful effects follow the term 'hypersensitive' is employed. Hypersensitivity reactions have been classified as:

(1) 'Immediate' reactions which are related to the presence of circulating antibodies.

(2) 'Delayed' reactions which occur where no obligatory role for circulating antibody can be demonstrated and altered reactivity of the tissues is associated with the presence of the lymphocyte and macrophage groups of cells. In the past, immune reactions have been commonly characterized as 'humoral' antibody dependent, or 'cellular' with respect to effector mechanisms. There is, however, evidence that an experimentally induced 'cellular' response will promote a superimposed plasma cell response [48] and it is now accepted that there is a degree of interdependence between 'humoral' and 'cellular' responses. Immune complexes may either enhance or block the cellular response [49].

Immediate hypersensitivity

A classification of immediate hypersensitivity reactions is shown in table 5.4.

ANAPHYLAXIS

A series of graded allergic responses to components of drugs or diet occur in some individuals, which may be mild, causing urticaria, hay fever or asthma but which sometimes lead to severe reactions terminating in death. The work of Landsteiner has shown that a complete antigen is not necessary and that incomplete antigen (hapten) can act as a sensitizing stimulus [50]. Different species react in different ways to the initial sensitizing stimuli and also when subsequently challenged. It is generally agreed that anaphylactic shock can be explained in terms of two tissue changes; damage to capillary endothelium, and contraction of smooth muscle. Anaphylaxis, although a generalized reaction, affects different parts of the body with varying severity. As a latent period is required between sensitizing and shocking doses, it appears that antibodies are a necessary prerequisite. During anaphylaxis the plasma fibrinolytic system may be activated, and the presence of an activated fibrinolytic enzyme in gingival fluid has been reported [51].

Fibrinolysis is the enzymatic breakdown of fibrin to fragments which are no longer able to form a coherent net [52]. *In vivo* this is produced by the enzyme plasmin, the proteolytic action of which is non-specific but which in the presence of inhibitors in the blood lyses only fibrin, to which it is adsorbed [53]. Fibrinolysis is determined primarily by the presence of plasminogen activators capable of converting plasminogen to plasmin [54 & 55]. Thus, the fibrinolytic system has four main components which are plasminogen, plasmin, activators and inhibitors. The interaction between these components will determine the rate and extent of fibrin dissolution and the production of unclottable fibrin/fibrinogen degradation products. Activators are present in blood, in tissues (cytofibrinokinase), milk, saliva and seminal fluid [56–60]. Certain exogenous bacterial enzymes (streptokinase and staphylokinase) are also activators (lysokinases) and some antigen-antibody interactions may cause activator activity [61, 62 & 63]. Fibrinolysis in the gingival sulcus is complex as many of these activators may be present. Gingival fluid which is an inflammatory exudate is one source of plasminogen. The consensus of current opinion is that proactivator is in fact predominantly plasminogen, possibly accompanied by a trace of an α_2 macroglobulin which may complex with streptokinase to form a minor activator of plasminogen [64–67]. Using a tanned red cell haemagglutinin inhibition immunoassay the mean level of plasminogen in stimulated mixed saliva is 0·05 caseinolytic units/ml and the difference in concentration between a dentate and an edentate population is not significant [68]. Thus, the source of plasminogen present in the fluid collected as gingival fluid may be two-fold, the relative contribution being dependent upon the degree of inflammation of the gingiva. Small quantities of plasminogen activator are present in saliva [59, 69 & 70] but it

has not been characterized nor has its significance been evaluated. Cytofibrinokinase is released from some cells following injury [57] and is thought to be closely related to the cell lysosomes [71]. Thus fibrinolytic activity can be produced by vascular endothelial cells [72], leukocytes [73] and desquamated epithelial cells of the oral mucosa [74]. Pandolfi *et al.* [75] using the fibrinolysis technique of Todd [72] found that chronically inflamed human gingival mucosa had substantially less fibrinolytic activity than normal mucosa. This reduction may be explained by the assumption that the blood vessels in chronically inflamed tissue continuously release plasminogen activator to remove fibrin deposits occurring in the interstitial spaces. This release reduces the enzyme content of the vessels and thereby the fibrinolytic activity of the tissues.

Recent work has gone a long way to elucidate the fibrinolytic pathway of human plasma [76–80].

There is an interphase between the components of gingival fluid and the constituents of mixed saliva including Hageman factor [81] in the region of the gingival sulcus. Hageman factor is a zymogen common to the coagulation system and fibrinolytic system alike. Saliva contains coagulant factors capable of coagulating the blood of haemophiliacs [81 & 82] and thus a complex interaction may be involved between gingival fluid and saliva. The nature of any postulated interaction, however, is obscured further by the presence of the oral commensal flora. Streptokinase is not generally considered to be produced by the commensal flora, being almost exclusively produced by β haemolytic streptococci. Gesner and Jenkin [83] showed that *Bacteroides melaninogenicus* has a heparinase and Reed *et al.* [84] demonstrated fibrinolysis from gas gangrene anaerobes. Recently Loesche *et al* [85] have shown that *Clostridium histolyticum* accounted for about 0·01–0·1 per cent of the bacteria of gingival plaque. This organism has collagenolytic properties and thus the thrombolytic and fibrinolytic activity of anaerobes isolated from gingival plaque will have to be evaluated. The processes which result in gingival haemorrhage are clearly complex and intricate and the significance of the component parts has yet to be evaluated.

Originally there was a controversy between those investigators of anaphylaxis who held that the effects were due to antibody reacting with antigen in the circulation, with the creation of a toxin called anaphylatoxin, and those who held that antibody must be fixed in the target tissues and that antigen-antibody interaction occurred peripherally. Both mechanisms obtain but the latter is usually dominant.

During anaphylaxis (fig. 5.4) four pharmacologically active agents are known to appear as a result of antigen-antibody interaction: hista-

mine, slow reacting substance of anaphylaxis (SRS-A), 5-hydroxytryptamine (serotonin) and the nona-polypeptide bradykinin. The results of anaphylaxis can be largely mimicked by histamine injection, and it has been shown that histamine is released from sensitized tissues immediately after addition of antigen. The main cell source of histamine and serotonin is the mast cell (fig. 5.4), a cell often occurring in gingival tissue. All antibody will not act to sensitize for anaphylaxis, as the reaction requires a type of immunoglobulin that will attach to tissue cells. Such homocytotropic antibody in man is of the IgE type. It has been proposed that

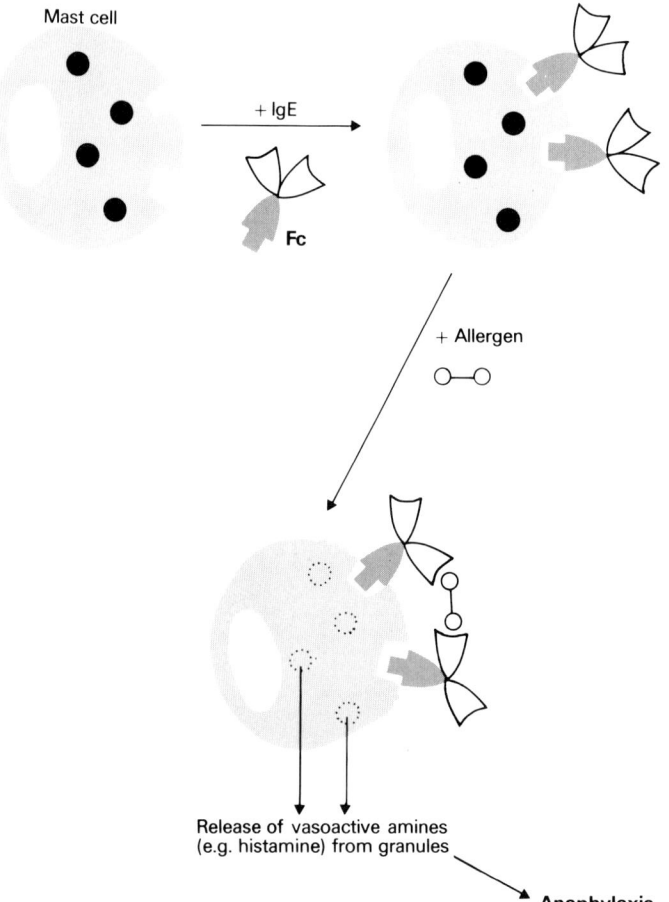

FIG. 5.4. Anaphylactic-type hypersensitivity. Mast-cell degranulation following interaction of antigen with bound homocytotropic (reaginic) antibodies. Slow reacting substance A (SRS-A) is released during anaphylaxis, but its origin is unknown. Courtesy of Dr Ivan M. Roitt (1974) *Essential Immunology*, 2nd Edition, p. 130. Oxford: Blackwell Scientific Publications.

gingivitis may have a component of immediate reagin-mediated hypersensitivity because a few IgE-immunocytes have been detected in the chronic inflammatory infiltrate (fig. 5.4) [86]. This immunoglobulin exhibits selective affinity for mast cells [87] which are abundant in the gingiva [88] and whose potent inflammatory mediators are released after degranulation. Antigen-antibody reaction involving IgE type mast cell cytotropic antibody fixed on mast cell surfaces can cause mast cell degranulation (fig. 5.4).

In cases of immediate hypersensitivity mediated by reaginic type antibody (atopy), it is difficult to detect antibodies *in vitro*. The presence of IgE type antibody can be demonstrated by its ability to passively sensitize a normal individual, e.g. Prausnitz–Kustner reaction.

The Prausnitz–Kustner reaction

The Prausnitz–Kustner reaction gets its name from Prausnitz who performed the experiment with the co-operation of Kustner who was hypersensitive to fish. When some of Kustner's serum was injected into the skin of Prausnitz's arm that area of the skin became hypersensitive to fish as was shown by subsequent intradermal injection of fish extract into the site. The antigen does not have to be injected, it may be taken by mouth and it will still cause the reaction. A varying period of up to 24 hours is necessary for the skin fixation of the antibodies to occur, but once fixed they remain there for at least 4–5 weeks. Immediate hypersensitivity can thus be transferred from one individual to another by serum alone, which confirms that it is mediated by humoral factors and not by cells. Serum sickness, the Arthus reaction and various drug and food hypersensitivities are also of the 'immediate' type.

COMPLEX MEDIATED HYPERSENSITIVITY (THE ARTHUS REACTION)

Arthus reactions occur when a soluble antigen is injected locally into animals that have complement fixing and precipitating antibodies usually of the IgM or IgG type in their circulation, and tissue fluids (fig. 5.5). Arthus injected monthly doses of horse serum subcutaneously into rabbits. Whereas the first injections were without effect, those following elicited a severe local reaction which appeared as an area of subcutaneous oedema and erythema which continued to increase for several hours, after which it began to gradually subside. The more antibody that was present in the rabbit the more intense the reaction and the longer it took to disappear. The antigen is deposited in the subcutaneous tissues and is

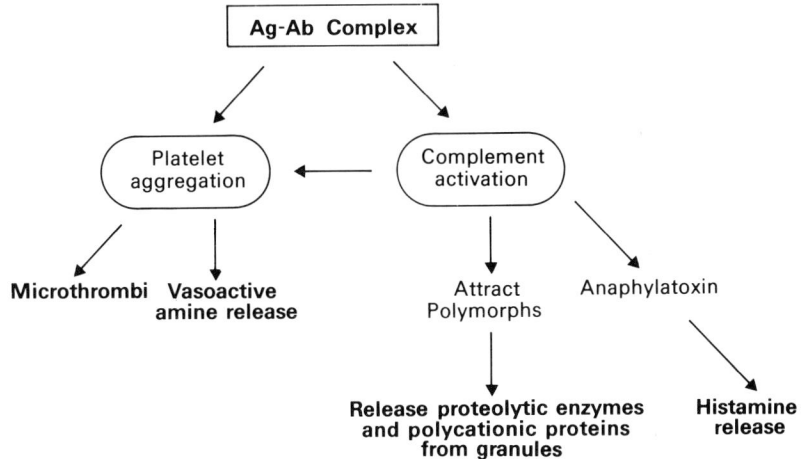

FIG. 5.5. Complex mediated hypersensitivity. Courtesy of Dr Ivan M. Roitt (1974) *Essential Immunology*, 2nd Edition, p. 131. Oxford: Blackwell Scientific Publications.

thus separated from the circulating antibody by the small blood vessel walls. Fluorescent antibody studies have shown that antigen-antibody complexes form in the subendothelial layer of venules in the injected area, presumably as a result of union of antibody in the blood with antigen diffusing from the local depot. The endothelial lining of the blood vessels swells, and platelets and neutrophils, including eosinophils, accumulate in the area. Stasis of blood, followed by thrombosis and necrosis, rupture of small vessels, haemorrhage and finally ulceration occur. The complexes are phagocytosed by granulocytes, including the eosinophils which arrive in large numbers. Many of these granulocytes are subject to sudden degranulation and cell death following ingestion of the immune complexes. Tissue damage could be the result of plugging of small vessels by vast numbers of polymorphs, the release of enzymes from ruptured lysosomes

following cell degranulation and death, or the induction by these cells of high local concentrations of lactic acid. Whatever the mechanism of tissue damage, the presence of large numbers of polymorphs is crucial to the Arthus reaction since it will not occur in rabbits deprived of granulocytes by treatment with nitrogen mustard.

LESIONS DUE TO ANTIBODIES AGAINST CELL OR TISSUE ANTIGENS (CYTOTOXIC TYPE HYPERSENSITIVITY)

Antibodies binding to antigen or cell surface cause (1) phagocytosis of the cell through opsonic (Fc) or immune (C3) adherence; (2) non-phagocytic cytotoxicity by killer (K) cells with receptors for IgFc and lysis for the full complement system up to C89 (fig. 5.6).

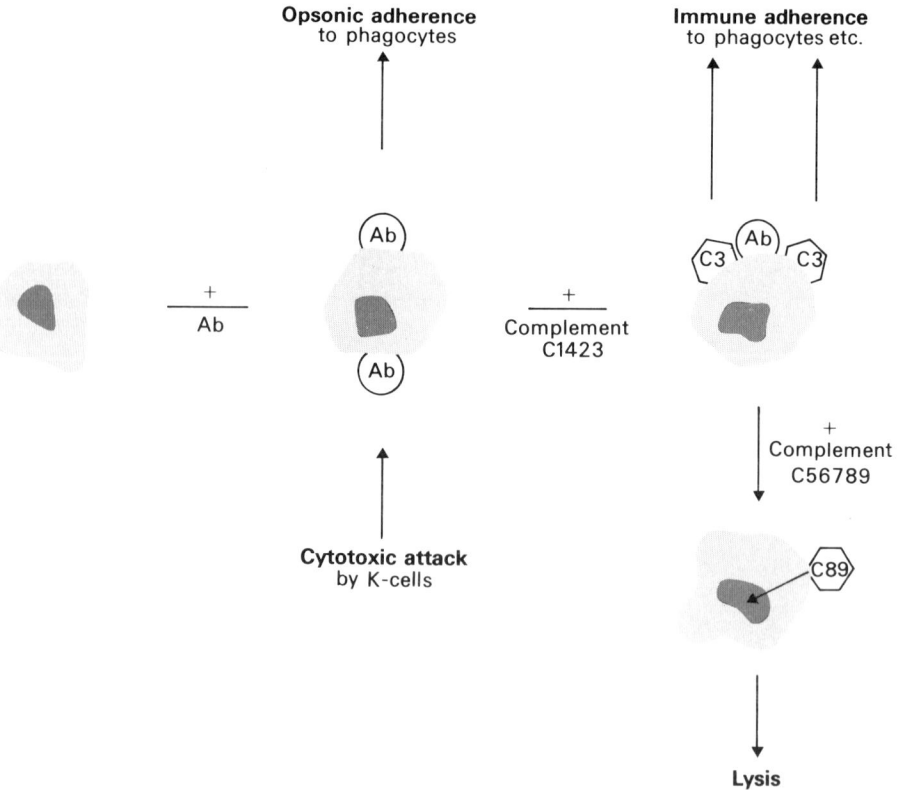

FIG. 5.6. Cytotoxic-type hypersensitivity. Lesions due to antibodies against cell or tissue antigens. Courtesy of Dr Ivan M. Roitt (1974) *Essential Immunology*, 2nd Edition, p. 131. Oxford: Blackwell Scientific Publications.

Several studies have emphasized the possibility that antibody mediated immunological mechanisms may be important in destructive gingival inflammation. Antibodies to oral bacteria have been demonstrated in human periodontal disease [59, 89 & 90]. A very large percentage of normal individuals have substantial serum antibody titres to many plaque organisms. These titres increase with age and the presence of these antibodies may prime an individual for immediate reaction to plaque antigens once these gain access to the gingival connective tissues. Gingival immunization has elicited humoral antibodies in rabbits [91] and guinea pigs [92] and it has been suggested that antibodies to bacterial products, irrelevant antigens, altered IgG, or to newly exposed tissue antigens exposed as the result of the inflammatory process, may all contribute to a continuous supply of immune complexes which may give rise to an Arthus type reaction in gingival tissues [93].

The role of antibody mediated mechanisms in the gingival tissue has been well summarized by Brandtzaeg [94]. In the oral cavity two distinct humoral effector systems contribute to the immunological protection of the host (fig. 5.7). A 'first line of defence' depends on gland associated immune responses mainly giving rise to dimeric IgA antibodies. These are selectively transferred through secretory epithelium by diffusion, and become complexed with a secretory component (SC) derived from the epithelial cells. SC is synthesized in excess of the IgA produced by the local immunocytes. About 50 per cent of the SC therefore occurs free in saliva but its function is unknown. The IgA conjugated SC probably serves to stabilize the secretory antibodies thereby rendering them resistant to degradation in the external milieu. There is evidence that secretory IgA may mediate external protection by several mechanisms (table 5.5). Deleterious effects of IgA antibodies have not been established. The possibility that such antibodies participate in bacterial plaque formation by contributing to the matrix should be considered; however, in the tissues IgA may exert blocking effects because of its lack of potent fixing properties. Although this may generally be conducive to health by slowing down deleterious consequences of antibody reactions involving IgM or IgG it may enhance the development of cancer. IgA antibodies to tumour antigens may coat the malignant cells and protect them against elimination by activated T lymphocytes (vide infra).

Immune responses associated with chronic inflammation proably represent a second line of defence against antigens penetrating the epithelium. The pattern of immunoglobulin synthesis mirrors that of secondary systemic immune responses with IgG and monomeric IgA as the major products. By passive diffusion, mainly through widened intercellular spaces in the cuff epithelium, some of the locally produced immunoglobulin enters gingival fluid and whole saliva. According to the concept of pathotopic potentiation this may reduce adverse effects of the bacterial plaque, but the ability of serum derived and locally produced IgG and monomeric IgA to function in the external milieu may be limited by enzymatic degradation. Their main function most likely takes place in the connective tissue and in the epithelium where they may mediate protection by several mechanisms (table 5.5). Recent studies have emphasized deleterious aspects of local IgG responses (table 5.5), although these to some extent may be moderated by a blocking effect of simultaneously formed IgA antibodies. Experimental models have suggested that an Arthus type reaction to a great extent may explain the destructive features of gingival inflammation. This is contrasted by the observation that individuals lacking functional B cells also respond to dental plaque with progressive gingival inflammation. Their inflamed gingivae are devoid of immunoglobulins but crowded with lymphocytes. It must be concluded that there is much to be learned about protective and destructive aspects of chronic inflammation with regard to the relative importance of humoral and cellular factors as well as interactions between B and T cells [94].

The evidence suggests, however, that when antigens from plaque gain access to gingival tissues immune complexes are formed. If these are large enough they will be deposited free in the tissues, or if they have an affinity for some tissue component they will localize to that com-

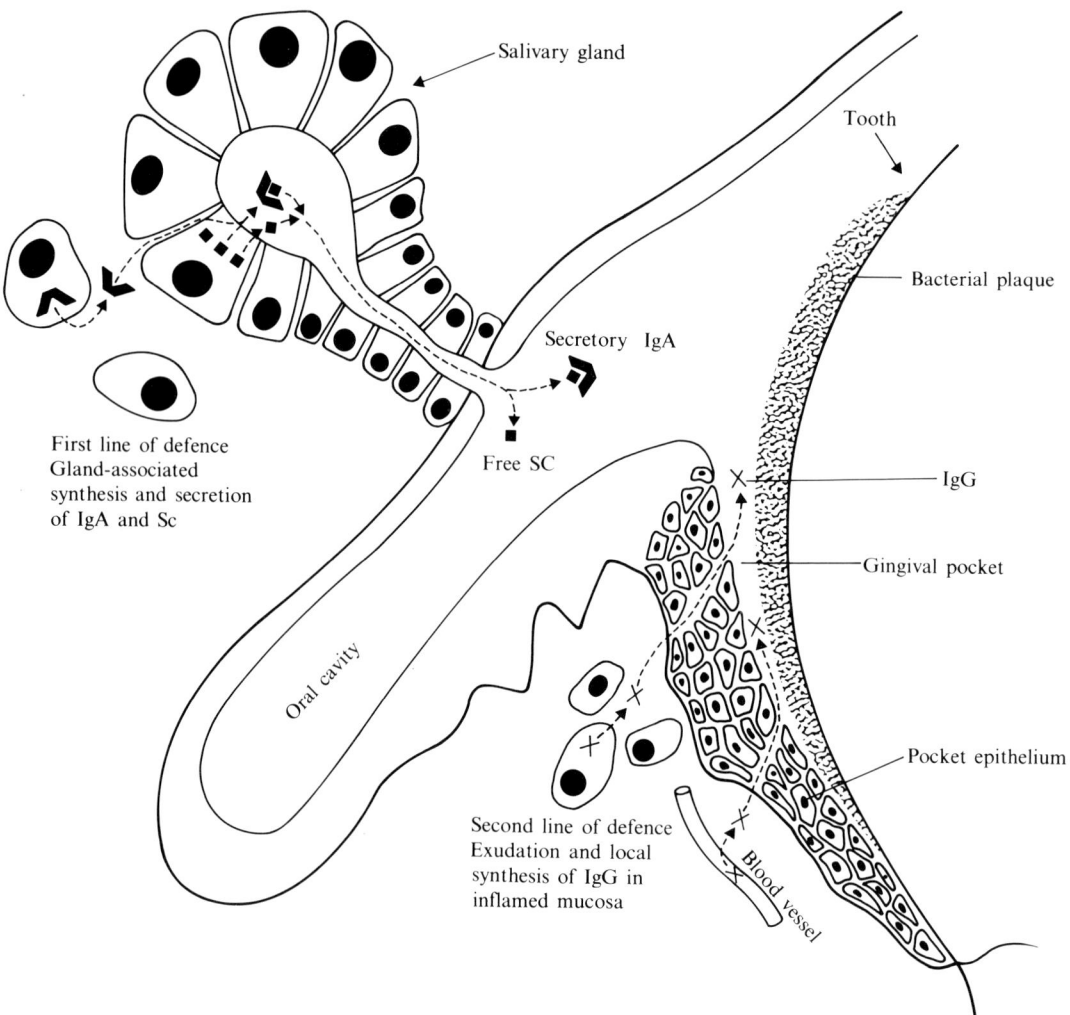

FIG. 5.7. Schematic representation of two major systems of host protection in the oral cavity. The 'first line of defence' primarily consists of secretory IgA which is produced as a dimer by immunocytes adjacent to glandular structures, conjugated with SC during selective transfer through secretory epithelium, and subsequently able to participate in external antibody functions. SC bound to IgA probably serves to stabilize the secretory antibodies, whereas the function of free SC is unknown. The 'second line of defence' is associated with local inflammatory reactions giving rise to exudation of serum antibodies and local formation of immunoglobulins, mainly IgG. This mechanism may contribute to external defence by passive diffusion of immunoglobulins through epithelia, but it is probably of greatest importance to antibody functions taking place in the tissue. Initially, complement-dependent consequences of IgG-reactions are most likely of great protective significance, but in the long run they may be deleterious. From Brandtzaeg P. (1973) Local formation and transport of immunoglobulins, in *Host Resistance to Commensal Bacteria. The Response to Dental Plaque*. Ed. MacPhee T. p. 140. Edinburgh: Churchill Livingstone.

TABLE 5.5. Postulated protective and deleterious consequences of local immune responses.

First Line of Defence The IgA response	Second Line of Defence The IgG response
Protective	*Protective*
Antigen trapping in mucous coat	Virus and toxin neutralization
Allergen blocking	Enzyme inhibition
Virus neutralization	Allergen blocking
Bacterial coating and aggregation	Bacteriolysis
Opsonization	Chemotaxis and opsonization
Bacteriolysis (?)	Inflammation due to immune complexes
Deleterious	*Deleterious*
Participation in dental plaque formation(?)	Release of pharmacologically active substances from bacteria and host cells
Enhancement of cancer(?)	Inflammation due to immune complexes (Arthus-type reaction)

From Brandtzaeg P. (1973) Local formation and transport of immunoglobulins, in *Host Resistance to Commensal Bacteria. The Response to Dental Plaque*. Ed. MacPhee T. p. 141. Edinburgh: Churchill Livingstone.

ponent. These complexes may activate the complement system leading to increased vascular permeability and a leucotactic response. Initially, complexing may be protective. Subsequently, phagocytosis of complexes may lead to degranulation and lysosomal release for phagocytic cells which may be related to tissue damage [95].

Delayed hypersensitivity

The three manifestations of delayed type or 'cell mediated' hypersensitivity (bacterial allergy, contact hypersensitivity and skin homograft reaction) differ from immediate or antibody dependent hypersensitivity states, principally in that these delayed hypersensitivity states cannot be transferred to an unsensitized animal by transfer of serum, but can be transferred only by means of lymphoid cells from spleen or lymph nodes of a sensitized animal. The study of tuberculosis has greatly increased understanding of chronic disease in general and of the phenomenon of delayed hypersensitivity in particular. The Koch phenomenon is taken as being typical of delayed hypersensitivity in the form of bacterial allergy. When tubercle bacilli are injected into a normal guinea pig, a small nodule develops at the injection site after 10 to 14 days. Ulceration follows and persists until the death of the animal. If, however, tubercle bacilli

are injected into an animal previously infected with this microorganism, a nodule appears within 1–2 days which then ulcerates and rapidly heals (Koch phenomenon). These two reactions differ in three respects. In a previously infected animal: (1) the lesion develops much more rapidly; (2) the lesion heals rapidly and (3) the lesion remains localized. These are features of an immune state. A similar altered tissue response can be demonstrated in a tuberculous animal by injecting dead bacilli or even extracts of bacilli. Injection of tuberculin or of purified tuberculin proteins derived from it is the basis of the Mantoux test, which is used clinically to detect previous contact with tubercle bacilli.

In man, the injection of white blood cells from a person with bacterial, fungal, viral or contact dermatitis types of hypersensitivity will cause the transfer of the condition. The subsequently passively induced delayed hypersensitivity appears within 24 hours and it may last for many months. It has been demonstrated by Raffel that the development of hypersensitivity in tuberculosis is independent of the degree of resistance to the disease [96]. The lesions are unaffected by antihistamines and are proliferative rather than exudative. Delayed hypersensitivity has been shown to develop in typhoid fever, undulant fever, chancroid, whooping cough, tularaemia and leprosy. Cat scratch fever yields a typical delayed skin response, as do the viral infections of psittacosis, trachoma and lymphogranuloma inguinale. Among the fungal diseases the delayed type of hypersensitivity is consistently present. It occurs, for example, in coccidiomycosis, blastomycosis, aspergillosis, candidosis and the dermatomycoses. The same reaction occurs in certain protozoal diseases [46]. The factors concerned in achieving the high levels of sensitivity of such diseases are largely unknown, but one common factor appears to be the persistent intracellular multiplication of these parasites especially within macrophages. Functioning of the immune mechanism in general, and of cell mediated delayed hypersensitivity reactions in particular, depends on co-operation between these two great cellular systems, the lymphoid system and the macrophage system. Aschoff formulated the concept of a system of macrophages throughout the body, the so-called reticuloendothelial system on the basis of the ability of such cells to take up injected particles. The cells of the reticuloendothelial system fall into two main classes, the sessile macrophages which line the sinuses of the spleen, lymph nodes and bone marrow and are stretched along the reticulum of these tissues, and the wandering macrophages (histiocytes) which are found scattered in the connective tissues throughout the body. In general, the phagocytes are divisable into the microphages, which are the granular leucocytes which derive from bone marrow, and the macrophages. The relative activities of these cells are not clearly understood. The microphages are the first cells to appear at a site of bacterial multiplication and invasion but are in general short-lived vulnerable cells. A high proportion are killed at the site of bacterial invasion so that it falls to the more slowly assembling macrophages to take up not only the bacterial invaders but also the cell debris of leucocytes.

In general, immunological responses occur in tissues provided with a component part of the reticuloendothelial system. However, oral tissues contain tissue macrophages (histiocytes), and virtually all tissues can mount a chronic inflammatory or granulomatous reaction if antigen remains for long enough locally, and antibody may be produced in the plasma cell component of any local granuloma. Immunologically com-

petent cells generally have the morphology of small lymphocytes. When these cells react to antigen they develop distinctive nuclear and cytoplasmic changes related to their projected function. For antibody production they become the immature and mature stages of the plasma cell, and for cell-mediated immunity they become large lymphocytes, which divide rapidly to form more small lymphocytes.

THE RESULTS OF THYMECTOMY

Lymphatic tissue of a neonatally thymectomized mouse becomes depleted in a characteristic way. The cortex of a lymph node with its germinal centres remains intact as does the medulla with its foci of plasma cells but there is striking depopulation of the paracortical area (fig. 5.8). Similarly, in the spleen, an area of the white pulp around the central arterioles becomes depleted of lymphocytes. These findings form the basis of the concept of the thymus dependent population of cells (T lymphocytes). While the thymus does not participate directly in the immune response it is very active in the production of lymphocytes. Some of these lymphocytes leave via efferent lymphatics to populate the thymus dependent areas of spleen and lymph

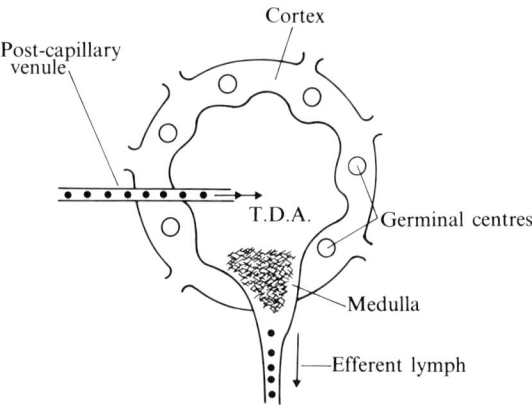

FIG. 5.8. Diagram of a lymph node to show the immunological compartments. T.D.A. = Thymus dependent area or paracortex. From White R.G. & Timbury M.C. (1973) *Essentials of Immunology and Microbiology*. London: Pitman Medical.

nodes (fig. 5.9). These lymphocytes are added
to the pool of cells which circulate from blood to
lymphatic tissues or via the thoracic duct when
they return by traversing the endothelium of the
post-capillary venules continuously to the same
area of lymphoid tissue.

Gowans, in his experiments on lymphocyte
turnover in rats [97], showed that when the
thoracic duct of a normal rat is cannulated and

continuously drained so that cells entering the
thoracic-duct lymph are lost from the body, the
initial high output of lymphocytes in the fluid
falls in a few days to low levels. This fall affects
almost exclusively the small lymphocytes, the
numbers of large and medium lymphocytes
(initially perhaps 5–10 per cent of the total cell
content) being maintained. Using an inbred rat
strain Gowans showed that the level of small

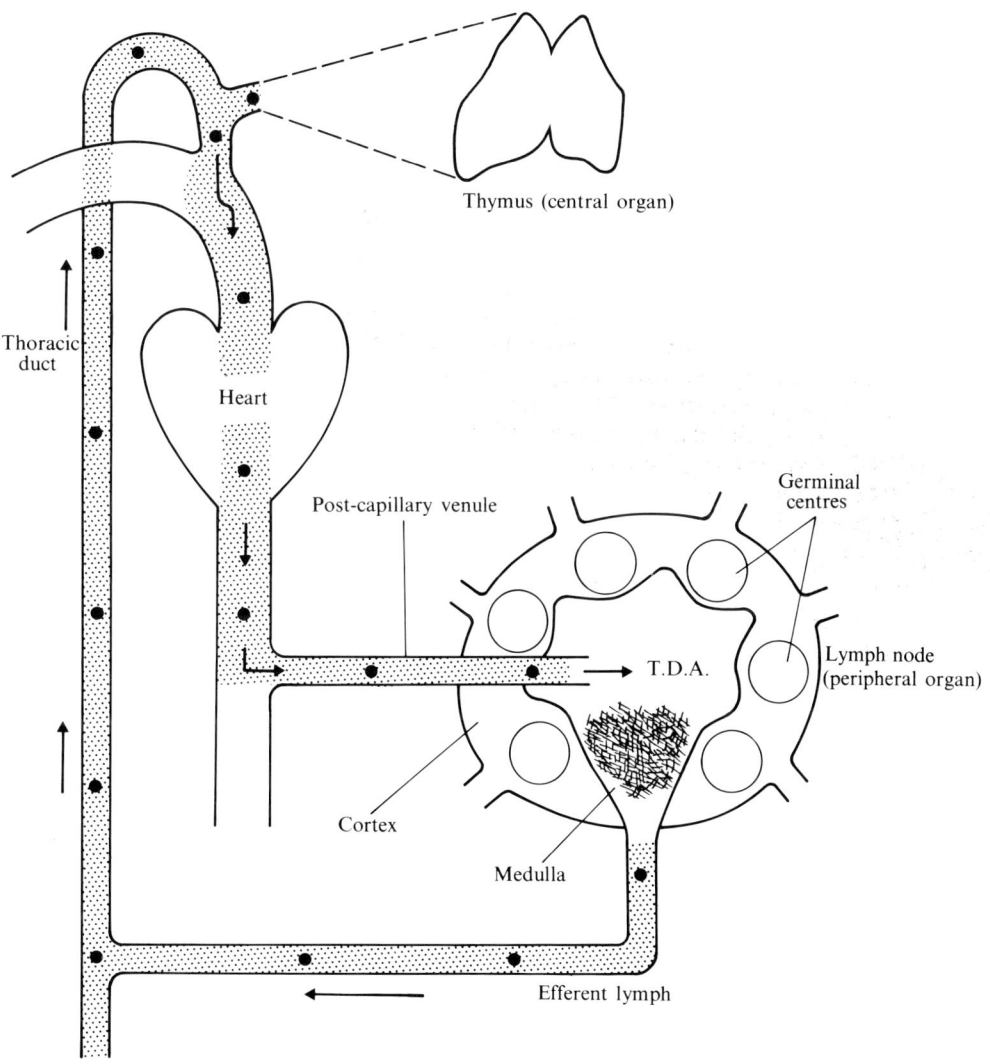

FIG. 5.9. Diagram of the circulatory pathway of small lymphocytes. T.D.A.=Thymus dependent area or paracortex.
After White R.G. & Timbury M.C. (1973) *Essentials of Immunology and Microbiology*. London: Pitman Medical.

lymphocytes is restored to normal in the draining thoracic-duct lymph by the intravenous infusion of lymphocytes similarly obtained from the freshly cannulated thoracic duct of a second rat of the same strain [98]. The restored level could be maintained for as long as fresh rats were recruited as donors.

By labelling the transfused cells *in vitro* (with a tritiated precursor of nucleic acid), Gowans showed that 80 per cent of them appeared in the recipient's thoracic-duct lymph; but labelling with H^3-thymidine *in vivo* revealed that the chronic drainage induced very little new formation of lymphocytes in the rat undergoing it, although most large and medium lymphocytes appearing in the duct lymph were labelled. It was clear that while the large and medium lymphocytes were maintained by cell division in the cannulated rat, the small lymphocytes were not. It was also clear that small lymphocytes (only some of them, for despite the depletion many remained fixed in the lymphoid tissues) recirculated freely from blood to lymph, at least in the rats under experiment. Autoradiography, in fact, showed that labelled small lymphocytes, infused intravenously, rapidly began to pass from the blood through the endothelial walls of post-capillary venules in the lymph nodes, spleen and Peyer's patches, although not in the thymus [99]. Large lymphocytes, in contrast, 'homed' chiefly to the gut where they apparently developed into plasma cells. Gut associated lymphoid tissue in man appears to be the equivalent of the Bursa of Fabricius in birds and is particularly associated with the B lymphocyte population. T lymphocytes are the immunologically competent cells of cell mediated immunity which can interact with antigen in the thymus dependent areas of spleen and lymph nodes. They multiply and form increased numbers of specifically reactive cells.

In contrast the B cells concerned in antibody responses are found infiltrating the medullary strands of lymph nodes and the red pulp of the spleen. The process of antibody production is always accompanied by germinal centre formation in the cortex of lymph nodes and in the white pulp of the spleen.

Following local application of contact sensitins or an allogenic skin-graft, the draining lymph node shows its response in the paracortical thymus dependent area as early as 12 hours after the stimulus, by the appearance of pyroninophilic blast cells. These cells do not contain demonstrable γ-globulin and are distinguishable from plasma cell precursors by their lack of endoplasmic reticulum in an electron-micrograph. By injecting tritiated thymidine during the response which becomes incorporated into newly made DNA, and preparing autoradiographs, it can be shown that these dividing blast cells give rise to labelled daughter cells which are small lymphocytes. These blast cells secrete a number of soluble factors (lymphokines) which function as mediators of cellular immune responses (see chap. 6).

Normally, the thymus acts to maintain the stock of small lymphocytes in the paracortical areas of lymph nodes. These cells are regarded as part of a recirculating pool of small lymphocytes (fig. 5.9) which are continuously entering the paracortical areas by specialized veins and leaving in the efferent lymph to rejoin the blood via the thoracic duct. Thus, the cell reactions for production of cell mediated hypersensitivity occur in a population of cells that are separate and distinct from that concerned in the elaboration of plasma cells and germinal centres [100].

REFERENCES

[1] BERVELL S.F.A. (1960) En ny teknikk ved bakteriologisk undersökelser av fysiologiske tannkjöttlommer. *Norske tannlaegeforen. Tid.* **70**, 425–433.

[2] EGELBERG J. & COWLEY G.C. (1963) The bacterial state of different regions within the clinically healthy gingival crevice. *Acta odont. scand.* **21**, 289–296.

[3] FISH E.W. (1939) Bone infection. *J. Amer. dent. Ass.* **26**, 691–712.

[4] FISH E.W. (1944) Location of bacteria in the oral tissues. *J. Canad. dent. Ass.* **10**, 385–393.

[5] WERTHEIMER F.W. (1964) A histologic study of microorganisms and human periodontal tissues. *J. Periodont.* **35**, 406–409.

[6] BECKWITH T.D., SIMONTON F.V. & WILLIAMS A. (1925) A histologic study of the gums in pyorrhea. *J. Amer. dent. Ass.* **12**, 129–153.

[7] BECKWITH T.D., SIMONTON G.W. & ROSE E.J. (1927) The presence of bacterial micro-organisms in human gingival tissue in gingivitis. *Dent. Cosmos* **69**, 164–171.

[8] BOX H.K. (1944) Can specific infective factors operate to deepen a pocket? *J. Canad. dent. Ass.* **10**, 427–435.

[9] HABERMAN S. (1959) Inflammatory and non-inflammatory responses to gingival invasion by micro-organisms. *J. Periodont.* **30**, 190–195.

[10] MACDONALD J.B., GIBBONS R.J. & SOCRANSKY S.S. (1960) Bacterial mechanisms in periodontal disease. *Ann. N.Y. Acad. Sci.* **85**, 467–478.

[11] NUCKOLLS J., DIENSTEIN B., BELL D.G. & RULE R.W. (1950) The periodontal lesion. I. The development of the lesion and the establishment and treatment of the periodontal pocket. *J. Periodont.* **21**, 7–18.

[12] BAER P.N. & KILHAM M.D. (1964) Rat virus and periodontal disease. III. The Histopathology of the early lesion in the first molar. *Oral Surg.* **17**, 116–124.

[13] FLEMING H.S. & SONI N.N. (1964) Polyoma virus and the periodontium. *Periodontics* **2**, 115–118.

[14] WESTPHAL O. & LUDERITZ O. (1954) Chemische erforschung von lipopolysacchariden gramnegativer bakterien. *Angew. Chem.* **66**, 407–417.

[15] THOMAS L. (1954) The physiological disturbances produced by endotoxins. *Ann. Rev. Physiol.* **16**, 467–490.

[16] BURNETT G.W. & SCHERP H.W. (1966) *Oral Microbiology and Infectious Disease*, 2nd Edition. Baltimore: Williams and Wilkins.

[17] ZWEMER J.D. & STENMAN R.R. (1960) Endotoxic activity of human saliva. *J. dent. Res.* **39**, 1074.

[18] RIZZO A.A. & MERGENHAGEN S.E. (1960) Local Schwartzman reaction in rabbit oral mucosa with endotoxin from oral bacteria. *Proc. Soc. exp. Biol. (N.Y.)* **104**, 579–582.

[19] MERGENHAGEN S.E., HAMPP E.G. & SCHERP H.W. (1961) Preparation and biological activities of endotoxins from oral bacteria. *J. infect. Dis.* **108**, 304–310.

[20] BORGLUM-JENSEN S. & MERGENHAGEN S.E. (1964) Influence of endotoxin on the dermal response of rabbits to human oral bacteria. *Arch. oral Biol.* **9**, 241–251.

[21] GUSTAFSSON G.T. & CRONBERG S. (1963) Effect of endotoxin on mast cells and the extension of the local Schwartzman reaction to the hamster. *Acta path. microbiol. scand.* **59**, 21–31.

[22] BAZIN S. & DÉLAUNEY A. (1957) Etudes sur la collagene. X. Modifications apportees aux combinaisons in vitro collagene—Mucopolysaccharides pardes polyosides bacteriens. *Ann. Inst. Pasteur* **92**, 459–465.

[23] CROMARTIE W.J., SCHWAB J.H. & CRADDOCK J.G. (1960) The effect of a toxic cellular component of Group A streptococci on connective tissue. *Amer. J. Path.* **37**, 79–99.

[24] SCHWAB J.H. & CROMARTIE W.J. (1960) Immunological studies on a C polysaccharide complex of Group A streptococci having a direct toxic effect on connective tissue. *J. exp. Med.* **111**, 295–307.

[25] STETSON C.A. (1961) Symposium on bacterial endotoxins. IV. Immunological aspects of the host reaction to endotoxins. *Bact. Rev.* **25**, 457–458.

[26] *World Workshop in Periodontics* (1966) Eds. Ramfjord S.P., Kerr D.A. & Ash M. Michigan: Ann Arbor.

[27] SCHULTZ-HAUDT S.D. & SCHERP H.W. (1955) Production of hyaluronidase and beta-glucuronidase by viridans streptococci isolated from gingival crevices. *J. dent. Res.* **34**, 924–929.

[28] SCHULTZ-HAUDT S.D. & SCHERP H.W. (1955) The production of chondrosulfatase by micro-organisms isolated from human gingival crevices. *J. dent. Res.* **34**, 725.

[29] DEWAR M. (1958) Bacterial enzymes and periodontal disease. *J. dent. Res.* **37**, 100–106.

[30] GIBBONS R.J. & MACDONALD J.B. (1961) Degradation of collagenous substrates by *Bacteroides Melaninogenicus*. *J. Bact.* **81**, 614–621.

[31] THONARD J.C., HEFFLIN C.M. & STEINBERG A.I. (1965) Neuraminidase activity in mixed culture supernatant fluids of human oral bacteria. *J. Bact.* **89**, 924–925.

[32] COWLEY G.C. (1966) Gingival inflammation. Thesis. University of Edinburgh.

[33] COWLEY G.C. (1967) The epithelium of the gingival crevice as a barrier, in *The Mechanisms of Tooth Support*. Ed. Anderson D.J. *et al.* Bristol: Wright.

[34] LUCAS R.B. & THONARD J.C. (1955) The action of oral bacteria on collagen. *J. dent. Res.* **34**, 118–122.

[35] FULLMER H.M. & GIBSON W. (1966) Collagenolytic activity in gingivae of man. *Nature (Lond.)* **209**, 728–729.

[36] BENNICK A. & HUNT A.M. (1967) Collagenolytic activity in oral tissues. *Arch. oral Biol.* **12**, 1–9.

[37] SCHULTZ-HAUDT S.D. (1958) Observations on the acid mucopolysaccharides of human gingiva. *Odont. T.* **66**, 3–98.

[38] LISANTI V.F. (1950) Hyaluronidase activity in human saliva. *J. dent. Res.* **29**, 392–395.

[39] THONARD J.C. & SCHERP H.W. (1962) Histochemical demonstration of acid mucopolysaccharides in human gingival epithelial intercellular spaces. *Arch. oral Biol.* **7**, 125–136.

[40] COURANT P.R., PAUNIO I. & GIBBONS R.J. (1965) Infectivity and hyaluronidase activity of debris from healthy and diseased gingiva. *Arch. oral Biol.* **10**, 119–125.

[41] TAKAHARA S., HAMILTON H.B., NEEL J.V., KOBARA T.Y., OGURA Y. & NISHIMURA E.T. (1960) Hypocatalasemia: a new genetic carrier state. *J. Clin. Invest. Derm.* **39**, 610–619.

[42] WORLD HEALTH ORGANISATION (1961) Report of an expert committee on dental health. No. 207.

[43] BURNET F.M. (1959) *The Clonal Selection Theory of Acquired Immunity*. Nashville: Vanderbilt Univ. Press.

[44] COONS A.H., LEDUC E.H. & CONNOLLY J.M. (1955) Studies on antibody production. I. A method for the histochemical demonstration of specific antibody and its application to a study of the hyper-immune rabbit. *J. exp. Med.* **102**, 49–60.

[45] ORTEGA L.G. & MELLORS R.C. (1957) Cellular sites of formation of gamma globulin. *J. exp. Med.* **106**, 627–639.

[46] HUMPHREY J.H. & WHITE R.G. (1970) *Immunology*

for Students of Medicine, 3rd Edition. Oxford: Blackwell Scientific Publications.

[47] MEDAWAR P.B. (1963) Introduction: Definition of the immunologically competent cell, in *The Immunologically Competent Cell*, Ciba foundation study group No. 16. London: Churchill.

[48] FLAX M.H., ELLIOTT J.H., DALY J.J., WILMS-FRETSCHMER K., MCCARTHY J.S. & LESKOWITZ S. (1969) Local plasmacytopoiesis in delayed hypersensitivity reactions. *J. Immunol.* **102**, 1214.

[49] OPPENHEIM J.J. (1972) Modulation in *in vitro* lymphocyte transformation by antibodies. Enhancement by antigen-antibody complexes and inhibition by antibody excess. *Excess Cell Immunol.* **3**, 41.

[50] LANDSTEINER K. (1945) *The Specificity of Serological Reactions.* Cambridge, Mass.: Harvard Univ. Press.

[51] GUSTAFSSON G.I. & NILSSON I.M. (1961) Fibrinolytic activity in fluid from gingival crevice. *Proc. Soc. exp. Biol. (N.Y.)* **106**, 277–280.

[52] VAN KAULLA K.N. (1963) Chemistry of thrombolysis. *Human Fibrinolytic Enzymes*, p. 7. Springfield, Ill.: Charles C. Thomas.

[53] RATNOFF O.D. (1953) Studies on a proteolytic enzyme in human plasma. IX. Fibrinogen and fibrin as substrates for the proteolytic enzyme of plasma. *J. Clin. Invest.* **32**, 475.

[54] ALKJAERSIG N., FLETCHER A.P. & SHERRY S. (1958) The activation of human plasminogen. 1. Spontaneous activation in glycerol. *J. Biol. Chem.* **233**, 81.

[55] ALKJAERSIG N., FLETCHER A.P. & SHERRY S. (1958) The activation of human plasminogen. II. A kinetic study of activation with trypsin, urokinase and streptokinase. *J. Biol. Chem.* **233**, 86.

[56] LEWIS J.H. & FERGUSON J.H. (1951) Studies on a proteolytic enzyme system of the blood. IV. Activation of profibrinolysin by serum fibrinolysokinase. *Proc. Soc. Exp. Bio. Med.* **78**, 184.

[57] ASTRUP T. & PERMIN P.M. (1948) Fibrinokinase and fibrinolytic enzymes. *Nature* **161**, 689.

[58] ASTRUP T. & STERNDORFF I. (1953) A fibrinolytic system in human milk. *Proc. Soc. Exp. Biol. Med.* **84**, 605.

[59] ALBRECHTSEN O.K. & THAYSEN J.H. (1955) Fibrinolytic activity in human saliva. *Acta Physiologica Scandinavica* **35**, 138.

[60] ALBRECHTSEN O.K. (1958) The fibrinolytic agents in saline extracts of human tissues. *Scand. J. Clin. & Lab. Invest.* **10**, 91.

[61] TILLET W.S. & GARNER R.L. (1933) The fibrinolytic activity of haemolytic streptococci. *J. Exp. Med.* **58**, 485.

[62] GERHEIM E.B. & FERGUSON J.H. (1949) Species reactivity to staphylokinase. *Proc. Soc. Biol. Med.* **71**, 261.

[63] UNGAR G., YAMURA T., ISOLA J.B. & KOBRIN S. (1961) Further studies on the role of proteases in the allergic reaction. *J. Exp. Med.* **113**, 359.

[64] REDDY K.N.N. & MARKUS G. (1972) Mechanism of activation of human plasminogen by streptokinase. Presence of an active centre in streptokinase-plasminogen complex. *J. Biol. Chem.* **247**, No. 6, 1683.

[65] TAKADA A., TAKADA Y. & AMBRUS J.L. (1972) Further studies of plasminogen proactivator. *Biochem. Biophys. Acta.* **263**, 610.

[66] WERKHEISER W.C. & MARKUS G. (1964) The interaction of streptokinase with plasminogen. II. The kinetics of activation. *J. Biol. Chem.* **239**, 2644.

[67] SUMMARIA L., HSIEH B., GROSKOPF W.R. & ROBBINS K.C. (1969) Direct activation of human plasminogen by streptokinase. *Proc. Soc. Exp. Biol. Med.* **130**, 737.

[68] MOODY G.H. (1974) Personal communication.

[69] SCHULTE W. (1968) Saliva and blood coagulation, in *Transactions of 3rd International Conference on Oral Surgery*, 1970, p. 494. Ed. Walker R.V. Edinburgh: Livingstone.

[70] NITTA H., SUGIE I., MORIMOTO S. & SATO S. (1967) Studies on physicochemical properties of the fibrinolytic substances in human saliva. *Nagoya Med. J.* **13**, No. 3, 151.

[71] LACK C.H. (1963) Origin of blood fibrinolytic activity. *Lancet* **ii**, 522.

[72] TODD A.S. (1959) The histological localization of fibrinolysin activator. *J. Path. & Bact.* **78**, 281.

[73] RIDDLE J.M. & BARNHART M.I. (1964) Ultrastructural study of fibrin dissolution via emigrated polymorphonuclear neutrophils. *Am. J. Path.* **45**, 805.

[74] WUNSCHMANN-HENDERSON B. & ASTRUP T. (1972) Relation of fibrinolytic activity in human oral epithelial cells to cellular maturation: the influence of smoking. *J. Path.* **108**, 293.

[75] PANDOLFI M., BJORLIN G. & NILSSON I.M. (1969) Decreased fibrinolytic activity in chronically inflamed tissue. *Odontologisk Revy.* **20**, 31.

[76] IATRIDIS S.G. & FERGUSON J.H. (1961) Effects of surface and Hageman factor on the endogenous or spontaneous activation of the fibrinolytic system. *Throm. Diath. Haemor.* **6**, 411.

[77] IATRIDIS S.G. & FERGUSON J.H. (1962) Active Hageman factor: A plasma lysokinase of the human fibrinolytic system. *J. Clin. Invest.* **41**, No. 6, 1277.

[78] OGSTON D., BENNET N.B., OGSTON C.M. & RATNOFF O.D. (1971) The assay of a plasma component necessary for the generation of a plasminogen activator in the presence of Hageman factor. (Hageman factor co-factor), *Brit. J. Haem.* **20**, 209.

[79] KAPLAN A.P. & AUSTEN F.K. (1972) The fibrinolytic pathway of human plasma. *J. Exp. Med.* **136**, No. 6, 1387.

[80] SCHREIBER A.D., KAPLAN A.P. & AUSTEN K.F. (1973) Plasma inhibitors of the components of the fibrinolytic pathway in man. *J. Clin. Invest.* **52**, 1394.

[81] DOKU H.C. (1960) The thromboplastic activity of human saliva. *J. Dent. Res.* **39**, No. 6, 1210.

[82] NOUR-ELDIN F. & WILKINSON J.F. (1957) The blood clotting factors in human saliva. *J. Physiol.* **136**, 324.

[83] GESNER B.M. & JENKIN C.R. (1961) Production of heparinase by bacteroides. *J. Bact.* **81**, 595.

[84] REED G.B., ORR J.H. & BROWN H.J. (1943) Fibrinolysins from gas gangrene anaerobes. *J. Bact.* **46**, 475.

[85] LOESCHE W.J., PAUNIO K.U., WOOLFOLK M.P. & HOCKETT R.N. (1974) Collagenolytic activity of

dental plaque associated with periodontal pathology. *I.A.D.R., Abstract J. Dent. Res.* **53**, 107.

[86] NISENGARD R.J., BEUTNER E.H. & GAUTO M. (1971) Immunofluorescence studies of IgE in periodontal disease. *Ann. N.Y. Sci.* **177**, 39.

[87] TOMOIKA H. & ISHIZAKA K. (1971) Mechanisms of passive sensitization. II. Presence of receptors for IgE on monkey mast cells. *J. Immunol.* **107**, 971.

[88] ZACHRISSON B.U. (1967) Mast cells in the human gingiva. II. Metachromatic cells at low pH in healthy and inflamed tissue. *J. Periodont. Res.* **2**, 87.

[89] LEHNER T. & CLARRY E.B. (1966) Acute ulcerative gingivitis. An immunofluorescent investigation. *Brit. Dent. J.* **121**, 366.

[90] WILTON J.M.A., IVANYI L. & LEHNER T. (1971) Cell-mediated immunity and humoral antibodies in acute ulcerative gingivitis. *J. Periodont. Res.* **6**, 9.

[91] RIZZO A.A. & MITCHELL C.T. (1966) Chronic allergic inflammation induced by repeated deposition of antigen in rabbit gingival pockets. *Periodontics* **4**, 5–10.

[92] THONARD J.C. & DALBOW M.H. (1965) Local cellular antibodies. I. Plaque formation by sensitized oral mucosal cells from conventional animals. *J. Immunol.* **95**, 209.

[93] COCHRANE C.G. (1967) Mediators of the Arthus and related reactions. *Progress in Allergy* **11**, 1.

[94] BRANDTZAEG P. (1973) Local formation and transport of immunoglobulins, in *Host Resistance to Commensal Bacteria. The Response to Dental Plaque*, p. 139. Ed. MacPhee T. Edinburgh: Churchill Livingstone.

[95] GENCO R.J., MASHIMO P.A., KRYGIER G., ELLISON S.A. (1974) Antibody-mediated effects on the periodontium. *J. Periodont.* **45**, 336–337.

[96] RAFFEL S. (1948) The components of the tubercle bacillus responsible for the delayed type of 'infectious' allergy. *J. infect. Dis.* **82**, 267–293.

[97] GOWANS J.L. (1959) The recirculation of lymphocytes from blood to lymph in the rat. *J. Physiol. (London)* **146**, 54.

[98] GOWANS J.L. (1957) The effect of the continuous re-infusion of lymph and lymphocytes on the output of lymphocytes from the thoracic duct. *Brit. J. Exp. Path.* **38**, 67.

[99] GOWANS J.L. & KNIGHT E.J. (1964) The route of re-circulation of lymphocytes in the rat. *Proc. Roy. Soc. (Biol.)* **159**, 257.

[100] WHITE R.G. & TIMBURY M.C. (1973) *Essentials of Immunology and Microbiology*, p. 160. London: Pitman Medical.

CHAPTER 6

Host–parasite interactions in gingivitis and periodontitis

The factors governing host resistance to dental plaque are not yet clearly defined. 'Epidemiological surveys have confirmed that serious metabolic disease and ageing are directly related to the severity of periodontal disease but do not explain the prevalence' [1]. 'Nutritional deprivation states particularly protein and ascorbic acid deficiency have tended to be associated with increased severity of periodontitis but have never been demonstrated to be the initiating factors' [2]. Similar conclusions may be reached by reviewing the data on the incidence and severity of periodontal disease in presence of particular systemic diseases such as diabetes [3], leukemia [4] and the hormonal shifts encountered commonly in puberty, pregnancy and menstruation [5, 6 & 7]. Reduction of host resistance to plaque may result from metabolic change at the cellular level not demonstrable by assay of circulating nutritional or hormonal factors in blood [8]. Numerous surveys have confirmed that homeostatic mechanisms are such that estimation of plasma levels of a particular factor such as albumen or total protein bear no direct relationship to whether a particular tissue is deprived or not. Experiment has shown that there is a consistent gingival repair potential independent of age both in young and mature rats [9, 10 & 11] which supports Waerhaug's earlier suggestion [12] that increased periodontal disease associated with ageing may represent an accumulative process rather than a direct cause and effect relationship.

Plaque is a normal finding in all mouths and the plaque/gingival tissue interphase is a constantly active homeostatic system in a dynamic equilibrium which in health is in favour of the host. Oral sulcular and junctional epithelia appear to represent no complete barrier to penetration of biologically active material from plaque. Experiments by Egelberg [13] with histamine have shown that at least small molecules can penetrate through intact cuff epithelium and Fine [14] has reported that carbon particles $1-3\mu m$ in diameter pass through cuff epithelium in normal gingiva into the underlying connective tissues. The results of such studies indicate that gingival connective tissue is subjected to continuous insult by bacterial products. Junctional epithelium acts as a two-way filter in that these stimuli result in the outflow of gingival fluid and Egelberg [15] described the environment of the crevice as 'here the environment must be governed primarily by factors such as gingival fluid, desquamated epithelial cells, and emigrated white blood cells. The gingival fluid as a substrate for bacterial growth is different from saliva. Gingival microbiota has to develop in co-existence with the crevicular leucocyte.'

The host resistance factors at the plaque–gingival interphase are summarized in fig. 6.1. Gingival fluid and leucocytes are the immediate environment of subgingival plaque which represents a non-invasive infection on the surface of oral sulcular epithelium and the sulcular surface of junctional epithelium. In terms of the classical theory of inflammation the leucocyte response to an irritant in the gingival sulcus should be a host defence measure aimed solely at destroying and eliminating injurious substances by a process of phagocytosis followed by intracellular digestion. While there is a lack of direct experimental evidence, electron microscope studies [16–19] and all indirect evidence suggests that the function of the large numbers of leucocytes in gingival fluid is to engulf foreign material at the plaque–gingival tissue interphase and at least partially degrade it by a process of enzymatic digestion. Since these cells have no intrinsic capacity to recognize a foreign particle, and a recognition of 'foreignness' leading to leucocyte migration and phagocytosis depends upon the interaction of antibody and complement with the foreign object [20], it seems quite clear that both the inflammatory mechanism and the immune response are active at the plaque–gingival tissue interphase. One of the prime functions of the immune response is to activate the inflammatory system; the two are closely interlinked. Both are homeostatic mechanisms which are normally successful in restoring and maintaining homeostasis, but a growing weight of evidence suggests that host resistance breakdown is a result of tissue injury brought about by mechanisms of chronic allergic inflammation, and that in these circumstances the inflammatory lesion of gingiva is no longer self limiting and becomes progressively tissue destructive. Dick and Trott [21] suggested that this could happen in two different ways.

(1) The immune system has no capacity to distinguish pathogenic from non-pathogenic antigens. In some individuals some indigenous oral bacterial antigens may give rise to an allergic reaction rather than an immune reaction. In this case a particular antigen would be the determinant; for example both the presence of serum antibodies and immediate hypersensitivity to actinomyces have been demonstrated in humans [22] and there are other similar examples.

(2) The presence of inflammation gives rise to varicose enlargement of the venular plexus underlying cuff epithelium. Immune reactions superimposed on this environment may be enhanced resulting in a destructive allergic reaction rather than healing. Inflammation may have a synergistic effect on the immune response resulting in allergy.

This work demonstrated that traumatically induced non-specific inflammation enhanced an Arthus phenomenon induced in the oral tissues of mice and it seems that both these concepts may be relevant to variation in host resistance to plaque throughout the population.

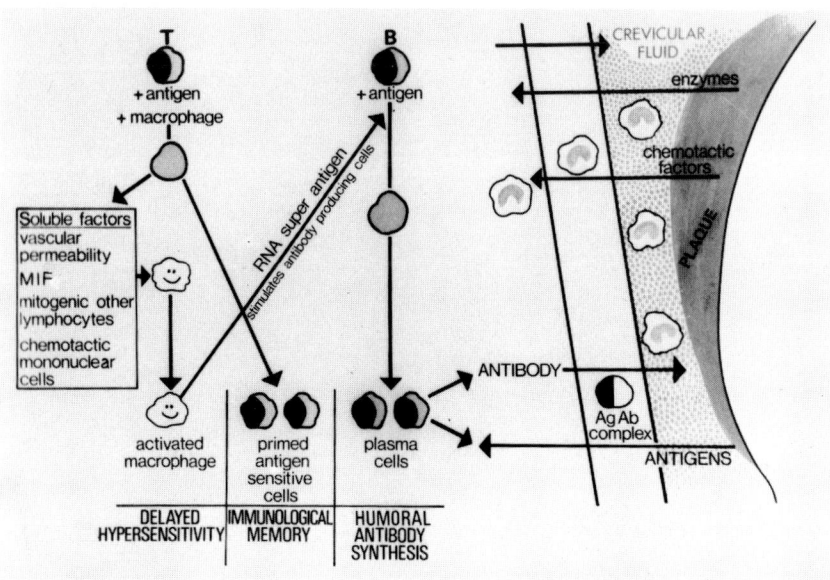

FIG. 6.1. Host resistance factors at the plaque gingival tissue interphase. From MacPhee T. (1973) Host resistance to dental plaque, in *Host Resistance to Commensal Bacteria. The Response to Dental Plaque.* Ed. MacPhee T. p. 4. Edinburgh: Churchill Livingstone.

The development of a local immune response in a site such as gingiva containing no lymphoid tissue is closely related to the prior infiltration of that tissue by polymorphonuclear leucocytes, and it is well recognized that the sequential changes in cell population characteristic of the immune response follow the presence of polymorphs in gingiva. It has been proposed as a general principle [23] that the extent of tissue damage which results from bacterial inflammation, surface or invasive, varies with the degree of hypersensitivity which the particular infection provokes and that since a hypersensitivity reaction has no specific antibacterial effects, blocking any hypersensitivity component may eliminate useless tissue destruction and increase the host's ability to deal with the invading bacteria. It is possible that such general mechanisms as development of hypersensitivity might account for variation in severity of periodontitis throughout the population.

Some of the host resistance factors of importance in this complex situation are shown in fig. 6.1. An inward diffusion of enzymes, chemotactic factors and antigens provokes emigration of polymorphs and outward diffusion of an immunoglobulin-rich inflammatory gingival exudate. Brandtzaeg [24] has pointed out that the biological significance of immunoglobulins synthesized in an inflammatory focus remains speculative. In the gingival connective tissue and epithelium they may in part represent protective antibodies which inactivate deleterious products of the bacterial plaque, promote phagocytosis, and initiate bacteriolysis. The pattern of immunoglobulin synthesis in gingival tissue is that of a secondary systemic immune response with IgG and monomeric IgA as the major products. By passive diffusion, mainly through widened intercellular spaces in oral sulcular and junctional epithelium, some of the locally produced immunoglobulin enters gingival fluid and whole saliva. This may to some extent reduce the damaging effects of bacterial plaque, but the ability of serum derived and locally produced IgG and monomeric IgA to function in the external milieu could be limited by enzymatic degradation. Their main function most likely takes place in connective tissue prior to exudation in gingival fluid. It seems clear,

however, that both the immunoglobulins and emigrated leucocytes of gingival fluid influence the ecology of subgingival plaque, and that there is a further contribution from factors such as lysozyme, and other anti-bacterial systems such as the peroxidase, thiocyanate, hydrogen peroxide system known to operate in saliva [25]. The presence of polymorphs in gingival tissues is shortly followed by the appearance of small lymphocytes, as in other tissues, in two distinct populations, the bursa equivalent B lymphocytes and the thymus dependant T lymphocytes. Both populations contain cells sensitive to plaque antigens, probably with specific antibody on their surface, and on contact with appropriate antigen the B lymphocytes differentiate, proliferate and mature through a blast phase into plasma cells which synthesize humoral antibody. T lymphocytes on contact with an antigen, which possibly has to be prior processed by a wandering macrophage, transform into large blast cells which subserve a number of functions associated with cell mediated immunity. Sensitized lymphocytes which have been immunologically activated by antigen will on encountering that antigen again give rise to at least three types of response.

(1) *Blast cell transformation*

In 1960, Nowell [26] demonstrated that an aqueous extract of the kidney bean, phaseolus vulgaris (phytohaemagglutinin or PHA), was able to produce large dividing blast-like cells in culture of human peripheral blood. A number of studies subsequently confirmed that the precursors of these blast cells were small lymphocytes. Many of the known lymphocyte activators have been classified into two groups: specific and non-specific. Non-specific activators, e.g. PHA, stimulate a sizeable proportion of the lymphocytes of all normal individuals and induce biochemical and physiological changes within one hour of being added to lymphocyte suspensions. Specific activators are antigens which stimulate only lymphocytes from individuals sensitized to that particular antigen. Blast cell transformation is assessed by measuring DNA or RNA synthesis using radioactive precursors such as C^{14} thymidine.

(2) *Cytotoxicity*

Sensitized lymphocytes are cytotoxic against unrelated target cells [27]. While antigen recognition by lymphocytes is specific, cytotoxicity against target cells is non-specific and fibroblasts and chicken red cells are some of the many cells used in experimental models. Since cytotoxicity against target cells is non-specific, damage may be caused to microorganisms and host tissues alike.

(3) *Lymphokines*

Activated lymphocytes secrete a number of soluble factors (lymphokines) which appear to function as mediators of cellular immune responses [28 & 29]. Lymphokines are soluble non-antibody products of lymphocyte activation by specific antigen which produce increased vascular permeability following intradermal injection, which increase tritiated thymidine incorporation by cultured lymphocytes, and which inhibit macrophage migration *in vitro* [30].

The biological and clinical importance of the cellular immune response lies in its role in maintaining resistance to facultative and obligate intracellular infection; in mechanisms of delayed hypersensitivity and allograft rejection; in restricting tumour growth; in its association with autoimmune disease; and in its role in facilitating antibody production (fig. 6.2). It is now customary to employ the term 'specific cell mediated immunity' (CMI) to denote those biological and clinical phenomena which seem to result from interaction between sensitized lymphocytes and specific antigen [31], and in which no obligatory role can be found for classical humoral antibodies [30].

It appears that various activities of sensitized lymphocytes may be partly expressed or amplified by means of soluble non-antibody mediators (lymphokines) appearing as a result of antigen lymphocyte interaction [32]. When lymphocytes from suitable animals or man are cultured with the sensitizing antigen, culture supernatants develop a number of biological activities (soluble factors, lymphokines) summarized in table 6.1. Lymphokines are to delayed hypersensitivity as the complement system is to antibody mediated immediate reactions. They fall broadly into two groups, lymphokines which affect other inflammatory cells, and lymphokines which affect target cells. One lymphokine from the attract group, eosinophil chemotactic factor, emphasizes the links between the antibody system and the lymphokine system in that it can only function after interacting with antigen-antibody complexes. Similarly, it seems that evidence is emerging that some complement

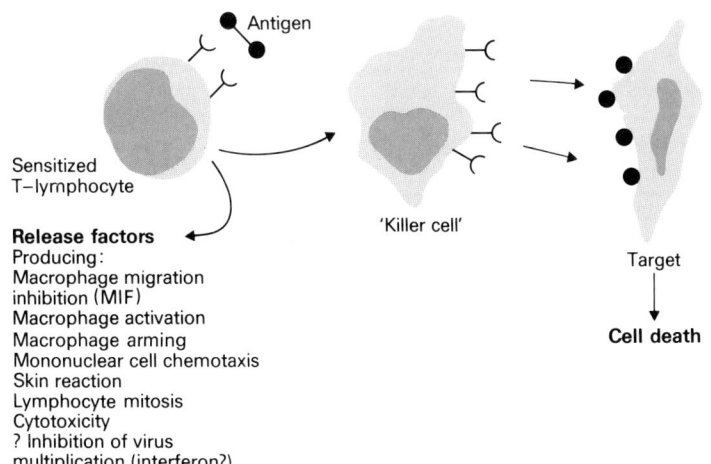

FIG. 6.2. Type IV—Cell-mediated (delayed-type) hypersensitivity. Courtesy of Dr Ivan M. Roitt (1974) *Essential Immunology*, 2nd Edition, p. 132. Oxford: Blackwell Scientific Publications.

TABLE 6.1. Some biological activities of non-antibody lymphocyte activation products.

Name (soluble factor) given to biological activity	Biological system revealing activity	Related feature of cellular immune response
Lymphocyte mitogenic factor	Enhancement of lymphocyte DNA synthesis (lymphocyte transformation)	Lymphocyte transformation
Inflammatory factor(s)	Clinical or isotope assay of inflammatory response to intradermal injection	Delayed-type hypersensitivity
Cytotoxic and cytopathic factor	Morphological or isotope evidence of cytotoxicity for fibroblast monolayers	Lymphocyte cytotoxicity
Migration-inhibition factor	Inhibition of polymorph or macrophage migration from cell explants in capillary tubes	Inhibition of leucocyte or macrophage migration
Macrophage-agglutinating factor	Agglutination of macrophage suspensions	Macrophage aggregation *in vitro* and *in vivo*
Macrophage-spreading factor	Inhibition of the spreading of macrophages on glass cover slips	Antigen-induced inhibition of macrophage spreading
Chemotactic factor	Accelerated passage of mononuclear cells through millipore membranes	Macrophage chemotaxis *in vitro* and *in vivo*
Lymph-node activating factor	Intra-lymphatic injection increases lymph-node weight, paracortical cellularity and induces lymphocyte plugging in cortico-medullary sinuses	Lymphoid cellular change during induction of delayed-type hypersensitivity
Macrophage-activating factor	Enhancement of metabolic phagocytic microbicidal capacity of cultured macrophages	Acquired cellular resistance of macrophages
Interferon-like factor	Interference with virus pathogenicity in cell culture	Non-specific resistance to viral infection

From Morley J., Wolstencroft R.A. & Dumonde D.C. (1973) The measurement of lymphokines, in *Handbook of Experimental Immunology*, 2nd Edition; Vol. 2, *Cellular Immunology*. Ed. Weir D.M. Oxford: Blackwell Scientific Publications.

fragments are chemotactic, some are cytotoxic and some may interact directly with macrophages and lymphocytes. The immune system and the inflammatory system function as one 'dual system' and not as two separate systems as has been the traditional view.

Lymphocytes from subjects with gingivitis and periodontitis activated by human plaque filtrates produce lymphokines which inhibit migration of macrophages, are cytotoxic for human gingival fibroblasts and activate osteoclasts to resorb bone. Horton *et al.* [33] have defined another lymphokine, lymphotoxin (L.T.), as being cytotoxic for human fibroblasts and have demonstrated a direct correlation between L.T. production and degree of periodontal disease in an affected population. Cultured lymphocytes from subjects with periodontal disease stimulated with filtrates of *Veillonella* produce a direct lymphocytotoxic activity.

Horton *et al.* [34] also defined the presence of an osteoclast activating lymphokine (O.A.F.) in individuals with periodontal disease generated by stimulation by plaque and this was clearly differentiated from parathormone active metabolites of vitamin D and other classical factors associated with bone resorption. These lymphocyte activation products appear to mediate the cellular immune response and may be involved in the inflammatory reaction.

The functions of the thymus dependent lymphocytes are briefly summarized in fig. 6.1.

(1) Thymus dependent lymphocytes divide to form an expanded population of primed antigen sensitive cells which provide immunological memory because of their long life span.

(2) They release a number of soluble factors (lymphokines, table 6.1) which increase vascular permeability, activate macrophages, are chemotactic for mononuclear cells, mitogenic for other lymphocytes, and perform a number of other functions associated with delayed hypersensitivity.

(3) They are directly cytotoxic to specific target cells (lymphocytotoxicity).

The functions of the activated macrophage (fig. 6.1) appear to be phagocytosis, degradation of antigen excess to prevent the induction of tolerance, and synthesis of RNA linked 'super antigen' for further stimulation of antibody producing cells.

Gingival tissue has frequently been described as being in a constant state of wound healing. There is a growing weight of evidence to support the concept that immediate hypersensitivity reactions are active in the initial stages of periodontitis, and that as the condition develops, delayed hypersensitivity contributes to the perpetuation of the lesion through its influence on mechanisms of tissue repair. The local formation of antigen-antibody complexes confers upon the antibody the property of activating the complement system. This results in the release of a wide range of biologically active proteins which induce, amongst other things, immune adherence of platelets and erythrocytes, virus neutralization, enhanced phagocytosis, increased vascular permeability, mast cell degranulation, leucocyte chemotaxis, and cytolysis of erythrocytes and bacteria.

COMPLEMENT

The important differences between one class of antibody and another reside not only in the nature of the antibody combining sites (the Fab portions) but in the Fc portions of the heavy chains which determine whether or not the antibody molecule can activate complement, whether it will attach to the surface membranes of certain cells, or whether it will cross the placental barrier. The biological consequences of antigen antibody interaction depend not only on the primary interaction between antigen and antibody but also on the secondary activation of the complement system which can result. While antigen can combine with antibody in the absence of complement in some circumstances, when the reaction takes place in fresh serum, complement components may add to the precipitate and may contribute up to a half of its weight at optimal proportions. Some serological reactions such as haemolysis and bacteriolysis are affected by and dependent upon the presence of complement. Complement has been shown to consist of a group of at least nine proteins and glycoproteins which become activated in a cascade or sequential manner by the primary union of antigen with antibody. Complement activity is involved in the killing of bacteria by serum antibodies, opsonization, phagocytosis and intracellular digestion, immune-adherence and conglutination, lysis of normal or tumour cells by antibody against antigen on their surface, and the activation of serum by antigen antibody complexes to cause inflammation or to produce anaphylatoxin (fig. 6.3).

Complement is often referred to by the abbreviated symbol C' and its various components are then known as $C'1$, $C'2$ etc. (fig. 6.3). The numerals indicate the order in which these components were discovered and do not correspond with the order in which they react. Most work on complement relates to the lysis of red cells using sheep red cells lysed by rabbit antibody in the presence of guinea pig complement. This illustrates the general truth that complement can react across species boundaries.

The reaction of complement components with antibody at the surface of a red cell results in damage to the cell membrane so that molecules leak in and out. The first evidence of the lesion can be seen in the electron microscope as holes in the erythrocyte membrane about 9 nm in diameter.

Mayer [35] took it as a starting assumption that lysis of the red cell could be the consequence of acquiring a single site of irreversible damage, or 'hit' at the cell surface which locally destroyed its osmotic properties. This would allow free diffusion of potassium out of the cell and sodium in and permit water to flow in to balance the very high colloid osmotic pressure of the haemoglobin. From a mathematical analysis of the rates of lysis of red cells treated serially with the known C' components it was possible to deduce that haemolysis must be due to a sequence of reactions, each of which was initiated by the one preceding it, and that the $C'3$ reagent which reacted last must itself be a complex of two or more active substances. It has subsequently been shown that the holes produced by the action of complement on other types of mammalian cell and on a bacterium are similar in size and appearance to those occurring

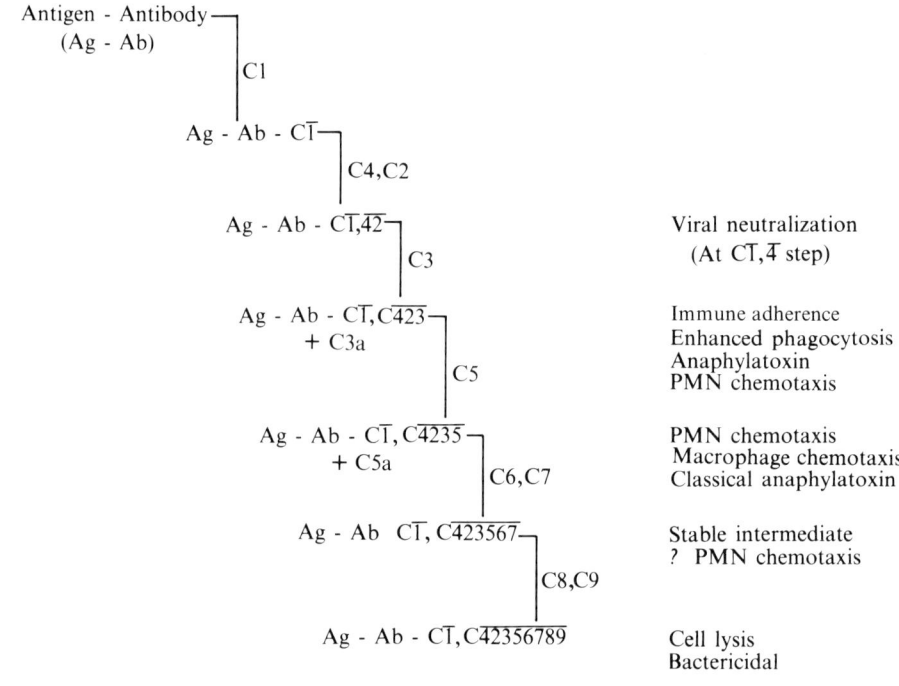

FIG. 6.3. Complement cascade and associated biological activities. From Mergenhagen S.E. (1973) A role for complement in host resistance, in *Host Resistance to Commensal Bacteria. The Response to Dental Plaque*. Ed. MacPhee T. p. 101. Edinburgh: Churchill Livingstone.

in a red cell system. The crucial step in the activation of the complement system by immune complexes is the reaction of the C′1 recognition unit with active sites formed in the antibody as a result of combination with specific antigen. It is now known that the C′1 recognition system comprises three different types of subunit which are thought to be present in the proportion of 1 : 2 : 4 for C′1q, C′1r and C′1s [36]. One molecule of IgM or two adjacent molecules of IgG antibody can be sufficient to initiate C′ activation. Non specifically aggregated IgA and probably IgE are capable of activating late components (C3) probably through an alternative pathway.

An essential step seems to be that the Fc parts of the H chains should become in some way distorted or exposed by combination with antigen, and that more than one pair of such H chains should be arranged at a suitably short distance apart. Thus, antigen-antibody com-

plexes activate C′ most efficiently when mixed at about equivalence ratio, but fail to do so when the antigen is present in such excess that no lattice structure is formed.

The first stage is attachment of C′1q to the Fc portion of the H chain followed by C′1r and C′1s. This requires the presence of calcium ions, and calcium probably acts as a link binding the whole C′1 complex together. As a consequence of the interaction between the Fc portion of the immunoglobulin and C1 an esterase activity (C′1a) is created which catalyses the formation of the C3 converting enzyme (C$\overline{42}$) which initiates consumption of C′3–C′9. The C′3, which is the most abundant component in human plasma, is converted by reactive C′42 complex to an active form which rapidly attaches itself to the adjacent cell membrane.

Relatively little is known at present about the way in which the next three components C′5, C′6 and C′7 act. There is some evidence that the activated C'7 acts directly on the cell membrane, without becoming permanently attached. The cell membrane is still intact at this stage. When the C' complex is activated as far as C'7 by antigen-antibody complex in serum a chemotactic factor is liberated. Following formation of the complex AgAb C$\overline{1, C423567}$, the last two identified components of C' (C'8 and C'9) act in turn, though little is known about how they do so. The end result is that the cell membrane is irreparably damaged, and that small molecules leak in and out. In the case of a red cell this leads to osmotic swelling and rupture, whereas in the case of other cells disorganization following disturbance of the internal environment leads to rupture of lysosomes and death without gross swelling. Gram-negative bacteria are both killed and rendered susceptible to digestion of the cell wall by lysozyme.

The lesions can be seen in the electron microscope as holes in the cell membrane, the diameter of which are about 10·3 nm with human C' and about 8·8 nm with guinea pig C'. These holes are a similar size and appearance whether they are formed by the action of C' on red cells, on tumour cells, or Gram-negative bacteria. They appear to be due to the local disruption of the continuous surface lipid layer by micelle formation, due to some alteration of the phospholipid component, but how this is brought about is still unknown [37].

Activation of complement by alternative pathways

While particular emphasis has been placed on systems involving the activation of complement via the C'1 recognition unit, it should be noted that both antigen-antibody complexes and non-specifically aggregated immunoglobulin have been observed to activate late components through alternative pathways. For example, it has been shown that pre-formed guinea pig Gamma 1 antibody-antigen precipitates, which are incapable of fixing complement through the classical pathway sequence, activate late components through an alternative pathway beginning at C'3 [38].

Alternative pathways for complement activation include:

(1) a direct enzymatic cleavage of complement components;
(2) an interaction of C'3 with aggregated Gamma 1 guinea pig immunoglobulins, certain polysaccharides, or lipo-polysaccharide endotoxins, in a manner which achieves sparing of C'1, C'4 and C'2; and
(3) by interaction of a cobra venom factor with a plasma protein co-factor to bypass the requirements for early acting complement components.

Alternative pathways of complement activation have been well reviewed by Götze and Muller-Eberhard [39].

Probably the major manifestations through which complement may participate in host resistance to commensal bacteria or their products is by the production of biologically active polypeptides which mobilize leucocytes from bone, chemotactically attract polymorphonuclear and mononuclear leucocytes, retard leucocytes by immune adherence and promote phagocytosis [40].

Complement deficiencies

It is uncertain in which cells or tissues most of the C' components are made. However, C'1 has been shown to be made in the human colon and ileum, probably by epithelial cells, and C'3 is certainly made largely or exclusively in the liver. C'3 exists in different allotypic forms, distinguishable by their electrophoretic mobility, which is characteristic for any given individual. C'2 is thought to be made by macrophages but also perhaps by other cells. C'1 deficiency, apparently due to the lack of C'1q component, has been found in an infant born with thymic alymphoplasia. A condition of hereditary deficiency in C'2 has been described in apparently healthy persons in whom haemolytic C' activity was found to be absent. A secondary C'2 deficiency occurs in subjects with hereditary angioneurotic oedema owing to continuous activation and spontaneous decay, due to the uninhibited action of C'1a.

An absolute C'6 deficiency has been found in an in-bred strain of rabbits, and an absolute C'5 deficiency occurs in certain in-bred strains of mice. There is evidence to suggest that the complement dependent chemotaxis of polymorphonuclear leucocytes has an important role in host defence mechanisms. Experiment has shown that a deficiency in generation of C′5 dependent chemotactic activity in C′5 deficient mice results in a deficient early accumulation of leucocytes which could account for the increased susceptibility of these animals to certain bacterial and mycotic infections [40].

The overall effect of complement activation may be increased permeability of gingival tissue allowing greater penetration of toxic products from plaque and a vicious circle may thus be established.

PERIODONTITIS AND CELLULAR IMMUNITY

In. vitro studies of lymphocyte transformation have clearly shown that cellular immunity may play a central role in chronic gingivitis and periodontitis (fig. 6.4). Ultrasonicates of *Veillonella alcalescens*, *Fusobacterium fusiforme*, *Bacteroides melaninogenicus* and *Actinomyces viscosus* have been used to study the response of lymphocytes from patients with increasing severity of gingivitis and periodontitis as graded according to the periodontal index [41] (fig. 6.4). The control subjects had a periodontal index of < 0.2 and *Lactobacillus acidophilus* and *Proteus mirabilis* were used as control organisms. A common pattern was established for the four organisms. A control base line with a stimulation index (SI) of < 2 was followed by significant rise in the SI in the gingivitis group $(P < 0.001 < 0.05)$ with a further rise in the mild and moderate periodontitis group and terminating by significant fall in patients with severe periodontitis $(P < 0.02$ and $< 0.05)$. The two control organisms *Lactobacillus acidophilus* and *Proteus mirabilis*

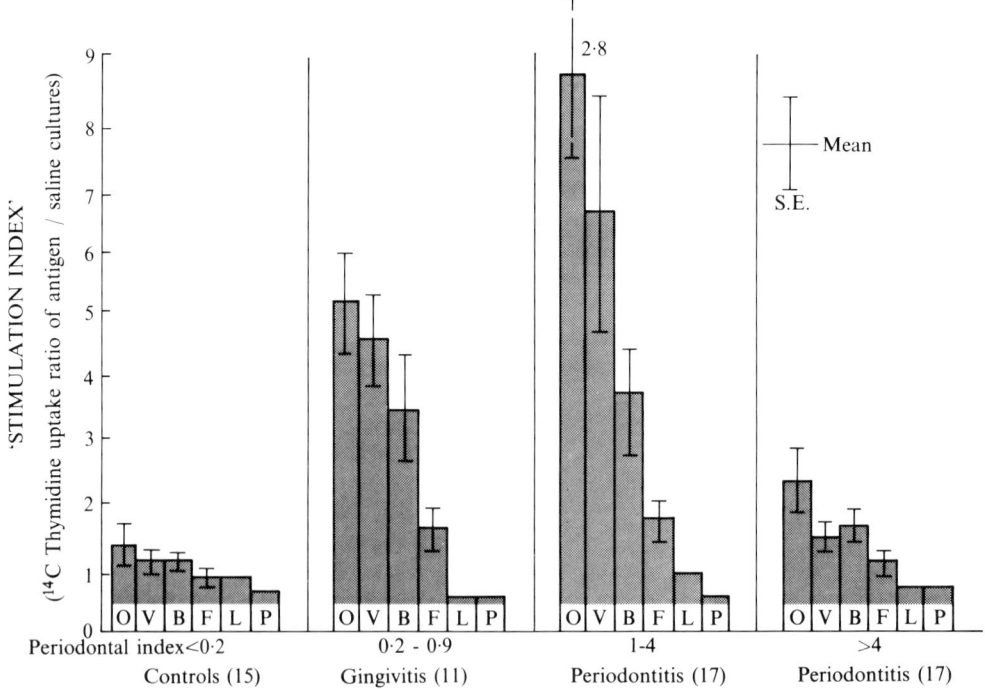

FIG. 6.4. Stimulation of lymphocyte transformation in patients with gingivitis, periodontitis and controls by ultrasonicates of *Odontomyces viscosus* (O), *Veillonella alcalescens* (V), *Bacteroides melaninogenicus* (B), *Fusobacterium fusiforme* (F), *Lactobacillus acidophilus* (L), and *Proteus mirabilis* (P). From Lehner T. (1973) Cellular immunity to oral infections, in *Host Resistance to Commensal Bacteria. The Response to Dental Plaque.* Ed. MacPhee T. p. 179. Edinburgh: Churchill Livingstone.

failed to stimulate lymphocyte transformation in any of the groups, and lymphocytes from control subjects responded only slightly more to the other four organisms than to saline.

In order to confirm that lymphocyte transformation in this system was a measure of CMI and to explore the relationship of other markers of CMI, the indirect macrophage migration inhibition test [42] and lymphocyte cytotoxicity against chicken red cells [27] were performed. Both tests showed a significant cytotoxic and migration inhibitory activity in gingivitis and all degrees of. severity of periodontitis and the results were negative in control subjects [43]. However, lymphocytes from patients with severe periodontitis showed only weak transformation but markedly raised cytotoxic and migration inhibition activity. The weak lymphocyte transformation in the severely affected group could be a result of a 'blocking' effect similar to that which may protect tumour cells from the cytotoxic effect of sensitized lymphocytes. Oppenheim [44] has reported that an excess of soluble antibody can block or modulate the response of sensitized lymphocytes to specific antigens, whereas antigen which is aggregated by antibody is able to enhance the lymphoproliferative response. It seems clear from these studies that lymphocyte transformation, cytotoxicity and migration inhibition tests represent cell mediated immunity in periodontal disease [45]. Although antigen recognition by lymphocytes is specific, the cytotoxic effect on target cells is non-specific [27]. This is consistent with the non-specific damage to gingival and cuff epithelium, periodontal membrane and bone in periodontal disease. The response of sensitization to some bacterial antigens is probably protective, preventing spread of microorganisms into deeper tissues. However, damage to adjacent tissues might be inevitable as the result of the immune and inflammatory reactions. Lehner [45] has further suggested that whilst gingivitis and various grades of periodontitis are generally considered as a continuous spectrum of disease, this concept may not be valid. A differentiation into several types of gingivitis and periodontitis might emerge. In a study of acute ulcerative gingivitis, however, the response of lymphocytes was similar to that found in chronic marginal gingivitis except for the significantly raised lymphocyte transformation stimulated by *F. fusiforme* [46].

Experiment has further shown that pasteurized saline extracts of plaque deposits stimulate lymphocytes *in vitro* from patients with periodontal disease, and that a direct correlation exists between the degree of periodontal disease and the degree of lymphocyte response to such plaque antigens [47]. While ultrasonicates of plaque deposits provided the most stimulating extracts, the exact nature of the stimulant was not defined in this study. All affected subjects, however, appeared to have similar stimulants deposited at the gingival margin since both autologous and pooled homologous plaque antigens stimulated the lymphocytes to the same extent.

It has been shown that lymphocytes from patients with periodontitis elaborate lymphotoxin when exposed to plaque antigen [33]. The production of lymphotoxin by *in vitro* leucocyte cultures was determined by assaying the inhibitory effect of leucocyte supernatants on protein synthesis of cell cultures of gingival fibroblasts or L cells. Inhibition was not produced by supernatants of unstimulated lymphocyte cultures from subjects with periodontitis, or from cultures of normal subjects stimulated with plaque antigens. Inhibition of protein synthesis as well as disruption of gingival fibroblasts or L cell mono-layers was produced by supernatants of lymphocyte cultures from periodontitis subjects when stimulated by plaque antigen.

The presence in the supernatant fluid of a soluble effector substance, osteoclast activation factor (OAF), from stimulated cultures of human peripheral blood leucocytes, that induces resorption of bone *in vitro*, has been reported [34]. This soluble mediator is elaborated in leucocyte cultures stimulated either by antigenic material present in human dental plaque or by the non-specific mitogen phytohaemagglutinin. Such *in vitro* studies suggest that immunologically specific reactions of the cell mediated type contribute to periodontitis and that tissue damage may be a function of 'the molecular pharmacology of cell mediated immunity'.

ENZYMIC BASIS OF HOST RESISTANCE

Studies of the effects of host resistance mechanisms on connective tissues have tended to concentrate on the extent to which phagocytic cells may react with immunologic stimuli to contribute to tissue breakdown, and the relationship of the enzyme systems within these cells which govern post-phagocytic events to known reduction in host resistance. In general terms, the sequence of events leading to degradation of phagocytosed material has been well demonstrated for polymorphonuclear leucocytes, and it is probable that similar mechanisms are active in the macrophage (fig. 6.5). Polymorphonuclear leucocytes contain particulate cytoplasmic particles known as 'primary lysosomes' [48] which contain something upwards of 20 acid hydrolases and at least two other antibacterial substances lysozyme and phagocytin [20]. Following ingestion of foreign material, the lysosomal membrane fuses with the membrane of the phagocytic vacuole, the contents of the lysosome are emptied into the vacuole and govern intracellular kill of ingested microorganisms, or degradation of biologically active proteins as the case may be. The cells also contain cytoplasmic particles called 'peroxy-

somes' [49] which contain a number of peroxidases, the most widely studied being myeloperoxidase, and catalase, which an increasing weight of evidence suggest have a role in resistance to infection. The present literature is to some extent conflicting as to the definition of the location of these enzyme systems within the cells, but it is clear that the peroxysomes are not the only possible intracellular site for peroxidases; catalase at least has been demonstrated in the non-particulate fractions of the cytoplasm of cells [50]. Following phagocytosis, some microorganisms are more easily destroyed than others, which may continue to multiply within the cytoplasm. The gonococcus and meningococcus, *Mycobacterium tuberculosis* and *Staphylococcus pyogenes* multiply within phagocytic cells and in such cases the cells may serve as a vehicle for dissemination of bacteria throughout the body. While it is known that a wide range of organisms possess this capacity, we have as yet no information as to intracellular survival of strains of organisms from human dental plaque. Much of the work designed to examine the role of intracellular enzyme systems in host resistance has been conducted using the capacity for intracellular kill of known strains of microorganisms as the experimental model. There is evidence that some phagocytic cells are capable

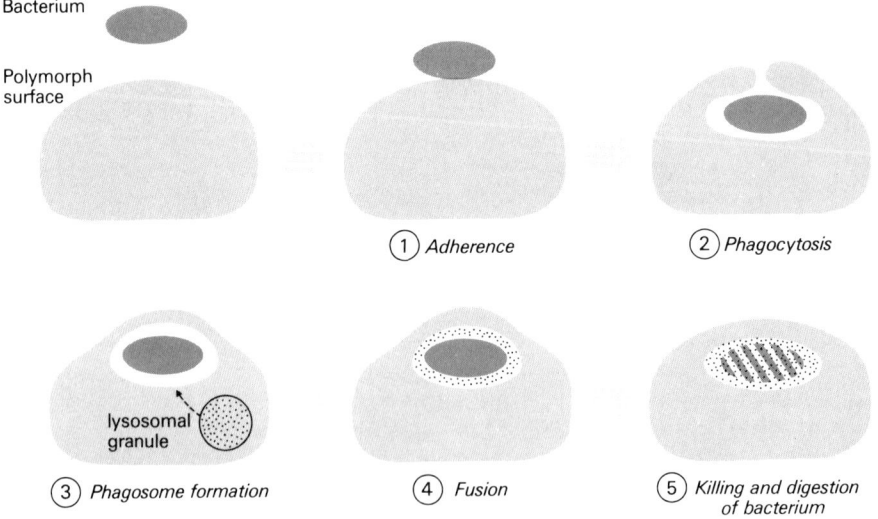

FIG. 6.5. Phagocytosis of bacterium by neutrophil leucocyte. Courtesy of Dr Ivan M. Roitt (1974) *Essential Immunology*, 2nd Edition. Oxford: Blackwell Scientific Publications.

of adaptive changes following repeated exposure to particular stimuli, which is manifested by increased phagocytic activity, increased enzyme synthesis, and changes in cellular morphology. The indications are that while these are clearly properties of the macrophage the polymorphonuclear leucocyte is an 'end cell' with a short life span. The evidence which might reflect intrinsic change in the polymorphonuclear leucocyte is the enhanced phagocytic activity following *in vitro* stimulation by endotoxin, which may be of particular importance in the gingival sulcus region, and their increased bacteriocidal capacity following multiple ingestion of staphylococci [51]. In contrast to this, the phenomenon of macrophage adaptation in immunity has been well demonstrated in the capacity of these cells to adapt not only to their particular environment, but also to the particular foreign materials introduced to that environment. It was demonstrated [52] that peritoneal macrophages from mice infected with BCG phagocytosed and killed virulent bacteria more effectively than peritoneal cells from normal mice. The effect was not limited to intracellular kill of tubercle bacillus, mice infected with BCG showed increased resistance to infection by salmonellae, and also cleared salmonellae from the circulation at an increased rate. Allison and his colleagues [53] found that after BCG vaccination, the increase in rabbit's resistance to infection with virulent tuberculosis was parallelled by an increase in the cell acid phosphatase levels, and also to some extent by increase in other enzymes in the cells. Similarly, other studies demonstrated that in-bred rabbits resistant to tuberculosis have macrophages with a higher acid phosphatase content than more susceptible strains of rabbits [54]. From this and other work arose the concept of the correlation between host resistance, the basic levels of acid hydrolases in non-adaptive cells such as polymorphonuclear leucocytes, and increased levels in macrophages demonstrating an adaptive capacity during cellular immunity. The evidence as to the role of intracellular lysosomal acid hydrolases in host resistance is to some extent conflicting. Bohme and his colleagues [55] studied the behaviour of the reticuloendothelial system in strains of mice genetically susceptible, or resistant, to infection with

Salmonella typhimurium. Acid phosphatase levels were found to have no predictive value for the outcome of the infection, and there was no evident significant difference in enzymatic changes in the cells during the period of infection. Similarly, Pavillard [56] compared the phagocytic and bacterial capacities of rat alveolar and peritoneal macrophages, and found that the peritoneal macrophages were less efficient despite their higher enzyme content. The position is complicated and the evidence which is presently available suggests that the absence of several lysosomal acid hydrolases from cells is associated more with the accumulation of metabolic products in the cell, as in generalized glycogen storage disease, rather than with lowered resistance to infection. While it is possible that localized pH changes within particular areas of a cell might allow acid hydrolases to act, these require such acid conditions for optimal activity that the cell would probably be dead or dying. It is probable that their effect is maximal at a late stage in tissue and microbial destruction. In contrast to this, the peroxidases have pH optima around neutrality, and it may be that these systems are of major significance in phagocytic activities at the plaque gingival tissue interphase.

In 1966 Klebanoff *et al.* [57] demonstrated the existence of a bacteriostatic system consisting of lactoperoxidase, hydrogen peroxide and thiocyanate, which had the capacity to inhibit the growth of streptococci in milk, and a similar system has been shown to be operative in saliva [25]. It was further found that a particular peroxidase obtained from leucocytes, myeloperoxidase, could substitute for lactoperoxidase in this system [57] and since it was known that increased respiratory activity during phagocytosis led to build up of hydrogen peroxide within the cell, studies were undertaken which confirmed the relationship of intracellular build up of hydrogen peroxide to the capacity for post-phagocytic killing of bacteria. Leucocytes phagocytosing organisms under anaerobic conditions which inhibited formation of hydrogen peroxide showed reduced bacteriocidal activity which was at least partially reversible by adding H_2O_2 to the system. The addition of exogenous catalase which breaks down H_2O_2 produced the same effect [58]. It has been suggested that the role of catalase in physiological terms is to prevent accumulation of hydrogen peroxide during phagocytosis to levels which would be toxic to the cell [59] or which would inhibit the activity of myeloperoxidase [60]. Plaque produces both catalase and hydrogen peroxide in fairly large quantities, and it is probable that the catalase-hydrogen peroxide-myeloperoxidase system is of particular importance in host resistance at the plaque/gingival tissue interphase both in terms of post-phagocytic events, and the possible effects on the ecology of subgingival plaque of bacteriostatic systems operating in gingival fluid, similar to those that have been demonstrated in milk and saliva. Evidence is accumulating that myeloperoxidase, besides catalysing oxidation of the classical substrates for peroxidases, also oxidizes amino acids in the presence of hydrogen peroxide, and is of particular importance in the degradation of bacterial toxins [57 & 61]. The pH of inflammatory foci corresponds to the optimal pH for enzymatic activity of myeloperoxidase. It has been suggested that the logical role of this enzyme may consist of decomposition of amino acids produced as a result of cytolysis in inflammatory processes [62].

There is some evidence that either absence or relative absence of components of these systems is associated with both general disease and periodontal disease in particular. For example, leucocytes from patients with chronic granulomatous disease are able to phagocytose bacteria readily, but are unable to kill the ingested organisms [63 & 64] because of lack of stimulation of hexose monophosphate shunt activity, and failure to show normal increments of hydrogen peroxide production during phagocytosis [58]. In 1952 Takahara [65] described oral ulceration and tooth loss due to grossly advanced periodontal disease relative to age in patients with an autosomal recessive deficiency of catalase. Studies [66] have suggested that patients with ulceromembranous gingivitis have reduced levels of erythrocyte catalase relative to a normal population. Such evidence as there is suggests that there is a relationship between erythrocyte catalase levels and periodontal disease, but this is difficult to define because of an apparent variation in intracellular catalase levels with time and the very wide ranges of normal which appear to exist. The situation is further complicated by the fact that there must be other enzyme systems capable of assuming the physiological role of catalase or any of the other enzyme systems which have been studied. Cohen and Hochstein [67], for example, have claimed that glutathione peroxidase may govern H_2O_2 levels in the erythrocyte in particular.

POTENTIAL OF PHAGOCYTIC CELLS TO CAUSE TISSUE DAMAGE

While experimental evidence has shown that the tissue damage of chronic periodontitis is to some extent a function of the molecular pharmacology of the sensitized lymphocyte population, there is also evidence to suggest that it may be a function of the activities of phagocytic cells. For example, it has been shown that lysosomal acid hydrolases of macrophages leak to the exterior in the course of phagocytosis [68] although the significance of this leakage on the integrity of normal tissue is still a matter of doubt. There is good evidence, however, that lysosomal enzyme secretion at cell surfaces may be involved in both physiological and pathological breakdown of connective tissue fibres. Woessner [69] concluded that collagen digestion begins extracellularly, involves either a collagenase or cathepsin, and is completed intracellularly while the components of ground substance may be broken down by lysosomal enzymes both extra and intracellularly. In theory, at least, lysosomes can induce tissue damage either through excess or deficiency of lytic activity.

In terms of excess of lytic activity, a variety of substances have been shown to have the potential to act as labilisers of lysosomal membranes resulting in cell death and massive extracellular extrusion of lysosomal enzymes. Streptolysin O and S, staphylococcal leucocidin, Hypervitaminosis, A, D, E, K and sterols, endotoxins, heterologous antibody and complement, and ultraviolet radiation have been shown to possess this property. It seems inevitable that plaque must be rich in lysosomal labilisers, most of which for the moment are largely unknown, but it is likely that the most important ones at the present stage are endotoxin known to be present in large quantities in the sulcus region, immune complexes, and complement.

It is well established that lysosomal enzymes of polymorphonuclear leucocytes are activated following ingestion of immune precipitates, and this activity is associated with degranulative changes and ultimately cell death and massive outpouring of lysosomes into the tissues. Once the inflammatory process is initiated in this way, it is probably self-perpetuating, as some of the liberated lysosomal proteins cause degranulation of mast cells and histamine release [70 & 71] while others maintain an inflammatory state without such mediators as histamine and serotonin.

This mechanism is known to be active in a wide variety of local inflammatory states, and electron microscope studies have confirmed the presence of increased numbers of free lysosomes in inflamed gingival tissue.

CONNECTIVE TISSUE ALTERATIONS

The nature of connective tissue alteration in chronic periodontitis has been well described by Page and Schroeder [72]. During the early stages of inflammatory gingival and periodontal disease, changes in the quality and quantity of the connective tissue components occur. A number of authors [73–76] have described morphologic features of altered collagen and others [75, 77 & 78] have reported changes in character of ground substance. Investigators comparing the collagen of normal and pathologically altered gingival tissues have shown a significant decrease in the total collagen content of affected tissues [79, 80 & 81].

Sun and Schneider [82], who used microdissection methods to separate the infiltrated and non-infiltrated connective tissue fractions of human biopsy specimens followed by biochemical analysis, demonstrated a reduction of 60 per cent in total collagen content of tissue fractions affected by the inflammatory response.

Similarly, Schroeder, Münzel-Pedrazzoli and Page [83], using morphometric point counting techniques, showed a reduction in total collagen of about 70 per cent in the infiltrated as compared with the non-infiltrated connective tissue. Not only are differences noted in the total amount of collagen present, but there is a marked reduction in the size of the acid soluble collagen compartment, in particular in surgically excised specimens of severely inflamed human gingivae. All experimental data shows that marked alterations in the quality and quantity of connective tissue components occur in inflammatory gingival and periodontal disease.

Mechanisms of the normal physiologic turnover of collagen and those which may be associated with its pathological alteration are as yet incompletely understood. Since the total amount of collagen present in a tissue is determined, at least in part, by the relative rates of production and degradation, an alteration in amount may result from an imbalance in these relative rates. Human periodontal tissues produce a specific endogenous collagenase (chap. 7). The enzyme is produced by epithelial cells, polymorphonuclear leucocytes, connective tissue cells, and by pieces of alveolar bone. In addition to such endogenous collagenases, bacterial collagenases are produced by some plaque organisms. While it is clear that there is degradation of collagen in excess of synthesis during the course of periodontal disease, there is no direct or indirect evidence that collagenases of bacterial origin are of significance. Such evidence as is available suggests that collagenase production associated with the presence of the local inflammatory and local immune response is primarily responsible for the reduction in collagen content of infiltrated tissue.

Experiments suggest that the loss of connective tissue substance in inflamed gingiva may be a consequence of depressed collagen production rather than enhanced collagen destruction. Gingival collagen may be unique biologically in that it may turn over at an inordinately high rate [84–87]. Studies of collagen turnover following the incorporation of C^{14} proline into collagen hydroxy-proline [81] have suggested that turnover of collagen in gingival tissue is very high in comparison to turnover in other tissues. It appears that insoluble gingival collagen is unusually labile and may turn over at an inordinately high rate, relative to other body tissues. If this is the case, relatively minor alterations in gingival collagen production or degradation may lead to dramatic changes in collagen content of gingivae as well as alteration in the size of various collagen compartments.

Morphometric analysis of human gingival biopsy specimens has suggested that reduced collagen production may be induced by the presence of dental plaque [88 & 89]. The fibroblasts present in the infiltrated connective tissue exhibited cytopathic alterations. These included abnormal nuclear electronlucency, swollen mitochondria, frequently without cristae, widely dilated cysternae of endoplasmic reticulum and ruptured plasma membranes. These alterations which are manifestations of dying or dead cells were not seen in fibroblasts of the non-infiltrated connective tissue nor in the non-fibroblasts of the infiltrated connective tissue. Lymphocytes and immunoblasts were the predominant infiltrating cells comprising 76·1 per cent of the total cell population in this study. Most of the lymphocytes were small or intermediate in size while 2 per cent exhibited morphologic features characteristic of cells undergoing blast transformation. There was a strong and positive correlation between the increasing fibroblast size and the numerical density of medium sized lymphocytes and immunoblasts. Taken over all, the data was consistent with the theory that cytopathic alteration of fibroblasts brought about by sensitized lymphoid cells may be responsible for the observed loss of connective tissue substance which is associated in the early gingival lesion. The observation that gingival collagen turns over at an inordinately accelerated rate and the demonstration of cytopathic alterations in gingival fibroblasts in inflamed tissues serve as a basis for a concept to account for the loss of connective tissue substance in periodontitis. In the early lesions, sensitized lymphoid cells responding to plaque antigen may induce cytopathic changes in fibroblasts and interfere with their normal functional capacity. The collagen loss, at least in the early gingival lesion, may result from lack of collagen production and maintenance, rather than col-lagen destruction. As the lesion develops, release of enzymes from macrophages and polymorphonuclear leucocytes and the action of bacterial collagenases may play an increasingly important role [72].

Cytopathic alterations in connective tissue fibroblasts have been demonstrated [72] and blastogenic type medium sized lymphocytes were seen intimately associated with the degenerating fibroblasts which suggests lymphotoxin mediated cytotoxicity or direct lymphocytotoxicity. Lymphokines may mediate collagenase release from macrophages [89] and neutrophils [90] which would contribute to further dissolution of collagen fibres. Production of osteoclast activation factor (O.A.F.) may account for the bone resorption in chronic periodontitis [34].

CONTAINED AND PROGRESSIVE LESIONS IN PERIODONTITIS

The plaque gingival tissue interphase is a homeostatic system within which a degree of tissue destruction is inevitable and normal except in artificially induced situations. Where the rate of destruction and repair are approximately in balance, there exists a contained lesion which may remain stable and non-progressive for very long periods of time. In some individuals at some points in time this stable lesion becomes converted into a slowly progressively destructive lesion for reasons which are not presently clear. While the evidence suggests that 'contained' gingivitis is virtually the norm particularly in the young individual, the probability is that the occurrence of the progressive lesion with increasing age is episodic and even well established periodontitis may have prolonged contained non-destructive phases.

A degree of general agreement has emerged that the microbial composition of a plaque and the host response that the particular composition evokes are unique to a particular site in the mouth at a particular point of time. Specific groups of micro-orgaisms which may emerge particularly in subgingival plaque may have the antigenic potential to induce local immune responses which may be variably tissue destructive. It has been suggested that variation in the response induced may be assessed on the basis of measure of alteration of the size of the area of inflamed connective tissue, the lymphocyte plasma cell ratios which are present [91], or the predominance of T or B lymphocytes in a particular area of inflamed connective tissue [92].

The development of chronic inflammatory periodontal disease under experimental conditions has been described as occurring in four stages [91].

The initial lesion is essentially an acute inflammatory response occurring within two to four days following the accumulation of plaque. The area of inflamed connective tissue is localized to the sulcus region and constitutes some 5 to 10 per cent of the gingival connective tissue. This acute vasculitis persists during the subsequent phases of development of the disease process.

The early lesion in humans appears at the site of the initial lesion within four to seven days following the beginning of plaque accumulation. The infiltrated area may come to occupy approximately 5 to 15 per cent of the marginal gingival connective tissue and lymphoid cells constitute approximately 75 per cent of the total cellular population. Within the reaction site collagen loss may reach 60 to 70 per cent.

The established lesion develops within two to three weeks following the beginning of plaque accumulation in adults. The distinguishing feature is the presence of a predominance of plasma cells within the affected connective tissue, in the absence of extensive bone loss. The plasma cells are not confined to the reaction site but appear in clusters along the blood vessels and between the collagen fibre bundles deep within the connective tissues. The established lesion is extremely widespread in humans and animals.

The clinical features of the advanced lesion are well known. The area of inflamed connective tissue is no longer localized and may extend apically and laterally to form a variably broad band around the necks and roots of the teeth. The lesion is characterized by a dense infiltrate of plasma cells, lymphocytes and macrophages superimposed upon the acute vasculitis which still persists. Many of the plasma cells appear to be degenerating.

The presently accepted view is that the initial, early and established lesions, represent stages in the development of contained gingivitis, and the advanced lesion progressive destructive periodontitis. In general the cellular composition, structure, size and location of the established and advanced lesion are essentially similar and the reason for the increased destructive capacity of the advanced lesion is not clear.

The association of a predominance of plasma cells with the established and the advanced lesion is well recognized and has been previously described [74, 93 & 94]. In contrast to this, periodontal disease associated with the deciduous dentition shows a predominance of lymphocytes with very few plasma cells present and then only at the edge of the lesion [95]. This lesion in children closely resembles the so-called early lesion in adults and does not seem to progress to the established or advanced lesion.

It has been demonstrated that following treatment of the established or advanced type of lesion in adults where plasma cells constituted close to 50 per cent of all the cells in the infiltrate, the cellular composition of the infiltrate was significantly altered. After treatment, lymphoid cells came to account for approximately 50 per cent of all the cells in the post treatment infiltrate with plasma cells present only occasionally [96].

At the present stage of knowledge there is good evidence that the progressive destructive lesion is a B cell lesion and more limited evidence to suggest that the contained stable lesion is a T cell lesion [97]. The cell types present in the advanced lesion have been extensively studied [98]. Using a variety of phenotypic markers, these workers have shown that the majority of lymphocytes present in the advanced lesion have the phenotype $IgM^+/Ia\text{-like}^+/HuTLA^-/T\text{-enzyme}^-.$* This phenotype is suggestive of B cells and as such the lesion should be considered a B cell lesion. While the results of these studies have shown that the advanced lesion in

---

* *IgM*: Immunoglobulin bearing. *Ia-like*: In the mouse antibodies directed against antigens coded for by genes in the I region (Ir gene) of the H-2 complex (Ia antigens) inhibit binding of immune complexes to B cells. *HuTLA*: Human thymus lymphocyte antigen. *T-enzyme*: Histochemical demonstration of the presence of enzymes such as acid phosphatase, β glucuronidase non-specific esterases etc.

humans should be considered predominantly a B cell lesion, cells with the phenotype of IgM$^-$/Ia-like$^-$/HuTLA$^+$/T-enzyme$^+$ have also been described [92, 98 & 99]. These cells are probably T cells and their occurrence in small numbers would seem to indicate that their primary role in progressive periodontal disease is one of 'helper activity' co-operating with macrophages in non-specific stimulation of B cells or in specific antigen presentation and hence antibody production.

Mackler *et al.* [100 & 101] have shown that mild gingivitis in adults as assessed by the Russell and Ramfjord indices is a lymphocyte dominated lesion while periodontitis as assessed by the same indices is a plasma cell dominated lesion. It was demonstrated that the majority of lymphocytes in the periodontitis group were immunoglobulin bearing, suggestive of B cells, but in the gingivitis group the lymphocytes were immunoglobulin negative and by exclusion T cells. Severe gingivitis appeared to be a transitional stage in that half the infiltrate lymphocytes possessed membrane bound IgG characteristic of a B cell population. These findings further support the hypothesis that the contained gingival lesion is probably a T cell lesion, while the progressive lesion is a B cell response.

It is possible to explain a stable T cell lesion in terms of negative feedback mechanisms in the presence of persistent antigens [92]. Lymphokines are widely regarded as mediators of the T cell response. It has been shown that prostaglandin PGE will inhibit both the production of lymphokines as measured by inhibition of macrophage migration and the transformation of lymphocytes [102 & 103]. It has been suggested that this mechanism affords a means of homeostatic control [92]. The production of PGE by macrophages activated by the lymphokine macrophage activating factor (MAF) would limit further lymphokine production. This negative feedback mechanism would then modulate the T cell response such that in terms of chronic inflammatory periodontal disease the lesion would remain stable.

The B cell progressive lesion would not be influenced by similar negative feedback control mechanisms. Stimulation of macrophages by immune complexes [104] might lead to an un-controlled production of PGE and hydrolytic enzymes. Persistent non-specific mitogenesis of B cells might also lead to the production of relatively large amounts of B cell lymphokines which could not be controlled by this feedback mechanism. It is possible that the uncontrolled production of lymphokines, prostaglandins and hydrolytic enzymes, postulated by Page and Schroeder [91] as being responsible for the tissue damage observed in the advanced lesion, could be explained in terms of a B cell response.

There is increasing evidence that the still prevalent view that dental plaque composition is reasonably consistent in health and disease and from site to site in the mouth is clearly not valid. Plaques have a variable tissue destructive capacity according to their microbial composition and are unique to a particular site in the mouth at any point in time. The immune response they evoke is probably unique to that site at that point in time. Different forms of periodontal disease probably have specific microbial aetiologies although these can only be identified in general terms at the present stage (see fig. 4.8, page 55).

Healthy periodontal tissues appear to be associated with a relatively scanty microbial flora located almost entirely supragingivally on the tooth surface, although even in health, there must be some subgingival plaque. Microbial cell accumulations are 1–20 cells in thickness made up mainly of Gram-positive coccal forms. The microorganisms commonly encountered in such sites in adults include *Streptococcus mitis*, *Streptococcus sanguis*, *Staphylococcus epidermis*, *Rothia dentocariosa*, *Actinomyces viscosus*, *Actinomyces naeslundii* and occasional species of *Nisseria* and *Veillonella* [105–108].

In experimental gingivitis there is an increase in the total mass of cell layers which often extend from 100–200 cells in thickness and is frequently attached to the tooth with a pallisade structure at right angles to the tooth surface. The increase in plaque mass is accompanied by an increase in the proportions of the members of the genus actinomyces. This group of organisms tends to be the dominant genus associated with supragingival plaque and gingivitis associated subgingival plaque frequently comprising of 50 per cent more of the isolates. The predominantly cultivable microbiota in developing plaques of this type is almost entirely Gram-positive and appears to represent an overgrowth of some of the forms found in plaque associated with healthy sites [106].

In long-standing gingivitis approximately 25 per cent of the microbiota may be Gram-negative including species of *Veillonella*, *Campylobacter*, *Fusobacterium* and *Spirochaeta* [107 & 109]. The structural organization becomes such that the Gram-negative cells and spirochaetes appear to be located primarily on the surface of the plaque immediately adjacent to the host tissues in subgingival sites.

Microbiological examination of subgingival plaque in rapidly destructive periodontitis has shown a largely motile plaque with predominance of Gram-negative rods [107]. A number of patterns of subgingival colonization has been observed. For example, one pattern appears to be dominated by *Bacteroides melaninogenicus asaccharolyticus* associated with large numbers of 6.12.6 axial-fibril rod spirochaetes.

A second pattern has been shown to consist of large numbers of monotrichously flagellated organisms and 'corroding bacteria' including an undescribed genes of anaerobic vibrios, *Bacteroides corrodens* and *Eikenella corrodens*. Other species associated with this pattern are *Fusobacterium nucleatum* and a recently described group of fusiform shape gelatine loving *Bacteroides* [105].

In the advanced lesion bacterial deposits are abundant and often consist in part of a zone of primarily Gram-positive organisms which are tooth attached and, between this zone and the epithelium, a zone of loosely free swimming Gram-negative organisms and spirochaetes which extend to the apical portion of the pocket.

It has been suggested [92] that this shift in the plaque microflora from an essentially Gram-positive population in health and early contained gingivitis, to one with increasing numbers of lipopoly saccharide bearing Gram-negative organisms is responsible for the emergence of the B cell lesion. On the other hand, the B cell mitogenic properties of *Actinomyces viscosus* have been recently demonstrated [110 & 111]. This organism forms a dominant part of plaques associated with gingivitis [112] and the *in vitro*

responses to the organism in terms of blast transformation relate more to gingivitis than to severe disease [113]. It has been suggested that the presence of *Actinomyces* organisms in plaque is responsible for the development of the initial B cell lesion which progresses creating conditions for the Gram-negative plaque to develop which in turn maintains the B cell lesion [92].

It is clear at the present stage that disease sites are predominated by microorganisms which are not dominant in supragingival plaque, but rather these less usual groups which emerge as a result of internal plaque growth in subgingival sites. There is no doubt that over the long term only cultural studies will provide the information which is necessary for truly selective disease control but there would appear to be little immediate prospect of developing a cultural technique suitable for widespread routine clinical diagnostic use.

Morphological techniques have for many years repeatedly indicated an association of certain microorganisms with periodontal disease. More than half a century ago, Kritchevsky and Seguin [114] recognized the association of spirochaetes with periodontal lesions and were able to distinguish three different types of spirochaetes in smears of bacteria from untreated pockets. They also presented data to show that anti-syphilitic therapy had a concomitant beneficial influence on the periodontal status of the patient. Rosebury *et al.* [115] noted that spirochaetes, vibrios and fusiform baccilli were found in much larger numbers in diseased sites than in healthy sites. Schultz-Haudt *et al.* [116] noted a dramatic increase in the relative proportion of spirochaetes from sites of health to disease from 0·6 per cent to 17 per cent in the presence of gingivitis and in the proportion of vibrios which increased from 1 to 11 per cent.

It has been suggested that by monitoring the proportions of bacteria present by phase contrast [117 & 118] or dark ground microscopy [119] it should be possible to decide the presence or absence of active disease, the prognosis or outcome of any therapy, and the frequency of recall which a particular patient requires.

The sampling technique is to clear any obvious supragingival bacterial deposits from the tooth and obtain a sample of the subgingival flora from the depths of the pocket with a curette. The sample is put in physiological saline containing 0·1 per cent gelatine and examined within one hour either by phase contrast or dark ground microscopy.

A standardized treatment programme for all patients in the care of the department of Periodontology of the Edinburgh Dental School was designed to be monitored by these techniques (see table 12.2, page 199). The patients are divided into three treatment streams according to the pocket depth criteria of the WHO 621 Report [120]. Treatment given is conventional with the exception that since it is clear that present methods of attempting to achieve control of periodontal disease are highly ineffective [121], there is a need to investigate means of increasing the time interval between appointments necessary for control of disease. The methods selected for investigation were subgingival flushing of 2 per cent chlorhexidine administered from a 10 ml syringe through a 23 gauge needle by an intracrevicular/pocket technique at four points around each tooth, and a patient self-administered 'salt out' technique using a mixture of baking soda, common salt and 3 per cent hydrogen peroxide as described by Keyes *et al.* [117 & 118].

Pocket depths of less than 3·5 mm were regarded as being within the general category of health and it was assumed that routine scaling, subgingival chlorhexidine flushing and self administered 'salt out' would achieve control in one to two visits. Patients with one or more pockets with a depth in excess of 3·5 mm were given a scaling, chlorhexidine flushing and 'salt out' programme of four visits extending over a period of approximately eight weeks. Any pocket remaining patent following this eight week programme was then treated by the modified Widman flap procedure [122] or by a conventional surgical pocket ablation technique. Where the microbiological picture maintains a disease pattern throughout the eight weeks, surgery is performed under antibiotic or metronidazole cover. At each visit sample pockets are monitored by phase contrast microscopy and a decision as to health or disease is made in the terms that health should be associated with a sparse population consisting predominantly of coccal forms and disease with the presence of large motile rods, spirochaetes, numerous leucocytes and a positive bleeding index.

While phase contrast microscopy proved convenient for routine clinical monitoring of large numbers of patients, it proved inadequate for a bacterial counting programme. Comparison of the same field under dark ground illumination and phase contrast microscopy showed that frequently large numbers of spirochaetes were present which were not evident to an experienced microbiologist under high quality phase contrast. The counting programme was based on a modification of the dark ground illumination technique described by Listgarten and Helden [119]. This technique was based on the classification of 1–200 bacteria from fields selected at random into nine morphological categories. Clear differences between the microbial populations in health and disease were demonstrated.

In health the proportion of coccoid cells is more than three times as high as in sites of disease and accounts for more than 75 per cent of the population.

The range of motility from health to disease was demonstrated as being from 1–50 to 1–1 and there was a 21-fold increase in the proportion of spirochaetes from health to disease [119].

On this basis it would appear that key parameters in the measure of health against disease by dark ground microscopy are the occurrence of motility and spirochaetes. The range of motility from 1–50 to 1–1 and the 21-fold increase in the number of spirochaetes constitute such large differences that it was assumed that these should be evident on a simpler scale designed for speed of counting for routine patient monitoring.

The clinical parameters chosen for comparison were pocket depth according to the criteria of the WHO 621 Report and Gingival Index [120 & 123]. The range of motility was expressed on a scale extending from 1–30 to 1–1, and the percentage of spirochaetes on a scale extending from 0–30 per cent for a random selected field on each smear (table 6.2).

Comparing GI against spirochaetes [124] on this scale it is clear that, as the GI increases, so do the number of spirochaetes. There is, how-

TABLE 6.2. Pilot study parameters.

WHO 621	Gingival Index	Motility	Spirochaetes %
< 3·5 mm	0	1–30	0
> 3·5 mm < 5·5 mm	1	1–20	5
> 5·5 mm	2	1–10	10
	3	1– 5	20
		1– 1	30

ever, considerable overlap. At a GI of 0 and 1, spirochaetes in the region of or in excess of 5 per cent are a relatively common finding and, at a GI of 3, some 20 per cent of the observations are in the no spirochaete range. Spirochaetes have been demonstrated to constitute approximately one-third of the subgingival flora in severely diseased sites [119]. It has been reported that in an infiltrate where the adjacent microbial population contains 5 per cent spirochaetes or less, the small lymphocyte is the dominant cell. Where it contains 5 per cent spirochaetes or more, the dominant cell is the plasma cell [96].

Comparing GI with motility, as the GI increases so does the motility but there is a degree of overlap. At GI 0 15 per cent of the observations are at 1 : 10 motility or more and at GI 3 almost 30 per cent of the observations are at 1 : 30 motility or less which should be firmly in the health range.

There is a poor correlation between pocket depth and the occurrence of spirochaetes. Forty per cent of the pockets of less than 3·5 mm depth have more than 5 per cent spirochaetes and about 50 per cent of the observations of 5·5 mm or more in depth have 5 per cent spirochaetes or less. The extent to which this overlap might represent variation in disease activity is unknown.

Motility does increase as the pocket depth increased but there is again a degree of overlap. While there is little 1–10 or greater motility at pocket depths of less than 3·5 mm, almost half the observations at pocket depths of 5·5 mm or more are well over towards the health end of the scale.

Following scaling, there is considerable reduction in the number of spirochaetes retrievable at the same visit but considerable rebound towards a disease pattern after one week. There is still however some evidence of improvement after two weeks.

In terms of motility there is a considerable reduction at the same visit following scaling which tends to be well maintained over two consecutive weeks.

Following scaling and chlorhexidine flushing, the number of spirochaetes is much reduced at the same visit but after two weeks only 17 per cent of the observations are in the 5 per cent spirochaetes or less range.

The change in motility following scaling and chlorhexidine flushing shows a similar pattern.

The change in spirochaete counts and motility is marginally in favour of scaling and chlorhexidine flushing as against scaling alone but the difference would appear to be relatively small. Some degree of rebound towards a disease pattern within two weeks appears to occur with both treatments.

There must be doubts as to the reproducibility of the sampling technique in terms of consistency of retrieval of organisms which are present. Taking a sample from a precise location such as the most apical part of a deep pocket while an idealized goal is a difficult task. The desired sample may occupy a band of less than 1 mm in diameter and must be approached through either an overlying tissue mass or the intervening pocket microbiotic [125].

The counting of percentages of 100–200 organisms in nine morphological categories as proposed by Listgarten and Helden [119] presents difficulties in terms of routine patient monitoring in that an output of six smears counted per hour may be reasonable for this technique. The modification of the counting technique to expressing motility ratio and percentage spirochaetes on the scales suggested allowed a throughput of fifteen smears per hour and the results generally accord with the concepts of health and disease expressed by Listgarten and Helden [119] in terms of these parameters.

The findings that 40 per cent of pockets of > 3·5 mm showed counts of 5 per cent spirochaetes or more and that almost 50 per cent of pockets < 5·5 mm showed counts of 5 per cent spirochaetes or less may have implications in terms of the reported relationship of ±5 per cent spirochaetes to the predominance of lympho-cytes and plasma cells in the associated infiltrate [96].

The presence of a predominantly lymphocyte infiltrate in mild gingivitis has been reported in a number of studies [91, 100, 101 & 126]. The extent to which this may be related to the low incidence of spirochaetes in young children is presently speculative [124].

It has been suggested that severe gingivitis may be a transitional stage to periodontitis in that it has been shown that at this stage half the infiltrating lymphocytes possessed membrane IgG [101]. This may be generally in accord with the relationship of GI to spirochaetes in this study [124].

There is no good evidence to the effect that rate of tissue destruction is directly related to extent of destruction as measured by pocket depth or similar criteria.

High rates of disease activity are probably episodic and it may be that clinical gingivitis may undergo periods of a high rate of tissue destruction and periodontitis 'contained' periods with no progressive tissue destruction.

There is a need to relate particular microbial populations to the cellular infiltrate of adjacent tissues at various stages in the disease process in a relatively large number of individuals. The extent to which periods of disease activity or quiescence are reflected by measurable change in the microbial population of a plaque or the cellular or humoral phases of the response evoked is still largely speculative.

(Pages 108–114 have been reproduced from MacPhee and Muir [124].)

SUGGESTED TEXTS

WARD F.A. (1970) *A Primer of Immunology*. London: Butterworths.

HOLBORROW E.J. (1968) *An A.B.C. of Modern Immunology*. London: The Lancet Ltd.

WHITE R.G. & TIMBURY M.C. (1973) *Essentials of Immunology and Microbiology*. London: Pitman Medical.

HUMPHREY J.H. & WHITE R.G. (1970) *Immunology for Students of Medicine*, 3rd Edition. Oxford: Blackwell Scientific Publications.

ROITT I.M. (1974) *Essential Immunology*, 2nd Edition. Oxford: Blackwell Scientific Publications.

REFERENCES

[1] LÖE H. (1963) Epidemiology of periodontal disease. *Odont. T.* **71**, 479.

[2] STAHL S.S. (1970) Host resistance and periodontal disease. *J. Dent. Res.* **49**, 248.

[3] RAY H.G. & ORBAN B. (1950) Gingival structures in diabetes mellitus. *J. Periodont.* **21**, 85.

[4] GLICKMAN I. (1958) *Clinical Periodontology*, 2nd Edition, p. 409. Philadelphia: W.B. Saunders Co.

[5] ZISKIN D.E. (1946) Pregnancy gingivitis. *Alpha Omegan* **40**.

[6] MAIER A.W. & ORBAN B. (1949) Gingivitis in pregnancy. *Oral Surg.* **2**, 334.

[7] LARATO D.C. *et al.* (1969) The effect of a prescribed method of toothbrushing on the fluctuation of marginal gingivitis. *J. Periodont.* **40**, 142.

[8] MACPHEE T. (1973) Host resistance to dental plaque, in *Host Resistance to Commensal Bacteria*. Ed. MacPhee T. Edinburgh: Churchill Livingstone.

[9] STAHL S.S. *et al.* (1968) Autoradiographic evaluation of gingival response to injury. I. Surgical trauma in young adult rats. *Arch. Oral Biol.* **13**, 71.

[10] TONNA E.A. *et al.* (1969) Autoradiographic evaluation of gingival response to injury. II. Surgical trauma in young rats. *Arch. Oral Biol.* **14**, 19.

[11] STAHL S.S. *et al.* (1970) Autoradiographic evaluation of gingival response to injury. III. Surgical trauma in mature rats. *Arch. Oral Biol.* **15**, 537.

[12] RAMFJORD S.P., KERR D.A. & ASH M. (1966) *World Workshop in Periodontics*. Michigan: Ann Arbor.

[13] EGELBERG J. (1963) Diffusion of histamine into the gingival crevice and through the crevicular epithelium. *Acta Odont. Scand.* **21**, 271.

[14] FINE D.H. *et al.* (1969) The penetration of human gingival sulcular tissue by carbon particles. *Arch. Oral Biol.* **14**, 1117.

[15] EGELBERG J. (1970) *Dental Plaque*, p. 13. Ed. McHugh W.D. Edinburgh: Churchill Livingstone.

[16] SCHROEDER H.E. (1970) The structure and relationship of plaque to the hard and soft tissues. Electron microscopic interpretation. *Int. dent. J.* **20**, 353–381.

[17] SCHROEDER H.E. (1973) Transmigration and infiltration of leucocytes in human junctional epithelium. *Helv. Odont. Acta* **17**, 6–18.

[18] LANGE D. & SCHROEDER H.E. (1971) Cytochemistry

and ultrastructure of gingival sulcus cells. *Helv. Odont. Acta* **15**, Suppl. **VI**, 65–86.

[19] FRANK R.M. & CIMASONI G. (1972) Electron microscopy of acid phosphatase in the exudate from inflamed gingivae. *J. Periodont. Res.* **7**, 213–225.

[20] SHANDS J.W. (1967) *Modern Trends in Immunology*, 2nd Edition, p. 87. Eds. Cruikshank R & Weir D.M. London: Butterworths.

[21] DICK H.M. & TROTT J.R. (1969) Immunity and inflammation as synergistic mechanisms in the pathogenesis of periodontal disease. *J. Periodont. Res.* **4**, 127.

[22] NISENGARD R.J. & BEUTNER E.H. (1970) Relation of immediate hypersensitivity to periodontitis in animals and man. *J. Periodont.* **41**, 223.

[23] BURKE J.F. (1971) Effects of inflammation on wound repair. *J. Dent. Res.* **50**, 296.

[24] BRANDTZAEG P. (1973) Local formation and transport of immunoglobulins, in *Host Resistance to Commensal Bacteria. The Response to Dental Plaque*, p. 139. Ed. MacPhee T. Edinburgh: Churchill Livingstone.

[25] KLEBANOFF S.J. & LUEBKE R.J. (1965) The antilactobacillus system of saliva. *Proc. Soc. Exp. Biol.* **118**, 483.

[26] NOWELL P.C. (1960) P.H.A., an initiator of mitosis in culture of normal human leucocytes. *Cancer Res.* **20**, 562.

[27] PERLMANN P. & HOLM G. (1969) Cytotoxic effects of lymphoid cells *in vitro*. *Adv. Immunol.* **11**, 117.

[28] DUMONDE D.C. (1970) Lymphokines, molecular mediators of cellular immune responses in animal and man. *Proc. Roy. Soc. Med.* **63**, 899.

[29] PICK E. & TURKE J.L. (1972) The biological activities of soluble lymphocyte products. *Clin. Exp. Immunol.* **10**, 1.

[30] MORLEY J., WOLSTENCROFT R.A. & DUMONDE D.C. (1973) The measurement of lymphokines, in *Handbook of Experimental Immunology*, 2nd Edition, vol. 2. Ed. Weir D.M. Oxford: Blackwell Scientific Publications.

[31] TURK J.L. (1967) Delayed hypersensitivity—specific cell-mediated immunity. *Brit. Med. Bull.* **23**, 1.

[32] LAWRENCE H.S. & LANDY M., Eds. (1969) *Mediators of Cellular Immunity*. New York: Academic Press.

[33] HORTON J.E., OPPENHEIM J.J. & MERGENHAGEN S.E. (1973) Elaboration of lymphotoxin by cultured human peripheral blood leucocytes stimulated with dental plaque deposits. *Clin. and Exp. Immunol.* **13**, 383.

[34] HORTON J.E., RAISZ L.G., SIMMONS H.A., OPPENHEIM J.J. & MERGENHAGEN S.E. (1972) Bone resorbing activity in supernatant fluid from cultured human peripheral blood leucocytes. *Science* **177**, 793.

[35] MAYER M.N. (1961) Complement, in *Experimental Immunochemistry*, 2nd Edition. Eds. Kabat & Mayer. Springfield, Ill.: Thomas.

[36] MÜLLER-EBERHARD H.J. (1971) Biochemistry of complement, in *Progress in Immunology*. Ed. Amos B. New York: Academic Press.

[37] HUMPHREY J.H. & WHITE R.G. (1970) *Immunology for Students of Medicine*, 3rd Edition, p. 195. Oxford: Blackwell Scientific Publications.

[38] SANDBER A.L., OSLER A.G., SHIN H.S. & OLIVERA B. (1970) The biologic activities of guinea-pig antibodies. II. Modes of complement interaction of gamma 1 and gamma 2 immunoglobulins. *J. Immunol.* **104**, 329.

[39] GÖTZE O. & MÜLLER-EBERHARD H.J. (1971) The C'3-activator system. An alternate pathway of complement activation. *J. Exp. Med.* **134**, Suppl. 905.

[40] MERGENHAGEN S.E. (1973) A role for complement in host resistance to commensal bacteria, in *Host Resistance to Commensal Bacteria. The Response to Dental Plaque*, p. 100. Ed. MacPhee T. Edinburgh: Churchill Livingstone.

[41] IVANYI L. & LEHNER T. (1970) Stimulation of lymphocyte transformation by bacterial antigens in patients with periodontal disease. *Arch. Oral Biol.* **16**, 1117.

[42] ROCKLIN R.E., MEYERS O.L. & DAVID J.R. (1970) An *in vitro* assay for cellular hypersensitivity in man. *J. Immunol.* **104**, 95.

[43] IVANYI L., WILTON J.M.A. & LEHNER T. (1972) Cell-mediated immunity in periodontal disease; cytotoxicity, migration inhibition and lymphocyte transformation studies. *Immunology* **22**, 141.

[44] OPPENHEIM J.J. (1972) Modulation of *in vitro* lymphocyte transformation by antibodies. Enhancement by antigen-antibody complexes and inhibition by antibody excess. *Cell Immunol.* **3**, 41.

[45] LEHNER T. (1973) Cellular immunity to oral infections, in *Host Resistance to Commensal Bacteria. The Responses to Dental Plaque*. Ed. MacPhee I.T. Edinburgh: Churchill Livingstone.

[46] WILTON J.M.A., IVANYI L. & LEHNER T. (1972) Cell-mediated immunity in *herpes virus hominis* infections. *Brit. Med. J.* **1**, 723.

[47] HORTON J.E., LEIKINS S. & OPPENHEIM J.J. (1972) Human lympho-proliferative reaction to saliva and dental plaque deposits: An *in vitro* correlation with periodontal disease. *J. Periodont.* **43**, 522.

[48] DE DUVE C. *et al.* (1955) Tissue fractionation studies. 6. Intracellular distribution patterns of enzymes in rat liver tissue. *Biochem. J.* **60**, 604.

[49] DE DUVE C. & BAUIDHUIN P. (1966) Peroxisomes (microbodies and related particles). *Physiol. Rev.* **46**, 323.

[50] MICHELL R.H. *et al.* (1970) The distribution of some granule associated enzymes in guinea-pig polymorphonuclear leucocytes. *Biochem. J.* **116**, 207.

[51] MELLY M.A. *et al.* (1960) Fate of staphylococci within human leukocytes. *J. Exp. Med.* **112**, 1121.

[52] JENKIN C. & BENACERRAF B. (1960) *In vitro* studies on the interaction between mouse peritoneal macrophages and strains of Salmonella and *Escherichia coli*. *J. Exp. Med.* **112**, 403.

[53] ALLISON M.J. *et al.* (1962) The correlation of a biphasic metabolic response in resistance to tuberculosis in rabbits. *J. Exp. Med.* **115**, 881.

[54] ALLISON M.J. *et al.* (1961) Metabolic studies on mononuclear cells from rabbits of varying genetic resistance to tuberculosis. I. Studies on cells of normal non-infected animals. *Amer. Rev. res. Dis.* **84**, 364.

[55] BOHME D. *et al.* (1961) Behaviour of acid phosphatase in the reticuloendothelial system of genetically susceptible and resistant mice infected with typhimurium. *Amer. J. Path.* **39**, 103.

[56] PAVILLARD E.R. (1963) *In vitro* phagocytic and bactericidal ability of alveolar and peritoneal macrophages of normal rats. *Aust. J. Exp. Biol. Med. Sci.* **41**, 265.

[57] KLEBANOFF S.J. *et al.* (1966) The peroxidase-thiocyanate hydrogen peroxide antimicrobial system. *Biochem. Biophys. Acta* **117**, 63.

[58] MCRIPLEY R.J. & SBÁRRA A.J. (1967) Role of the phagocyte in host-parasite interactions. XI. Relationship between stimulated oxidative metabolism and hydrogen peroxide formation and intracellular killing. *J. Bact.* **94**, 1417.

[59] RECHCIGL M. Jr. & EVANS W.H. (1963) Role of catalase and peroxidase in the metabolism of leucocytes. *Nature (Lond.)* **199**, 1001.

[60] EVANS W.H. & RECHCIGL M. Jr. (1967) Factors influencing myeloperoxidase and catalase activities in polymorphonuclear leukocytes. *Biochem. Biophys. Acta* **148**, 243.

[61] AGNER K. (1950) Studies on peroxidative detoxification of purified diphtheria toxin. *J. Exp. Med.* **92**, 337.

[62] ZGLICZYNSKI J.M. *et al.* (1968) Myeloperoxidase of human leukaemic leucocytes. Oxidation of amino acids in the presence of hydrogen peroxide. *Europ. J. Biochem.* **4**, 540.

[63] HOLMES B. *et al.* (1966) Fatal granulomatous disease of childhood. An inborn abnormality of phagocytic function. *Lancet* **i**, 1225.

[64] QUIE P.G. *et al.* (1966) Decreased bactericidal activity of polymorphonuclear leukocytes in children with chronic granulomatous disease. *J. Clin. Invest.* **45**, 1058.

[65] TAKAHARA S. (1952) Progressive oral gangrene probably due to lack of catalase in blood (acatalasaemia). *Lancet* **ii**, 1101.

[66] NICOL A.D. *et al.* (1971) Erythrocyte catalase activity in human ulceromembranous gingivitis. *Arch. Oral Biol.* **16**, 21.

[67] COHEN G. & HOCHSTEIN P. (1963) Glutathione peroxidase: the primary agent for the elimination of hydrogen peroxide in erythrocytes. *Biochemistry (Washington)* **2**, 1420.

[68] COHN Z.A. & WIENER E. (1963) The particle hydrolases of macrophages. II. Biochemical and morphological response to particle ingestion. *J. Exp. Med.* **118**, 1009.

[69] WOESSNER J.F. Jr. (1965) Acid hydrolases of connective tissue. *International Review of Connective Tissue Research* **3**, 201.

[70] JANOFF A. *et al.* (1965) Mediators of inflammation in leucocyte lysosomes. II. Mechanism of action of lysosomal cationic protein upon vascular permeability in the rat. *J. Exp. Med.* **122**, 841.

[71] SEEGERS W. & JANOFF A. (1966) Mediators of inflammation in leucocyte lysosomes. VI. Partial purification and characterization of a mast cell-rupturing component. *J. Exp. Med.* **124**, 833.

[72] PAGE R.C. & SCHROEDER H.E. (1973) Biochemical aspects of the connective tissue alterations in inflammatory gingival and periodontal disease. *Int. Dent. J.* **23**, 455.

[73] TALBOT E.S. (1899) Interstitial gingivitis or so-called pyorrhoea alveolaris. Philadelphia: S.S. White Dental Hyg. Co.

[74] JAMES W.W. & COUNSELL A. (1927) Histological investigation of so-called pyorrhoea alveolaris. *Brit. Dent. J.* **48**, 1237.

[75] FULLMER H.M. (1961) A histochemical study of periodontal disease in maxillary alveolar processes of 135 autopsies. *J. Periodont.* **32**, 206.

[76] MELCHER A.H. (1967) Some histological and histochemical observations on connective tissues of chronically inflamed human gingiva. *J. Periodont. Res.* **2**, 127.

[77] CABRINI R.L. & CARRANZA F.A. (1966) Histochemistry of periodontal disease. A review of the literature. *Int. Dent. J.* **16**, 466.

[78] BALAZS E.A. & RODGERS H.J. (1965) The amino sugar-containing compounds in bones and teeth. *The Amino Sugars* **IIA**, 263.

[79] SCHULTZ-HAUDT S.D. & ASS E. (1960) Observations on the status of collagen in human gingiva. *Arch. Oral Biol.* **2**, 131.

[80] DE RYSKY S., CATTANEO V. & MONTANARI M.C. (1969) Determination quantitative des exasamines et de l'hydroxyproline dans les inflammations gingivates chroniques. *Bull. Group Int. Res. Sci. Stomatol.* **12**, 359.

[81] PAGE R.C. (1972) Macromolecular interactions in the connective tissues of the periodontium, in *Developmental Aspects of Oral Biology*. Eds. Slaukin H. & Bavetta L. New York: Academic Press.

[82] FLIEDER K.E., SUN C.H. & SCHNEIDER B.C. (1966) Chemistry of normal and inflamed human gingival tissues. *Periodontics* **4**, 302.

[83] SCHROEDER H.E., MUNZEL-PEDRAZZOLI S. & PAGE R.C. (1973) Correlated morphometric and biochemical analysis of gingival tissues. The early gingival lesion in man. *Arch. Oral Biol.* **18**, 899.

[84] SKOUGAARD M.R., LEVY B.M. & SIMPSON J. (1969) Collagen metabolism in skin and periodontal membrane of the marmoset. *J. Periodont. Res.*, Suppl. **4**, 28.

[85] CARNEIRO J. (1965) Synthesis and turnover of collagen in periodontal tissues. *Sym. Int. Soc. Cell Biol.* **4**, 247.

[86] CRUMBLEY J.P. (1964) Collagen formation in normal and stressed periodontium. *Periodontics* **2**, 53.

[87] CLAYCOMB C.K., SUMMERS G.W. & DIVORAK E.M. (1967) Oral collagen biosynthesis in the guinea-pig. *J. Periodont. Res.* **2**, 115.

[88] SCHROEDER H.E. & PAGE R.C. (1972) Lymphocyte-fibroblast interaction in the pathogenesis of inflammatory gingival disease. *Experientia* **28**, 1228.

[89] ROBERTSON P.G., SHYU K.W., VAIL M.S., TAYLOR R.E. & FULLMER H.M. (1973) Collagenase. Demonstration in rabbit macrophages. *J. Dent. Res.* (Special Issue) **189**, (Abs. 522).

[90] LAZARUS G.S., BROWN R.S., DANIELS J.R. & FULLMER H.M. (1968) Human granulocyte collagenase. *Science* **159**, 1483.

[91] PAGE R.C. & SCHROEDER H.E. (1976) Pathogenesis of inflammatory periodontal disease. A summary of current work. *Lab. Invest.* **33**, 235.

[92] SEYMOUR G.J., POWELL R.N. & DAVIES W.I.R. (1979) Conversion of a stable T cell lesion to a progressive B cell lesion in the pathogenesis of chronic inflammatory periodontal disease: a hypothesis. *J. Clin. Periodont.* **6**, 267.

[93] FREEDMAN H.L., LISTGARTEN M.A. & TAICHMAN N.S. (1968) Electron microscopic features of chronically inflamed human gingiva. *J. Periodont. Res.* **3**, 313.

[94] ZACHRISSON B.W. (1972) Gingival condition associated with orthodontic treatment. II. Histologic findings. *Angle Orthodontist* **42**, 352.

[95] LONGHURST P., JOHNSON N.W. & HOPPS R.M. (1977) Differences in lymphocyte and plasma cell densities in inflamed gingiva from adults and young children. *J. Periodont.* **48 (11)**, 705.

[96] LISTGARTEN M.A., LINDHE J. & HELLDEN L. (1978) The effect of tetracycline and/or scaling on human periodontal disease. Clinical microbiological and histological observations. *J. Clin. Periodont.* **5: 4**, 246.

[97] SEYMOUR G.J., DOCKRELL H.M. & GREENSPAN J.S. (1978) Enzyme differentiation of lymphocyte subpopulations in sections of human lymph nodes, tonsils and periodontal disease. *Clin. and Exp. Immunol.* **32**, 169.

[98] SEYMOUR G.J. & GREENSPAN J.J. (1979) The phenotypic characterisation of lymphocyte subpopulations in established human periodontal disease. *J. Periodont. Res.* **14**, 39.

[99] SEYMOUR G.J. (1978) The immunopathogenesis of chronic inflammatory periodontal disease in man: phenotypic characterisation of lymphoid cell subpopulations using enzyme and surface antigen markers. Ph.D. Thesis, University of London.

[100] MACKLER B.F. *et al.* (1977) Immunoglobulin bearing lymphocytes and plasma cells in human periodontal disease. Lymphoid cells in periodontal disease. *J. Periodont. Res.* **12**, 37.

[101] MACKLER B.F. *et al.* (1978) IgG subclasses in human periodontal disease. I. Distribution and incidence of IgG subclass bearing lymphocytes and plasma cells. *J. Periodont. Res.* **13**, 109.

[102] MORLEY J. (1976) Prostaglandins as regulators of lymphoid cell function in allergic inflammation: a basis for chronicity in rheumatoid arthritis, in *Infection and Immunology in Rheumatic Diseases.* Ed. Dumonde D.C., pp. 511–517. Oxford: Blackwell Scientific Publications.

[103] SMITH J.W. *et al.* (1971) Human lymphocyte metabolism. Effects of cyclic and non cyclic nucleotides on stimulation by phytohaemoglutinin. *J. Clin. Invest.* **50**, 442.

[104] CARDELLA C., DAVIES P. & ALLISON A.C. (1974) Immune complexes induce selective release of lysosomal hydrolases from macrophages. *Nature* **247**, 46.

[105] SOCRANSKY S.S. (1977) Microbiology of periodontal disease—present status and future considerations. *J. Periodont.* **48: 9**, 497.

[106] LISTGARTEN M.A., MAYO H.E. & TREMBLAY R. (1975) Development of dental plaque on epoxy resin crowns in man. A light and electron microscope study. *J. Periodont.* **46**, 10.

[107] LISTGARTEN M.A. (1976) Structure of microbial flora associated with periodontal disease and health in man. A light and electron microscope study. *J. Periodont.* **47**, 1.

[108] SLOTS J. (1977) The microflora in the healthy gingival sulcus in man. *Scand. J. Dent. Res.* **85**, 247.

[109] VAN PALENSTEIN HELDERMAN W.H. (1976) Total viable count and differential count of vibrio (campylobacter) sputorum, fusobacterium nucleatum, selenomonas sputigena, bacteroides ochraceous and veillonella in the inflamed and non inflamed human gingival crevice. *J. Periodont. Res.* **10**, 294.

[110] ENGEL D. *et al.* (1977) Mitogenic activity of actinomyces viscosus. I. Effects on murine B and T lymphocytes and partial characterisation. *J. Immunol.* **118**, 1466.

[111] BURKHARDT J., GUGGENHEIM B. & HEFTI A. (1977) Are actinomyces viscosus antigens B cell mitogens? *J. Immunol.* **118**, 1460.

[112] LOESCHE W.J. (1976) Chemotherapy of dental plaque infections. *Oral Sci. Rev.* **9**, 65.

[113] SMITH F.N. & LANG N.P. (1977) Lymphocyte blastogenesis to plaque antigens in human periodontal disease. II. The relationship to clinical parameters. *J. Periodont. Res.* **12**, 310.

[114] KRITCHEVSKY B. & SEGUIN P. (1918) The pathogenesis and treatment of pyorrhoea alveolaris. *Dental Cosmos.* **60**, 781.

[115] ROSEBURY T. *et al.* (1950) A bacteriological survey of gingival scrapings from periodontal infections by direct examination, guinea pig inoculation and anaerobic cultivation. *J. Dent. Res.* **29**, 718.

[116] SCHULTZ-HAUDT S.D., BRUCE M.A. & BIBBY B.G. (1954) Bacterial factors in non specific gingivitis. *J. Dent. Res.* **33**, 454.

[117] KEYES P.H., WRIGHT W.E. & HOWARD S.A. (1978) The use of phase contrast microscopy and chemotherapy in the diagnosis and treatment of periodontal lesions—an initial report (1). *Quintessence International* **1**, Report 1590, 51.

[118] KEYES P.H., WRIGHT W.E. & HOWARD S.A. (1978) The use of phase contrast microscopy and chemotherapy in the diagnosis and treatment of periodontal lesions—an initial report (I). *Quintessence International* **2**, Report 1590, 69.

[119] LISTGARTEN M.A. & HELDEN L. (1978) Relative distribution of bacteria at clinically healthy and periodontally diseased sites in humans. *J. Clin. Periodont.* **5**, 115.

[120] WORLD HEALTH ORGANIZATION (1978) Epidemiology, etiology and prevention of periodontal diseases. *Technical Report Series 621.* Geneva.

[121] AXELSSON P. & LINDHE J. (1978) Effects of controlled oral hygiene procedures on caries and periodontal disease in adults. *J. Clin. Periodont.* **5: 2**, 133.

[122] RAMFJORD S.P. & NISSLE R.R. (1974) The modified Widman flap. *J. Periodont.* **48(8)**, 601.

[123] LOE H. & SILNESS J. (1963) Periodontal disease in pregnancy. I. Prevalence and severity. *Acta Odont. Scand.* **21**, 533.

[124] MACPHEE I.T. & MUIR K.F. *European Commission Symposium on Efficacy of Treatment of Periodontal Disease.* In press.

[125] TANNER A.C.R. *et al.* (1979) A study of the bacteria associated with advancing periodontitis in man. *J. Clin. Periodont.* **6: 6**, 278.

[126] PAYNE W.A. *et al.* (1975) Histopathologic features of the initial and early stages of experimental gingivitis in man. *J. Periodont. Res.* **10**, 51.

CHAPTER 7

Central factors

CENTRAL FACTORS GOVERNING METABOLISM OF TISSUES WHICH MAY CONDITION THE HOST RESPONSE TO LOCAL IRRITATION

There is as yet no clear evidence demonstrating a direct relationship between the systemic control of tissue metabolism and the prevalence of periodontitis. Control of tissue metabolism is a complex phenomenon related to heredity, age, sex, endocrine control, psychosomatic factors and nutrition. All such factors may potentially be related to alteration of tissue resistance relative to the commensal population of the mouth. There is no indication that any single factor is responsible for a biochemical lesion, universally expressed in the mouth as periodontitis.

Traditionally, the mouth has been considered as an indicator of general health and nutritional state. If known systemic factors are associated with the initiation and prevalence of periodontitis, this should be demonstrable by epidemiological analysis (see chap. 16). Epidemiological surveys have confirmed that serious metabolic disease and ageing are directly related to the degree of severity of periodontal disease, but they do not explain the prevalence [1]. Physical examination of severely affected groups of the population has provided no clear evidence of specific systemic upset which would account for the increased severity within the group, and has led the World Health Organization to state:
'Epidemiological studies have failed to detect any systemic factors that are a significant primary cause of chronic periodontal disease, but some have demonstrated certain hormonal, metabolic, genetic, and nutritional variables that modify the progress of the disease' [2].

It seems probable that reduction of tissue resistance may result from metabolic change at the cellular level, which is not demonstrable at the present time, by assay of the level of circulating nutritional or hormonal factors in the blood. Reduction of tissue resistance may follow alteration of the dynamic equilibrium of epithelium or connective tissue. This may be the result of a change in utilization or availability of metabolites rather than a primary deficiency of metabolites.

Dynamic equilibrium of epithelium

The dynamic equilibrium of the epithelial sheath is such that there is a constant progression of cells from basal to surface layers, whereby the cell population of adult skin is renewed every 32–36 days. The rate of renewal of the cell population of gingival epithelium in mice is of the order of 10–12 days, and of junctional epithelium 2–5 days [3] (fig. 7.1). In epithelium the turnover rate is increased by age, keratin loss, increase in O_2 tension, increase in glucose level, administration of oestrogen and testosterone and the presence of inflammation. There is a decrease in rate of cell turnover in the presence of insulin induced hypoglycaemia, increased adrenalin or with the administration of cortisone. The presence of an endogenous mitotic inhibitor (Chalone), which is thought to exert some control of mitotic activity by forming a complex with adrenaline, has been demonstrated in epithelium [4].

There is considerable variation in the degree of keratinization of oral mucous membrane throughout the mouth (fig. 1.9). The degree of keratinization of epithelium is in part inherent to any particular region, but it is also related to function, to the rate of turnover of the cell population and to the presence or absence of inflammation [5]. The higher the rate of turnover of the cell population due to frictional loss of superficial layers, the less the time available for the process of keratinization to become complete. In the presence of inflammation the rate of cell turnover is increased, the probability of complete keratinization reduced, and in the region of the junctional epithelium in particular, the gingival tissue may be considered to be in a continuous phase of wound healing.

Dynamic equilibrium of connective tissue

Connective tissue may be regarded as a pool of polysaccharide–protein complexes, called the intercellular ground substance, which contains various types of vessels, nerves, fibres and cells. It is the medium through which water, salts, gases, nutrients, metabolic products and internal secretions must diffuse, and it is the site of the inflammatory reaction. The ground substance is condensed to a variable degree to form the fibrous elements of individual tissues. The degree of condensation may vary from the solid translucent material of hyaline cartilage to the fluid of synovial joints.

COLLAGEN

Collagen is the main fibrous protein of connective tissue and constitutes about one third of the total protein in the body. Skin, tendon, bone, cartilage, teeth, periodontal membrane and gingiva all contain collagen.

Collagen is synthesized by specialized connective tissue cells (fibroblasts) and the molecules are released into the intercellular spaces. The collagen molecule consists of three polypeptide chains each containing about 1000 amino acid residues. Each chain twists itself into a left handed helix and then three chains intertwine to form a right handed super helix, which is the tropocollagen molecule (fig. 7.2). Many tropocollagen molecules line up in a staggered fashion, overlapping one another by one quarter of their length, to form a fibril [6]. Fibrils in tissue are often stacked in layers, with groups of fibrils aligned at right angles. Groups of fibrils are seen in the optical microscope as bundles of collagen.

In most types of collagen, two of the polypeptide chains ($\alpha 1$) are identical in amino acid composition, whilst the third ($\alpha 2$) has a different composition. Collagen is subjected to the activity of several enzyme systems that modify the molecules during and after their synthesis. Hydroxylation of the lysyl and prolyl residues is carried

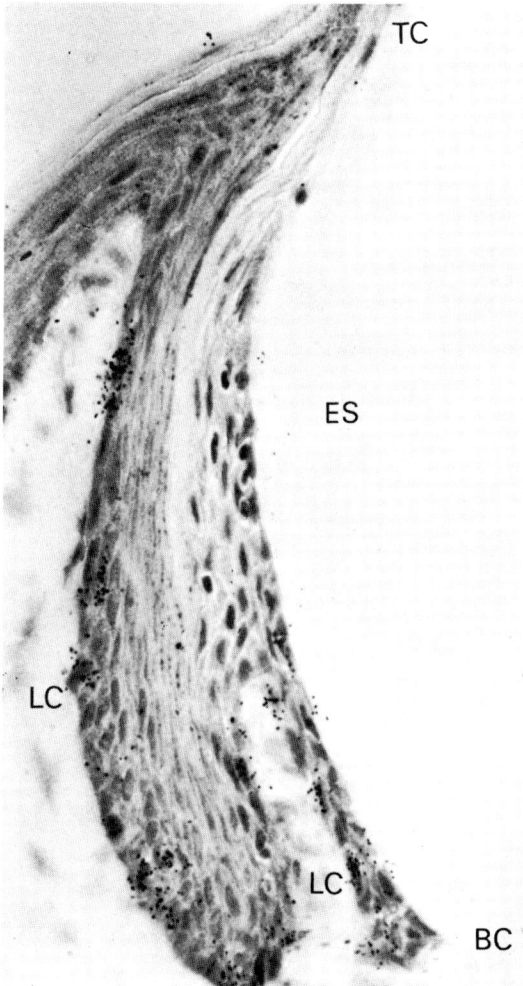

FIG. 7.1. Autoradiograph of cuff epithelium of mouse previously injected with H^3 thymidine; TC, top of cuff; BC, base of cuff. Labelled cells (LC) indicating dividing cells are present in the basal layers and in the epithelium contiguous to enamel space (ES). Courtesy of Professor G. S. Beagrie.

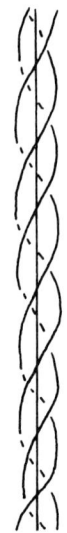

FIG. 7.2. Tropocollagen. Three helical polypeptide chains wound round a common axis.

out by specific enzyme systems located in the microsomes. Subsequently the chains are acted on by a glycosyl transferase system that catalyses glycosylation of some hydroxylysyl side chains. After extrusion to the extracellular space, tropocollagen molecules are acted upon by lysyl oxidase, which initiates the maturation and stabilization process.

The form of collagen containing two $\alpha 1$ and one $\alpha 2$ chains per molecule is the major molecular form present in most connective tissues (Type 1) but it is now apparent that other molecular types exist. A form of collagen with three $\alpha 1$ chains which are homologous to, but not identical with, the $\alpha 1$ chains described, has been isolated from cartilage and it now appears that additional molecular species may be present in basal lamina and as a minor component in other connective tissues (Types II, III and IV). A recent paper has suggested Type I collagen is the principal constituent of human gingival connective tissue but that 5 to 30 per cent is Type III. Fibroblasts from diseased gingiva were found to synthesize a collagen of $(\alpha 1)_3$, probably of Type I [7].

Collagen stability

The stability of collagen fibres is a function of the degree of covalent interchain crosslinking. Evidence is rapidly accumulating to support the concept that the degree of crosslinking in the collagenous component of the gingiva is much less than that seen in other mature connective tissues [8]. Newly synthesized collagen molecules aggregate very rapidly into fibrils, and in most connective tissues undergo stabilization by covalent interchain crosslinking within a matter of hours. Extraction of tissues with dilute saline solutions at neutral pH and 4°C removes the newly synthesized noncrosslinked collagen and, therefore, serves as a simple way to measure the size of the unstabilized collagen compartments. In comparison with skin, human gingiva contains an inordinately large pool of recently synthesized unstable collagen [8].

Collagen turnover

Collagen exhibits different rates of turnover from species to species and from organ to organ within the same animal. In the rat for example, collagen in the aorta and tendons is relatively inert; in bone there is a moderate turnover; in liver or gut, replacement occurs in 30–50 days; and in the dermis 50 per cent of labelled collagen is present after 300 days. In most connective tissues, the rates of synthesis and degradation of collagen decrease markedly as the animal reaches adulthood. Current evidence suggests that the turnover of the collagenous component of the gingiva may remain high, even in the adult. Experiments using radioactive labelled precursors in various animals, including young adult marmosets, lend support to the concept that the collagenous component of the normal noninflamed primate gingiva undergoes an inordinately rapid rate of synthesis relative to other mature adult tissues [8].

Collagen breakdown and the role of inflammation

Under homeostatic conditions, collagen is highly resistant to the proteolytic enzymes found in tissue fluid, and for many years it was the view that there did not exist in mammalian tissue an enzyme that was capable of digesting collagen at physiological pH. However, under certain circumstances, such as an involuting uterus or an area of inflamed tissue, collagen can be rapidly removed from an area.

Recently, proteolytic enzymes that have collagen breakdown as a specific mode of action were isolated from several sources and have been classified as collagenases. In metamorphosing tadpoles, a collagenase plays an essential role in the resorption of its tail. The granules of polymorphonuclear leukocytes and macrophages have the property of degrading collagen and therefore contain collagenase. Endogenous collagenases have now been identified in many different tissues and it seems likely that they play an important role in the removal or remodelling of collagen. In collagen breakdown the susceptible bonds are the intra and intermolecular crosslinkages within collagen molecules. The collagen molecule is in intimate association with polysaccharide molecules and it seems possible that these molecules shield the collagen molecules from the action of other proteolytic enzymes that are usually present in tissue fluids. Lapiere and Gross [9] have suggested that early in the destruction of collagen there is an increase in the water concentration in the area, which brings about a loosening of the fibre bundles and facilitates the migration of cells to the area with subsequent elaboration of a collagenase. This shift in water is a reflection of the altered integrity of the ground substance, which plays a vital role in the binding of water of hydration in collagen molecules. This separation of fibres and fibrils has been noted at the ultrastructure level in tissue taken from patients with periodontal disease [10]. Resorbtion and remodelling of alveolar bone are accepted functions of the osteoclast and osteoblast and there is now evidence that the fibroblast has the dual ability to synthesize and to degrade collagen at any one time [11].

It is probable that there exists between collagen and the carbohydrate-protein complexes of the ground substance, an involved inter-relationship that is vital for the maintenance of both.

RETICULIN FIBRES

Reticulin fibres are in many respects similar to collagen. They exhibit the same periodicity in electron microscope preparations, and show the same x-ray diffraction pattern. These fibres stain faintly with Van Gieson's stain and eosin, but they differ from mature collagen fibres in that they stain an intense black with silver impregnation techniques (argyrophilia). In granulation tissue the first formed fibres are reticulin, and it is possible that these may represent an early stage in the process of maturation of collagen, although not all unbranched argyrophilic fibres develop into collagen [12 & 13]. It has, therefore, been suggested that the term reticulin, or reticular fibres, be reserved for the fine branching fibres which do not develop into collagen [14].

ELASTIC FIBRES

Elastic fibres are large branching refractile structures that do not show the characteristic periodicity of collagen and reticulin. They stain deep red with eosin and dark brown with orcein. Elastic fibres are sparsely distributed in gingival tissue but are more numerous in alveolar mucosa.

GROUND SUBSTANCE

The polysaccharide–protein pool of ground substance is the direct environment of the cells, nerves, vessels and fibres of the organism. It constitutes the extracellular, extravascular tissue zone, and it stabilizes the spatial relationships of cells. Interchange of oxygen and waste products between cells and the blood vessels takes place across the ground substance. Alteration of the state of aggregation of the ground substance influences the water binding capacity of the tissue and the distribution of electrolytes. The main components of ground substance are derived from blood, parenchymal cells and connective tissue cells (table 7.1). Ground substance contains approximately one third of the total body water with all its normal constituents. Electron microscope studies have revealed a degree of organization of ground substance, which appears as a series of submicroscopic vacuoles believed to contain chiefly water, surrounded by denser walls rich in protein.

The functions of ground substance [15]

(1) Ground substance is the actual environ-

ment of most cells of the organism and determines the relative concentration of water, ions and metabolites around the cells. It is the chief mechanism for homeostasis of the cellular environment.

(2) Ground substance is the 'mother liquor' from which are extracted the components which form collagen, and reticulin fibres, and the denser organic components of cartilage, dentine and bone.

(3) Ground substance is the seat of the inflammatory reaction and is critically important in protecting the organism against bacterial invasion.

(4) Ground substance plays a part in the changes which occur during growth, differentiation, regeneration and ageing.

(5) Ground substance reacts to hormones (*vide infra*).

(6) The nature of ground substance is altered in various pathological conditions, e.g. inflammation, oedema, rickets, scurvy, arterio-sclerosis and some of the collagen diseases.

(7) In sites such as cartilage and bone, ground substance becomes calcified and serves as part of the hard endoskeleton.

Chemical change in the ground substance may be caused or reflected by change in metabolic function of the cell. It is in dynamic equilibrium with both the tissue cells and the intravascular fluid. There must, therefore, be a mechanism to explain the equilibrium which exists between tissues of widely differing colloid, electrolyte and water content, and blood which is relatively constant in composition. A simple equilibrium in terms of direct osmotic gradients would not account for the hydration of some, but not all, tissues under physiologic conditions, which occurs following oestrogenic or androgenic stimulation. Some explanation is required to account for the independent alterations in water content of individual tissues in an organism which is presumably in overall equilibrium with plasma. It has been shown that in a heterogeneous colloidal system consisting of a colloid-rich, water-poor phase, co-existing with a water-rich colloid-poor phase, the composition of the two phases in terms of chemical potentials of water and electrolytes remains constant within narrow limits, for wide variations in the amounts of these phases. In such a system the ionic environment of the cell may remain constant for large changes in the proportion of the two phases, which may alter the characteristics of the tissue in terms of consistency, mass and total volume. A two phase colloidal system is the minimal sufficient condition to show these properties; the possibility exists that the system is polyphasic [15].

Ground substance is a reservoir from which the stored nutritional requirements of cells are selectively available. The equilibrium between ground substance and blood is two-way, in the sense that depletion of stored nutritional factors may take place to maintain intravascular levels in dificiency. Alteration in the composition of ground substance, which may be sufficient to cause alteration in metabolic function of the

TABLE 7.1. Components of the ground substance. After Schultz-Haudt & Aas.

1	2 A high molecular weight component		3 A low molecular weight component
	Locally formed	Derived from plasma	
	Polysaccharide-protein complexes containing: acid mucopolysaccharides; heteropolysaccharides; sialic acid	Albumins Globulins Hormones	Water Inorganic ions Glucose, etc. Metabolic products
Submicroscopic fibrils	Soluble collagen Enzymes Immunoglobulins Other proteins		

cells, is not likely to be demonstrable by change in the level of the humoral elements in blood, except in extreme cases. This may account for the lack of evidence of demonstrable systemic change in blood, to account for the prevalence of periodontal disease.

If a biochemical lesion in tissue resistance to account for the high prevalence of periodontal disease does exist, the possibilities are that there may be:

(1) alteration in utilization of available metabolites by the cell.

(2) alteration in availability of metabolites due to change in the equilibrium between ground substance and blood, not reflected by change in the level of humoral elements except in extreme cases.

THE BASEMENT MEMBRANE

A fine membrane, the basement membrane, is situated at the junction between gingival epithelium and the underlying connective tissue [16–20]. Under the light microscope, and using suitable stains, e.g. periodic acid–Schiff, it can be seen as a magenta zone at the dermo-epidermal junction. In electron micrographs this zone appears as an electron dense line, much thinner than when seen under the light microscope, and it has been termed the lamina densa by Kurtz [21]. The exact relationship between these two structures remains in doubt, and there is little known about the structure or physical properties of the lamina densa, or the material in the zone between it and the epithelial cells. Although traditionally basement membranes have been considered to be connective tissue structures, many papers have presented evidence suggesting that the lamina densa, at least in some instances, is a product of epithelial cells [22–31].

The basement membrane zone changes during maturation, ageing and in certain pathological conditions, such as the presence of inflammation, desquamative gingivitis and invasive tumour growth. Exchanges between blood plasma, ground substance and epithelium must take place through two basement membranes, one related to the blood vessel wall and the other at the dermoepidermal junction. Placing of micro-pore filters between the basal layers of the epithelium and connective tissue has confirmed that the equilibrium of epithelium may be mediated by humoral factors from the connective tissue [32]. Epithelium and connective tissue, therefore, appear to function as an integrated dynamic system.

Effect of hormones on tissues

In a multicellular organism the cells are organized into tissues and in order for each tissue to perform its role, the component cells must function in a co-operative fashion. For a considerable period, there has been great interest in the way in which tissue functions are controlled, providing the organism with the flexibility it needs to adapt to a changing environment. It is now clear that among the primary controllers are the hormones; thus, whereas genes control the activities of individual cells, these same cells constitute the tissues that respond to the influence of hormones. Hormones of the most diverse sources, molecular structure and physiological influence, appear able to rapidly alter the pattern of activity in the cell responsive to them [33]. The endocrine and nervous systems together form a complex unit of great flexibility which enables transient or long-lasting adjustments in metabolism to be made in response to internal bodily or external environmental changes. The interactions between the endocrine system and both the central and peripheral aspects of the nervous system are very close. For example, the hypothalamus, which is part of the central nervous system, controls the anterior pituitary which itself controls production of many of the other endocrines. The effects of hormones are not limited to specific organs. Some hormones affect all cells and tissues more or less directly. For example, insulin and somatotrophic hormone influence all cells and much of the intercellular ground substance of the body.

SEX HORMONES

The specific stimulating effect of oestrogens and androgens is exerted particularly on those organs which mediate the development of male or female sex characteristics. These are not the only effects of sex hormones, as generalized anabolic effects also occur.

Androgens cause retention of nitrogen, phosphorus and potassium and stimulate protein formation. They are anabolic agents and promote growth of muscle and deposition of bone. Gingival biopsies from humans receiving testosterone propionate show more marked keratinization than normal, epithelial hyperplasia and increased mitotic activity [34].

Oestrogens have widespread anabolic effects. They promote nitrogen retention and protein synthesis, water retention in connective tissues, and deposition of glycogen. Administration of oestrogen causes an increase in acid mucopolysaccharides in connective tissue ground substance of human oral mucosa and thickening of stratified squamous epithelium with hyperkeratinization.

Progesterone produces dilatation of the gingival microvessels which has been shown to increase susceptibility to injury and exudation [35]. Exacerbation of gingivitis has been shown to follow the use of hormonal contraceptives [36 & 37]. Relaxin levels rise steeply during pregnancy reaching a peak at or just before parturition and decline rapidly in the few hours thereafter. Relaxin appears either to enhance the effect of oestrogen or to render tissues more responsive to the action of oestrogen. It has also been reported to cause depolymerization of connective tissue fibres.

ADRENAL CORTICOSTEROIDS

The steroid hormones of the adrenal cortex are secreted under the influence of the regulatory hormone ACTH of the anterior pituitary. Corticosteroids greatly influence the balance of electrolytes in the body, the metabolism of carbohydrates and the function of the sex organs. Cortisone, and its metabolic product cortisol, have an important inhibitory effect upon the inflammatory process. Cortisol acts to stabilize the lysosomal and possibly other membranes of the cell. In culture it has been shown to inhibit the breakdown of cells, whether this is caused by the addition of vitamin A or other means. In addition to their anti-inflammatory effect, glucocorticoids influence enzymes important in carbohydrate, lipid and protein metabolism. The systemic administration of cortisone in experimental animals results in osteoporosis of alveolar bone, capillary dilation and engorgement, with reduction in the number of collagen fibres in the periodontal membrane and increased destruction of the periodontal tissues associated with local inflammation [38]. In humans, systemic administration of cortisone and ACTH appears to have no effect on the incidence and severity of gingival and periodontal disease [39].

ADRENAL MEDULLARY HORMONES

Adrenaline is synthesized and stored in the chromaffin cells of the body sited in the adrenal medulla, peripheral sympathetic ganglia and other organs. The effects of injected adrenaline mimic the effects of stimulation of the sympathetic nervous system causing peripheral vasoconstriction, and dilation of the arterioles supplying muscles.

INSULIN

Insulin is secreted by the β cells in the pancreas. It affects the entry rate of carbohydrates, amino acid, cations and fatty acids into cells. It promotes protein synthesis and affects glycogen synthetic activity. It also stimulates the synthesis of fat and acid mucopolysaccharides.

THYROID HORMONES

Thyroid hormones effect the metabolic rate, growth, water and ion excretion. They promote protein synthesis and are required for normal muscle function. They probably affect all tissues and particularly affect carbohydrate levels, transport and synthesis.

PARATHYROID HORMONE

Parathyroid hormone promotes the release of calcium from bone, increased excretion of phosphate by the kidney and increased absorption of calcium by the gut.

ANTERIOR PITUITARY HORMONES

The principal hormones of the anterior pituitary

are: growth or somatotrophic hormone (STH), adrenocorticotrophic hormone (ACTH), thyroid stimulating hormone and the pituitary gonadotrophins. STH causes skeletal and visceral growth and probably affects all cells in the body. Its effect is an anabolic one and it stimulates formation of protein and retention of nitrogen, probably through control of RNA synthesis. ACTH stimulates the adrenal cortex, stimulates fat breakdown and inhibits protein synthesis in adipose tissue.

REFERENCES

[1] Loë H. (1963) Epidemiology of periodontal disease. *Odont. T.* **71**, 479–503.

[2] World Health Organization (1978) Epidemiology, etiology and prevention of periodontal diseases. Report of a WHO Scientific Group. *Technical Report Series 621.*

[3] Beagrie G.S. & Skougaard M. (1962) Observations on the life cycle of the gingival epithelial cells of mice as revealed by autoradiography. *Acta. odont. scand.* **20**, 15–31.

[4] Bullough W.S. (1964) Mitotic control by Chalone-adrenaline complexes. *J. exp. cell. Res.* **33**, 176–194.

[5] Mackenzie I.C. (1972) Does toothbrushing affect gingival keratinization? *Proc. Roy. Soc. Med.* **65**, 39.

[6] Kuhn K. (1969) The structure of collagen, in *Essays in Biochemistry*, Eds. Campbell P.M. & Grevile G.D. New York: Academic Press.

[7] Narayanan A.S. & Page R.C. (1976) Biochemical characterization of collagens synthesised by fibroblasts derived from normal and diseased human gingiva. *Journal of Biological Chemistry*, **251**, 5464–5471.

[8] Page R.C. (1972) Macromolecular interactions in the connective tissues of the periodontium, in *Developmental Aspects of Oral Biology*, Eds. Slavkin H.C. & Bavetta L.A. New York: Academic Press.

[9] Lapiere C.M. & Gross J. (1963) Animal collagenase and collagen metabolism, in *Mechanisms of Hard Tissue Destruction*, Ed. Sognnaes R.F. Washington D.C., Amer. Ass. Advan. Sci. Pub. No. 75.

[10] Selvig K.A. (1966) Ultrastructural changes in cementum and adjacent connective tissue in periodontal disease. *Acta odont. scand.* **24**, 495.

[11] Ten Cate A.R. & Deporter D.A. (1975) The degradative role of the fibroblast in the remodelling and turnover of collagen in soft connective tissue. *The Anatomical Record*, **182**, 1–14.

[12] Jackson D.S. & Williams G. (1956) Nature of reticulin. *Nature (Lond.)*, **178**, 915.

[13] Robb-Smith A.H.T. (1958) The relationship of reticulin to other 'collagens', in *Recent Advances in Gelatin and Glue Research*, Ed. Stainsby G. London: Pergamon.

[14] Melcher A.H. (1963) Argyrophilic fires of human gingival connective tissue. *Arch. oral Biol.* **8**, 397–406.

[15] Gersh I. & Catchpole H.R. (1960) The nature of ground substance of connective tissue. *Perspect. Biol. Med.* **3**, 282–319.

[16] Themann H. (1958) Elektronenmikroskopische Untersuchungen der normalen und der pathologisch veränderten Mundschleimhaut. *Fortschritte der Kiefer-und Gesichts-Chir*, **4**, 390–398.

[17] Laurenza A. (1959) La guinzione dermo-epidermica nella gengiva umana normale e patologica al microscopico electronico. *Minerva Stomatol.* **8(8)**, 511–517.

[18] Kurahashi Y. & Takuma S. (1962) Electron microscopy of human gingival epithelium. *Bull. Tokyo Dent. Coll.* **3**, 29–43.

[19] Listgarten M.A. (1964) The ultrastructure of human gingival epithelium. *Amer. J. Anat.* **114**, 49–69.

[20] Stern I.B. (1965) Electron microscopic observations of oral epithelium I. Basal cells and the basement membrane. *Periodontics*, **3**, 224–238.

[21] Kurtz S.M. (1961) The fine structure of the lamina densa. *Lab. Invest.* **10**, 1189–1208.

[22] Pease D.C. (1960) The basement membrane: Substratum of histological order and complexity. *Fourth Int. Conf. on electron microscopy. Berlin 1958*, **2**, 139–155, Berlin: Springer-Verlag.

[23] Weiss P. & Ferris W. (1956) The basement lamella of amphibian skin. Its reconstitution after wounding. *J. biophys. biochem. Cytol.* **2**, 275–282.

[24] Salpeter M.M. & Singer M. (1960) Differentiation of the sub-microscopic adepidermal membrane during limb regeneration in adult triturus, including a note on the term basement membrane. *Anat. Rec.* **136**, 27–32.

[25] Vernier R.L. & Birch-Anderson A. (1962) Studies of the human fetal kidney. *J. Pediat.* **60**, 754–767.

[26] Vernier R.L. & Birch-Anderson A. (1963) Studies of the human fetal kidney. II. Permeability characteristics of the developing glomerulus. *J. Ultrastruct. Res.* **8**, 66–88.

[27] Kurtz S.M. & Feldman J.D. (1962) Experimental studies on the formation of the glomerular basement membrane. *J. Ultrastruct. Res.* **6**, 19–27.

[28] Pierce G.B. Jr., Midgley A.R. Jr., Sri Ram J. & Feldman J.D. (1962) Parietal yolk sac carcinoma due to the histogenesis of Reicherts membrane of the mouse embryo. *Amer. J. Path.* **41**, 549–566.

[29] Pierce G.B., Midgley A.R. & Sri Ram J. (1963) The histogenesis of basement membranes. *J. exp. Med.* **117**, 330–347.

[30] Mukerjee H., Sri Ram J. & Pierce G.B. (1965) Basement membranes. V. Chemical analysis of neoplastic basement membrane mucoprotein. *Amer. J. Path.* **46**, 49–58.

[31] Hay E.D. & Revel J.P. (1963) Autoradiographic studies of the origin of the basement lamella in ambystoma. *Devel. Biol.* **7**, 152–168.

[32] Dodson J.W. (1967) The differentiation of epidermis. I. The interrelationship of epidermis and dermis in embryonic chicken skin. *J. Embryol. exp. Morph.* **17**, 83–105.

[33] Davidson E.H. (1968) Hormones and genes, in *The Molecular Basis of Life*, pps. 254–263. San Francisco: W.H. Freeman & Co.

[34] Ziskin D.E. (1941) Effect of the male sex hormones on the gingivae and oral mucous membranes. *J. dent. Res.* **20**, 419.

[35] Hugoson A. (1970) Gingival inflammation and female sex hormones. A clinical investigation of pregnant women and experimental studies in dogs. *J. periodont. Res.* Suppl. **5**. 1.

[36] Lindhe J. & Björn A.L. (1967) Influence of hormonal contraceptives on the gingiva of women. *J. periodont. Res.* **2**, 1.

[37] Lynn B.D. (1967) The pill as an etiologic agent in hypertrophic gingivitis. *Oral Surg.* **24**, 333.

[38] Glickman I., Stone I.C. & Chawla T.C. (1953) The effect of cortisone acetate upon the periodontium of white mice. *J. Periodont.* **24**, 161.

[39] Krohn S. (1958) The effect of the administration of steroid hormones on the gingival tissues. *J. Periodont.* **29**, 300.

SUGGESTED ADDITIONAL READING

Anderson D.J. *et al.* (1967) *The Mechanisms of Tooth Support: a Symposium.* Bristol: Wright.

Schroeder H.E. & Theilade J. (1966) Electron microscopy of normal human gingival epithelium. *J. periodont. Res.* **1**, 95–119.

Schultz-Haudt S.D. & From S. (1961) Dynamics of periodontal tissues. 1. The epithelium. *Odont. T.* **69**, 431–460.

Schultz-Haudt S.D. & Aas E. (1962) Dynamics of periodontal tissue. 2. The connective tissue. *Odont. T.* **70**, 389–428.

CHAPTER 8

Classification of periodontal disease

CLINICAL FEATURES OF PERIODONTAL DISEASE

It is an essential part of the study of any disease process that there should be standardized terminology and a generally recognized classification to define the clinical conditions which are commonly seen. The fact that there is at present no classification which is in general use, is symptomatic of the confusion which has clouded the issues with regard to the aetiology of periodontal disease. The majority of classifications are based on aetiology, and since it is clear that the disease involves a wide range of host–parasite interactions, classification on this basis is necessarily complex. Similarly, clinical appearance as a basis for classification is imprecise, as widely differing pathological processes tend to produce similar clinical appearances, in so far as the common tissue response is an increase in the general level of nonspecific inflammatory change. For practical purposes the most acceptable form of classification at the present time is a modification of that proposed in the 1961 World Health Organization Technical Report on Periodontal Disease [1], which is based on the general pathological features of the disease.

The changes occurring most frequently with chronic periodontitis have been described in chap. 3. These changes usually occur in combination, but one or other tissue reaction may be predominant in a particular mouth. Pathological change and deviation from normal anatomical form of the gingival tissues may be:

(1) Predominantly inflammation and oedema, associated with disaggregation of the gel structure of connective tissue, and hyperplasia of the epithelial tissues resulting in pocket formation (fig. 8.1).

Such change may be a limited reaction to bacterial plaque, thus essentially of local origin, or may be secondary to alteration in tissue metabolism, and reduction in host resistance (see chap. 13).

(2) Predominantly hyperplasia of the connective tissues of the gingivae. This may or may not be associated with hyperplasia of the epithelial tissues and pocket formation (fig. 8.2).

The most frequently occurring form of gingival hyperplasia is of inflammatory origin. In chronic periodontal disease, an alternating process of tissue destruction and repair occurs, and the presence of hyperplasia may represent an exaggerated phase of repair, particularly in a young patient. It may be a response to mouth breathing, a high rate of plaque formation or

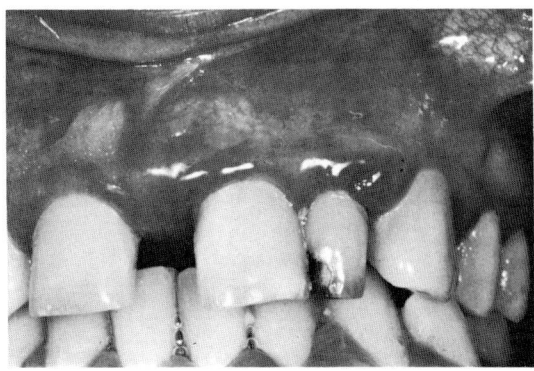

FIG. 8.1. Predominantly inflammation and oedema associated with disaggregation of connective tissue and hyperplasia of epithelial tissues resulting in pocket formation.

any form of local irritant. Hyperplasia of inflammatory origin may be associated with a variable degree of clinically evident inflammation. Typically the tissue is to some degree oedematous, and reddish in colour, as a result of the vascular change. On occasion, hyperplasia occurs secondary to low grade chronic inflammation which is histologically, but not clinically, apparent (fig. 8.2a). The enlarged tissue has minimal clinical signs of oedema or vascular change. Histologically the bulk of the tissue is mature collagen.

Inflammatory hyperplasia may be modified by alterations in tissue metabolism. These modifications of host resistance are conditioned by endocrine, allergic or tissue intoxicating factors (see chap. 13). Gingival hyperplasia may be

genetically determined [2 & 3], and such enlargement has been termed gingivomatosis (hereditary gingival fibromatosis).

This condition is characterized by diffuse enlargement of the gingivae on both the medial and lateral aspects of the alveolar crest (fig. 8.3). It is

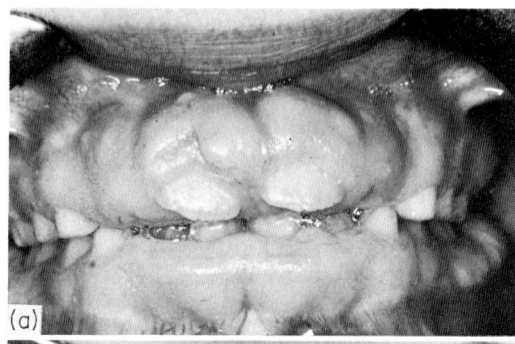

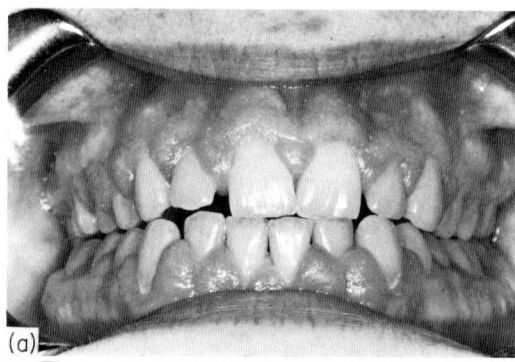

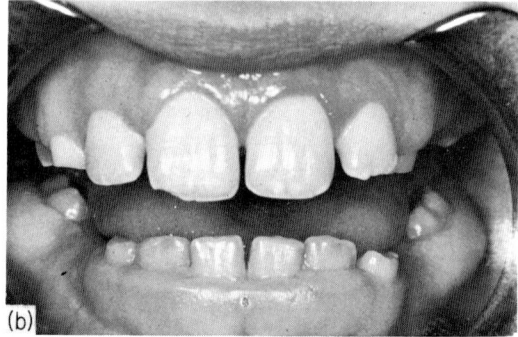

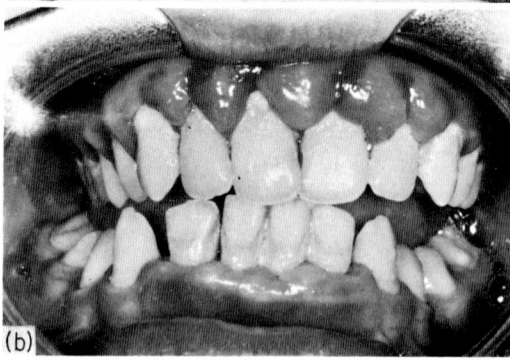

FIG. 8.2. (a) Hyperplasia of connective tissue not associated with hyperplasia of epithelial tissues and true pocket formation (limited hyperplastic gingivitis). No clinically evident inflammation. (b) Hyperplasia of connective tissue and hyperplasia of epithelial tissues resulting in formation of true pockets. Gingival hyperplasia associated with established periodontitis. Marked clinically evident inflammation associated with obvious deposits on teeth.

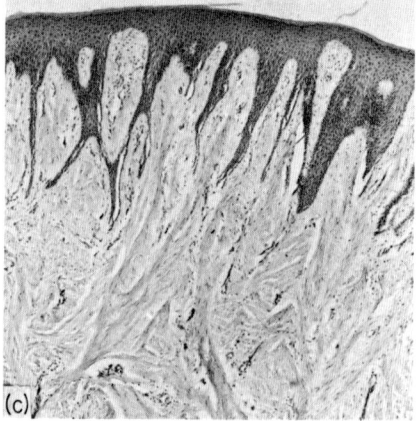

FIG. 8.3. Hereditary gingival fibromatosis (a) in a child age 8; (b) same child aged 9 following gingivectomy around maxillary anterior teeth, compare with mandibular incisors; (c) enlarged tissue composed of mature collagen with minimal signs of inflammation.

generally accepted that inflammation is not a characteristic feature unless it results from plaque formation following distortion of gingival form. The enlarged tissue consists of dense white collagenous connective tissue (fig. 8.3c), which clinically may be paler in colour than the adjacent normal mucosa. The disease occurs early in life, and the clinical manifestations may become more pronounced during puberty.

(3) Predominantly recession and atrophy of the epithelial and connective tissue elements around the tooth (fig. 8.4).

Generalized atrophic change of the gingival tissues, and mucosa of lips, cheeks and tongue, is commonly seen in relation to old age, and to menopausal hormonal effects. Localized atrophic change may occur in the periodontium of a nonfunctional tooth where the lamina dura

becomes thinner, the periodontal membrane reduced in width and the connective tissues of the membrane less well organized (see chap. 14). In hyperfunction, pressure ischaemia from excessive lateral forces on a tooth may give rise to sterile ischaemic necrosis of bone, which in association with toxic factors from plaque at the cervical margin may result in dehiscence (fig. 8.5a) (chap. 15). Recession and atrophy of the marginal tissue is a common feature of the crowded mouth, particularly where teeth are buccal to the dental arch (fig. 8.5b). This has given rise to speculation as to the adequacy of the blood supply to the gingival tissues, where there is a large tooth volume in relation to a relatively smaller volume of supporting bone [4]. The reduction, with age, of approximately 1 cm in the anteroposterior dimension of the arch,

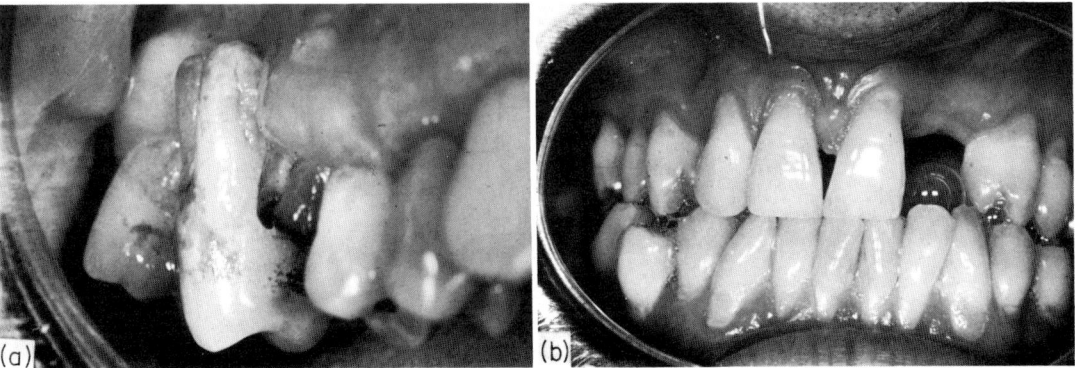

FIG. 8.4. Predominantly recession and atrophy of epithelial and connective tissues around the tooth.

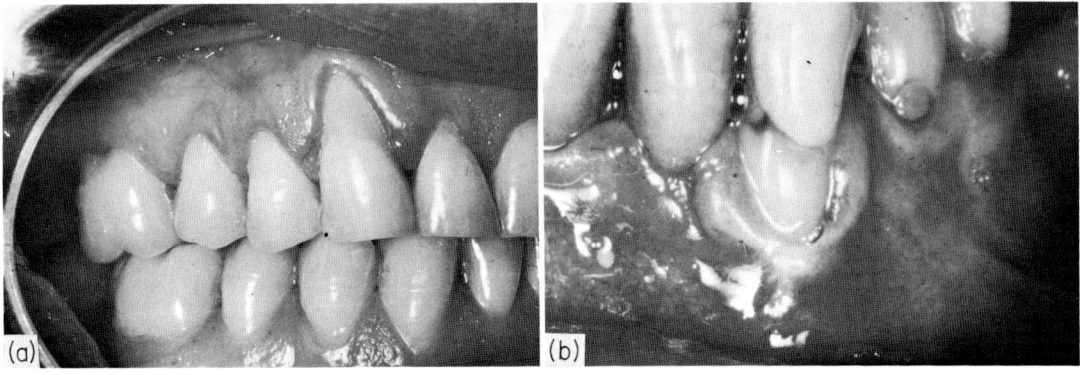

FIG. 8.5. (a) Recession and atrophy of marginal tissues. This may result from excessive lateral force on a tooth, particularly in presence of gnashing or grinding of teeth. Note excessive attrition of 3/ (see chap. 14). (b) Recession and atrophy of marginal tissues around a tooth which is buccal to the arch. The rolled gingival margin, which has been described as a 'McCalls Festoon', is not particularly associated with excessive occlusal forces.

which resulted from interstitial contact point wear, does not occur to the same degree with modern low friction diets (fig. 2.5).

The presence of low grade inflammation may produce alteration in the milieu of tissue cells which may be reflected as atrophic or degenerative change. Gingival tissue may recede from plaque at the cervical margin.

Atrophy of the gingival tissues is a complex phenomenon, which frequently produces distortion of gingival form, resulting in plaque accumulation. In the majority of cases atrophic gingivitis is seen in association with a variable amount of inflammation which is histologically, if not clinically, evident. It is at present impossible to establish to what extent atrophy is of local as against systemic origin, except where it results from misuse of a toothbrush (fig. 8.6).

CLASSIFICATION

Periodontal disease is defined as being all those pathological processes which involve the periodontium. Most periodontal disease is limited to the periodontium, but in some cases it may be a manifestation of general disease of other organs. Three fundamental types of pathological process differing distinctly in character, origin and course can be recognized [1].

Inflammatory processes

Inflammation occurs whenever an irritant affects the integrity of the tissues by physical or by chemicoinfectious action. It is a type of reaction

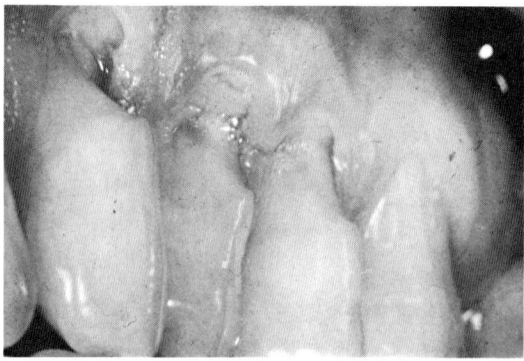

FIG. 8.6. Recession, atrophy and cervical abrasion resulting from misuse of a hard toothbrush.

and repair involving primarily the differentiated connective tissue, and its circulatory system. The calcified connective tissue, e.g. bone, cartilage, cementum and dentine, may subsequently undergo secondary change.

Degenerative processes

The term degenerative is applied to regressive conditions related to general or local metabolic deviation. They are caracterized by structural changes resulting in the disappearance from the histological picture of certain elements, or the appearance of substances foreign to the normal composition of cells and tissues.

Neoplastic processes

The periodontium may be the site of primary neoplasms derived from its various constituent tissues. It may also rarely be the site of metastases from neoplasms elsewhere. Reference should be made to a textbook of oral pathology for a classification of tumours.

The relationship of inflammatory and degenerative processes

It is inherent in the concept of the mouth as a host–parasite system tending towards balance, that inflammatory and degenerative processes rarely, if ever, occur in a pure form. Pathological change, and deviation from the normal anatomical form of the tissues of the periodontium, is always accompanied by a variable degree of inflammation (chap. 3), and there is little evidence to support the concept that degenerative change is particularly associated with general metabolic deviation. It is clear that degenerative change may occur as a result of local deviation in cellular metabolism induced by local factors (chaps. 4 & 7). There is insufficient evidence to support the concept of the term periodontosis, denoting a primary degenerative process, which is distinct from disease of inflammatory origin. Evidence to support the conventional concept of periodontosis is unsubstantiated. It was the consensus of the World Workshop in Periodontics 1966: 'that the term periodontosis is ambiguous and should be eliminated from periodontal nomenclature' [5]. They did, however, suggest that evidence exists to indicate that a clinical entity different from adult periodontitis, occurs in adolescents and young adults [6].

The problem of classification is simplified if it is accepted that the bulk of periodontal disease is classifiable as nonspecific inflammatory change, both in its clinical appearance and in the direct mechanism of its cause. In a small percentage of cases, laboratory procedures may define an alteration in host resistance such as a blood dyscrasia, which may be a factor, or the presence of infection predominantly by one particular group of organisms, e.g. coccal gingivitis. In the majority of these instances the clinical picture is not specifically recognizable as being related to the established cause. On this basis periodontal disease may be classified as follows.

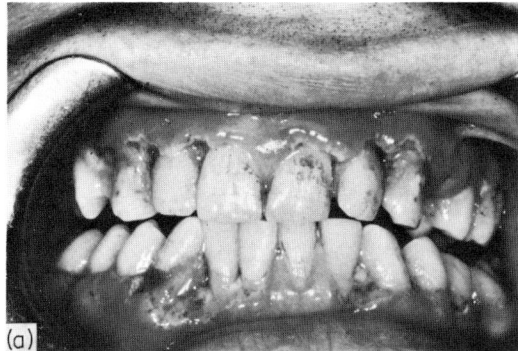
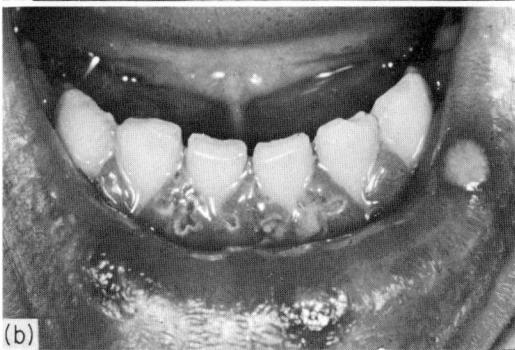
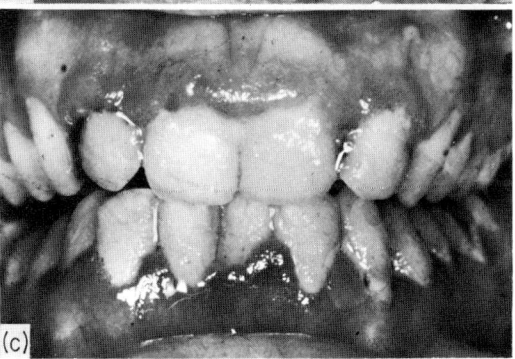

FIG. 8.7. (a) Acute ulceromembranous gingivitis characterized by 'crater' ulceration of papillae and ulceration of gingival margins (chap. 11). (b) Primary herpetic stomatitis characterized by punched out ulceration of gingivae, lips, cheeks and tongue (chap. 11). (c) Acute coccal gingivitis characterized by 'beefy' red oedematous enlargement of gingivae and haemorrhagic exudate at gingival margin; no frank ulceration (chap. 11).

Gingivitis

ACUTE

Acute specific gingivitis

There are three forms of acute specific gingivitis that are clinically distinguishable, the diagnosis of which can be supported to some extent by laboratory procedures:

(1) acute ulceromembranous gingivitis (fig. 8.7a),

(2) acute herpetic gingivitis (fig. 8.7b),

(3) acute coccal gingivitis (fig. 8.7c).

Acute nonspecific gingivitis (fig. 8.8)

All other cases of acute gingivitis are clinically indistinguishable from each other and should be classified as acute nonspecific gingivitis. Laboratory investigation may subsequently reveal an

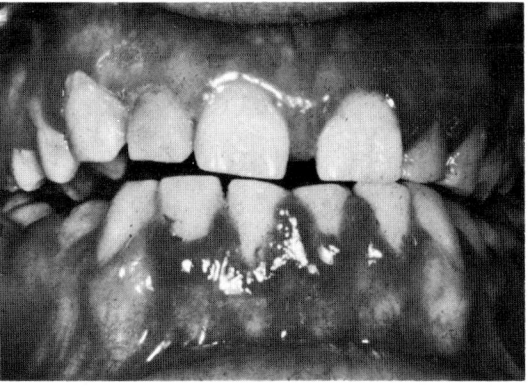

FIG. 8.8. Acute nonspecific gingivitis. Generalized nonspecific inflammation and oedema of gingival tissues of sudden onset (chap. 11).

aberrant factor in host resistance, or the presence of organisms which may be contributory to the condition in a small proportion of cases.

CHRONIC

Chronic nonspecific gingivitis

See fig. 8.9 and table 8.1.

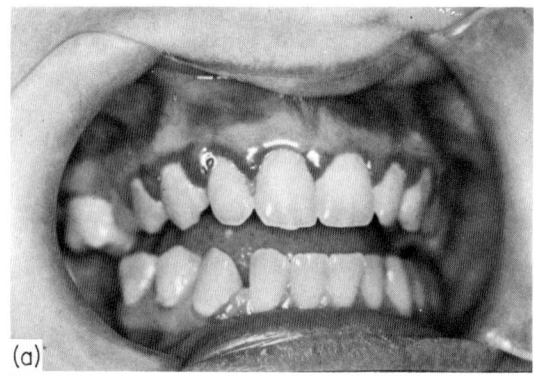

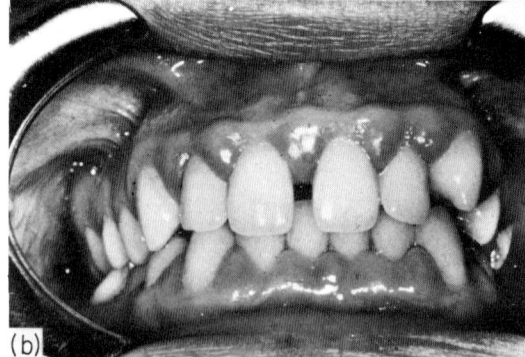

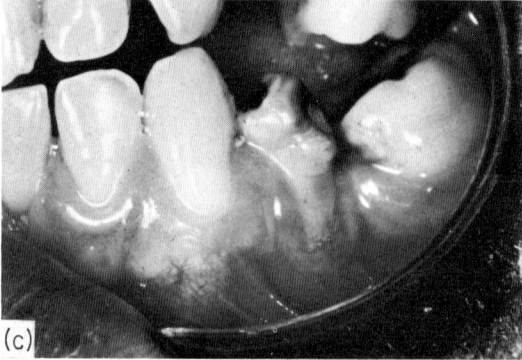

FIG. 8.9. (a) Chronic oedematous gingivitis (chap. 12). (b) Chronic hyperplastic gingivitis (chap. 12). (c) Chronic atrophic gingivitis (chap. 12).

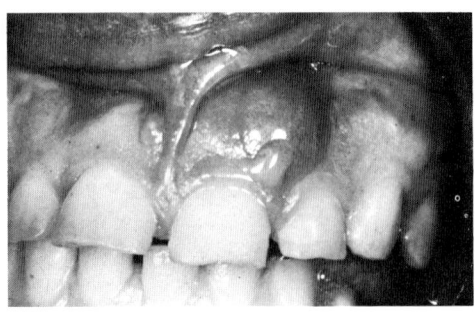

FIG. 8.10. Periodontal abscess. Localized swelling discharging pus from a small sinus (chap. 11).

Periodontitis

Acute nonspecific periodontitis (periodontal abscess, fig. 8.10)

Chronic nonspecific periodontitis

(1) Periodontitis simplex is characterized by pocket formation of regular depth throughout the mouth and a horizontal pattern of bone resorption (fig. 8.11).

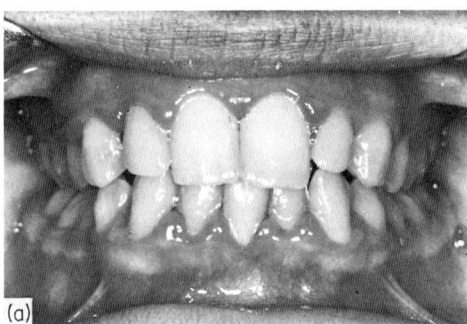

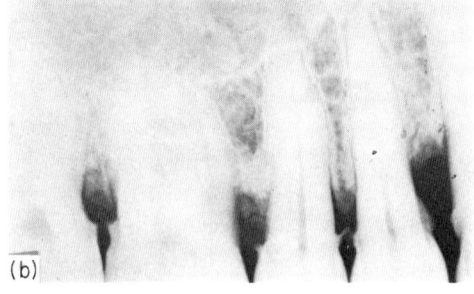

FIG. 8.11. (a) Periodontitis simplex characterized by pocket formation of fairly regular depth throughout the mouth and a degree of tissue destruction in phase with the age of the patient. (b) X-ray periodontitis simplex showing typical horizontal bone resorption and deposits of calculus and plaque on the teeth.

(2) Periodontitis complex is characterized by advanced tissue destruction relative to the age of the patient, pocket formation of irregular depth throughout the mouth and irregular vertical bone resorption (fig. 8.12).

All conditions may be exacerbated by systemic disease, by hormonal factors, or by drugs such as diphenylhydantoin (chap. 13).

Little acceptable evidence has been put forward to confirm the traditional concept that periodontitis simplex is local factor in origin, and that periodontitis complex is related to reduction in tissue resistance of systemic origin. The terms should be used to describe the pattern of tissue destruction, and the extent of tissue destruction relative to the age of the patient. They have no meaning in relation to aetiology.

All periodontitis is a complex phenomenon involving a wide range of interaction between the parasitic population of the mouth, and the host tissues.

A summary of the classification appears in table 8.1.

Rate of progression of periodontitis is not linear and evidence suggests that changes in rate of progression may be associated with changes in the infectivity of plaque, the hypersensitivity component of the host response to plaque and perhaps to changes in occlusal function.

While the term 'juvenile periodontitis' describes a high rate of activity of progression of periodontitis in the young individual, it cannot be applied to the adult who has had a stable,

TABLE 8.1. Classification of periodontal disease. All conditions may be exacerbated by systemic factors. (See chap. 13 for systemic factors which may condition and exacerbate pre-existing inflammation.)

GINGIVITIS

ACUTE GINGIVITIS

Acute specific
Ulceromembranous gingivitis
Herpetic gingivitis
Coccal gingivitis.

Acute nonspecific
Acute gingivitis which does not present the features characteristic of ulceromembranous gingivitis; herpetic or coccal gingivitis.

CHRONIC GINGIVITIS

Chronic nonspecific
Chronic oedematous gingivitis
Chronic hyperplastic gingivitis
Chronic atrophic gingivitis.

PERIODONTITIS

Acute nonspecific
Periodontal abscess.

Chronic nonspecific
Periodontitis simplex
Periodontitis complex.

virtually non-progressive degree of periodontitis for many years which suddenly enters a period of high activity. In our opinion, a highly active, destructive periodontitis in a patient of any age merits the term 'periodontitis complex' or 'precocious periodontitis'.

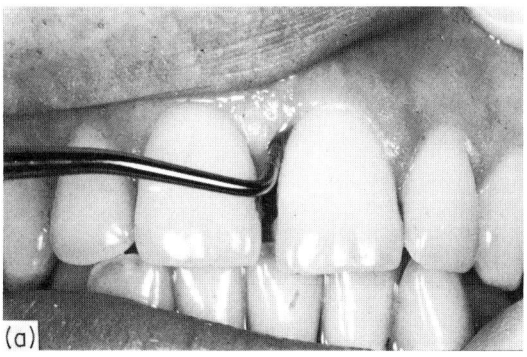 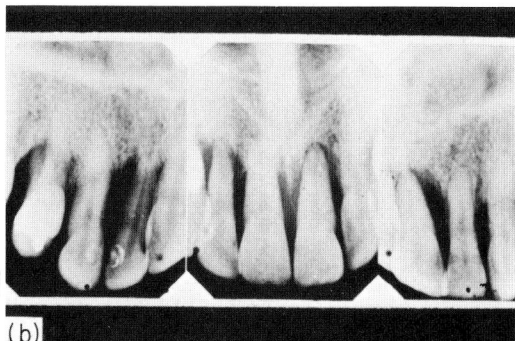

FIG. 8.12. Periodontitis complex. (a) Advanced tissue destruction and pocket formation in 15-year-old boy; note minimal clinical signs of inflammation (chap. 12). (b) X-ray showing advanced tissue destruction relative to age and irregular vertical bone resorption (chap. 12).

REFERENCES

[1] WORLD HEALTH ORGANIZATION (1961) Report of an Expert Committee on Dental Health No. 207.

[2] RUSHTON M.A. (1957) Hereditary or idiopathic hyperplasia of the gums. *Dent. Practit. dent. Rec.* **7**, 136–146.

[3] FLETCHER J.P. (1966) Gingival abnormalities of genetic origin: A preliminary communication with special reference to hereditary generalized fibromatosis. *J. dent. Res.* **45**, 597–612.

[4] LAMMIE G.A. (1965) *Dental Orthopaedics*, p. 242. Oxford: Alden Press.

[5] *World Workshop in Periodontics* (1966) Eds. Ramfjord, Sigurd P., Kerr, Donald A. & Ash Major M., p. 123. Michigan: University of Michigan.

[6] BAER P.N., STANLEY H.R., BROWN K., SMITH L., GAMBLE J. & SWERDLOW H. (1963) Advanced periodontal disease in an adolescent (Periodontosis). *J. Periodont.* **34**, 533–539.

CHAPTER 9

The general principles of periodontal therapy

The treatment of periodontitis is largely empirical, and it is limited to treatment of the signs and symptoms of the disease complex, rather than of the direct cause. Prevention is superior to any form of treatment, and it can only be achieved by a high standard of patient self-care from the time of eruption of the teeth. Since it has been shown that the main factors accounting for the prevalence of periodontitis throughout the population are quantitative, and to some extent qualitative, change in the commensal population of plaque, it follows that the first essential of any course of therapy is to reduce the bacterial population of the cuff region. Plaque left undisturbed on a tooth surface for 24 hours can become fixed to a degree that it is impossible for the patient to completely remove it with a toothbrush; it must, therefore, be removed by scaling and polishing. This finding forces the adoption of a rigid system of patient discipline, whereby all treatment is based on a high standard of self-care by the patient at all stages of therapy.

It is convenient to consider the principles of therapy in general terms under three headings ('3 R's of Therapy').

(1) Remove the cause by reducing the local irritants and gaining control of the bacterial population of the cuff region.

(2) Raise the resistance of the tissues by the elimination of stagnation areas, correcting intra- and interocclusal relationships, and the creation of as functional and self-cleansing a mouth as possible.

(3) Remove the effects by treating the local tissue destruction caused by the disease complex.

These basic principles should be applied by means of a programme of definite phases of treatment followed out in a logical order.

The hygiene phase

This includes the scaling and polishing of teeth and establishing a high standard of patient self-care.

Control of infection is the first consideration in treatment and in some cases may necessitate drug therapy, but all treatment must involve scaling and polishing and instruction of the patient in effective oral hygiene methods. Drugs should never be administered in isolation from hygiene phase therapy.

The corrective phase

(1) Correction of tooth relationships; the objective being to create the most functional occlusion possible by means of restoration or replacement of decayed teeth, correction of occlusal disharmony or orthodontic movement of teeth.

(2) Surgical correction of tissue relationships; the objective being the elimination of pockets by surgery and the restoration of soft tissue and bone architecture to a functional anatomical form.

The maintenance phase

Present methods of treatment do not alter the fact that periodontitis is likely to recur in patients who are unable to prevent the accumulation of bacterial deposits on their teeth. The aim of treatment is to achieve reduction of the level of inflammation present, and to repair the damage which has been caused. Thereafter, the mouth will require regular hygiene phase care, to prevent recurrence.

Systemic treatment, if indicated, should be conducted concurrently with the three basic phases outlined above. Invariably systemic therapy should be carried out in conjunction with these three phases of treatment and should never be performed in isolation.

To achieve acceptable results a patient who does not meet the exacting standards of the hygiene phase should not be allowed to pass to the corrective phase, and treatment should be planned to progress by stages towards advanced procedures, which must never be performed on a patient not proved suitable during the initial phases of treatment.

CHAPTER 10

Hygiene phase therapy

The hygiene phase is divided into two equally important parts: the patient's self-care, and the practitioner's care of the patient.

PATIENT SELF-CARE

The responsibility for the reduction and control of superficial inflammation lies as much with the patient as with the practitioner. The patient should be made familiar with the anatomy of his mouth and should be taught to adapt his toothbrushing technique to any irregularities of his own dentition.

The general requirements of a toothbrush are firstly, it should be small; a large brush tends to create problems of access and to miss the irregularities of the dentition which may be the main stagnation areas (fig. 10.1). Secondly, it should be of such a texture as to clean adequately, without damaging either the tooth or the periodontium. Provided that the brush is allowed to dry thoroughly between times of use, bristles or synthetic filaments of medium stiffness should be recommended for routine use. The brush should be applied to the gingival tissues primarily to control plaque deposition at the cervical margin, and secondarily to stimulate circulation in the connective tissues.

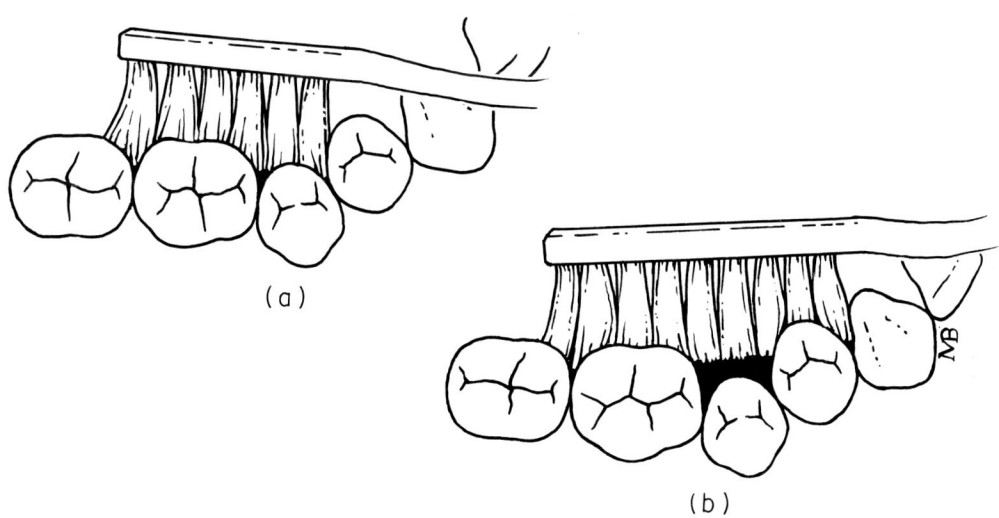

(a)

(b)

FIG. 10.1. A toothbrush should be small (a), a large brush (b) tends to create problems of access and miss the irregularities of the dentition.

Toothbrushing

There are several methods of toothbrushing, all of which are variants of three basic techniques.

The physiological downstroke technique (fig. 10.2)

The brush is placed at an angle to the tooth and is carried down over the gingival margin towards the buccal or lingual sulcus in an attempt to reproduce a frictional action, similar to that obtained from the mastication of fibrous foods.

This technique gives adequate cleansing and stimulates circulation in the soft tissues. It is suitable only for the anatomically normal mouth. Where there is an existing pocket, movement of the brush from the tooth to soft tissue tends to strip the tissue away from the tooth and to pack debris into the open pocket.

The vibratory technique (fig. 10.3)

The Charter's technique is performed by placing the bristles on enamel, at 45° to its surface, pointed occlusally. Pressure is applied to the bristles as they are vibrated gently over a short distance. The sides of the bristles press against, and massage, the gingival margins, and the tips of the bristles are worked into the embrasures.

This technique is generally satisfactory, and it provides soft tissue stimulation and adequately cleans the teeth. It is not, however, well performed by patients.

~ The Bass technique is a variant of the vibratory technique whereby the bristles are applied to the tooth at a 45° angle pointed apically, so that the bristle tips enter the gingival sulcus. The brush is then activated with a slight vibratory motion.

The roll technique (fig. 10.4)

The bristles of the brush are placed on the alveolar mucosa as far away from the occlusal surface as possible, with the side of the bristles resting against the gingivae. With a rolling motion, the bristles are swept across the tissue towards the clinical crown, and this action is repeated ten to twelve times in each area of the mouth.

'Though there are remarkably few published reports of studies which have attempted to evaluate the effectiveness of the various methods advocated for toothbrushing, it appears that the roll technique is the one most often recommended. The method and toothbrush of choice depends on the patient's oral health, manual dexterity, personal preference and his ability and desire to learn and follow prescribed procedures. No definite superiority has been shown for either natural or synthetic bristles' [1].

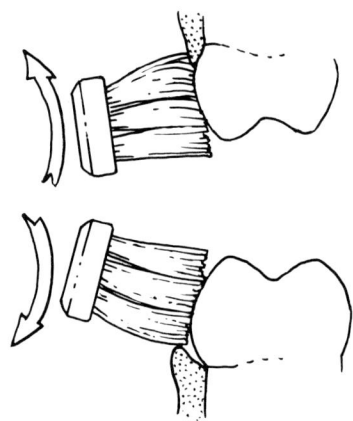

FIG. 10.2. Physiological downstroke. Where there is an existing pocket movement of the brush from tooth to soft tissue tends to displace the tissues from the tooth and pack debris into the open pocket.

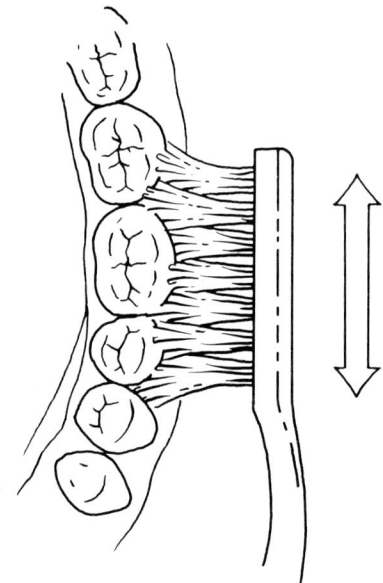

FIG. 10.3. Vibratory technique. Brush placed on enamel at 45° to its surface pointed occlusally and vibrated gently.

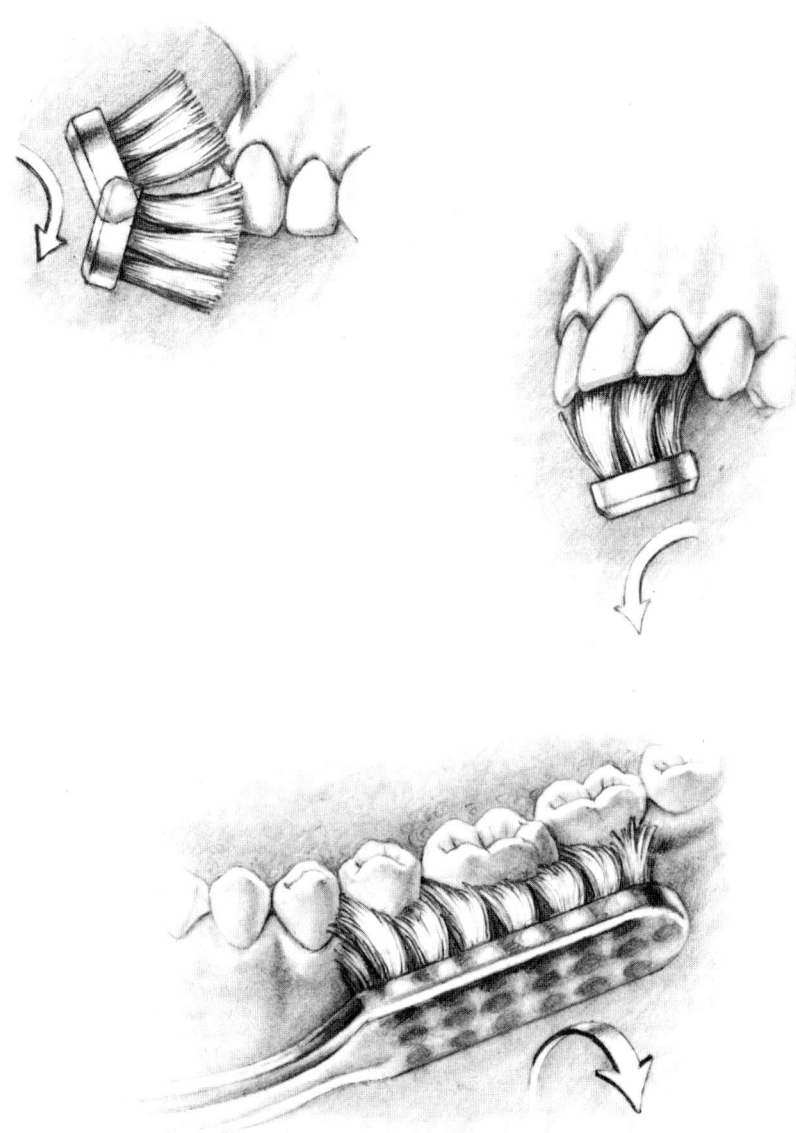

FIG. 10.4. The roll technique. Brush placed on alveolar mucosa and swept towards the clinical crowns of the teeth. This technique is widely recommended and well performed by patients.

INSTRUCTION OF THE PATIENT

The unidirectional movement of the brush from soft tissue to tooth (the roll technique) is probably the safest and most effective method of application of a toothbrush for a mouth with an existing periodontitis, and therefore for general application throughout the population as a whole. There is no risk of the patient packing debris into an open pocket, and the technique is easily acquired and performed. Studies by Hansen and Gjermo [2] and Frandsen *et al.* [3] suggested that the roll technique might not be the method of choice as this technique was associated with the highest mean plaque score in trial groups. A trial of the scrub brush technique [4] (haphazard brushing in all directions) suggested that this might be the method of choice for the primary dentition, but there is insufficient evidence to suggest that a particular toothbrush or brushing technique is clearly superior. It is insufficient to indicate the method verbally, in general terms. The patient should be formally instructed with the use of a suitable brush and models. Each arch should be divided into twelve areas (fig. 10.5), and the brush applied on the basis of a minimum of ten to twelve strokes per area. The occlusal

surfaces of the teeth should be cleaned by the scrub brush technique (fig. 10.6). It should be emphasized at this stage that it is insufficient to keep the mouth clear of obvious deposits, debris and calculus, and that the accumulation of bacterial plaque, which may not be clinically evident, will cause tissue damage. Disclosing tablets, or a suitable stain, e.g. alcoholic fuchsin, should be used to demonstrate the presence of plaque in the apparently superficially clean mouth, by staining the deposits so that they are clearly visible to the patient [5]. It should be emphasized that the disease may arise from such hidden deposits (fig. 10.7). Where it is at all possible, the point should be illustrated with photographs, taken before and after the establishment of an adequate regimen of tooth-brushing, and the patient should be given disclosing tablets for use at home. At the time of the second visit, it will have become evident that certain areas in relation to restorations or irregularities in the dentition present a problem of access and may require the use of a special brush. The interspace brush provides a convenient answer to the majority of such problems and is used in localized areas to supplement the normal brush (fig. 10.8).

THE ELECTRIC TOOTHBRUSH

Electric toothbrushes have been described and used for a considerable number of years, and a wide range of devices is now commercially available. Review of the literature suggests that the electric toothbrush is superior to the manual

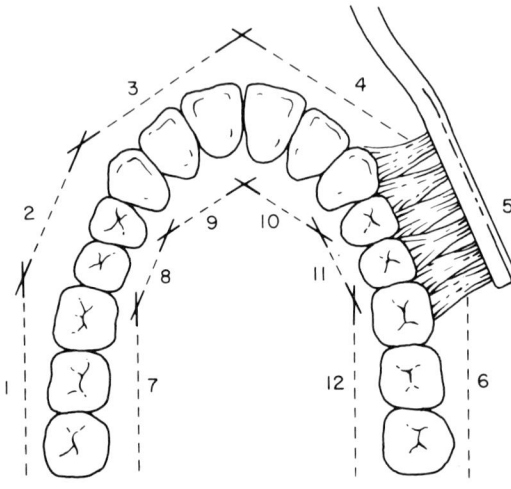

FIG. 10.5. Each arch should be divided into twelve areas, and the brush applied by the roll technique on the basis of a minimum of ten to twelve strokes per area.

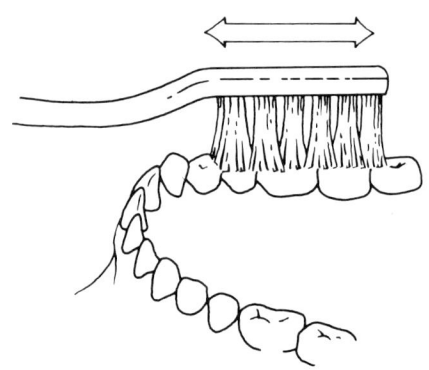

FIG. 10.6. Cleansing of occlusal surfaces by scrub brush technique.

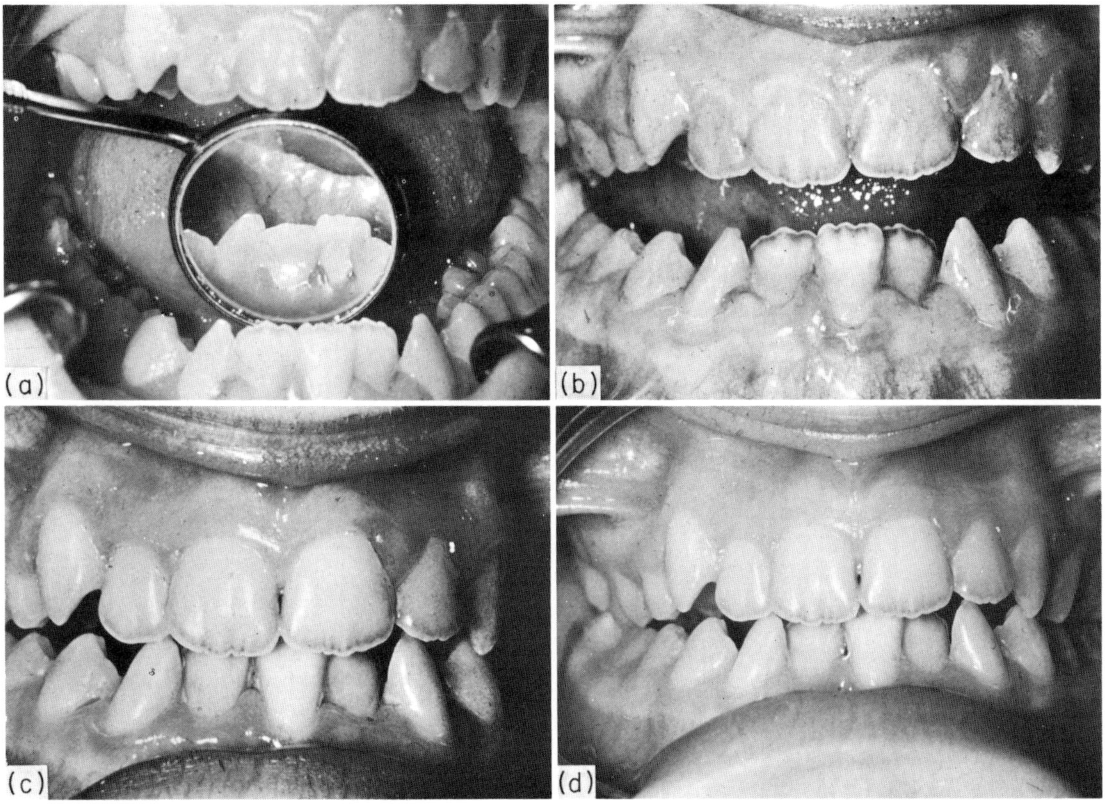

FIG. 10.7. (a) Oedematous gingivitis. (b) Mouth disclosed by erythrosin tablet. (c) Following 7 days correct tooth-brushing. (d) Complete resolution following 2 weeks correct toothbrushing.

brush when used by handicapped individuals unable to manipulate a manual brush. There is less general agreement where non-handicapped individuals are concerned. In some studies electric toothbrushes have been found to be superior to the manual brush in plaque removal,

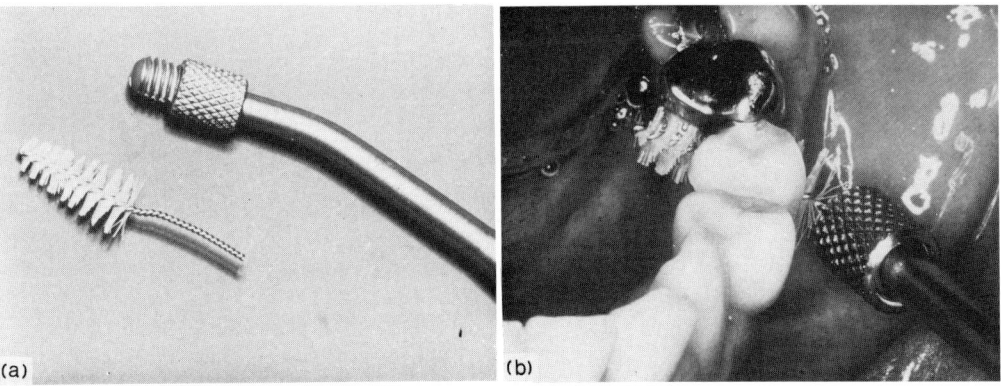

FIG. 10.8. Interspace brush used to cleanse areas where there is a problem of access. (Courtesy of Mr K. W. Stephen.)

while in others no significant advantage was noted. For example, the electric brush has been shown to be the equal of the natural bristle manual brush, in removing plaque from the teeth of non-handicapped adults, regardless of whether the subjects were instructed, or had received no instruction in the use of the brush [6]. On the other hand, in children of the 5–12 year age group, electric toothbrushes have been shown to be more effective in removing plaque and debris than the manual brush [7]. There is no evidence that the electric brush is less effective than the manual brush in removal of deposits from the teeth, or that it is more damaging to the soft tissues. Studies into the effects of excessive brushing with an electric brush have shown no clinical evidence of a harmful effect on the gingival tissues [8]. Following the use of an electric brush on the gingival tissues for 30 seconds each day for 30 days, a significant rise in the proportion of keratinized cells at the gingival surface was claimed [8]. Histological studies have shown that there is a significant increase in the number of cell layers in keratinized or parakeratinized epithelium following the use of electric and manual brushes. No difference was found in the ability of electric or hand toothbrushes to bring about this change [9].

The reports of studies comparing the effectiveness, and effects, of the manual and electrically powered toothbrushes, when considered collectively, lead to the following conclusions:

(1) The automatic toothbrush and the manual brush can be used with equal effectiveness for removing and preventing the formation of dental plaque, and for removing debris and materia alba.

(2) Neither the manual nor the automatic toothbrush is clearly superior with respect to cleansing ability or potential for stimulating gingival keratinization, or for causing damage to the tissue and tooth surfaces.

(3) The electrically operated brush may be especially useful in the oral health care of handicapped persons [1].

The use of woodsticks

Soft woodsticks are a valuable adjunct to therapy after the initial stage of the hygiene

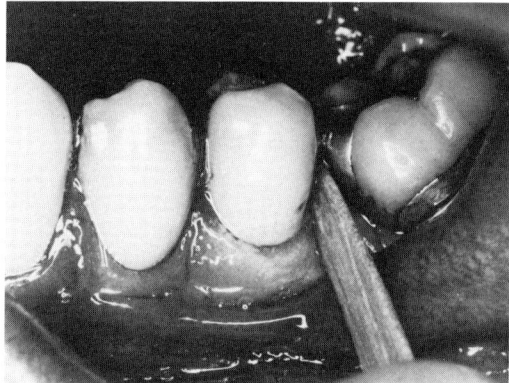

FIG. 10.9. A wood point should be placed at an oblique angle to the tooth so that the point passes through the embrasure without impacting against the lingual papillae.

phase has been completed. Misapplication of woodsticks is potentially damaging. The essential functions of woodstick therapy are cleansing of the embrasure and, to a lesser extent, reshaping of the soft tissues to a functional form. Some degree of increased keratinization of the col may follow the use of woodsticks. Woodstick therapy in the presence of subgingival calculus may cause breach of the cuff epithelium, and it may exacerbate existing inflammation. It should be emphasized that the sticks are not intended as toothpicks. They should be placed at an oblique angle to the tooth, so that the point passes through the embrasure without impacting against the lingual papillae (fig. 10.9). The functional parts of the stick are the sides, which remove plaque from the proximal surfaces of the teeth in the depth of the embrasure, and the base, which shapes the buccal wall of the papilla to form an interdental sluice.

Dental floss or tape

Several studies have shown that periodontal disease is most extensive in the interdental areas, where the use of the toothbrush alone leads to incomplete plaque remov.l [10 & 11]. It has been shown that dental floss is more effective in removing plaque on proximal tooth surfaces than woodsticks [12] but its use is more time consuming. The use of dental floss (fig. 10.10) or tape has been widely advocated [13].

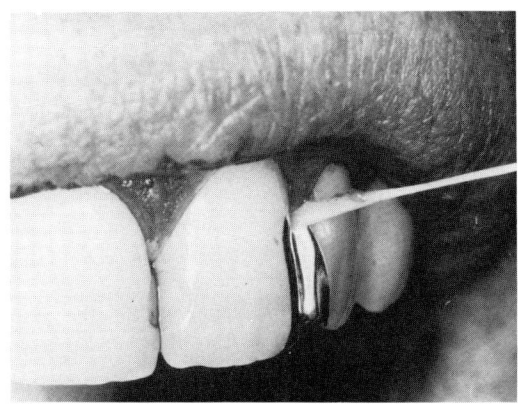

FIG. 10.10. Dental floss or tape tends to be misused by patients and is potentially damaging. It can remove plaque from areas not reached by other aids.

Many authors have stressed that damage can occur through the improper use of dental floss [14 & 15]; thus careful instruction of patients is important and it is essential to monitor the patient at regular intervals.

Dentifrices

A dentifirice is a substance used with a toothbrush for the purpose of cleaning accessible surfaces of teeth. Commercial dentifrices are available in both paste and powder forms and contain, in addition to flavouring, colouring agents, medicaments, foaming agents, water, various abrasives for cleaning or polishing. The latter must be able to polish the teeth, i.e. remove plaque and pellicle, without leaving a rough surface liable to encourage subsequent plaque retention. Chalk has been most frequently used for this purpose, but alumina and zirconium silicate are also used. Toothpaste containing fluoride would seem desirable to reduce enamel solubility, and in cases where exposed dentine at the neck of the tooth interferes with effective cleaning, a toothpaste containing a desensitizing agent might prove helpful. Where the patient is unable to obtain relief, desensitizing can also be undertaken by the dentist. Many agents have been used for this purpose, including zinc chloride and formaldehyde, but sodium fluoride paste consisting of 10 gm each of sodium fluoride and kaolin mixed into a stiff paste with glycerine is usually effective and can be stored for long periods without deterioration. The tooth surface must be thoroughly cleaned and dried and the paste applied for 2 mins before being washed off with warm water.

THE PRACTITIONER'S CARE OF THE PATIENT

The responsibility of the practitioner during the hygiene phase is to assist the patient in reducing the level of inflammation present in the mouth, by scaling and polishing the teeth, by the use of packs, or by instituting drug therapy where presence of acute inflammation justifies its use. Any cavities present in the mouth should be dressed to prevent food stagnation.

Scaling and polishing

Scaling and polishing of teeth is amongst the most demanding and important aspects of periodontal therapy. It should be remembered that bacteraemia is a virtually inevitable consequence of all except the most superficial scalings, and that prophylactic antibiotics should be administered in cases of rheumatic fever, congenital or acquired cardiac defects, or where the patient's medical history suggests that tissue resistance might be impaired (see p. 202). To perform a scaling properly requires a high degree of skill and a large measure of self-discipline. It is totally insufficient only to remove the obvious deposits with gross scalers. Superficial scaling does not constitute an adequate basis for corrective phase periodontal therapy. It is essential that following instrumentation the mouth should be completely free of supra and subgingival calculus and bacterial plaque. To achieve this result requires an intelligent choice of instruments and a systematic approach to the procedure. Disclosing tablets or solutions and a calculus probe (fig. 10.11) should be used to define the location of deposits before instrumentation is commenced. The prime essential of good periodontal practice is to acquire a systematic technique of scaling and polishing which is effective, and which will give the maximum result for the minimum of effort on time and motion study principles. The choice of instruments and the technique which may be adopted to achieve this ideal are highly personal, and the description which follows is the routine which is currently in use in the authors' clinics. This is by no means the only, and perhaps not even the best, routine which is available, and it is reproduced to illustrate the principles which are involved and the need for a systematic approach. Supragingival scaling and the removal of obvious deposits can be performed with many instruments and presents no particular problem. The

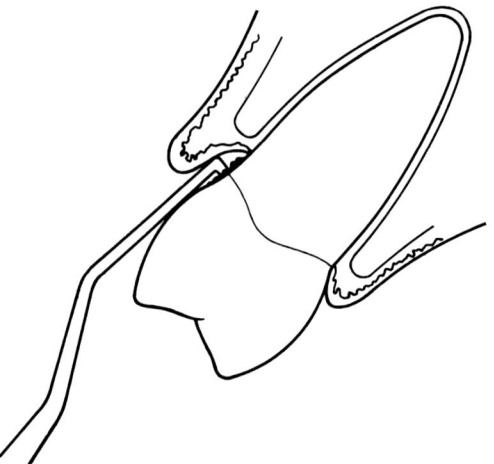

FIG. 10.11. Cross calculus probe used to detect subgingival deposits. Courtesy of Miss Jenny Mitchell.

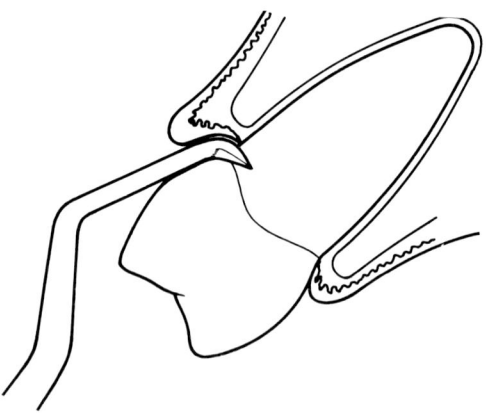

FIG. 10.12. The essential factors in the design of scalers are the degree to which the shape of the instrument conforms to the tooth surface and the size of the working head relative to the space available within the crevice. Courtesy of Miss Jenny Mitchell.

essential factors which govern the design of instruments for the removal of subgingival deposits are the degree to which the shape of the instrument conforms to the curvature of the tooth surface and the size of the instrument relative to the space available within the pocket (fig. 10.12).

GENERAL PRINCIPLES OF INSTRUMENTATION

Force applied to an instrument in the mouth must be applied about a fulcrum. The finger used as a fulcrum should be placed on tooth or bone close to the point of application of the force.

There are two grips by which an instrument should be held.

The modified pen grasp

The instrument is gripped between the thumb and forefinger, the shank rests against the middle finger, the ball of which serves as the finger rest and the fulcrum (figs. 10.13, 15 & 16).

The palm and thumb grasp

The handle of the instrument is held in the cupped second, third and fourth fingers; the thumb acts as a fulcrum as the blade engages the tooth surface (fig. 10.14).

There are four basic movements in the practice of scaling [16].

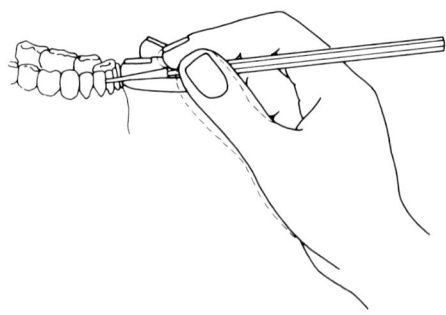

FIG. 10.13. The modified pen grasp using a Cushing's chisel scaler with a digital movement.

Digital movement

This involves sliding a chisel scaler in short smooth strokes in continuous contact with the tooth, by movement of the index finger and thumb across a middle finger fulcrum (fig. 10.13).

Wrist drop

An instrument used in the vertical plane by wrist action (fig. 10.15).

Wrist roll

An instrument used through the rotation of the wrist in the horizontal plane (fig. 10.14).

A combination of the three above (fig. 10.16)

During application of these movements the left hand serves to hold the mirror and to control the lips, cheeks and tongue. It must also support the mandible during scaling (fig. 10.17).

INSTRUMENTS

A minimum practical group of instruments which are suitable for the scaling procedure might be as follows.

125–126 large excavator (fig. 10.18a)

This instrument is a useful multipurpose scaler

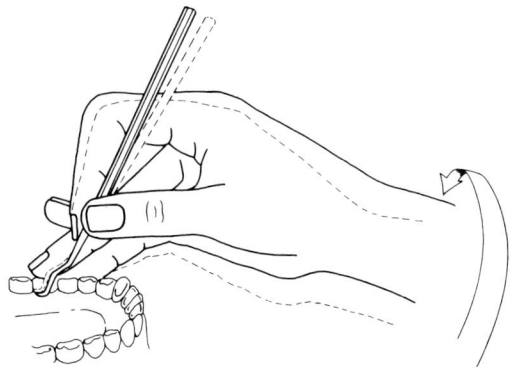

FIG. 10.16. Combination of digital movement, wrist drop and wrist roll using Jaquette scaler.

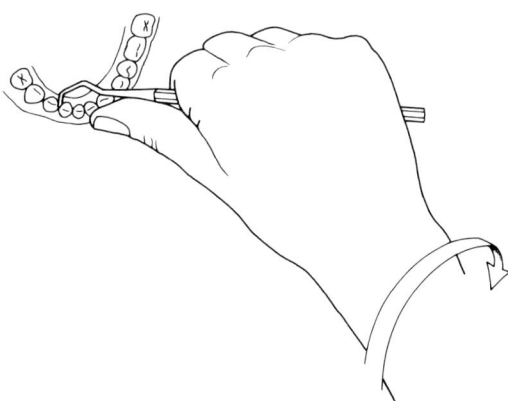

FIG. 10.14. Palm and thumb grasp using a Younger–Good scaler with wrist roll movement.

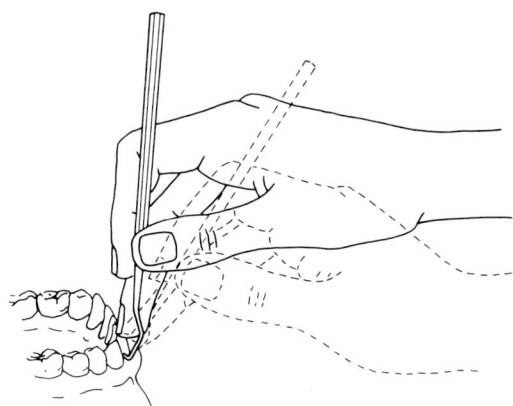

FIG. 10.15. Wrist drop movement using a Jaquette scaler.

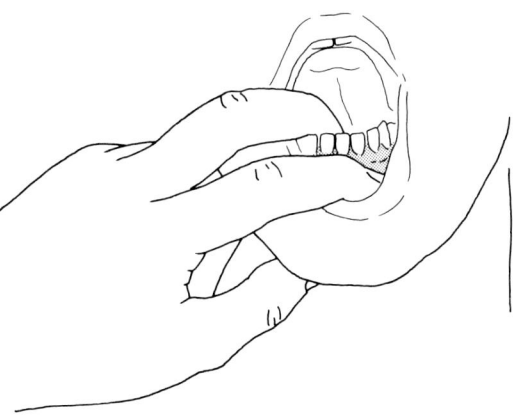

FIG. 10.17. Left hand control of lips, cheeks and tongue, and support of the mandible, for scaling of mandibular incisors when seated in front of the patient.

for speedy and convenient removal of supra-gingival stains and deposits from all areas of the mouth.

Cushing's chisel, watchspring scaler (fig. 10.18b)

This chisel scaler is particularly designed to remove calcified deposits from the embrasure. The edge of the chisel is placed against the tooth surface (fig. 10.13) and lateral pressure applied to

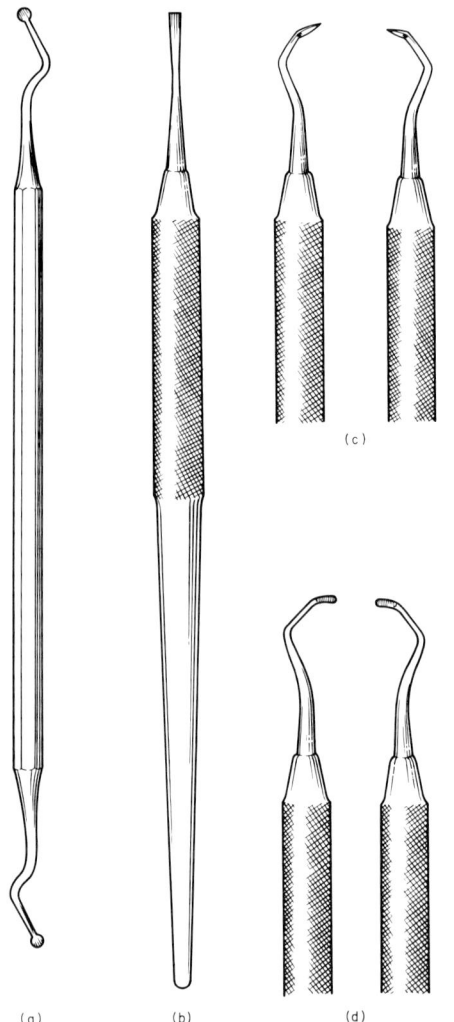

FIG. 10.18. (a) 125–126 Excavator. (b) Cushing's chisel. (c) Jaquettes 2 and 3. (d) Younger-Good 72 and 73.

the working edge. The spring in the tempered blade impacts the edge against the tooth surface and the instrument is passed through the embrasure by digital pressure, stripping the tooth surface of any deposit. This instrument is of particular value in the mandibular incisor region to clear the embrasure of heavy deposits of calculus prior to using finer scalers. It may also be used to remove interproximal calculus from posterior teeth where there is adequate access.

Jacquette scalers (fig. 10.18c)

Jacquettes are robust triangular bladed scalers which are at the upper limit of size for sub-gingival scalers. The instrument should be positioned so that the curve of the tooth crown accords with the curved shank of the instrument and manipulated by a wrist movement so that the point always moves towards and into an embrasure (fig. 10.16).

Younger–Good curettes (fig. 10.18d)

Younger–Good curettes are medium sized scalers particularly suited to subgingival scaling of the incisor and canine regions. The instrument has two cutting edges; the upper edge of the curved working point towards the shank and the spoon shaped tip. The curved upper edge may be used by manipulating the instrument with a wrist movement for sub- and supra-gingival scaling of the margins and interproximal surfaces of incisor teeth in particular (fig. 10.20d). The spoon shaped tip may be used with a palm grip to instrument the lingual surface of incisors and canines (fig. 10.14).

These curettes are at the upper limit of size for subgingival scalers, and it is desirable to add to this minimum instrument kit, fine curettes such as Gracey curettes for subgingival scaling.

McCall's curettes (fig. 10.19a)

McCall's curettes are suitable for use as sub-gingival scalers in all areas of the mouth on the same principles of positioning and movement as are applicable to the Jaquettes and Younger-Goods. The tungsten carbide tipped version of this instrument is also suitable for curettage of

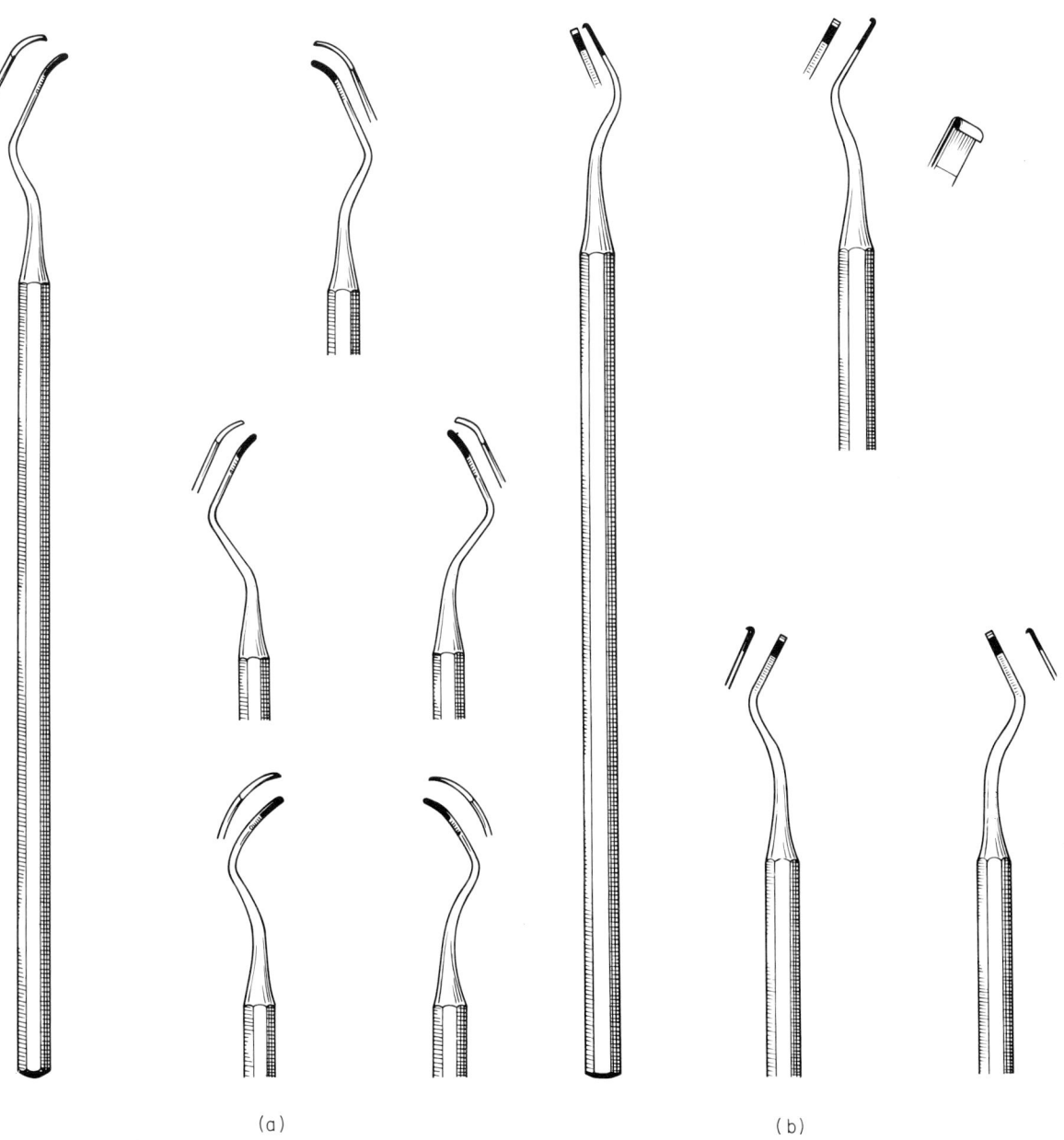

(a) (b)

FIG. 10.19. (a) McCall's curettes. (b) Periodontal hoes.

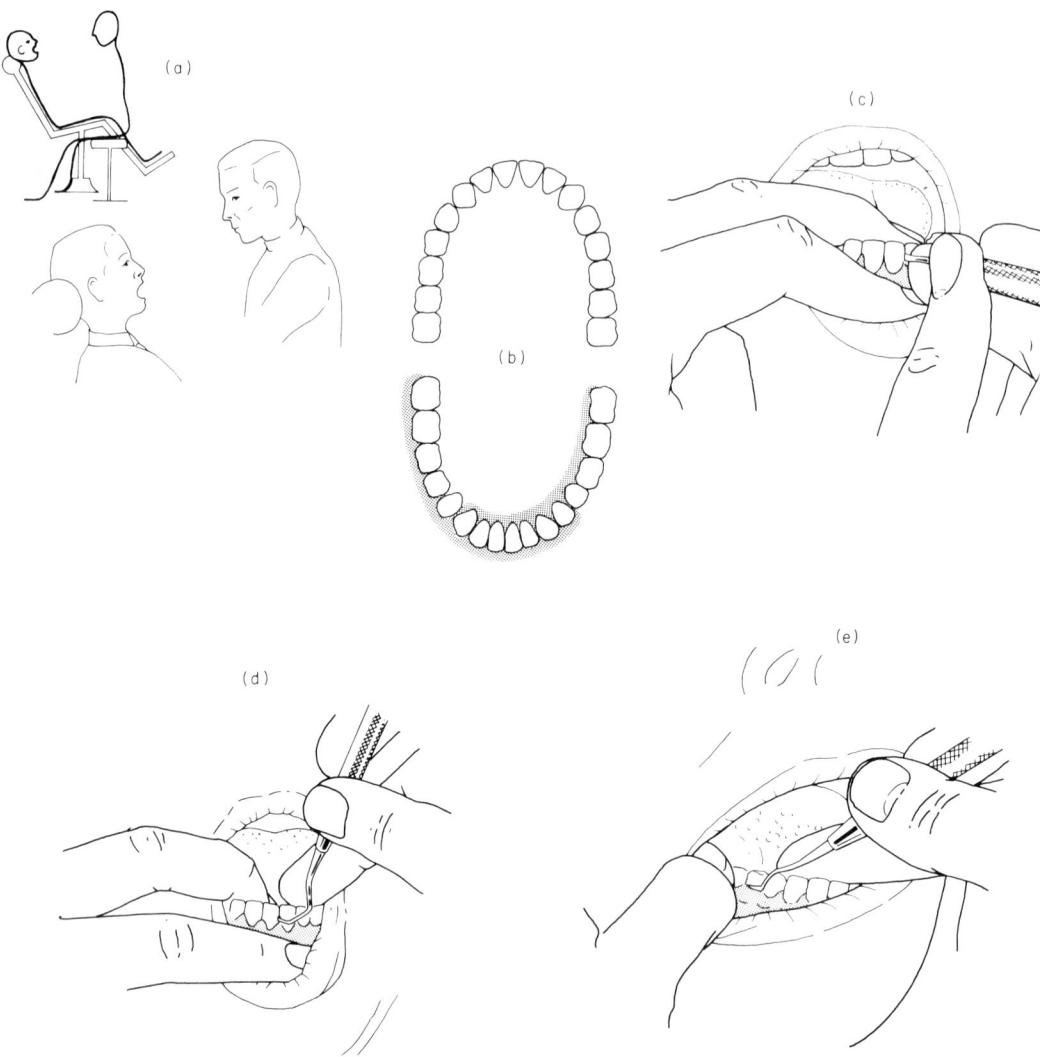

FIG. 10.20. (a) Patient-operator positions working from the front. Chair positioned 10° to vertical, occlusal plane of mandibular teeth at biceps level. (b) Areas of the mouth to be scaled while seated in front of the patient. (c) The use of Cushings chisel to clear deposits from embrasures between anterior teeth. Note use of middle finger as fulcrum and left hand control. (d) The use of a Younger–Good 73 with pen-grasp and middle finger fulcrum to scale the labial surfaces of the anterior teeth, the distal embrasure surfaces of $\overline{321}/$ and the mesial embrasure surfaces of $/\overline{123}$. The same instrument is used to scale the lingual surfaces of $\overline{321/123}$ with a palm-grasp and thumb fulcrum (fig. 10.14). The mesial embrasure surfaces of $\overline{321}/$ and the distal embrasure surfaces are scaled with the Younger–Good 72. (e) The use of a Jaquette 2 to scale towards the distal embrasure surfaces on the buccal surface of mandibular right posterior teeth. The same instrument is used to scale towards the distal embrasure surfaces on the lingual surface of mandibular left posterior teeth. The mesial embrasure surfaces are scaled by the Jaquette 3 on the same principle.

the soft tissue walls of a periodontal pocket (chap. 15). For this procedure the complete set of six curettes is desirable.

Periodontal hoes (fig. 10.19b)

Periodontal hoes are amongst the most effective subgingival scalers. The instrument is placed with the shank parallel to the long axis of the tooth and withdrawn from the full depth of the pocket with a digital movement (fig. 10.12). The tungsten carbide tipped cutting edge effectively planes the tooth surface free from all deposits. This instrument is also used for root planing during subgingival curettage, for which procedure the complete set of four hoes is desirable (chap. 15).

SYSTEMATIC SCALING

To ensure that all areas of the mouth are thoroughly scaled with the minimum of effort, instrumentation of the mouth should be carried out in a precise order as a matter of routine. Most operative procedures should be performed from the seated position, and there is some variation in the working routine according to the particular type of equipment which is being used. One standard routine is used in the authors' clinics for the older types of dental chair, and this is modified for the modern equipment where all operating is performed with the patient position virtually horizontal. An attempt was made by Beagrie to standardize the teaching of scaling to undergraduates by means of a colour code

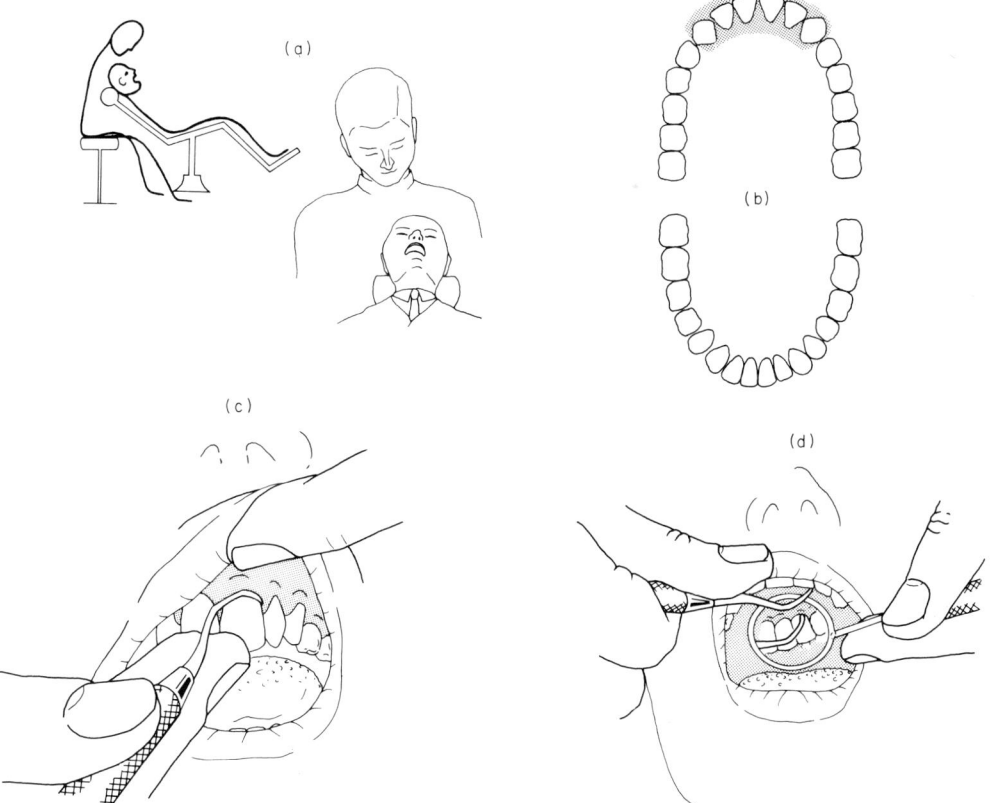

FIG. 10.21. (a) Patient-operator positions working from the rear. Chair position 45° to vertical and patient's head at operator's shoulder level. (b) Area of the mouth to be scaled with patient's head remaining in midline. (c & d) The use of Younger–Good curettes to scale the maxillary incisors from the rear.

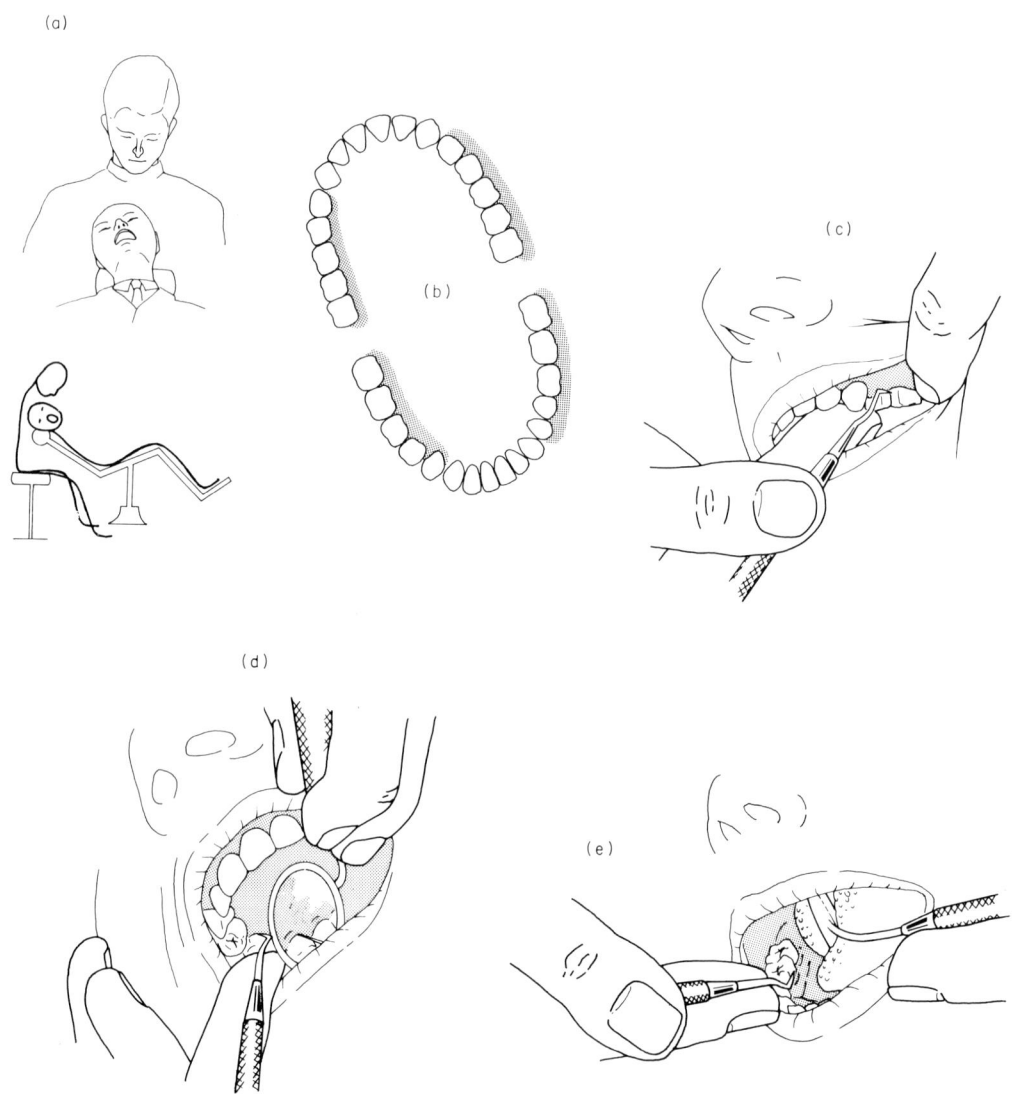

FIG. 10.22. (a) Working from the rear with patient's head turned to the right. (b) Areas of the mouth to be scaled from this position. (c) The use of a Jaquette 3 scaler on the buccal surface of the maxillary left molars by direct vision. (d) The use of a Jaquette 2 on the palatal surface of the maxillary right posterior teeth using a mirror. (e) The use of a Jaquette 3 on the lingual surface of the mandibular right posterior teeth.

system [16], and it is a modification of that system which is described here.

With the older type of dental chair where the patient is treated at an angle rarely less than 45° to the horizontal, it is possible to scale the mouth moving only once from in front of the patient to behind the chair. The simple sequence of patient operator movements is shown in figs. 10.20, 21, 22 & 23.

(1) Seated in front of the patient, who is positioned 10° to vertical with the head turned towards the operator (fig. 10.20a), instrument all surfaces of $\overline{321}/\overline{123}$, the lingual surface of mandibular left molars and the buccal surface of the mandibular right molars (fig. 10.20). The relevant instruments are the Cushing's chisel, the younger–Good curettes, and the Jaquettes, as indicated in figs. 10.20c, d & e. Habit and custom largely govern the ability of the individual to scale from a particular position relative to the patient.

In our experience these are the only areas of the mouth where the student gains a direct advantage in working from the front, from which position he acquires an effective technique most readily. All other areas of the mouth are scaled from behind the patient.

(2) Move behind the patient and tilt the chair

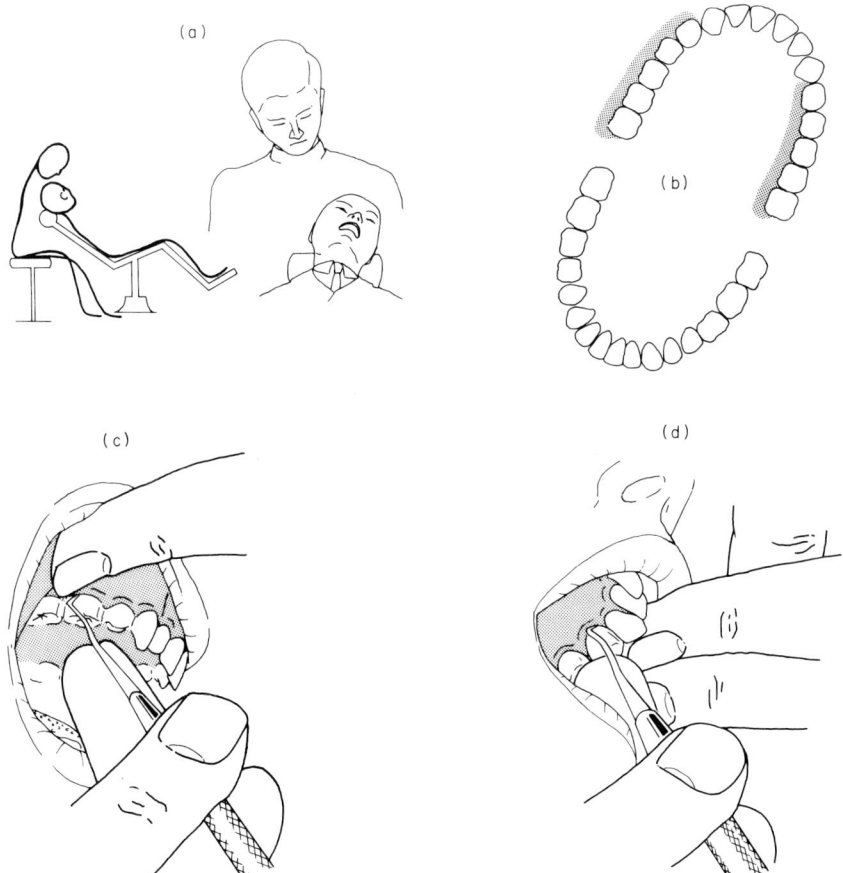

FIG. 10.23. (a) Patient–operator position to gain access to the buccal surface of the maxillary right posterior teeth and the palatal surface of the maxillary left posterior teeth. (c & d) The use of Jaquettes in the areas defined in (b).

back to approximately 45° to the horizontal (fig. 10.21a). With the patient's head remaining in the midline position, scale all surfaces of 321/123 with the Younger–Good curettes on the principle adopted for the mandibular incisors (fig. 10.21b, c & d).

(3) Move the patient's head to the right (fig. 10.22a) when the areas accessible for scaling are the buccal surface of maxillary and mandibular left posterior teeth, the palatal surface of the maxillary right posterior teeth and the lingual surface of the mandibular right posterior teeth (fig. 10.22b). The relevant instruments are the Jaquettes, the McCall's curettes and the periodontal hoes.

(4) Move the patient's head to the left and scale the buccal surface of the maxillary right molars and the palatal surface of the maxillary left molars with the same instruments (fig. 10.23 a & b).

Systematic instrumentation of the mouth is thus completed from the seated position with the minimum of unnecessary physical effort moving only once from in front of the patient to behind. The mouth may be subsequently polished in exactly the same sequence, with the exception that it is convenient to polish the buccal surface of mandibular left molars and the lingual surface of the mandibular right molars from the front. This is simply a matter of access. It is convenient to polish the surface of lower molars from the front, which were instrumented from behind, and vice versa.

The suggested routine does not imply that one should never instrument the lingual surface of 321/123 from behind the patient and it should not be interpreted too rigidly. It represents only the nearest approach to a disciplined system of scaling and polishing which we have been able to establish.

With modern chairs, where the patient is positioned approximately horizontally for all procedures, the complete operation can be performed from behind the patient.

ULTRASONIC SCALING

Ultrasonic dental equipment was first used for cavity preparation, and shortly following its introduction, a series of reports confirmed the potential of such equipment to produce disturbance of amelogenesis, severe pulp changes and alterations in dentine formation [17]. The ultrasonic scaler was produced in the U.S.A. as a development of this original machine, and it is now fairly widely used in Dental Schools and to an increasing extent in general practice. The original Cavitron 30 unit has been superseded by the Cavitron 700 (fig. 10.24a), a much smaller, but essentially similar, machine. The handpiece consists of a 'stack' of ferromagnetic metal which changes in size due to magnetostriction, induced by the magnetizing effect of an alternating electric current [18]. A 25 kilocycle current is converted through the handpiece to 25 000 mechanical strokes per second, the working

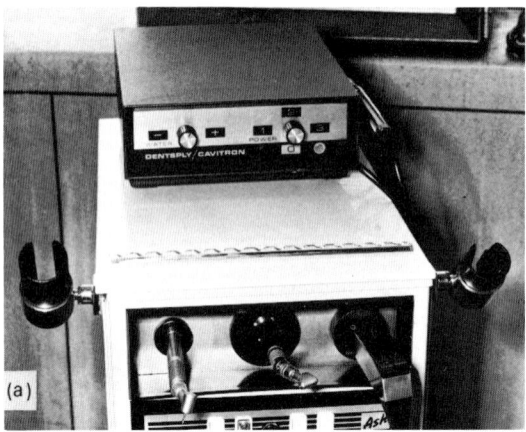

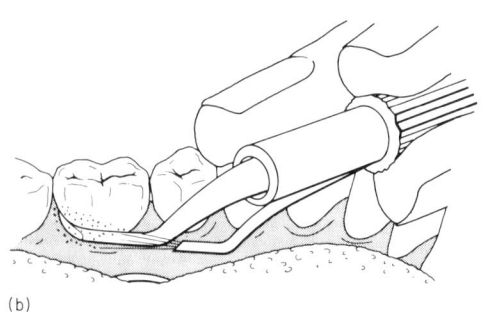

FIG. 10.24. (a) Cavitron 700 Ultrasonic Scaling Unit. (b) Curette type Cavitron working point.

point moving through approximately 1/1000 of an inch with each stroke. The tip action is thus neither radiant nor electrical, but mechanical in action. The most generally useful shape of working point is the curette type (fig. 10.24b).

Water is passed through the handpiece for cooling purposes, and to contribute to the scaling procedure. The water emerges from the handpiece as a fine jet, which on striking the vibrating tip is converted into a spray of fine bubbles. The scaling action of the instrument is a combination of the mechanical action of the tip, and the effects of the formation and violent collapse of small bubbles, the cavitation effect. Apart from the mechanical cleansing action, cavitation is associated with complex physical, chemical and biological phenomena, the significance of which are by no means fully understood. In principle, cavitation may be associated with local pressures of thousands of atmospheres, local temperatures of hundreds of degrees, and local oxidative changes [19]. The potential of this instrument to reduce gingival inflammation results from the mechanical action of the tip, and the mechanical cleansing and biologic effects of cavitation.

A number of investigators have reported favourably on the results of ultrasonic scaling, and they have found no adverse effects on the tissue of the periodontium [20 & 21]. Ultrasonic curettage is an effective method of debridement of the soft tissue walls of periodontal pockets, and histological studies of tissue excised after curettage have shown that healing occurs by epithelialization of the sulcular surface and resolution of inflammation in the gingival corium [22]. Experience with the Cavitron over a number of years confirms the finding that the ultrasonic technique is equally as effective as conventional hand instrumentation in calculus removal, but less effective in stain removal [23], and the instrument does not remove entirely the need for hand instrumentation. There has been some dispute as to whether scaling by the ultrasonic technique is more rapid than hand instrumentation, although no report has suggested that it is less rapid. In the hands of an experienced operator, a saving in time of 20 per cent has been reported [17], but it should be stressed that speed is by no means the only advantage of the ultrasonic technique. There is no doubt at present that this machine is a valuable addition to the armamentarium of the periodontist, and it has the potential to contribute largely to the reduction of acute and chronic inflammation during the hygiene phase (fig. 10.25).

In a study of 240 scaling procedures carried out by dental technicians in the American Air Force, it was concluded that ultrasonic scaling was just as effective as hand scaling and was learned more readily, and that most patients preferred the ultrasonic instrument [23]. Stende and Schaffer observed in a study of 150 teeth that had been scaled ultrasonically, and by hand, that there was no essential difference in the removal of calculus, but that the ultrasonic instrument was not as efficient in root planing [24] (chap. 15). It has been reported, however, that ultrasonic scaling leaves a polished surface on the roots and crowns of teeth [25].

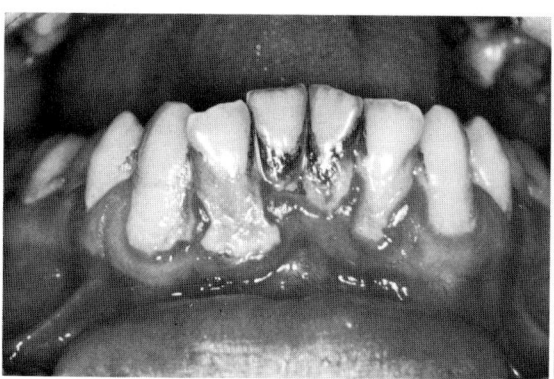 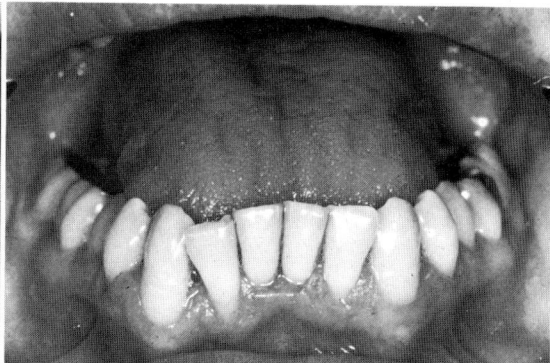

FIG. 10.25. Before and after cavitron.

It has been reported [26 & 27] that the aerosol produced by ultrasonic scalers is heavily contaminated by bacteria and constitutes a potential hazard to the dentist, nursing staff and patients. Marked increases in numbers of airborne bacteria were noted in samples collected from a periodontal clinic when 12 ultrasonic scalers were in use compared with the numbers obtained from the same or similar clinics in which no ultrasonic scalers were being used. A considerable microbial challenge was also noted in the immediate vicinity of individual patients receiving treatment with an ultrasonic scaler.

The use of portable high efficiency electrostatic precipitators was demonstrated to control cumulative aerosol contamination. Chlorhexidine mouthwashes (0·2 per cent) before operation were shown to offer an effective alternative method of control of this contamination and all staff should be masked.

Packs and splints

Nonspecific inflammation of the gingival tissues may prove slow to resolve during hygiene phase therapy, in spite of thorough scaling and polishing and an adequate standard of patient self-care. Resolution of inflammation may be expedited by the use of a periodontal pack. Following scaling and polishing of the teeth, the role of a pack is to protect the swollen tissues from trauma of normal function. The following is a suitable, low cost, all purpose periodontal pack with sufficient power of retention to remain in position for periods up to seven days:

Powder	Zinc oxide	40%
	Resin powder	40%
	Alum. sil. hyd.	3%
	Acid tannic	7%
	Cotton wool	10%
	Carmine	q.s.
Liquid	Thymol	2%
	Clove oil	98%

When mixed properly, two drops of liquid will absorb several spatulas of powder, to form a stiff dry mix which sets hard and dry within minutes of being placed in position (fig. 10.26). The thymol acts as an accelerator, and therefore the speed of setting can be adjusted to suit the convenience of the individual operator. The dressing should be positioned, by packing each embrasure firmly, to obtain retention, and by

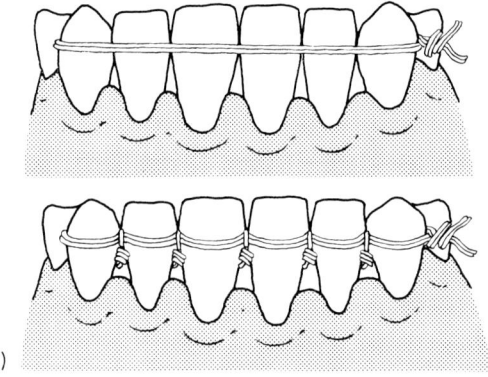

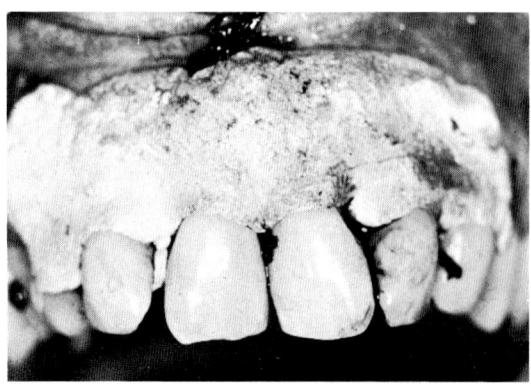

FIG. 10.26. Pack in position.

(a)

(b)

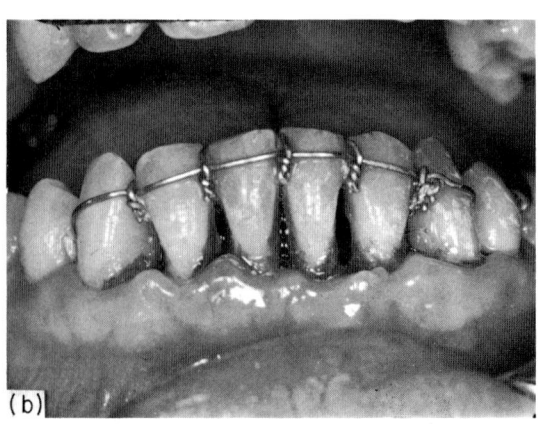

FIG. 10.27. Wire splint (a) technique, (b) in position.

placing a strip of pack across the whole field, which becomes bonded to the packed embrasures. Experience is necessary to time the mix correctly, but this pack has the advantage that it has considerable powers of retention when properly positioned. It is relatively inert with respect to the soft tissues, and it is easy to remove cleanly. There is an increasing tendency to replace the use of pressure packs with chemotherapeutic plaque control agents such as 0·2 per cent chlorhexidine mouthwashes (see p. 262).

TEMPORARY SPLINTS

The instability of proximal contacts of excessively mobile teeth which are poorly supported may cause low grade inflammation to persist during hygiene phase therapy by disseminating toxic factors from plaque throughout the periodontal tissues. Stabilization of such teeth by some simple form of temporary splinting may contribute to the speed of resolution of inflammation. The most convenient and generally useful type of splint for this purpose is formed from an arch wire stabilized by embrasure wires placed around each contact point (fig. 8.27). Additional stability may be gained by covering the wire with cold cure acrylic.

The arch wire is placed in position, the two ends joined opposite an embrasure on the buccal side, but not drawn tight until the embrasure wires have been placed in position. Wires are passed through each embrasure passing apical to the arch wire buccally and lingually and loosely joined buccally so that the occlusal part of the loop lies above the contact point. Working alternately from each end of the splint towards the centre, the embrasure wires are drawn tight so that the occlusal part of the loop wedges in the contact point. The last wire to be fully tightened should be the main arch loop. All joins are cut off on the buccal side and the points turned into the embrasures.

A periodontal pack may be subsequently placed over the splint, and a combination of pack and splint may be used to reduce inflammation, particularly in relation to mobile lower incisors. While it has been reported that wire ligatures are an undesirable form of temporary splinting since they may induce active forces on the ligated teeth, causing them to be moved into new positions [28], temporary splinting of excessively mobile teeth may improve oral hygiene through closure of loose contacts between adjacent teeth, and contribute to reduction of inflammation. Such splints are gradually being replaced by direct bonding to enamel.

REFERENCES

[1] RAMFJORD S.P., KERR D.A. & ASH M. (Eds) (1966) *World Workshop in Periodontics.* Michigan: University of Michigan.

[2] HANSEN F. & GJERMO P. (1971) The plaque-removing effect of four toothbrushing methods. *Scand. J. dent. Res.* **79**, 502.

[3] FRANDSEN A.M., BARBANO J.B., SUOMI J.D., CHANG J.J. & BURKE A.D. (1970) The effectiveness of the Charters' Scrub and Roll methods of toothbrushing by professionals in removing dental plaque. *Scand. J. dent. Res.* **78**, 459.

[4] McCLURE D.B. (1966) A comparison of toothbrushing techniques for the pre-school child. *J. Dent. Child.* **33**, 205.

[5] ARNIN S.S. (1963) The use of disclosing agents for measuring tooth cleanliness. *J. Periodont.* **34**, 227–245.

[6] BEUBE F.E., SCHWARTZ M. & THOMPSON R.H. (1964) Comparison of effectiveness in plaque removal of an electric toothbrush. *Periodontics.* **2**, 71–75.

[7] CONROY O. & MELFI O. (1966) Comparison of automatic and hand toothbrushes; cleaning effectiveness for children. *J. Dent. Child.* **33**, 219–225.

[8] TOTO P.D. (1966) Electric toothbrush effect upon keratin formation. *Periodontics,* **4**, 332–333.

[9] BELCHLEM D.N., SAXE S.R. & STERN I.B. (1965) The effect upon the gingivae of using an electric toothbrush in the presence of marginal periodontitis. *Periodontics,* **3**, 90–94.

[10] LOVDAL A., ARNO A. & WAERHAUG J. (1958) Incidence of clinical manifestations of periodontal disease in light of oral hygiene and calculus formation. *J. Am. dent. Assn.* **56**, 21–33.

[11] LINDHE J. & KOCH G. (1966) The effect of supervised oral hygiene on the gingivae of children. *J. periodont. Res.* **1**, 260–267.

[12] GJERMO P. & FLÖTRA L. (1970) The effect of different methods of interdental cleaning. *J. periodont. Res.* **5**, 230.

[13] PIERRE FAUCHARD ACADEMY (1956) Use of floss or tape recommended routinely by majority of dentists. *Dent. Sur.* **32**, 1167–1169.

[14] EVERETT F.G. & KUNKELL P.W. (1953) Abrasion through the abuse of dental floss. *J. Periodont.* **24**, 186–187.

[15] LEGGET L.M. & PATERSON L.N. (1958) Dental injury from floss: case report. *Acad. Rev. Calif. Acad. Periodont.* **6**, 93.

[16] BEAGRIE G.S. (1960) Pre-clinical teaching in periodontology. *Brit. dent. J.* **109**, 168–172.

[17] FORREST J.O. (1967) Ultrasonic scaling: A five year assessment. *Brit. dent. J.* **122**, 9–14.

[18] GREEN G.H. & SANDERSON A.D. (1965) Ultrasonics and periodontal therapy, a review of clinical and biologic effects. *J. Periodont.* **36**, 232–238.

[19] WEISSLER A. (1953) Sonochemistry. The production of chemical changes with sound waves. *J. acoust. Soc. Amer.* **25**, 651–657.

[20] ZINNER D.D. (1955) Recent ultrasonic dental studies: including periodontia without the use of an abrasive. *J. dent. Res.* **34**, 748–749.

[21] MALLERNEE R.E. (1958) Effect of ultrasonic energy on the periodontal membrane, alveolar bone, and gingivae. *J. prosth. Dent.* **8**, 147–152.

[22] GOLDMAN H.M. (1960) Curettage by ultrasonic instrument. *Oral Surg.* **13**, 43–53.

[23] McCALL C.M. & SZMYD L. (1960) Clinical evaluation of ultrasonic scaling. *J. Amer. dent. Ass.* **61**, 559–564.

[24] STENDE G.W. & SCHAFFER E.M. (1961) Objective evaluation of ultrasonic and hand scaling. *J. Periodont.* **32**, 312–314.

[25] JAMES E. (1960) Ultrasonics in periodontal therapy (clinical observations). *J. Mich. dent. Soc.* **42**, 472–474.

[26] HOLBROOK W.P., MUIR K.F., MacPHEE I.T. & ROSS P.W. (1978) Bacteriological investigation of the aerosol from ultrasonic scales. *Brit. Dent. J.* **144**, 245.

[27] MUIR K.F., KOWOLIK M.J. & MacPHEE I.T. (1978) Bacterial aerosol from ultrasonic scales. *Brit. Dent. J.*, **145**, 3, 76–78.

[28] SATUREN B. (1960) Wire ligature: An undesirable form of temporary splinting. *J. Periodont.* **31**, 37–39.

CHAPTER 11

The reduction of acute inflammation

ACUTE SPECIFIC GINGIVITIS

Acute ulceromembranous gingivitis

Acute ulceromembranous gingivitis is characterized by ulceration of the gingival papillae and margins of sudden onset, frequently following debilitating illness, or occurring in association with periods of emotional stress or crowded living conditions. The exact aetiology of the disease is unknown, but evidence suggests an association with the fusospirochaetal complex [1 & 2] and other bacilli which are commensal in the mouth [3]. The disease appears to result from imbalance of the host–parasite relationship, following alteration in host resistance to organisms indigenous to the mouth. The condition is characterized by an increase in the number of fusospirochaetal organisms, in the affected area.

Such an ulcerative gingivitis was described amongst soldiers in the fourth century B.C. [4], and in modern times during World War II [5]. While the disease is apparently infectious, it is not clear to what extent it is communicable [6].

CRITERIA FOR DIAGNOSIS

The criteria used to diagnose acute ulceromembranous gingivitis (fig. 11.1) are:

(1) necrosis and ulceration of the interdental papillae,

(2) typical punched out crater ulcers which involve the papillae and/or gingival margins,

(3) an ulcer surface covered by a grey pseudomembranous slough, demarcated from the surrounding mucosa by a linear erythema,

(4) a history of soreness and bleeding of the gingivae following minor trauma.

There is evidence of considerable misdiagnosis of ulceromembranous gingivitis [6, 7 & 8]. Other clinical signs and symptoms which have

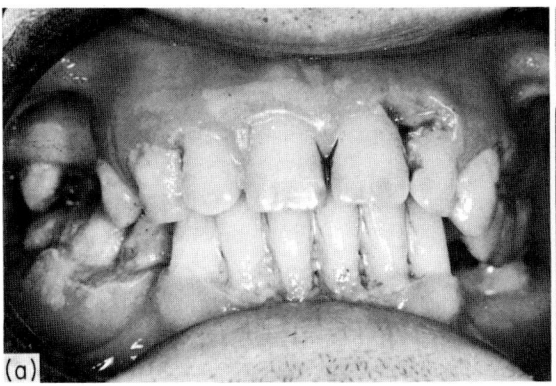 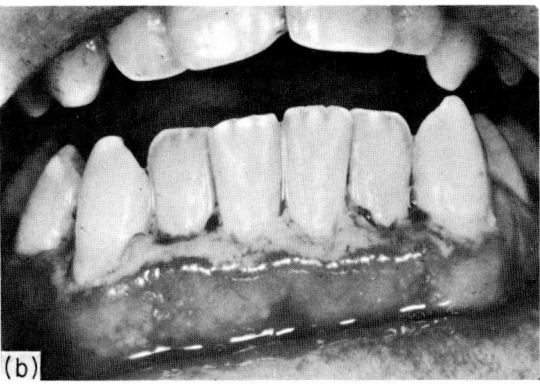

FIG. 11.1. Acute ulceromembranous gingivitis. (a) Typical punched out crater ulcers which involve the papillae and/or gingival margins. (b) Ulceration demarcated from normal tissue by a linear erythema.

been said to be associated with the disease include increased salivation, a characteristic foetid odour, spontaneous gingival haemorrhage, lymphadenopathy, fever and malaise [9]. These may be general signs and symptoms of infection in the mouth and are not specific to ulceromembranous gingivitis. It has been stated that fever and malaise in particular are not characteristic of ulceromembranous gingivitis [6], but suggest the presence of primary herpetic stomatitis, or a mixed herpetic and fusiform stomatitis. The relationship between herpetic and fusospirochaetal infection is further supported, in that a serological study suggested that primary herpetic infection: 'must frequently initiate, or recently precede, acute ulcerative gingivitis or cancrum oris', in Nigerian children [10].

AETIOLOGY

Role of microorganisms

The fact that the acute signs and symptoms of ulceromembranous gingivitis respond dramatically to administration of penicillin and broad spectrum antibiotics, leaves little doubt that bacteria are directly associated with the lesions. It is not clear to what extent the fusospirochaetal organisms present on a direct smear (fig. 11.2) initiate the disease, since the presence of an overgrowth of a particular bacterial species indigenous to the area does not indicate a direct cause and effect relationship with any disease process which may be present [11]. Histopathological studies [1] have demonstrated that fusiform bacilli and spiral organisms are present in

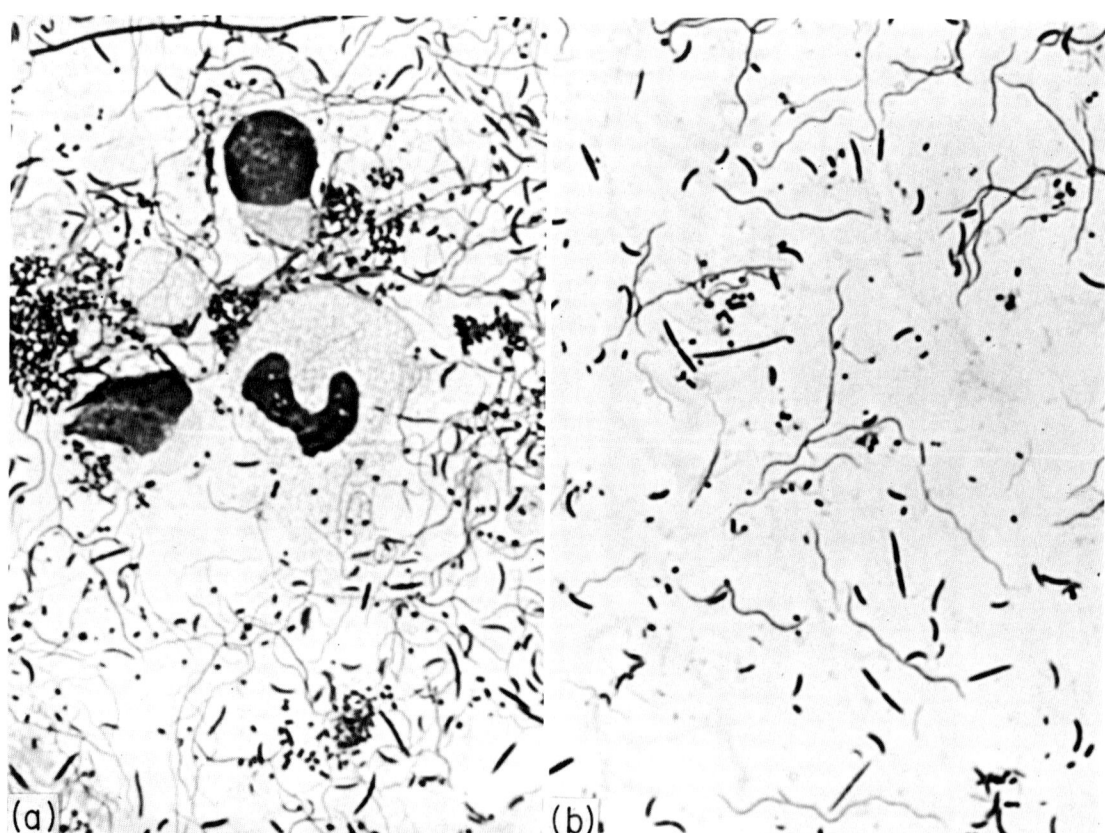

FIG. 11.2. (a) Smear showing organisms from fusospirochaetal complex and inflammatory cells. Spirochaetes, coccal organisms, vibrios and fusiform bacilli are predominant. (b) High power of (a) showing cigar shaped fusiform bacilli and spirochaetes.

the necrotic material, and that the spiral forms appear to invade the tissue in advance of the bacilli (fig. 11.3). Electron micrographs of thin sections of ulcerated gingivae have demonstrated compact masses of spirochaetes and fusiform bacilli invading the intercellular spaces of still vital epithelium [2]. It has been shown that *Treponema microdentium* in particular produces an endotoxin [12], and that injections of live or dead spirochaetes into rabbits produce abscesses [13]. Such studies confirm the potential pathogenicity of the fusospirochaetal complex but not the capacity to produce disease in man. There is indirect evidence as to the role of spirochaetes; studies have confirmed that the antispirochaetal agent metronidazole is as effective as penicillin in treating the disease [14–21]. With the exception of work carried out using the guinea pig as an experimental model, attempts to transmit repeatedly the condition by injection of all, or part, of the mixed flora which is present in association with these lesions have failed. A typical experimental fusospirochaetal infection

has been induced in the guinea pig groin by a minimum combination of four oral organisms, two bacteroides, a motile Gram-negative anaerobe and a facultative diphtheroid, although this is not necessarily the only combination of microorganisms which may be capable of transmitting the infection. The presence of fusiform bacilli or spirochaetes was not required either to initiate or maintain the infection [22]. Further work with this experimental model suggested that the primary pathogen may be *Bacteroides melaninogenicus*, which produces an enzyme thought to be capable of attacking native collagen [23].

The concept has developed that ulceromembranous gingivitis is an endogenous infection which follows alteration of tissue resistance. The onset of the disease represents a change in the host–parasite equilibrium, which favours commensal organisms. To what extent a particular organism, or group of organisms, from the oral commensal population is primarily involved is not clear.

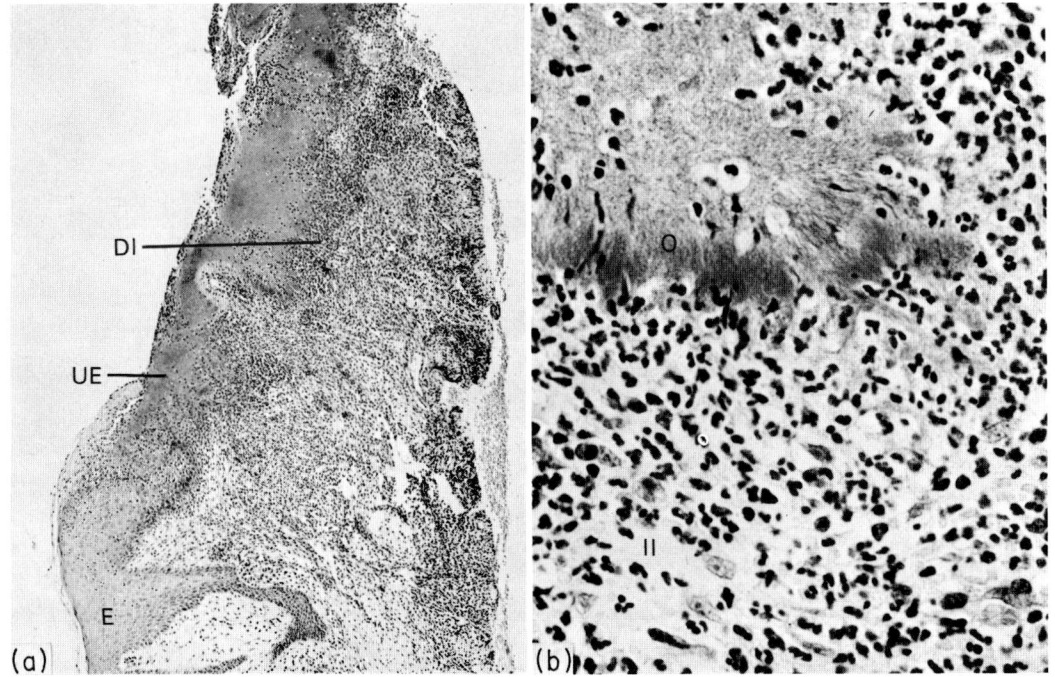

FIG. 11.3. (a) Biopsy of marginal tissue from patient with acute ulceromembranous gingivitis; E, normal gingival epithelium; UE, ulcerated epithelium; DI, dense inflammatory infiltrate or acute inflammatory cells. (b) High power view showing inflammatory infiltrate (II) and mesh work of organisms (O) at ulcer base.

Host resistance

The mechanisms whereby various factors can cause a symbiotic host–parasite relationship to become parasitic are not known. It has been suggested that intrinsic conditions such as nutritional deficiencies [24], debilitating disease [25] or psychological stress [26 & 27] may predispose the patient to the local condition. In Europe and the United States ulceromembranous gingivitis is usually considered a disease of limited consequences (fig. 11.4a). In developing countries the appearance of ulcerative gingivitis in young children is frequently associated with predisposing systemic disease, such as measles, smallpox, malaria and secondary anaemia [10], and the condition often progresses to cancrum oris (fig. 11.4b). In general the most conspicuous predisposing factors are tobacco smoking, pre-existing gingivitis or local trauma, in association with acute psychological disturbance which may precipitate the disease in susceptible individuals [6].

The possibility of a direct relationship between the necrosis of ulceromembranous gingivitis and change in gingival circulation has been considered [28]. It is well recognized that stress can result in the production of adrenaline from the adrenal medulla, and that nicotine is one of the most effective compounds inducing release of adrenaline from the adrenal glands [29]. It has been further shown that small doses of endotoxin from Gram-negative bacteria cause marked enhancement of vasoconstrictor reactions to adrenaline. Clinical experience suggests that the distribution of necrosis in ulceromembranous gingivitis bears a relationship to the distribution of the major gingival blood vessels. There are

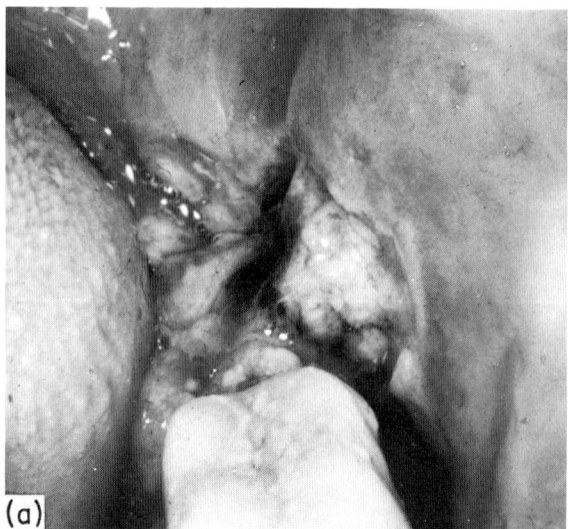
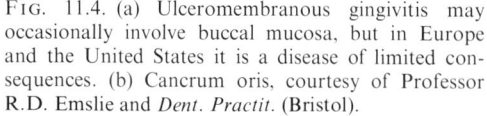
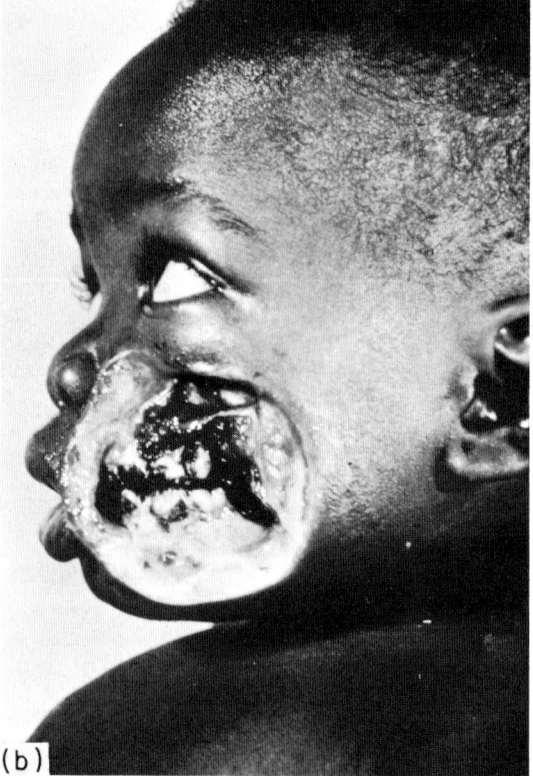

FIG. 11.4. (a) Ulceromembranous gingivitis may occasionally involve buccal mucosa, but in Europe and the United States it is a disease of limited consequences. (b) Cancrum oris, courtesy of Professor R.D. Emslie and *Dent. Practit.* (Bristol).

different degrees of lateral ulceration; necrosis may be limited to the papilla tip (fig. 11.5a) or may involve a variable proportion of the buccal surface of the papilla, and the gingival margin, extending on occasions across the width of the attached gingivae to involve the alveolar mucosa (fig. 11.5b). In contrast to this, deep necrosis of the tissues of the embrasure may occur with minimal involvement of the lateral surface of the papillae and margins (fig. 11.5c). It has been suggested that these patterns of necrosis are related to the fact that the major blood supply to the two areas is different [28]. The gingival tissues are supplied with blood from two main sources (chap. 1). The major blood supply arises from vessels lying above the periosteum which supply the attached gingivae, lateral margins and lateral parts of the papillae, while the interdental col and body of the papillae derive a capillary network from the intra-alveolar and main periodontal vessel (fig. 11.6). It has been stated that inflammation tracks through connective tissue along the line of the blood vessels [30 & 31]. While it is accepted that there is considerable anastomosis between the vessels lateral to the periosteum and the intra-alveolar and main periodontal vessels, it is possible that local accumulation of endotoxins, or other toxic factors from plaque, may alter vasoconstrictor activity, and cause localized ischaemic necrosis. Lateral ulceration involving primarily the buccal wall of the papillae, margins, and possibly the attached gingivae, occurs in the distribution of the lateral blood supply. Deep ulceration involving primarily necrosis of the tissues of the

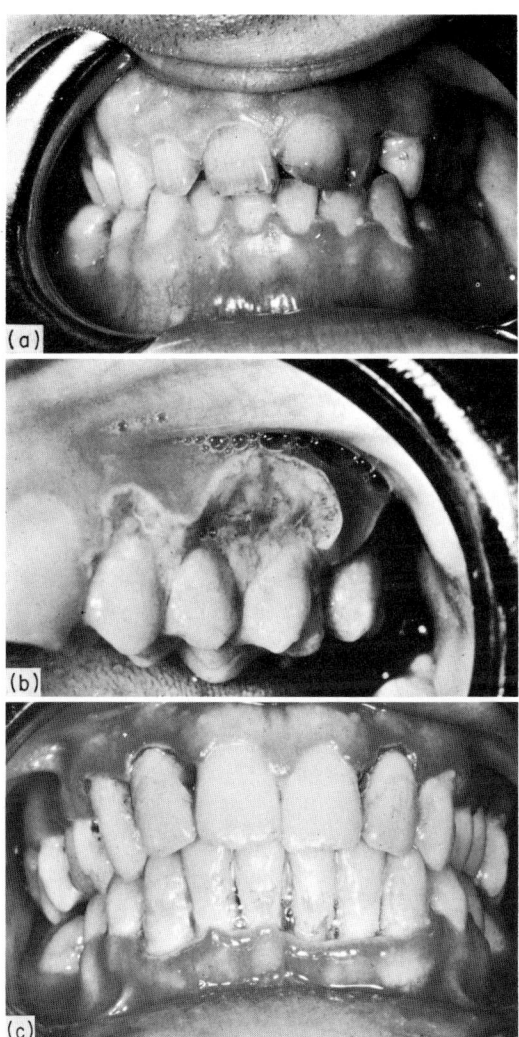

(a)

(b)

(c)

FIG. 11.5. (a) Ulceration limited to the tips of the papillae. (b) Ulceration extending across the attached gingivae, to involve the reflected mucosa, courtesy of *Brit. dent. J.* (c) Deep crater ulceration of the embrasure.

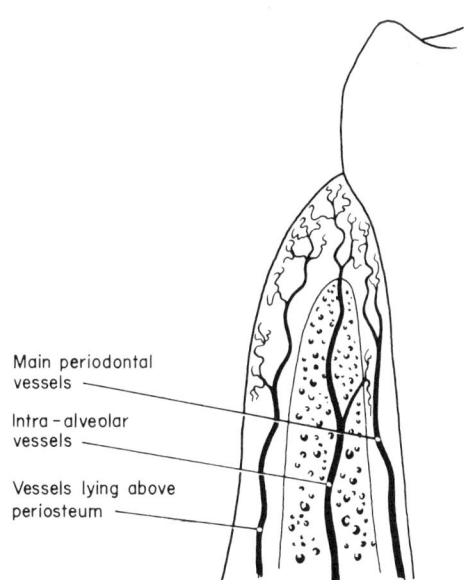

Main periodontal vessels

Intra-alveolar vessels

Vessels lying above periosteum

FIG. 11.6. Blood supply to gingivae.

embrasure, giving rise to the typical truncated papillae, occurs in the distribution of the intra-alveolar and main periodontal vessels. The pattern of necrosis which is present is of significance in the approach to treatment (*vide infra*).

Lateral ulceration

Lateral ulceration is characterized by tissue necrosis extending from the papilla tip and margin, a variable distance down the lateral surface of the papilla, to involve the attached gingiva and occasionally the alveolar mucosa (fig. 11.7). Such a lesion differs widely in its character and in its sequelae from deep ulceration of

the embrasure region. Lateral ulceration is less common than deep ulceration of the tissues of the embrasure and tends to occur in mouths where there has not been an established periodontitis. In general, little permanent damage follows an episode of this type provided it is controlled quickly, since the destruction of tissue is initially superficial and in the contour of the normal gingivae. Regeneration and healing may restore the gingival tissue to an acceptable functional form. Superficial and deep ulceration frequently occur in different areas of the same mouth. Where treatment is inadequate, either form of ulceration may result in permanent damage (fig. 11.8).

Deep ulceration of the embrasure region

Clinically this is an interpapillary lesion, and necrosis is essentially limited to the interstitial tissues of the embrasure (fig. 11.9). In general, but not always, this type of ulceration is seen where there has been pre-existing chronic periodontitis. The area of necrosis within the pocket may be extensive, but due to its deep position not immediately apparent. The general direction of tissue loss is vertical and from within the pocket outwards, resulting in loss of functional anatomical form. The main clinical significance of this lesion is that irrespective of the method of treatment during the acute phase, the

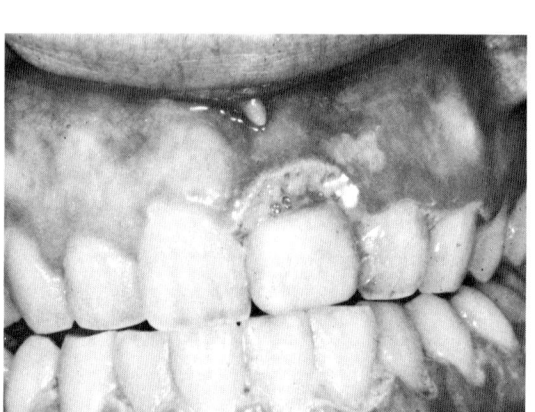

FIG. 11.7. Lateral ulceration.

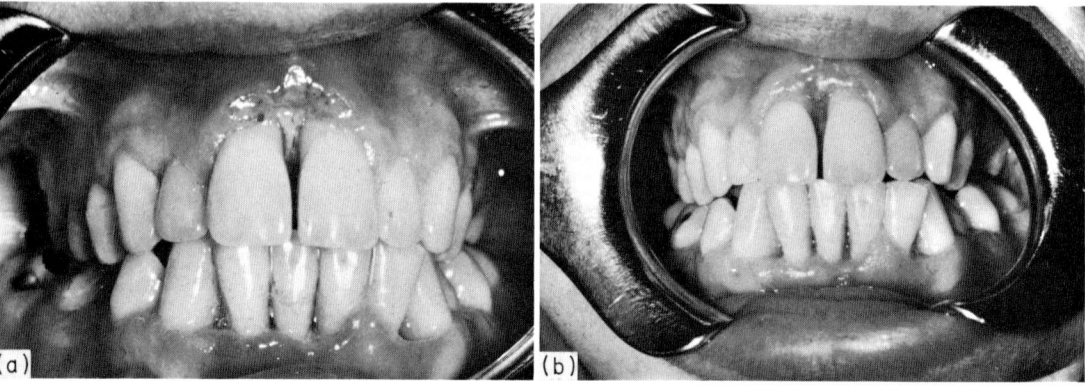

FIG. 11.8. (a) Lateral and deep embrasure ulceration occurring in the same mouth. The untreated lateral ulceration has denuded and exposed alveolar bone. (b) Following treatment the lateral ulceration has healed and regenerated to something approximating to a functional form without surgical intervention. The deep embrasure ulceration in the mandibular incisor region requires surgical correction of gingival form.

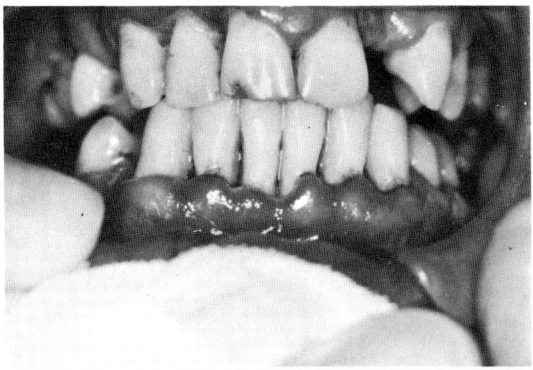

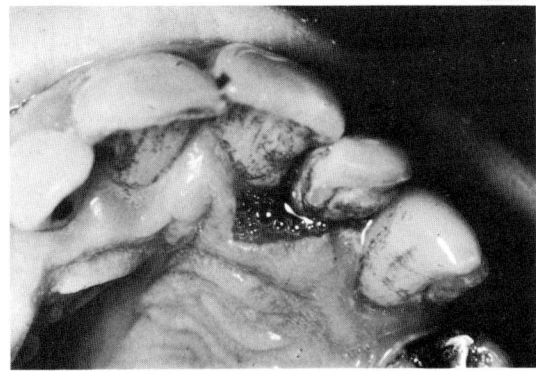

FIG. 11.9. Deep ulceration of the embrasure. Following the acute phase this often results in flat shelving, or crater formation, of the interdental area, which promotes food stagnation. Subsequent surgical correction of gingival form is frequently obligatory.

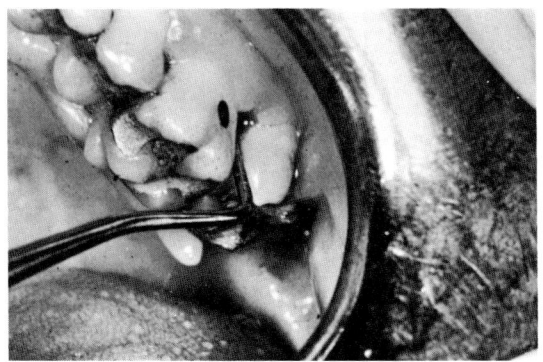

FIG. 11.10. Distortion of gingival form following a minor episode of deep ulceration of the embrasure region.

result of the necrosis is flat shelving or crater formation in the interdental area promoting food stagnation. Some degree of regeneration of tissue does take place during healing, but the common sequellae are progressive pocket formation and chronic periodontitis (fig. 11.10).

TREATMENT

Acute phase

The first essential of treatment of infection of the mouth is scaling and polishing and the establishment of an effective regimen of patient self-care. Drugs should never be administered in isolation from hygiene phase therapy (chap. 10). At the time of admission, the mouth should be as thoroughly scaled as the patient's discomfort will allow, all carious cavities should be dressed and the patient instructed in the proper use of a toothbrush. The majority of patients, particularly those with predominantly lateral ulceration, respond dramatically to local hygiene measures alone, and the importance of early local cleansing and maintenance of oral hygiene has been established [32 & 33] (fig. 11.11). It has been stressed that every endeavour should be made to promote early healing and the minimum of gingival deformity [34]. The supportive use of drugs may be necessary, particularly in patients with deep ulceration of the embrasure region where the lesion is not comparably accessible to local measures. Having instituted hygiene phase control the need for drug therapy should be assessed.

Drug therapy

Survey of the literature shows that a legendary number of drugs have been used in the treatment of ulceromembranous gingivitis. At the present time the following methods of treatment are still widely used, although there is now little justification for direct application of oxygen releasing agents and, since the development of metronidazole, a much reduced indication for the use of antibiotics.

Oxygen releasing agents. (1) Direct application of hydrogen peroxide, aqueous solutions of chromic acid or sodium perborate mixed with distilled water.

(2) Oxygen releasing agents and mucin solvents used as mouthwashes.

Oxygen releasing agents are widely used in the treatment of ulceromembranous gingivitis. Where they are used at all the use of sodium perborate should be discarded in favour of hydrogen peroxide, over which sodium perborate has no apparent clinical advantage [35]. It has been stated that it is doubtful whether the amounts of oxygen released by hydrogen peroxide have a significant action on the metabolism of anaerobic organisms during the short period of exposure [36], although oxygen releasing agents may affect bacterial metabolism in other ways [36]. Hydrogen peroxide is most probably of advantage only as a mechanical cleansing agent. Chromic acid acts as a protein precipitant and obtundent, its function being to cover the cleansed surface of the ulcer with a layer of precipitated protein.

There is no direct evidence of tissue damage resulting from the use of direct application of Solution of Hydrogen Peroxide B.P. diluted, equal parts with water, provided this is limited to the ulcerated surface. The diluted solution may be applied directly to the ulcer surface by means of the capillarity of college dressing tweezers. Direct application of chromic acid at any dilution causes severe tissue damage and should not be used for treatment of infections of the mouth.

Oxygen releasing agents and mucin solvents used as mouthwashes may be valuable adjuvants

to treatment. Wade has reported that a sodium peroxyborate preparation (Bocasan, Knox Laboratories) and hydrogen peroxide (0·3 per cent) were effective in reducing the severity of the acute phase of ulceromembranous gingivitis in a sufficiently high proportion of cases to recommend them as alternatives to antibiotic therapy [37]. He has reported that there was no statistically significant difference in the effectiveness of metronidazole (200 mg three times per day) and peroxyborate preparations [19].

Antibiotics. (1) Topical applications of penicillin or tetracycline.

(2) Penicillin lozenges or chewing gums.

(3) Antibiotics administered systemically.

Administration of antibiotics inevitably disturbs the bacterial flora in the human host, so that organisms insensitive to the particular drug being given will colonize and sometimes infect [38]. If antibiotics are to be used at all they should be administered in a sufficient dosage, for an adequate length of time, to minimize the risks of sensitization of the patient and the production of resistant strains of organisms [39]. If these principles are adhered to, the widespread and indiscriminate use of antibiotics will not occur, which will reduce the risk of producing a large population of antibiotic resistant microorganisms, and diminish the incidence of fatal side effects to treatment. Feinberg *et al.* estimated that there had been more than 1000 deaths due to penicillin anaphylaxis [40]. It has been estimated the death rate is 0·1 for each million injections [41], and that at the Mayo Clinic almost

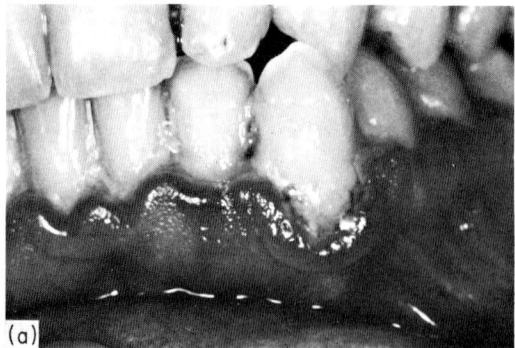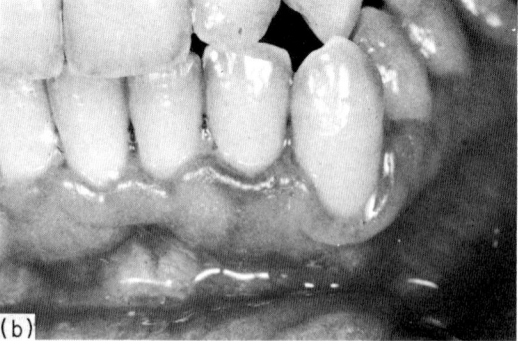

FIG. 11.11. (a) Predominantly lateral ulceration. (b) Resolution following 3 day oral hygiene control without drug therapy.

1 per cent of the patients receiving penicillin had reactions [42].

Ideally the organisms should always be identified and their susceptibility to antibacterial drugs ascertained before treatment is given [38].

The use of antibiotics in the treatment of ulceromembranous gingivitis does not accord with these principles. It has been shown that metronidazole administered either locally or systemically is equally as effective as penicillin in treatment of ulceromembranous gingivitis. In view of the relative absence of side effects following administration of metronidazole, there seems no present justification for the use of antibiotics in treatment of ulceromembranous gingivitis.

Metronidazole. 1–B–hydroxyethyl–2–methyl–5–nitroimidazole (Flagyl–May and Baker). Dose: 200 mg three times daily for 3 days.

Shinn observed that, in a patient taking metronidazole for trichomonal infection of the vagina, a rapid improvement occurred in a concurrent acute ulcerative gingivitis [14]. It has since been clearly demonstrated that metronidazole is effective in treatment of the acute phase of ulceromembranous gingivitis, whether administered systemically [14–20] or locally [21].

The drug appears to be relatively nontoxic and can be used during pregnancy, though it is probably wise to avoid the use in early pregnancy. Its chemical composition suggested that blood dyscrasias might result from its use, but in prac-tice these have not been observed, even with high and prolonged dosage [43].

As a result of its present lack of side effects, this drug has supplanted antibiotics in the treatment of ulceromembranous gingivitis.

Rehabilitation of mouth

Following treatment of the acute phase, scaling and polishing of the mouth should be completed, and the patient instructed in interdental cleaning. Further treatment should be directed towards creation of a functional arch form and elimination of stagnation areas from the mouth. This should embrace restoration of carious teeth and redesigning of any fillings present which are functionally inadequate from the point of view of food shedding. Flaps over partially erupted third molars, or anatomically grossly misplaced teeth, should be removed and bite reconstruction carried out, particularly where, over the long term, tooth drift is likely to lead to formation of further stagnation areas. Where the disease has caused distortion of gingival form, or where there has been a pre-existing periodontitis, the final phase of treatment should involve surgical elimination of pockets, and restoration of soft tissue and bone architecture to a functional anatomical form (chap. 15) (fig. 11.12).

Primary (acute) herpetic gingivostomatitis

Primary herpetic gingivostomatitis is an acute infectious disease usually occurring in young

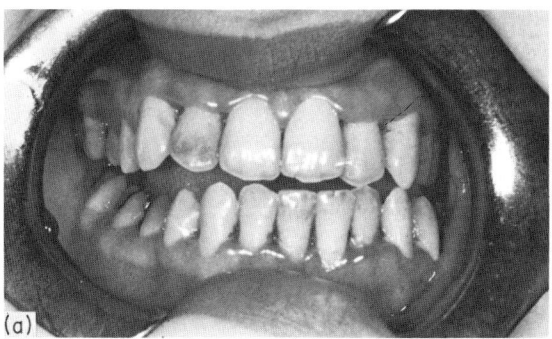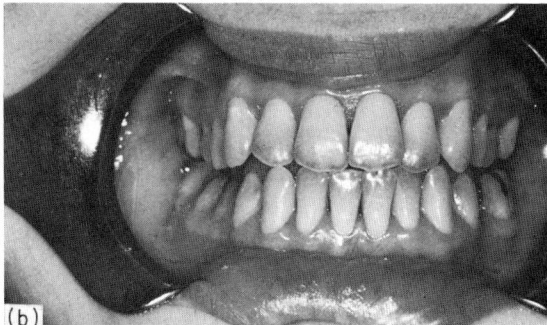

FIG. 11.12. (a) Distortion of gingival form following deep ulceration of the embrasure region. (b) Following surgical correction by gingivectomy.

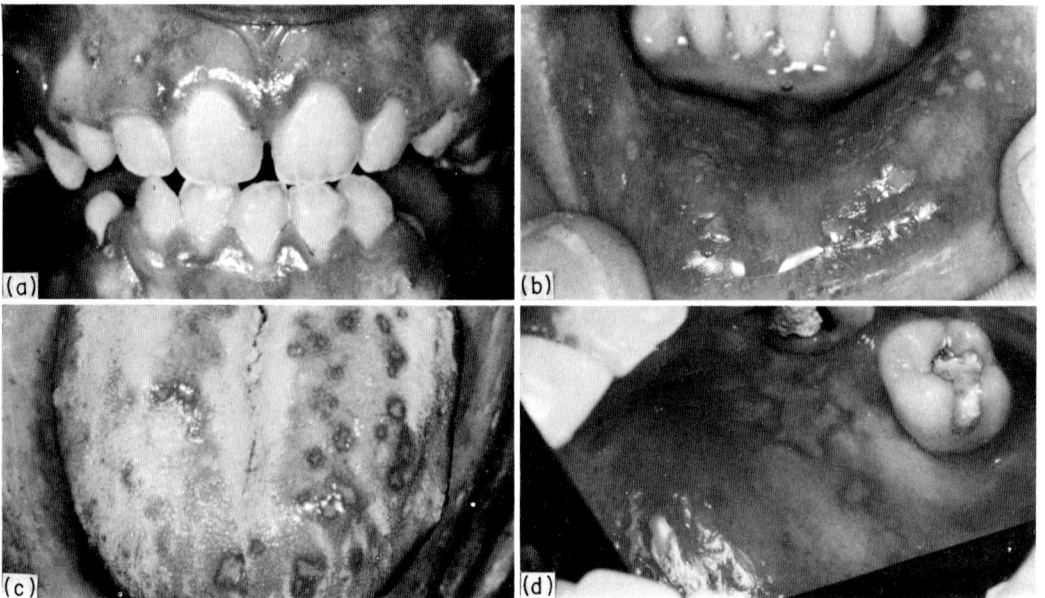

FIG. 11.13. Primary herpetic stomatitis ulceration of (a) gingivae, (b) lips, (c) tongue and (d) palate.

children as a result of the first exposure to *Herpesvirus hominis*. A greater proportion of the population has an acquired immunity to the virus than a history of an episode of acute gingivostomatitis. This suggests that the results of initial infection may be subclinical in a proportion of the population. The first exposure usually causes an acute systemic upset with fever, malaise, lymphadenitis and severe local discomfort due to ulceration of oral mucous membrane (fig. 11.13). Subsequently, either by activation of virus lying dormant in the host tissues or re-infection, a recurrent form of the disease may ensue (recurrent herpes labialis) (fig. 11.14), but this is clinically quite distinct from the primary infection and is usually localized to the muco-cutaneous junction of the lips. It is generally agreed that acute herpetic stomatitis is not recurrent [44, 45 & 46].

Herpesvirus hominis is very widely distributed in man; more than 97 per cent of persons in an urban area over the age of 60 years have been infected with the virus [47]. Overcrowding increases the incidence markedly, and the percentage of persons with herpetic antibodies is higher in urban communities than in rural areas. Infection is transmitted by contact with a carrier who is excreting the virus in secretions from the oropharynx, eyes or genitalia.

CLINICAL FEATURES

The clinical appearance is usually quite characteristic and, in the majority of instances, a definite diagnosis can be made on the basis of the history and the clinical features alone without resorting to laboratory procedures. In many instances a history of recent contact with an

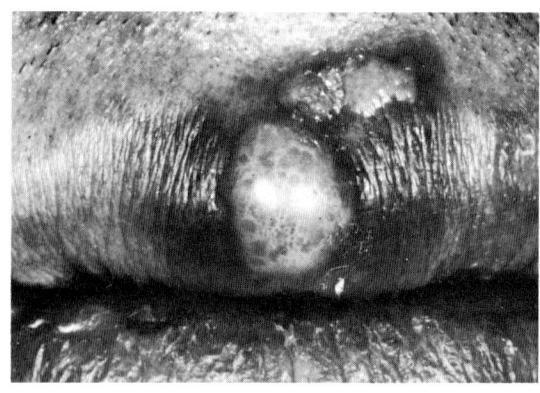

FIG. 11.14. Recurrent herpes labialis.

individual having a herpetic infection can be elicited. The condition is characterized during the initial stages by the formation of discrete spherical grey vesicles which rupture after a few hours to form ulcers. The ulcers may appear on the lips, cheeks, tongue, sublingual mucosa and palate (fig. 11.13). The gingiva may also be diffusely inflamed and ulcerated. The ulcers are painful, small and shallow, with a halo-like margin and a yellowish or greyish white base. The condition usually appears as an acute febrile disease with temperatures varying from 100° to 103°F, accompanied by general malaise and marked cervical lymphadenitis. The tongue is frequently coated, and the patient may complain of foul breath.

Such an episode runs a course of 7–18 days and is considered to be the result of the first exposure of a person to the virus where there has been no pre-existing immunity. Where there is a degree of acquired immunity, the typical lesion is a 'cold sore' which is situated at the mucocutaneous junction of the lip, and which is frequently recurrent (fig. 11.14).

Maternal antibodies are present during the first few months of life, and young babies seldom develop the infection. Primary infection has been reported to occur most commonly in children between the ages of 1–8 years [48], although a subsequent investigation has suggested that a greater proportion of young adults is at risk than has hitherto been realized [47]. Only 40 per cent of medical students in Oxford and Edinburgh, and 48 per cent of student nurses were found to

have had contact with the virus, as evidenced by serological investigation. In this selected group of the population some 60 per cent appear to be still at risk. This finding may also be of importance to dental personnel, where there is a danger of contracting a herpetic whitlow (fig. 11.15) or keratoconjunctivitis when working in an infected mouth.

DIAGNOSIS

In the majority of cases a diagnosis can be made from the history and clinical features alone, but where there is a doubt, supportive data may be obtained from laboratory investigation.

Cytological smears

The diagnosis of acute primary herpetic stomatitis may occasionally be confirmed by examination of material from the base of the vesicles. The base of the vesicle is scraped with a scalpel or plastic instrument, and a smear prepared from the scrapings. The slide should be fixed in alcohol and stained by haematoxylin and eosin or with giemsa stain. Epithelial cells producing virus protein and nucleic acid show grossly enlarged and bizarre nuclear patterns, and they are frequently multinucleated (fig. 11.16). Such cells have been described as mulberry cells [49 & 50]. This test is of limited assistance in confirming the diagnosis of herpetic stomatitis, since 'mulberry' cells are usually only demonstrable from scrapings taken during the early stages. Eosinophilic intranuclear inclusion bodies may also occasionally be seen.

Virus isolation

During the first week, swabs from the base of the lesion will frequently yield virus particles which can be grown in suitable living cells *in vitro*, and it is possible to demonstrate a cytopathic effect of the virus on such cells. Intracerebral inoculation of suckling mice can also be used to demonstrate the presence of virus. It is possible to identify a virus by mixing it with a specific anti-serum of known anti-viral activity. Where known neutralizing antibody, specific to the virus, is present in the mixture, the capacity

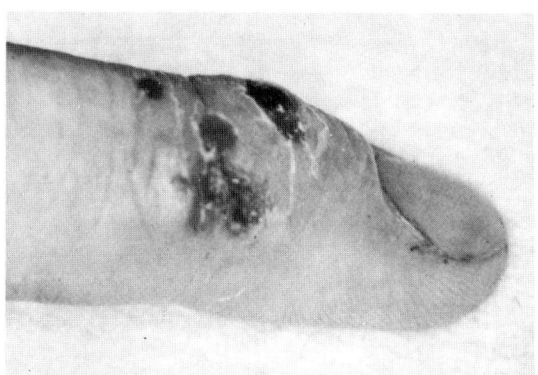

FIG. 11.15. Herpetic whitlow contracted by a dental student.

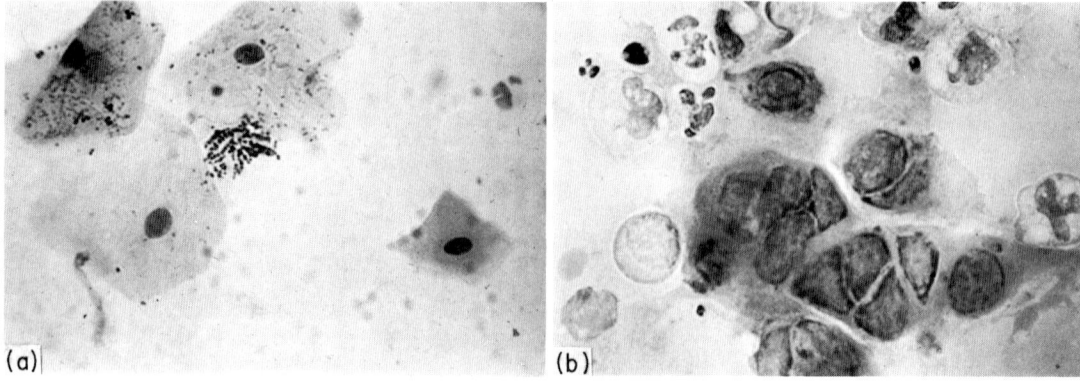

FIG. 11.16. (a) Smear of normal epithelial cells. (b) Typical 'mulberry' cells from vesicles of primary herpetic stomatitis.

of the virus to infect living cells is reduced or completely inhibited.

Serological investigation

Investigation of acute phase and convalescent sera may also yield supportive evidence. In the case of primary herpetic stomatitis, acute phase serum should be negative, both for neutralizing and complement fixing antibody, whilst subsequent examination of convalescent serum should yield demonstrable antibody.

In the case of recurrent herpes labialis, both acute phase and convalescent sera should show antibody, but the titre is not increased in the convalescent serum. Thus, serum antibodies seem unable to protect some patients from recurrent herpetic infections and it has been suggested that cell mediated immunity might be involved [51]. In a parallel investigation of cell mediated and antibody responses in patients with recurrent herpetic infections, stimulation of lymphocyte transformation with *Herpesvirus hominis* type 1 and the complement fixing antibody titre did not differ significantly between patients and controls. However, macrophage migration inhibition and lymphocyte cytotoxicity were significantly impaired in affected patients [51].

DIFFERENTIAL DIAGNOSIS

Acute herpetic stomatitis should be distinguished from the following.

Acute ulceromembranous gingivitis

At the stage of ulceration it can be difficult on occasion to distinguish acute herpetic stomatitis from acute ulceromembranous gingivitis. Herpetic ulceration of the gingivae can occur without the obvious presence of ulceration of the lips, cheeks, tongue or reflected mucosa (fig. 11.17). Similarly, mixed herpetic and fusiform infections are more common than has been previously thought. The presence of a significantly elevated temperature, generalized malaise and cervical lymphadenitis suggest the presence of acute herpetic stomatitis, rather than acute ulceromembranous gingivitis.

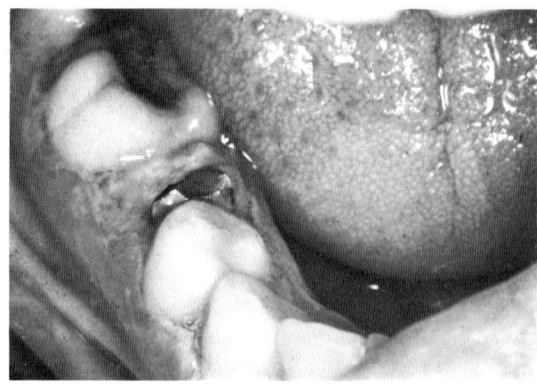

FIG. 11.17. Herpetic ulceration of gingivae in the absence of involvement of lips, cheeks, tongue or palate.

Erythema multiforme

The vesicles of erythema multiforme are generally more extensive than those in acute herpetic stomatitis, and they may form bullae which show a tendency towards crust formation on the lips (fig. 11.18). There is no marked lymphadenitis except where there is associated secondary infection. Oral involvement in erythema multiforme may or may not be accompanied by lesions on the skin or other mucous membranes (chap. 13).

Aphthous stomatitis

There has been a considerable misuse of the term aphthous stomatitis, and at least eleven synonyms for the condition have been recorded [52]. Conditions which have been generally described as aphthous ulceration have been classified into four groups by Kramer [53].

(1) Patients who experience recurrent crops of one to four ulcers affecting the nonkeratinized mucosa only, and lasting from 7–14 days. This has been described as 'minor' aphthous ulceration (fig. 11.19).

(2) Patients who have recurrent attacks of herpetiform stomatitis in which there are twenty or more ulcers at a time, and which may not be confined to the nonkeratinized parts of the mouth (fig. 11.20). This condition is not caused by *Herpesvirus hominis*.

(3) Patients who suffer recurrent attacks where there are usually one or two ulcers at a time, but these are deep, destructive and may take 6 or more weeks to heal. This condition is described as periadenitis mucosa necrotica recurrens but is best referred to as 'major' aphthous ulceration (fig. 11.21).

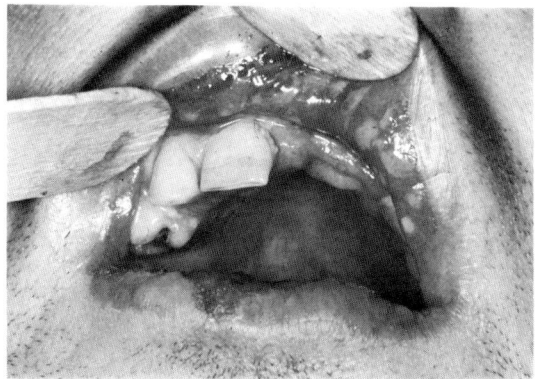

FIG. 11.18. Erythema multiforme (chap. 13).

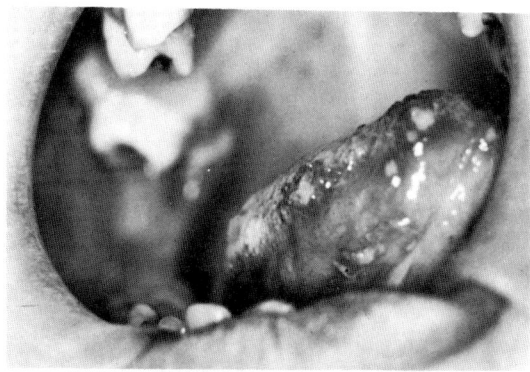

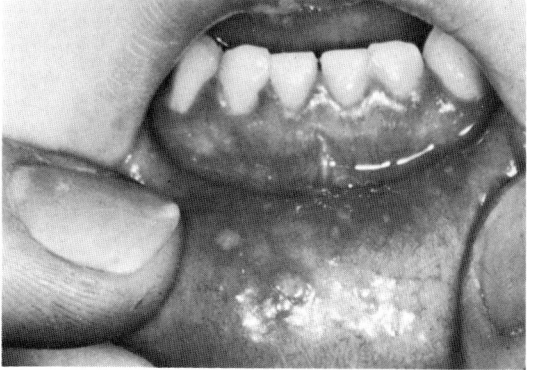

FIG. 11.20. Recurrent herpetiform stomatitis.

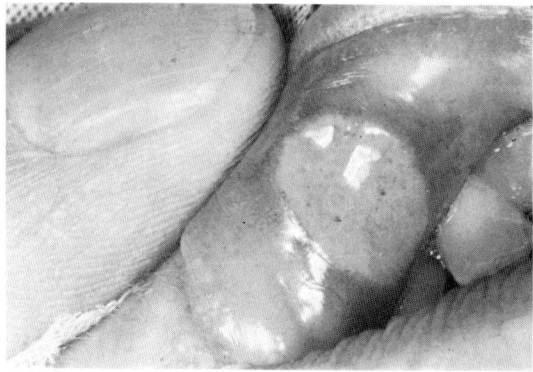

FIG. 11.19. Aphthous ulcer traumatized by sharp lateral incisor.

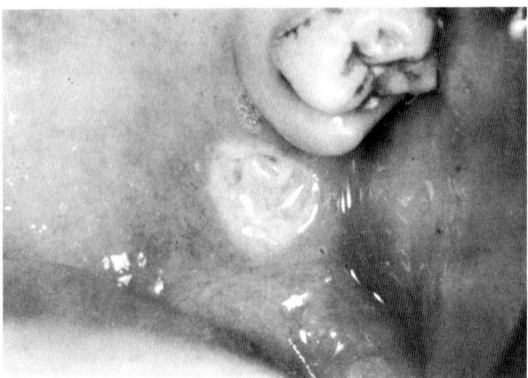

FIG. 11.21. Periadenitis mucosa necrotica recurrens.

(4) Patients who have ulceration in the mouth accompanied by similar ulcers of genital mucosa and skin (fig. 11.22).

Considerable difficulty may arise in drawing a purely clinical distinction between recurrent herpetiform stomatitis and acute herpetic stomatitis. Recurrent herpetiform stomatitis occurs in the older age groups, and the distinction is clear from the history in so far as recurrent episodes of acute herpetic stomatitis do not occur.

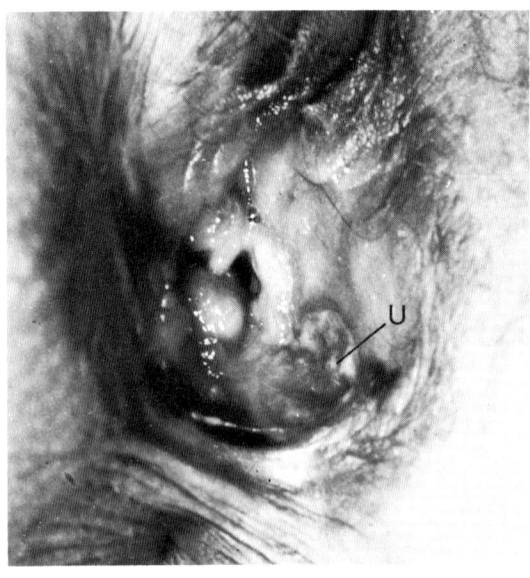

FIG. 11.22. Ulceration (U) of genital mucosa occurring in association with mouth ulceration, courtesy of Dr W. Sircus.

Herpangina

This term is used to describe vesiculation and ulceration of the tonsils, pillars of the fauces and soft palate (fig. 11.23), associated with the presence of the Coxsackie A virus [54]. Lesions may occur in sites other than the palate, pharynx and tonsils, and stomatitis, from which the Coxsackie A virus is subsequently isolated, may be clinically indistinguishable from acute herpetic stomatitis. Serological investigation may assist to differentiate herpetic infections from those caused by the Coxsackie virus.

TREATMENT

At the present time there is no treatment which has been unequivocally shown to alter significantly the course of acute herpetic stomatitis. Claims that encouraging results have followed administration of gammaglobulin [55] or trypsin [56] have not subsequently been fully supported. To produce infection the DNA core of the virus must gain access to the host cell. The herpes virus is capable of entering into an integrated relationship with the host cell, leading to the production of further virus nucleic acid and protein. As this method of intracellular reproduction is fundamentally different from bacterial reproduction, antibiotics, which interfere with bacterial enzyme systems, cannot be expected to prevent virus multiplication. The use of antibiotics is to be discouraged for treatment of virus infection, except where secondary bacterial infection has occurred, or possibly where

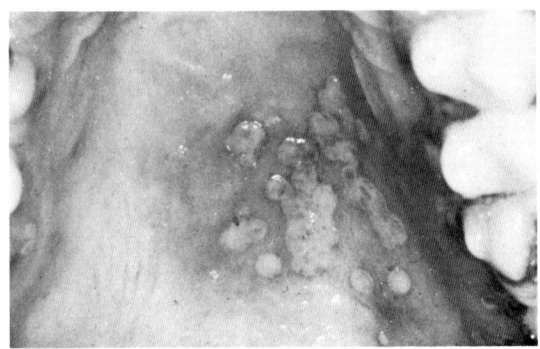

FIG. 11.23. Herpangina.

there is infection of the host by a virus and bacterial combination, where the bacteria have a potentiating effect upon the virus. Reports have indicated that *Trichomonas tenax* may have such a potentiating effect on *Herpesvirus hominis*, and it is of interest that metronidazole, which is active against trichomonas, has been reported to reduce the symptoms of acute herpetic stomatitis [57 & 58].

There is evidence that the administration of antiviral agents such as 5-iodo-2-deoxyuridine are effective [59 & 60], but the virus has been shown to develop resistance to the drug.

The principles of treatment are based on the control of secondary infection and the establishment of an adequate standard of oral hygiene. The patient should be instructed in the use of bland mouthwashes and a soft toothbrush. It has been suggested that herpetic ulcers respond to tetracycline, or chlortetracycline, used as a mouthwash [57]. The recommended dosage is one 250 mg capsule dissolved in one fluid ounce of warm water used as a mouthwash three times daily for 3 days. There is probably no advantage over a 0·2 per cent chlorhexidine mouth rinse.

Acute coccal gingivitis

Acute coccal gingivitis [61] is relatively rare and occurs much less frequently than ulceromembranous gingivitis or acute herpetic gingivostomatitis.

CRITERIA FOR DIAGNOSIS

Acute coccal gingivitis may occur in association with streptococcal infection of the throat. The condition is characterized by a diffuse, beefy red erythema of the gingival tissues, and it may be accompanied by exudation of blood and pus stained fluid from the gingival margins (fig. 11.24). Necrosis and frank ulceration are not evident at any stage, but oedematous enlargement is consistently present. Bacterial smears show a predominance of coccal forms (fig. 11.25).

Cocci are found in all smears taken from the mouth, and it is possible that acute coccal gingivitis occurs as an endogenous infection, associated with imbalance of the host–parasite system, in relation to groups of alpha haemolytic streptococci, commonly streptococcus viridans. Occasionally the condition may occur following infection by an exogenous β haemolytic streptococcus.

TREATMENT

The aim of treatment should be quantitive reduction of the bacterial population of the mouth, which is achieved by scaling and polishing the teeth, and the use of mouthwashes as supportive agents. Swabs should be sent for culture and antibiotic sensitivity tests at the time of the patient's initial visit, so that information as to sensitivity is available should subsequent antibiotic therapy prove necessary. Arbitrary administration of large doses of penicillin suppresses most of the

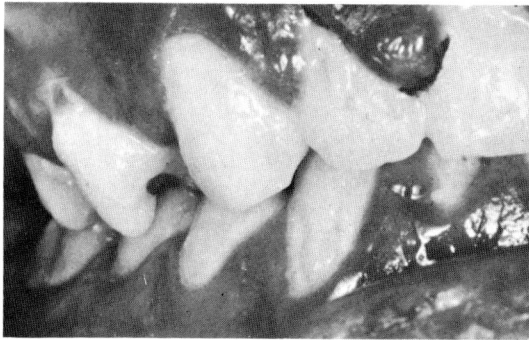

FIG. 11.24. Acute coccal gingivitis characterized by beefy red gingivae and exudation of blood stained fluid from the gingival margin.

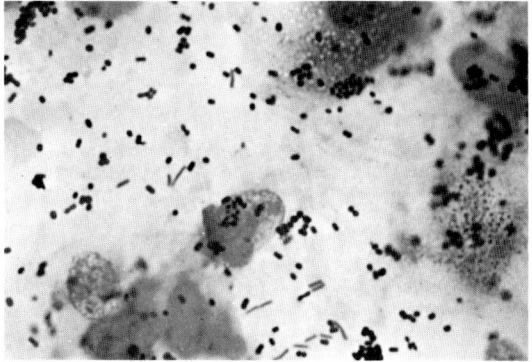

FIG. 11.25. Smear from coccal gingivitis showing predominance of coccal organisms.

streptococci in the mouth, but the resulting flora includes many strains of streptococci which are penicillin resistant. It is possible that the infection may have been initially due to the predominance of penicillin resistant groups, and indiscriminate administration of penicillin may render subsequent treatment more difficult. If an antibiotic is to be administered before culture and sensitivity reports are available, the drug of choice is tetracycline.

ACUTE NONSPECIFIC GINGIVITIS

Acute nonspecific gingivitis is an acute inflammatory condition which is the result of change in the oral flora associated with accumulation of dental plaque. The condition is characterized by bleeding, oedema and swelling of the tissues in the absence of frank ulceration, necrosis or any of the characteristics which have defined the acute specific gingivitis (fig. 11.26). The aim of treatment should be removal of bacterial deposits by scaling and polishing, and the establishment of a high standard of patient self-care. In the presence of an adequate standard of hygiene phase control, drug therapy in any form is rarely, if ever, necessary.

Reduction of oedema may be further promoted by the use of pressure packs following initial scaling and polishing. Complete control of superficial inflammation should be achieved within 1 week of commencing treatment. Should the acute inflammation persist beyond this time, arrangements should be made for general examination of the patient to exclude the possibility that imbalance of the host-parasite system is of systemic origin.

ACUTE NONSPECIFIC PERIODONTITIS

Periodontal abscess

A periodontal abscess is an area of the periodontium where localized acute inflammation has resulted in necrosis of tissue and formation of pus. Periodontal abscesses occur:

(1) in a pre-existing periodontal pocket (fig. 11.27) where imbalance of the host–parasite system is such that necrosis of tissue and pus formation result; this may occur as a direct effect of the virulence of toxic factors from plaque, or secondary to reduction in host resistance during debilitating disease;

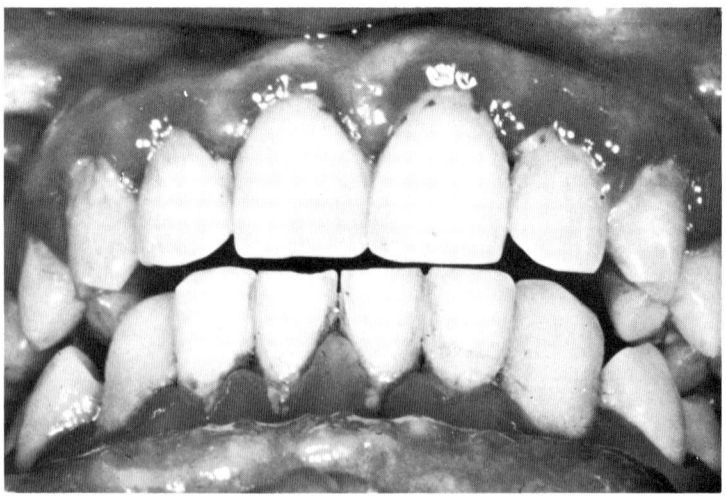

FIG. 11.26. Acute nonspecific gingivitis characterized by oedema, erythema, and bleeding of the tissues, in the absence of frank ulceration, necrosis, or of any of the characteristics which define the acute specific gingivitis.

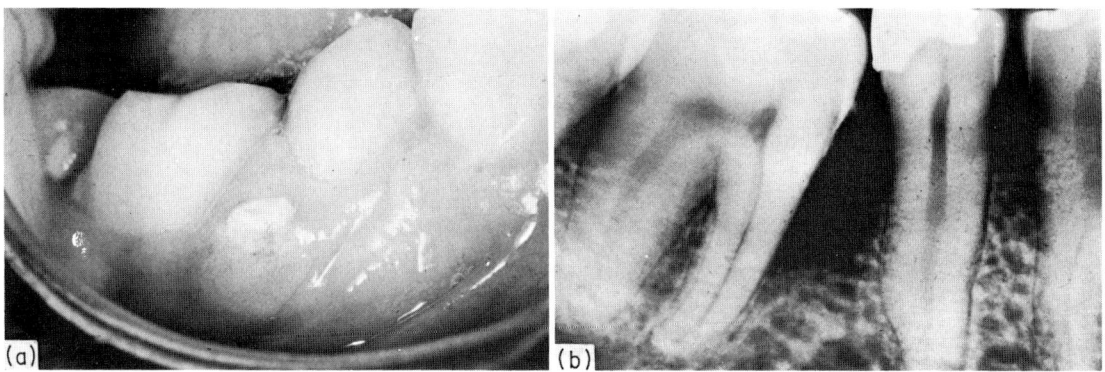

FIG. 11.27. (a) Acute periodontal abscess. (b) Radiograph of (a) showing presence of true pocket.

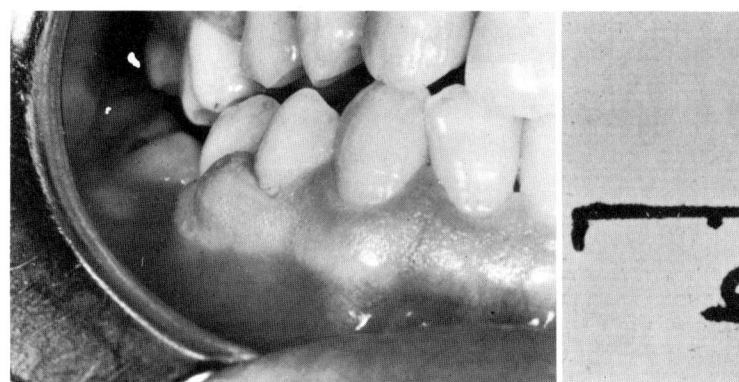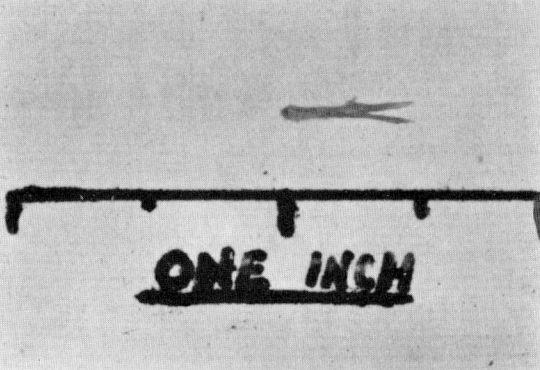

FIG. 11.28. Acute periodontal abscess caused by toothbrush bristle impacted in the tissues.

(2) following traumatic injury to a tooth;

(3) as a result of introduction of a foreign body into the periodontium (fig. 11.28);

(4) as a result of infection introduced during endodontic therapy.

Periodontal abscesses may be acute or chronic. An acute abscess may burst, drain spontaneously and resolve, or it may subsequently persist in a chronic state (fig. 11.29). A chronic abscess may develop without a preceding acute phase, but chronic lesions commonly undergo acute exacerbation.

ACUTE PERIODONTAL ABSCESS

An acute periodontal abscess appears as a discrete fluctuant swelling of the gingivae of sudden onset. The overlying tissue is oedematous and red with a smooth shiny surface. The swell-ing is accompanied by a localized throbbing pain. The teeth associated with the swelling are tender to percussion, may be mobile and in

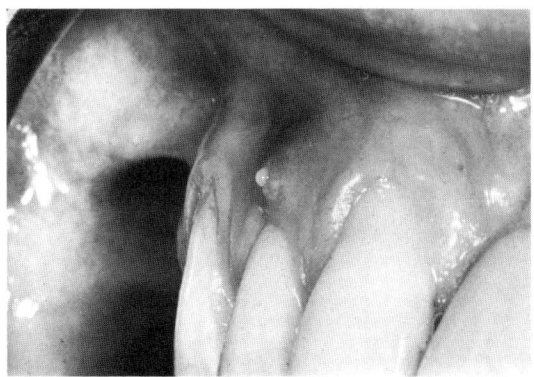

FIG. 11.29. Chronic periodontal abscess.

supraocclusion as a result of oedema of the supporting tissues. The patient may complain of malaise, lymphadenitis and a degree of fever and leucocytosis may be present.

Treatment

The immediate treatment of an acute abscess is to establish drainage. The abscess should be incised at its most dependent point and the incision developed with artery forceps (fig. 11.30). Where the abscess has already pointed, the incision should be extended from the sinus to the most dependent point of the swelling.

It has been widely held that where a tooth is in supraocclusion, the occlusal surface may be ground to relieve trauma, but in practice this may be difficult to achieve without grinding away excessive amounts of tooth substance. A hot mouthwash should be regularly used during the period of drainage. There is no indication for local or systemic use of antibiotics unless justified by the presence of systemic disease.

CHRONIC PERIODONTAL ABSCESS

A chronic periodontal abscess may present as a sinus on the gingival mucosa from which there may be intermittent discharge of pus. A chronic persistent periodontal abscess suggests the presence of a foreign body or an established periodontal pocket. Chronic abscesses are frequently associated with periodontal pockets, which involve the bifurcation or trifurcation of multi-rooted teeth (fig. 11.27). In these circumstances the patient should be advised to use a hot mouthwash to increase the rate of drainage, and the local pocket should be treated subsequently as part of the treatment of the general periodontitis (chap. 12).

RADIOGRAPHIC APPEARANCE

An acute periodontal abscess resulting from trauma, or introduction of infection into a healthy periodontium, shows no radiographic signs with the possible exception of slight widening of the periodontal space.

An acute or chronic periodontal abscess, in association with a pre-existing pocket, will be characterized by radiographic evidence of bone resorption (fig. 11.28). Since a radiograph of a tooth and its supporting structures is a two-dimensional representation of a three-dimen-

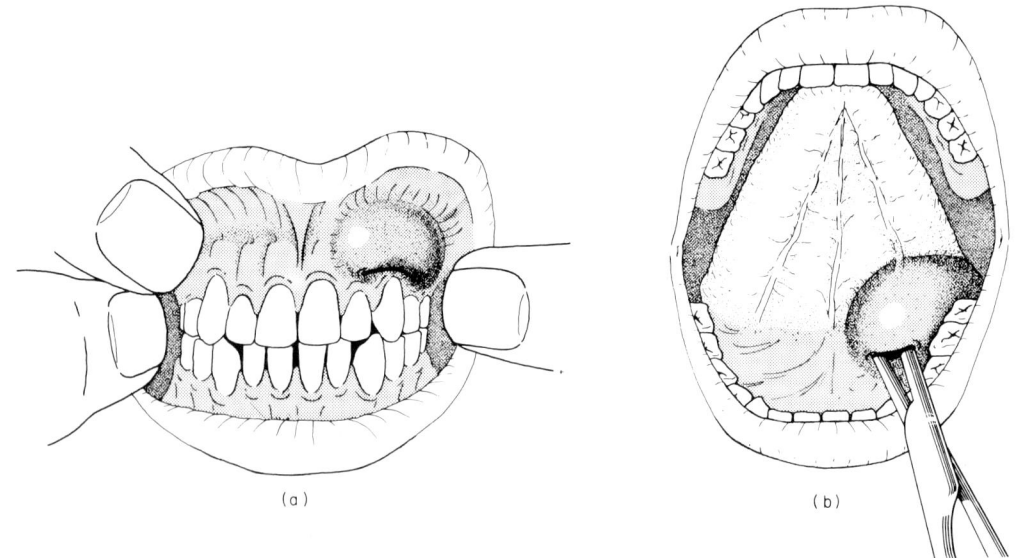

(a)   (b)

FIG. 11.30. (a) Periodontal abscess showing the line of incision for drainage. (b) The use of artery forceps to develop drainage tract.

sional structure, a radiograph is not a reliable guide as to the presence of small areas of bone resorption which may be concealed by the image of the root.

DISTINCTION FROM AN APICAL ABSCESS

The main distinction from an apical abscess is that a periodontal abscess is usually associated with a vital tooth. An apical abscess may occasionally track along the lateral surface of a root to drain from the gingival margin. As a generalization, when the apex and the lateral surface of the root are involved in a lesion, which can be probed from the gingival margin, the lesion is most likely to have originated as a periodontal abscess.

Pericoronitis

Pericoronitis denotes inflammation of the soft tissues around the crown of a tooth, which has not reached a fully functional position in the mouth. Erupting or impacted mandibular third molar teeth are most commonly involved. A flap of gingiva overlying the occlusal surface may persist after complete eruption. The flap is particularly vulnerable to irritation, either directly from the opposing tooth during closure or from stagnation of food debris and overgrowth of microorganisms between the soft tissue and the underlying tooth. It is difficult for a patient to exert adequate oral hygiene control in such an area, and this predisposes to inflammation.

The tissues swell as a result of the inflammatory reaction and become more likely to be traumatized by opposing teeth. Should the infection spread, the patient may experience difficulty in opening the mouth.

If adequate treatment is not instituted, the infection may spread to involve the masseteric, peritonsillar or parapharyngeal spaces, and muscle spasms become so marked that opening of the mouth is severely limited.

MANAGEMENT

The clinical management can be divided into two phases:
  (1) management of the acute phase,
  (2) eradication of the stagnation area.

Management of the acute phase

The aim of treatment is relief of pain and the control of infection. The area should be gently debrided, and the space under the flap irrigated with warm saline. If localization and formation of pus has occurred, the swelling should be incised at its most dependent point and drained. Trauma from any opposing tooth must be eliminated, either by reducing the height of offending cusps or extracting the opposing tooth. The principles of treatment are irrigation and free drainage from the area. The use of packs inserted under the flap is to be avoided as these may obstruct drainage.

The patient should be instructed in oral hygiene measures, and if the pain is severe an analgesic prescribed (chap. 15). In almost all cases benefit will be derived by prescribing a hot saline mouthwash taken every few hours.

Eradication of the stagnation area

Once the acute phase has been controlled, the mouth should be assessed to determine whether or not the third molar teeth should be retained. If partially erupted third molars are to be retained, the flap should be excised to expose the crown of the tooth and to eliminate the stagnation area. Where a third molar is to be removed, consideration must be given to the desirability of retaining the other wisdom teeth present, whether erupted or unerupted. Overeruption of third molars following extraction of the opposing tooth is a common cause of occlusal interference (chap. 14).

REFERENCES

[1] WEAVER G.H. & TUNNICLIFF R. (1907) Noma (Gangrenous stomatitis; water cancer; scorbutic cancer; gangrena oris; gangrene of the mouth.) *J. infect. Dis.* **4**, 8–35.

[2] HEYLINGS R.T. (1967) Electron microscopy of acute ulcerative gingivitis (Vincent's type). Demonstration of the fuso-spirochaetal complex of bacteria within the pre-necrotic gingival epithelium. *Brit. dent. J.* **122**, 51–56.

[3] MacDonald J.B., Sutton R.M., Knoll M.L., Madlener E.M. & Grainger R.M. (1956) The pathogenic components of an experimental fuso-spirochaetal infection. *J. infect. Dis.* **98**, 15–20.

[4] Hirschfeld I., Beube F. & Siegal E.H. (1940) The history of Vincent's infection. *J. Periodont.* **11**, 89–98.

[5] Schluger S. (1943) Vincent's infection. *J. Amer. dent. Ass.* **30**, 524–532.

[6] Goldhaber P. & Giddon D.B. (1964) Present concepts concerning the aetiology and treatment of acute necrotizing ulcerative gingivitis. *Int. dent. J.* **14**, 468–496.

[7] Schluger S. (1949) quoted in Goldhaber P. & Giddon D.B. Present concepts concerning the aetiology and treatment of acute necrotizing ulcerative gingivitis. *Int. dent. J.* **14**, 468–496.

[8] Carter W.J. & Ball D.M. (1953) Results of a three year study of Vincent's infection at the Great Lakes Naval Dental Department. *J. Periodont.* **24**, 187–194.

[9] Barnes G.P., Bowles W.F. & Carter H.G. (1973) Acute necrotizing ulcerative gingivitis: A survey of 218 cases. *J. Periodont.* **44**, 35–42.

[10] Emslie R.D. (1963) Cancrum oris. *Dent. Practit. Bristol*, **13**, 481–495.

[11] Burnett G.W. & Scherp H.W. (1962) *Oral Microbiology and Infectious disease*, 2nd Edition. Baltimore: Williams and Wilkins.

[12] Mergenhagen S.E., Hamp E.G. & Scherp H.W. (1961) Preparation and biological activities of endotoxins from oral bacteria. *J. infect. Dis.* **108**, 304–310.

[13] Hampp E.G. & Mergenhagen S.E. (1961) Experimental infections with oral spirochaetes. *J. infect. Dis.* **109**, 43–61.

[14] Shinn D.L.S. (1962) Metronidazole in acute ulcerative gingivitis. *Lancet*, **i**, 1191.

[15] Shinn D.L.S., Squires S. & McFadzean J.A. (1965) The treatment of Vincent's disease with metronidazole. *Dent. Practit. dent. Rec.* **15**, 275–280.

[16] Duckworth R., Waterhouse J.P., Britton D.E.R., Nuki K., Sheiham A., Winter R. & Blake G.C. (1966) Acute ulcerative gingivitis. A double blind controlled clinical trial of metronidazole. *Brit. dent. J.* **120**, 599–602.

[17] Glenwright H.D. & Sidaway D.A. (1966) The use of metronidazole in the treatment of acute ulcerative gingivitis. *Brit. dent. J.* **121**, 174–177.

[18] Stephen K.W., McLatchie M.S., Mason D.K., Noble H.W. & Stevenson D.M. (1966) Treatment of acute ulcerative gingivitis (Vincent's Type). *Brit. dent. J.* **121**, 313–322.

[19] Wade A.B., Blake G.C. & Mirza K.B. (1966) Effectiveness of metronidazole in treating the acute phase of ulcerative gingivitis. *Dent. Practit. dent. Rec.* **16**, 440–443.

[20] Fletcher J.P. & Plant C.G. (1966) An assessment of metronidazole in the treatment of acute ulcerative pseudo-membranous gingivitis (Vincent's disease). *Oral Surg.* **22**, 729–736.

[21] Emslie R.D. (1967) Treatment of acute ulcerative gingivitis. A clinical trial using chewing gums containing metronidazole or penicillin. *Brit. dent. J.* **122**, 307–308.

[22] Macdonald J.B., Gibbons R.J. & Socransky S.S. (1960) Bacterial mechanisms in periodontal disease. *Ann. N.Y. Acad. Sci.* **85**, 467–478.

[23] Gibbons R.J. & MacDonald J.B. (1961) Degradation of collagenous substrates by *Bacteroides melaninogenicus*. *J. Bact.* **81**, 614–621.

[24] Kirkpatrick R.M. & Clements F.W. (1934) Diet in relation to Vincent's infection: Preliminary report. *Aust. dent. J.* **6**, 371–372.

[25] Cautley R.L. (1943) Vincent's infection. *Brit. dent. J.* **74**, 34–37.

[26] Moulton R., Ewen S. & Thieman W. (1952) Emotional factors in periodontal disease. *Oral. Surg.* **5**, 833–860.

[27] Goldberg H., Ambinder W.J., Cooper L. & Abrahams A.L. (1956) Emotional status of patients with acute gingivitis. *N.Y. St. dent. J.* **22**, 308–318.

[28] MacPhee I.T., Beagrie G.S. (1962) Treatment of ulcero-membranous gingivitis. *Brit. dent. J.* **113**, 107–111.

[29] Watts D.T. (1960) The effect of nicotine and smoking on the secretion of epinephrine. *Ann. N.Y. Acad. Sci.* **90**, 74–80.

[30] Macapanpan L.C. & Weinman J.P. (1954) Influence of injury to the periodontal membrane on the spread of gingival inflammation. *J. dent. Res.* **33**, 263–272.

[31] Glickman I. & Smulow J.B. (1962) Alterations in the pathway of gingival inflammation into the underlying tissues induced by excessive occlusal forces. *J. Periodont.* **33**, 7–13.

[32] Oliver W.M. & Fletcher J.P. (1959) Oral hygiene in the treatment of acute ulcerative gingivitis. *Brit. dent. J.* **106**, 177–180.

[33] Fitch H.B., Alling C.C., Bethart H. & Munns C.R. (1963) Acute necrotising ulcerative gingivitis. *J. Periodont.* **34**, 422–426.

[34] Wade A.B., Blake G.C., Manson J.D., Berdon J.K., Mathieson F. & Bate D.M. (1963) Treatment of acute phase of ulcerative gingivitis (Vincent's type). A comparative assessment of the use of sodium peroxyborate monohydrate and penicillin. *Brit. dent. J.* **115**, 372–375.

[35] *Accepted Dental Remedies* (1960) 25th Edition. Chicago: American Dental Association.

[36] Knighton H.T. (1940) The effect of oxidising on certain spore-forming anaerobes. *J. dent. Res.* **19**, 429–439.

[37] Wade A.B. & Mirza K.B. (1964) Relative effectiveness of sodium peroxyborate and hydrogen peroxide in treating acute ulcerative gingivitis. *Dent. Practit. dent. Rec.* **14**, 185–187.

[38] Murdoch J.Mc. (1966) Antibiotics and chemotherapy, in *Textbook of Medical Treatment*, 10th Edition. Dunlop D. & Alstead S. (eds), pp. 53–85. Edinburgh: Livingstone.

[39] Kramer I.R.H. (1956) Antibiotic therapy in dental practice. *Brit. dent. J.* **100**, 69–80.

[40] Feinberg S.M., Feinberg A.R. & Moran C.F. (1953) Penicillin anaphylaxis: Non fatal and fatal reactions. *J. Amer. Med. Ass.* **152**, 114–119.

[41] Guthe T., Idsoe O. & Wilcox R.R. (1958) Untoward penicillin reactions. *Bull. Wld. Hlth. Org.* **19**, 427–501.

[42] Corr D.J. & Wellman W.E. (1956) Reaction to peni-

cillin. Review of the literature concerning severe reactions (England & North America). *Minn. Med.* **39**, 599–610.

[43] LEES R. (1966) Venereal diseases, in *Textbook of Medical Treatment*, 10th Edition, Eds. Dunlop D. & Alstead S. pp. 171. Edinburgh: Livingstone.

[44] BLANK H., BURGOON C.F., CORIELL L.L. & SCOTT T.F.M. (1950) Recurrent aphthous ulcers. *J. Amer. med. Ass.* **142**, 125–126.

[45] DODD K. (1950) Herpes simplex virus not the etiologic agent of recurrent stomatitis. *Pediatrics*, **5**, 883–887.

[46] MCCARTHY P.L. & SHKLAR G. (1964) *Diseases of the Oral Mucosa.* New York: McGraw-Hill.

[47] SMITH J.W., PEUTHERER J.F. & MACCALLUM F.O. (1967) The incidence of *Herpesvirus hominis* antibody in the population. *J. Hyg. (Lond.).* **65**, 395–408.

[48] BUDDINGH G.J., SCHRUM D.I., LANIER J.C. & GUIDRY D.J. (1953) Studies on the natural history of herpes simplex infections. *Pediatrics*, **11**, 595–609.

[49] TZANCK A. & ARON-BRUNETIERE R. (1949) Le 'cyto diagnostic immediat' des dermatoses bulleuses. *Gaz. méd port.* **2**, 667–675.

[50] COOKE B.E.D. (1958) Epithelial smears in the diagnosis of herpes simplex and herpes zoster affecting the oral mucosa. *Brit. dent. J.* **104**, 97–99.

[51] LEHNER T. (1973) Cellular immunity to oral infections in *Host Resistance to Commensal Bacteria.* Ed. MacPhee I.T. pp. 176–189. Edinburgh: Churchill Livingstone.

[52] SIRCUS W., CHURCH R. & KELLEHER J. (1957) Recurrent aphthous ulceration of the mouth. A study of the normal history, aetiology and treatment. *Quart. J. Med.* **50**, 235–249.

[53] KRAMER I.R.H. (1965) Aphthous and herpetic lesions of the oral mucosa. *Proc. Roy. Soc. Med.* **58**, 458–462.

[54] HUEBNER R.J., COLE R.M., BEEMAN E.A., BELL J.A. & PEERS J.H. (1951) Herpangina, etiologic studies of a specific infectious disease. *J. Amer. med. Ass.* **145**, 628–633.

[55] STREAN L.P., WILLIAMS B.H. & PRITCHARD J. (1958) Oral herpetiform lesions treated with gamma globulin. *Oral Surg.* **11**, 266–274.

[56] INERFIELD I., ANGUS A., SCHWARTZ A. & RUGIERIO W. (1953) Intravenous trypsin, its effects upon intravascular thrombi and acute inflammatory reactions. *Surg. Forum*, 526–530.

[57] KAY L.W. (1967) New drugs. *Brit. J. Oral Surg.* **5**, 120–134.

[58] MCGUIRE W.F. & GOLDBERG H.R. (1965) Viral stomatitis: A treatment for viral stomatitis. *J. Kans. Med. Soc.* **66**, 545.

[59] KAUFMAN H.E., NESBURY A.B. & MALONEY E.D. (1962) IDU therapy of herpes simplex. *Arch. Ophthal.* **67**, 583–591.

[60] JAFFE E.C. & LEHNER T. (1968) Treatment of herpetic stomatitis with idoxuridine. *Brit. dent. J.* **125**, 392–395.

[61] TYLDESLEY W.R. (1973) Oral medicine for the general practitioner: Infections of the oral mucosa. *Brit. dent. J.* **135**, 449–455.

CHAPTER 12

Chronic gingivitis and periodontitis

At the present time, imprecise terminology tends to discriminate against a systematic approach to the treatment of chronic gingivitis and periodontitis.

The periodontium consists of bone, cementum, periodontal membrane and the investing sheath of gingivae and mucous membrane. It follows that the term periodontitis implies inflammation of any or all of the individual tissues of the periodontium; it may describe any stage in the progression of periodontitis, from the earliest superficial inflammatory change with little or no destruction of the deeper tissues to destruction extending to the apical region of the root.

The term gingivitis implies inflammation of the gingival tissue, and it is frequently used to describe inflammatory change of the marginal and papillary tissues, which may or may not be associated with a degree of destruction of the deeper supporting tissues of the tooth. Gingivitis is present at all stages in the progressive destruction of the periodontium. It may be evident as superficial inflammatory change around a fully supported tooth (fig. 12.1a) or as superficial inflammatory change around a tooth which is almost totally unsupported (fig. 12.1b).

Corrective therapy must be based on a precise assessment of the condition of the supporting tissues, and it is therefore necessary to use descriptive terms which accurately convey the form and extent of any disease present.

From the point of view of treatment, it is helpful to divide the progression of inflammatory periodontal disease in the first instance into the following parts.

Gingivitis
(The gingivally contained lesion)

Limited superficial inflammation of the gingival tissues, where the base of the pocket remains

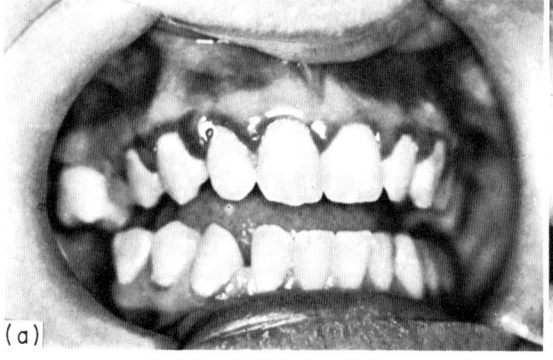 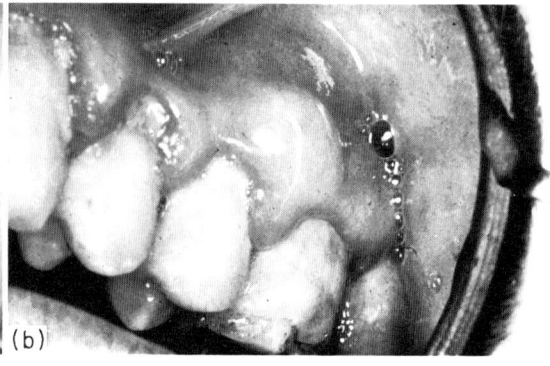

(a)   (b)

FIG. 12.1. Clinically evident superficial inflammation: (a) around a fully supported tooth (limited gingivitis), (b) in presence of inflammatory destruction of tissues of the periodontium apical to the amelocemental junction (established periodontitis), and abscess formation.

situated at the amelocemental junction, and increase in pocket depth beyond the 2 mm generally accepted as normal, is caused by occlusal proliferation of the gingival tissues (false pocket, fig. 12.2).

The term 'gingivally contained' implies limited involvement of marginal and papillary tissues in the absence of alveolar bone resorption and destruction of the deeper tissues. Any pockets present are therefore false pockets. Typically the gingivally contained lesion shows inflammation and oedema of the papillae and marginal tissues. Hyperplasia of the gingivae may also give rise to a gingivally contained lesion, but may be associated with destruction and disorganization of the deeper supporting tissues. A clear distinction must be made between limited and nonlimited gingivitis before the correct approach to treatment can be selected. Nonlimited gingivitis is associated with destruction of tissues apical to the amelocemental junction and is best described as periodontitis.

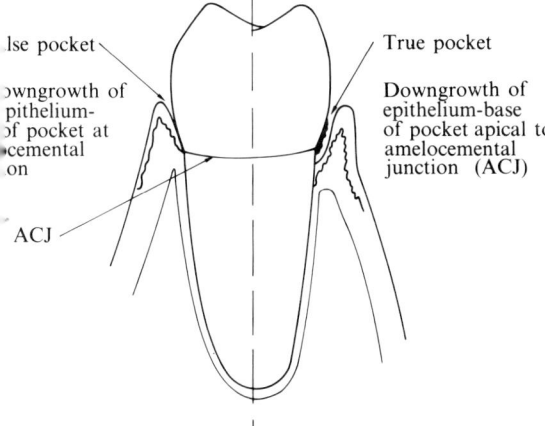

FIG. 12.2. False pocket. Limited superficial inflammation of the gingival tissues where the base of the pocket remains situated at the amelocemental junction. The increase in depth results from occlusal proliferation of gingival tissues.
  True pocket. Nonlimited inflammation of the periodontium where the base of the pocket is apical to the amelocemental junction and increase in pocket depth is largely caused by destruction of main fibre bundles of the marginal ligament followed by apical proliferation of the cuff epithelium in an attempt to seal the breach.

Periodontitis
(The nongingivally contained lesion)

Nonlimited inflammation of the periodontium, where increase in pocket depth apical to the amelocemental junction is caused by destruction of main fibre bundles of the marginal ligament, followed by apical proliferation of the cuff epithelium in an attempt to seal the breach (true pocket, fig. 12.2).

It should be appreciated that in the case of a true pocket, it is possible to have a variable degree of occlusal proliferation of gingival tissue at the same time as extension of the base of the pocket apical to the amelocemental junction.

The term nongingivally contained means the presence of alveolar bone resorption, loss of attachment and disorganization of the collagen bundles attaching tooth to bone. True pockets are always present, and such destruction of the deeper tissues will be associated with a variable degree of clinically evident inflammation of the superficial gingivae.

The term periodontitis simplex is used to describe a nongingivally contained lesion which is associated with the presence of local irritants in the mouth, and the presence of inflammatory destruction of the supporting tissues of the teeth (fig. 12.3). The condition is typically associated with a history of gingivitis over a long

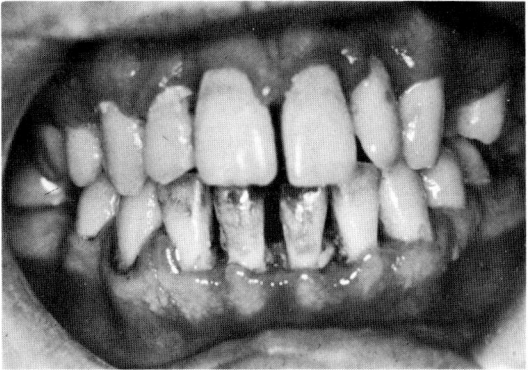

FIG. 12.3. Periodontitis simplex. Inflammatory destruction of tissue apical to the amelocemental junction associated with the presence of obvious deposits on the teeth; patient aged 30 years.

period and gradually progresses towards loss of the dentition in the 35–45 year age group.

The concept of periodontosis describing degenerative destruction of the periodontium arose in an attempt to explain advanced alveolar resorption seen in young patients, typically, but not always, in the absence of clinically evident inflammation and of obvious local irritants (fig. 12.4). The assumption was made that, initially at least, the condition resulted from a systemic alteration of bone, cementum or collagen metabolism that resulted in degeneration of one or more of these tissues. Following the initial degeneration, which was described as periodontosis, inflammation supervened, and the combined degenerative and inflammatory processes were described as periodontitis complex.

The first formal description of such apparently noninflammatory periodontal disease was published by Gottlieb, in 1920, who defined the condition as: 'diffuse atrophy of alveolar bone', followed by secondary failure of the other supporting tissues [1 & 2]. In 1942, Orban and Weinmann coined the term periodontosis, based on their observations in human jaws at autopsy, of a condition which appeared to be degenerative [3].

Three stages in the process were described:

(1) degeneration of the principal fibres of the periodontium leading to cessation of cementum formation,

(2) rapid migration of epithelium along the

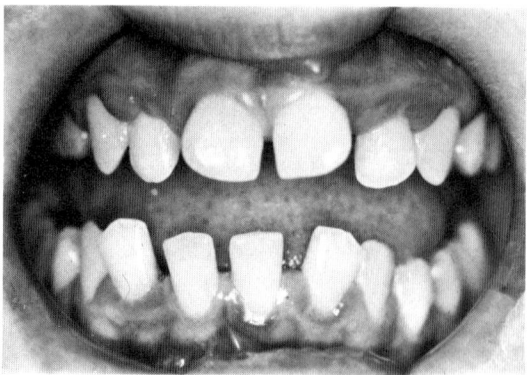

FIG. 12.4. Advanced alveolar resorption and drifting of the dentition in child aged 14 years, in presence of minimal clinically obvious inflammation.

affected cementum, at which stage the first signs of inflammation became evident,

(3) degeneration of the epithelial tissues at the base of the crevice, which allowed access of toxic factors from mouth bacteria; following this the primary signs of degeneration were obliterated by inflammation.

It is this third stage of systemically determined degeneration, and local inflammation, which has been called periodontitis complex.

It is inherent in the concept of the host–parasite system of the mouth, that all periodontitis is a complex phenomenon involving a wide range of interaction between the tissues of the host and the commensal population of the mouth. A wide range of systemic factors and conditions may influence the response of the host tissues to local irritants in the mouth (chap. 13), but there are few known systemic diseases associated with specific periodontal changes. Notable amongst these are the advanced periodontitis associated with the presence of hyperkeratosis palmoplantaris (Papillon Lefèvre syndrome) [4] and the change of orientation and thickening of the fibres of the periodontal membrane associated with scleroderma ([5].

If the anatomical barrier (chap. 4) is breached by degenerative or other change inflammation immediately supervenes, and the condition becomes indistinguishable from any other periodontitis. Epidemiological surveys have confirmed that the severity of periodontitis is directly associated with age, emotional stress, dental plaque and calculus [6] and possibly with educational level and income [7]. Few workers claim that there is any direct evidence to support the concept of periodontosis, or of periodontitis complex, being entirely of systemic origin [8]. There is no evidence at present to suggest that advanced destruction of the supporting tissues in young adults represents anything other than gross imbalance of the host–parasite system. It is possible that degenerative change such as described by Orban and Weinmann [3] could result from local alteration in the *milieu* of cells, in the absence of gross morphological changes associated with inflammation (chap. 3). The term periodontosis should be discarded as it is the source of unnecessary complication. The terms periodontitis simplex and periodontitis complex may be used to describe clinical findings, without implicating any particular aetiology, beyond the host response to the presence of dental plaque.

PERIODONTITIS SIMPLEX

Periodontitis simplex is the typical classic pro-

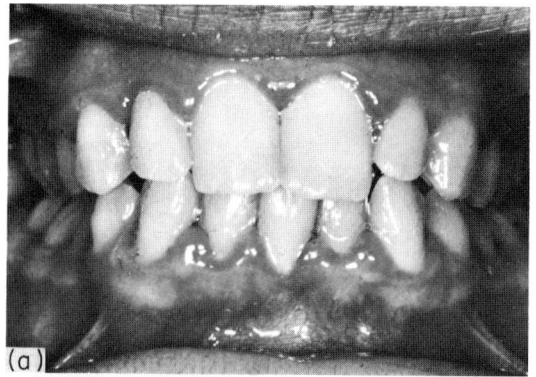

gression of periodontitis described in chap. 3, which accounts for over 95 per cent of cases. The condition is associated with changes in colour, texture and form of the gingival tissues which accompany the presence of long term chronic inflammation. There is frequently a clear history of pre-existing gingivitis for a considerable period of time, and the condition pursues a slow, often symptomless, progression with age, towards loss of the dentition in the 35–45 year age group. 'In developed communities caries is responsible for somewhat more than 40 per cent of total tooth mortality and is the primary cause of tooth loss prior to the age of 30 years. Periodontal disease is responsible for something less than 40 per cent of total tooth mortality and is the dominant cause of tooth loss after the age of 40 years. More than 10 per cent of teeth are extracted for orthodontic, prosthetic or other reasons. In less developed communities, and

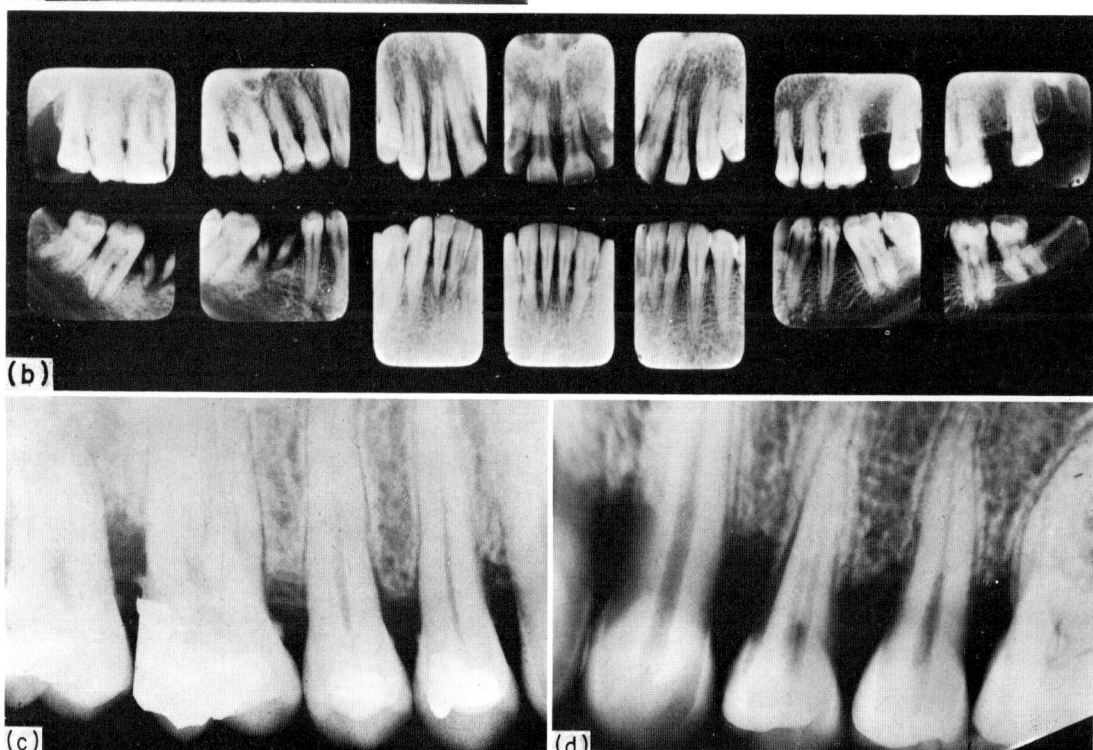

FIG. 12.5. Periodontitis simplex. (a) Typically the stage of progression of periodontitis is approximately the same in all areas of the mouth (b), and in phase with the age of the patient. The pattern of alveolar resorption in the early stages is horizontal (c) but tends to become irregular and vertical as the condition progresses (d).

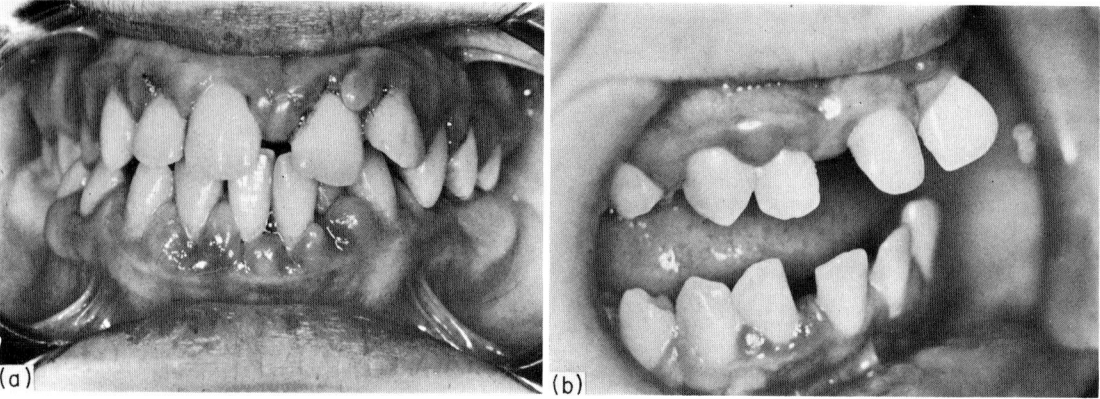

FIG. 12.6. Periodontitis complex. (a) In 15-year-old girl presenting as advanced destruction of the supporting tissues associated with the presence of severe inflammation and gingival hyperplasia. (b) Periodontitis complex in 14-year-old girl presenting as change in alignment and drifting of the teeth.

therefore on a world wide basis, periodontal disease is quite obviously the dominant factor in tooth mortality' [9].

Typically, in periodontitis simplex, the stage of progression of periodontitis is approximately the same in all areas of the mouth, except where obvious local factors account for a more advanced condition (fig. 12.5). On radiographic examination the typical pattern of alveolar resorption is horizontal (fig. 12.5c) and there may be evidence of sclerosis or an attempt at repair of the resorbing bone, in some areas.

The degree of bone loss is in phase with the age of the patient towards loss of the dentition in the 35–45 year age group.

PERIODONTITIS COMPLEX

Periodontitis complex occurs infrequently. It may present as a bizarre exaggerated hyperplasia of the gingivae in a patient, associated with severe inflammation and advanced destruction of the supporting tissues (fig. 12.6a). Conversely, there may be little superficial evidence of inflammation, and the gingival tissues may present an acceptable colour, texture and form. The presenting signs and symptoms may be change in alignment and drifting of the teeth (fig. 12.6b), or a complaint of cyclical loosening and tightening of the teeth. Clinical and radiographic examination of the mouth reveals a degree of tissue destruction that is gross in proportion to the age of the patient. Pocket

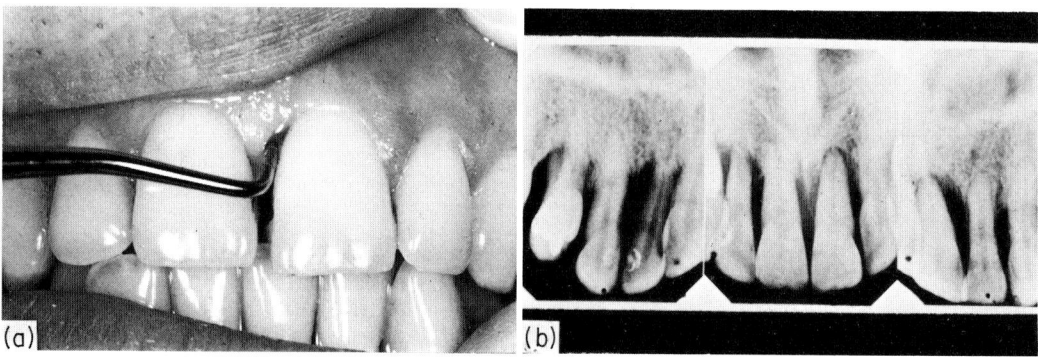

FIG. 12.7. (a) Periodontitis complex in 15-year-old boy. (b) Radiograph of (a); note extensive vertical bone resorption and advanced alveolar destruction relative to the age of the patient.

depth is irregular throughout the mouth without any obvious relationship to local factors. The pattern of bone resorption is typically vertical (fig. 12.7), and the most advanced degree of pocket formation may be associated with groups of teeth by developmental age. Examination may reveal extensive alveolar resorption associated with first molars, or a group of incisors, in an otherwise normal mouth. There is frequently no radiographic evidence of sclerosis in areas, to suggest an alternating pattern of tissue destruction and repair.

The importance of making a clear distinction between periodontitis simplex and periodontitis complex lies in assessing the probable response to treatment. The 'complex' type of lesion in a young patient is evidence of a degree of imbalance of the host–parasite system, which may prejudice the response to treatment. These cases should be approached with caution, and the response to hygiene phase therapy particularly carefully assessed, before attempting surgical intervention.

Treatment of chronic gingivitis and periodontitis

ASSESSMENT AND TREATMENT PLANNING

The morphological changes which are associated with the presence of chronic gingivitis or periodontitis have been described in chap. 3. Successful treatment of these conditions depends on the ability to make an accurate assessment of the degree and pattern of destruction of the supporting structures, and subsequently to institute appropriate treatment. This is a highly subjective judgement, and at the present time there is no generally accepted method of examining the mouth and charting the condition of the supporting tissues, which is widely accepted as a basis for treatment planning. As has been stated previously, there is considerable variation and confusion in the terminology used to describe the stages in the gradual progression of gingivitis and periodontitis. An adequate treatment plan for any patient [10] is based on a knowledge of:
(1) the caries incidence of the patient,
(2) the condition of the supporting structures of the teeth, and knowledge of the extent and

pattern of any destruction of the supporting tissues which may be present,
(3) the degree of superficial inflammation of the gingivae at the time of the initial visit; this should become a declining index as treatment progresses, and superficial inflammation should be completely controlled at the end of the hygiene phase before the patient is accepted for corrective phase therapy.

METHOD OF EXAMINATION

Systems of assessing and recording the caries incidence are well established, but there is less general agreement as to an acceptable method of examination of the supporting tissues. In general it is customary to assess the periodontal condition by measurement of pocket depth at one or more points around the circumference of the tooth. The essential objections to the use of pocket depth as the only basis of assessing the stage of development of periodontitis, for purposes of treatment planning, are that pocket depth at one or two points around the circumference of the cuff is not necessarily a true reflection of the total support of the tooth, and that the time taken to examine the mouth adequately on this basis is long. An accurate and quickly performed assessment of the periodontal condition may be made on the basis of the appearance of the tissues and on the information gained from a percussion test. Accurate measurement of pocket depth, type and extent, should subsequently be carried out to provide detailed information in relation to the specific areas of the mouth requiring treatment, as indicated by these primary criteria. Detailed examination of pocket morphology is mandatory immediately prior to surgical intervention (fig. 12.9). At the stage of treatment planning it is sufficient to define the lesion as limited to superficial tissues suitable for treatment by superficial excision procedures, or involving bone to an extent necessitating flap surgery and correction of bone architecture. Detailed examination of pocket morphology at the initial treatment planning stage is unnecessary duplication of work. On this basis the speed of assessment is increased without loss of accuracy. The gradings suggested by WHO (see chap. 16) using a probe with

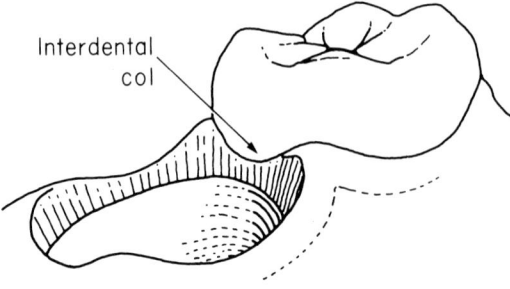

Fɪɢ. 12.8. Normal relationship of epithelial cuff to tooth.

calibrated markings for pocket-depths of 3·5 mm, 5·5 mm, 8·5 mm and 11·5 mm might well prove a useful clinical aid in preliminary determinations of periodontal status.

The appearance of tissues

The normal tooth–tissue relationship has been described as the epithelial cuff being closely adapted to the tooth in the region of the amelo-cemental junction and intact epithelium covering the interdental col through the embrasure (fig. 12.8) (chap. 1).

Visual criteria which are important in assessing the stage of progression of periodontitis are as follows.

(1) The presence of superficial inflammation, oedema or hyperplasia of the tissues (figs. 8.1 & 8.2). A record of the degree of superficial gingival inflammation which is present at the time of the initial visit has a two-fold advantage. Firstly, it is essential that there should be an adequate standard of patient self-care established during the hygiene phase before the patient is accepted for corrective phase therapy. This is known to be established if the initial index of gingival inflammation shows a distinct decrease. Where large numbers of patients are under treatment, memory is not a sufficiently reliable guide. Should the index not decrease in the presence of adequate patient care, a physical examination is indicated to exclude the possibility of general disease. Secondly, the distribution of residual inflammation after completion of the hygiene phase may highlight particular factors contributing to the progression of periodontitis. For example, persistent residual inflammation may result from the presence of undetected subgingival calculus, or hyperfunction which is exacerbating the periodontitis in that area. The most informative method of recording the distribution and extent of gingival inflammation is a modification of the PMA Index of Massler and Schour [11]. The presence of inflammation is recorded as papilla (P), margin (M), and attached (A) on the appropriate area of the chart (see fig. 12.23). For the general purposes of treatment planning there is no necessity for numerical expression of

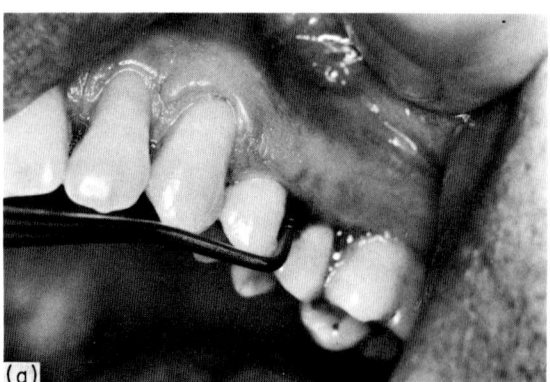

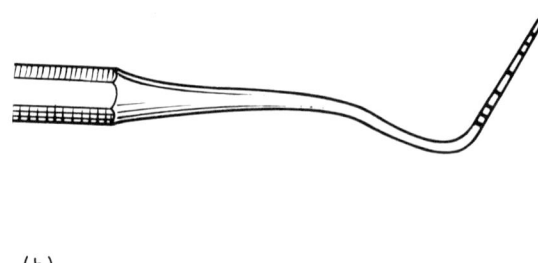

Fɪɢ. 12.9. Loss of adaptation of epithelial cuff to tooth apical to amelocemental junction and ulceration of interdental col. (b) Williams graduated probe.

the PMA Index, or the overall periodontal score (*vide infra*), as has been recommended for purposes of epidemiological survey.

(2) Loss of adaptation of the epithelial cuff to the tooth apical to the amelocemental junction as demonstrated by use of a probe or an air syringe (fig. 12.9).

(3) Loss of continuity of epithelium through the embrasure as shown by obvious splitting of the papillae from buccal to lingual and by bleeding from the embrasure with gentle probing (fig. 12.10).

(4) Changes in the normal anatomical form of attached gingivae. Loss of stippling and inflammation of attached gingivae may indicate that oedema from superficial inflammation has tracked between mucoperiosteum and bone, or that there has been localized resorption of the buccal plate of bone in that region. A percussion test (*vide infra*) will clearly indicate the distinction. Thickening and change in texture of the attached gingivae suggests the presence of long term chronic inflammation, which has caused disorganization of the deeper tissues (fig. 12.11).

(5) The presence of recession of tissue apical to the amelocemental junction (fig. 12.12). It is convenient and simple to note the significant visual signs while charting the caries incidence in a particular quadrant. The tooth and its supporting structures should always be examined as an integral unit, and it should be possible to

assess the approximate stage of the progression of periodontitis in a quadrant on the basis of the appearance of the tissues alone, although no firm conclusion should be drawn at this stage.

The technique of percussion test

A percussion test carried out by gently striking the tooth with the handle of a mirror, with one finger of the left hand held against the tooth to register movement (fig. 12.13), gives an indication of the degree of destruction of the supporting tissues. This is based on the percussion note and the degree of vibration of the percussed

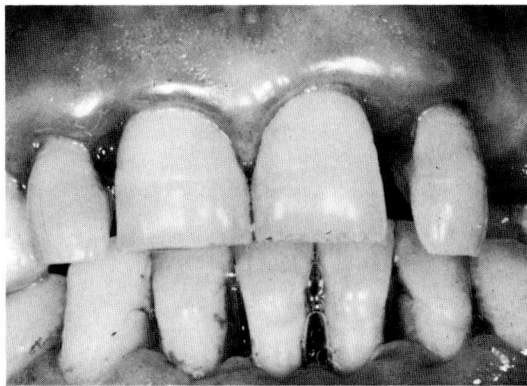

FIG. 12.11. Thickening and change in texture of the attached gingivae may suggest the presence of long term chronic inflammation which has caused disorganization of the deeper tissues.

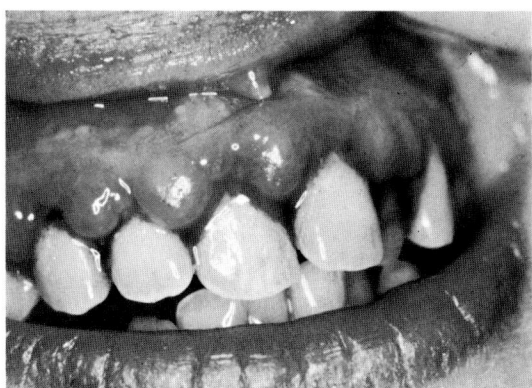

FIG. 12.10. Loss of continuity of epithelium through the embrasure as shown by obvious splitting of the papillae from buccal to lingual.

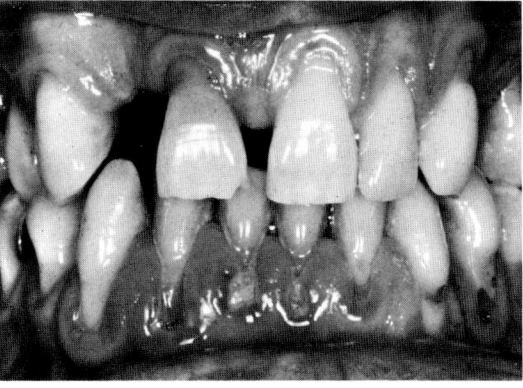

FIG. 12.12. The presence of recession of tissue apical to the amelocemental junction.

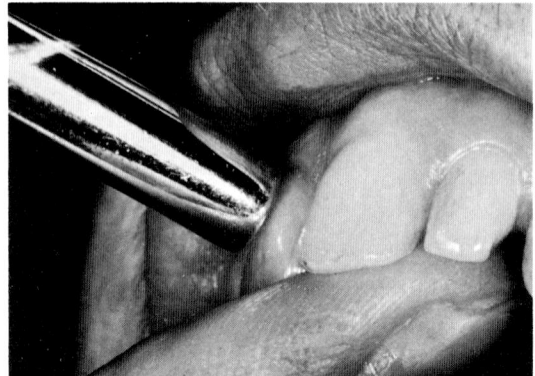

FIG. 12.13. Technique of percussion test.

tooth. The percussion note increases in pitch in proportion to the degree of destruction of the supporting tissues, and in proportion to the degree of inflammation and oedema of these tissues. The degree of vibration which registers against the finger of the left hand increases in proportion to the extent of destruction of the supporting tissues.

Mobility of a tooth is not of itself a reliable guide. The stability of a tooth is in part a function of the extent of inflammation of the supporting connective tissues, and it is not directly related to the degree of alveolar resorption around the tooth. The presence of inflammation and oedema of the surrounding connective tissues may cause a considerable degree of mobility of a tooth which is quantitively well supported. Similarly, a tooth which has loss of the supporting tissues in excess of half the length of the roots of the tooth may be perfectly stable if there is no inflammation of the remaining supporting tissues. Assessment on the basis of percussion note and degree of vibration of the percussed tooth gives a more generally accurate indication of the quantity and quality of support than can be based on examination for mobility alone. Mobility of a tooth may be simply an expression of the width of the periodontal membrane.

Stages in progression

GINGIVITIS

The term gingivitis is commonly used to describe superficial inflammation or hyperplasia in the presence of an established periodontitis, where the lesion is not gingivally contained. This causes unnecessary confusion, and it is convenient to distinguish these by referring to the gingivally contained lesion as a limited gingivitis.

LIMITED OEDEMATOUS GINGIVITIS

A limited oedematous gingivitis exists where

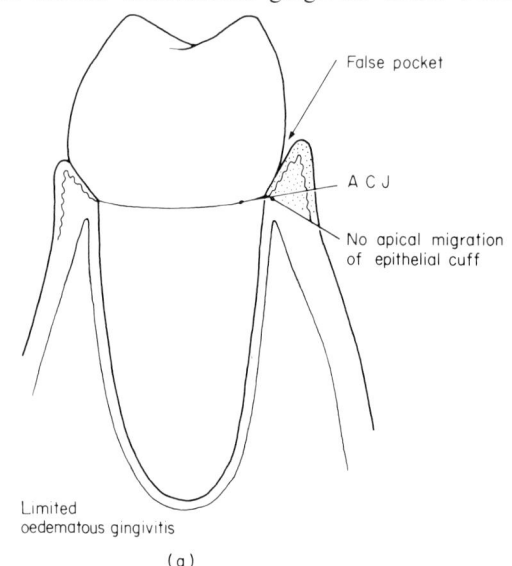

(a)

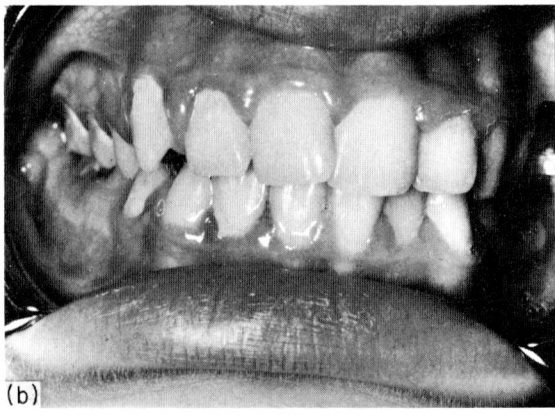

FIG. 12.14. (a) Limited oedematous gingivitis. (b) The anatomical structure of the collagen bundles of the marginal ligament and the deeper tissues of the periodontium remains intact.

there is increase in the volume of the tissues due to local exudation of fluid and cells as a result of inflammatory change in the connective tissues of the papillae and the margins (fig. 12.14a). The lesion is gingivally contained, and the anatomical structure of the collagen bundles of the marginal ligament and the deeper tissues of the periodontium remain intact (fig. 12.14b). There may be a breach in the continuity of epithelium through the embrasure, shown by bleeding following the gentle insertion of a blunt probe, but no hyperplasia of cuff epithelium apical to the amelocemental junction. Any increase in the depth of the pocket is the result of occlusal increase in the volume of the tissues and not a result of migration of the gingival cuff apical to the amelocemental junction (false pocket, fig. 12.14a).

Principles of treatment

A limited oedematous gingivitis is a tissue change which is reversible following hygiene phase therapy and is not associated with permanent change in the anatomical form of the tissues if treated at an early stage. If this condition is allowed to persist there will be a variable increase in the amount of collagen formed during phases of repair (fibrous gingivitis), and eventual progression of inflammation resulting in destruction of tissues apical to the amelocemental junction.

LIMITED FIBROUS GINGIVITIS

A limited fibrous gingivitis exists where enlargement of tissues is due primarily to increase in the content of formed collagen. The lesion is comparable to a limited oedematous gingivitis in so far as it is gingivally contained, and the anatomical integrity of the collagen bundles of the marginal ligament remains intact (fig. 12.15a). The hyperplasia may be accompanied by a variable degree of inflammation and by breach of continuity of epithelium through the embrasure. There is no hyperplasia of cuff epithelium apical to the amelocemental junction, and pocket formation is the result of occlusal enlargement of the tissues to form a false pocket (fig. 12.15b). Where enlargement of

the tissue is a result of a mixture of oedema and hyperplasia, it is convenient to estimate the amount of oedema which is present by applying pressure to the tissues to displace the oedema and reveal the degree of fibrosis.

Principles of treatment

A limited fibrous gingivitis represents a tissue change which is not reversible by hygiene phase therapy alone, but which requires subsequent

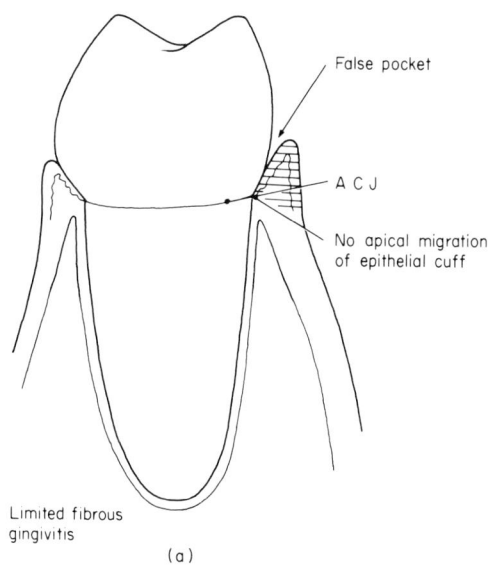

False pocket

A C J

No apical migration of epithelial cuff

Limited fibrous gingivitis

(a)

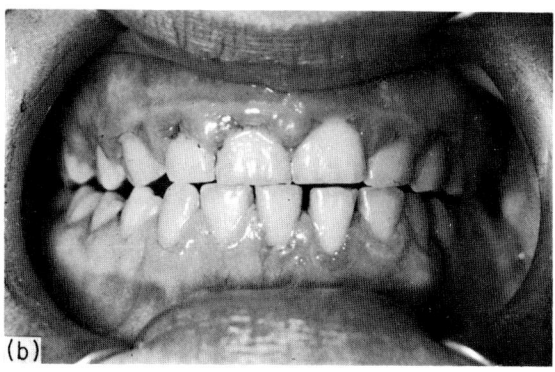

(b)

FIG. 12.15. (a) Limited fibrous gingivitis. (b) Hyperplasia of supracrestal connective tissues without apical proliferation of cuff epithelium.

surgical removal of the hyperplastic tissue. If the condition is allowed to persist, distortion of gingival form will result in increased plaque accumulation and eventual progression of inflammation, resulting in destruction of tissues apical to the amelocemental junction. Gingival fibrosis may be present at any stage of destruction of the supporting tissues.

PERIODONTITIS

Initial stage

The initial stage of periodontitis exists when there is:

(1) hyperplasia of cuff epithelium apical to the amelocemental junction giving rise to the presence of true pockets.

(2) disaggregation and loss of attachment of the collagen bundles of the marginal ligament to the tooth and the alveolar crest, which allows hyperplasia of the cuff epithelium apical to the amelocemental junction to cover cementum from which the connective tissues have become detached.

(3) early resorption of the alveolar crest occurring partly under the influence of toxic factors from the mouth causing osteoclasia, and partly from loss of functional stimulation after detachment of the collagen bundles of the marginal ligament.

In the presence of a true pocket there is no prospect of reattachment of the connective tissues to the root surface until the pocket epithelium has been removed. This is a basic principle of the surgical treatment of true pockets.

At this stage the pattern of bone resorption is generally horizontal, and the pocket has soft tissue walls and a bone base. Using the probe suggested by the WHO (fig. 12.16) such pockets would not extend deeper than the 5·5 mm mark. For practical purposes the base of the pocket is coronal to the alveolar crest (fig. 12.17). Such a pocket may be described as a simple, true pocket. The formation of simple true pockets represents a permanent change in the tooth–tissue relationship that is not reversible without

surgery. Simple true pockets can usually be eliminated by superficial excision procedures (chap. 15), as the lateral walls are of soft tissue.

It is convenient to divide the further progression of periodontitis into arbitrarily chosen ranges of tissue destruction according to the amount of tooth support which has been lost.

(1) An established periodontitis with pockets greater than 5·5 mm, but not exceeding 8·5 mm on the probe (fig. 12.18).

(2) An advanced periodontitis with indicated probing greater than the 8·5 mm mark (fig. 12.19).

Pattern of bone resorption

In the healthy mouth the compact bone forming the lamina dura of the sockets is continuous across the interdental crest between adjacent

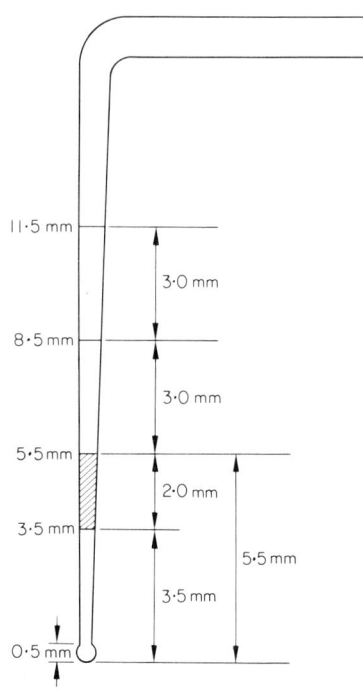

FIG. 12.16. Instrument suggested for measurement of pockets and probing for subgingival calculus and gingival bleeding. From WHO (1978) Technical Report Series No. 621, p. 37.

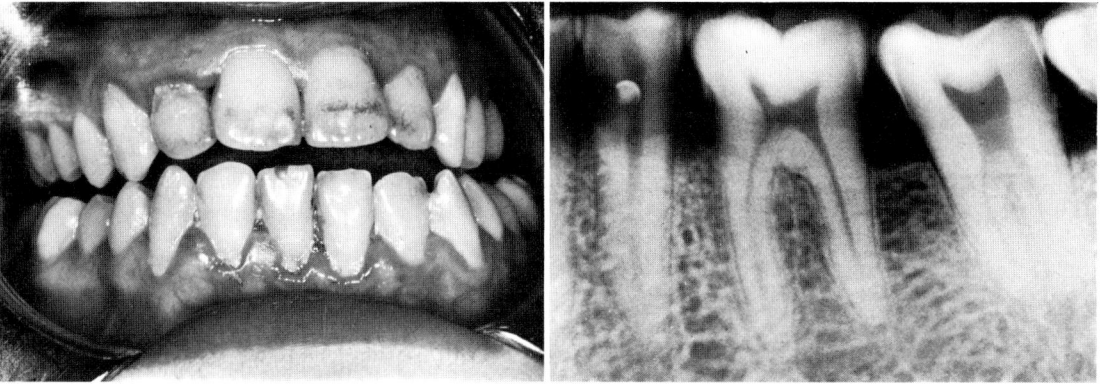

FIG. 12.17. Early periodontitis.

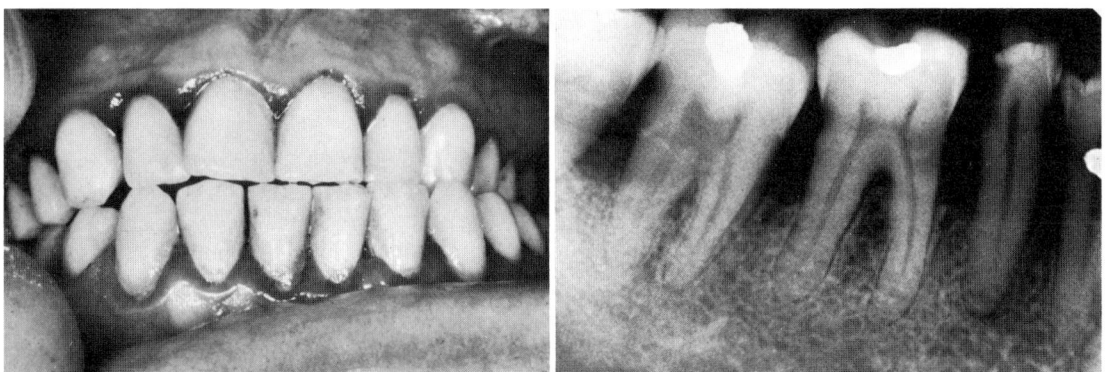

FIG. 12.18. Established periodontitis.

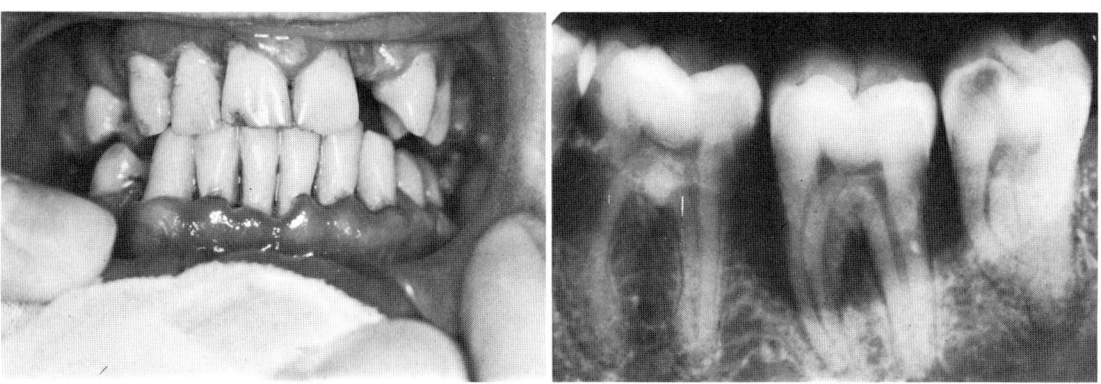

FIG. 12.19. Advanced periodontitis.

teeth (fig. 12.20). Following early resorption of the alveolar crest and loss of attachment of the collagen bundles of the marginal ligament, resorption may proceed more quickly in the central area of the crest or on the tooth side of the crest than laterally (fig. 12.21). The result may be the formation of a pocket which has a base apical to the alveolar crest; this is termed a compound or infra-bony pocket. A compound pocket may be defined as a pocket where the base is apical to the alveolar crest and which has one or more bone walls.

Periodontitis is characterized by tissue destruction with periodic attempts at repair (chap. 3). The rate of progression is governed by the degree of imbalance between local irritants in the mouth, and the factors which govern tissue resistance (chaps. 4 & 7). There may be excessive production of collagen during phases of repair, producing a fibrous gingivitis, and there may be a variable sclerosis and thickening of the alveolar crest, in response to toxic factors from the mouth. As a result of such thickening, compound pocket formation may occur at an early stage in the progression of periodontitis, particularly in relation to posterior teeth. The comparatively broad interdental table of bone between posterior teeth is commonly associated with central resorption and peripheral thickening

of bone leading to the formation of compound pockets at an early stage (fig. 12.21). The pointed interdental spine between anterior teeth is more likely to be resorbed as a whole, in the initial stages of periodontitis, giving rise to the presence of simple true pockets. In general the tendency towards irregular vertical resorption of bone increases as the periodontitis progresses.

As a matter of routine, full mouth radiographic examination should be carried out before commencing corrective phase therapy, to confirm the pattern and extent of bone resorption (fig. 12.22). Problems of shortage of attached gingivae may be associated with pockets of any depth and should always be considered with care; see chap. 15.

Principles of treatment

Well developed compound pockets with one or more bone walls cannot be eliminated by superficial excision of soft tissue. Correction of bone architecture should be carried out by a flap technique (chap. 15).

With adequate treatment, the prognosis is usually good up to pockets indicated by the 8·5 mm mark, except in the young adult with advanced vertical alveolar resorption relative to age.

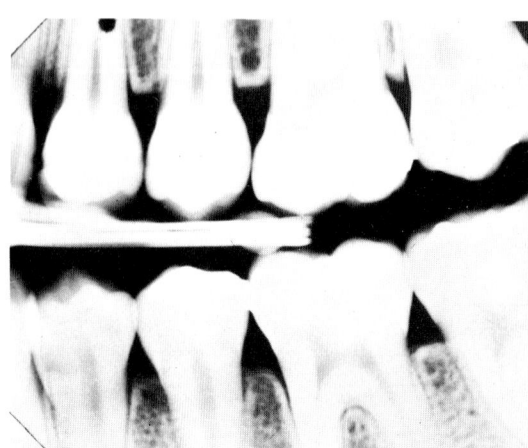

FIG. 12.20. Radiograph of a normal mouth. The lamina dura of adjacent teeth appears to be continuous across the interdental crests, courtesy of Mr A.R. Bradshaw.

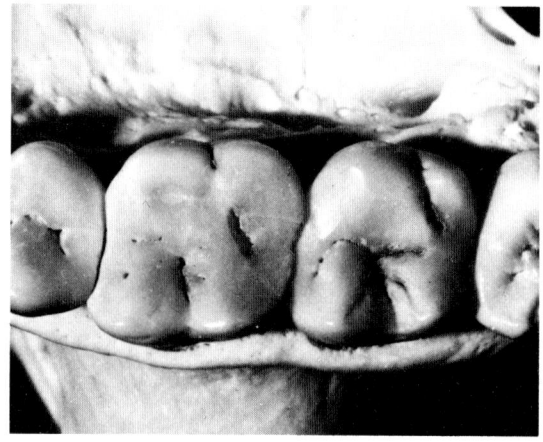

FIG. 12.21. Resorption may proceed more quickly in the central area of the crest, than laterally (dried skull).

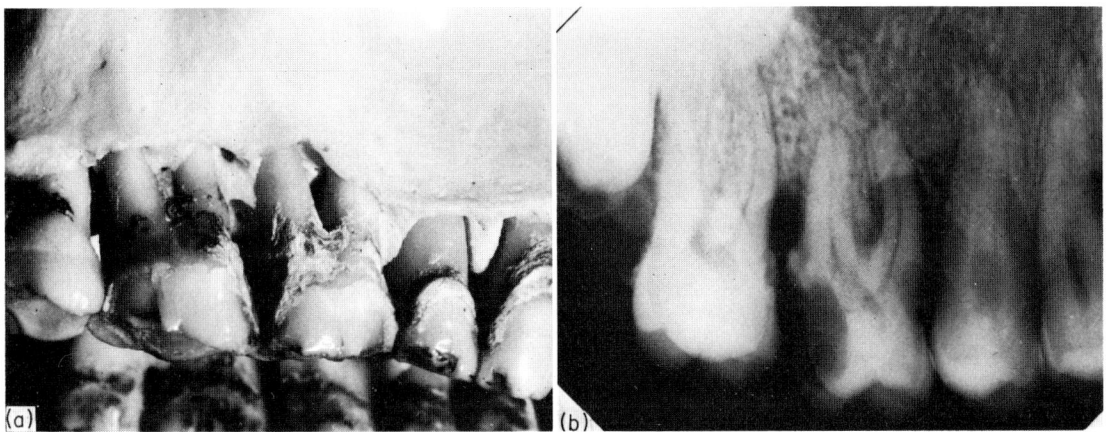

FIG. 12.22. Compound pocket formation. (a) note tortuous pocket morphology due to involvement of multi-rooted teeth (dried skull), (b) Compound pocket, X-ray trifurcation involvement of maxillary molar.

Above 8·5 mm, the long term prognosis is less certain, and such patients should not be subjected to radical corrective phase therapy unless there is a clear indication for keeping the teeth.

The relationship of the progression of periodontitis to the types of pocket which are likely to be present, and to the treatment which is appropriate, is summarized in table 12.1.

When planning reconstruction of an occlusion, it is immaterial whether the loss of support is the result of pocket formation or recession of supporting tissues from the tooth.

ing of pockets have a grid system to indicate pocket depth. Position of bone and gingival margins can be recorded separately to give a visual record of the type and extent of problem. It is convenient to record the caries incidence, and findings of the percussion test in terms of vibration or mobility, beside the crown and the PMA findings alongside the neck.

It is undesirable and unnecessary to examine for individual characteristics in separate circuits of the mouth. Each tooth and its supporting tissues should be examined as a functional unit in a single circuit of the mouth.

Patient record chart

Many different forms of chart suitable for record-

TABLE 12.1. The relationship of stages in the progression of periodontitis to appropriate treatment.

Stage in progression of periodontitis	Range of therapy	Type of pocket
Limited oedematous gingivitis	Controlled oral hygiene, oral toilet	False, simple
Limited fibrous gingivitis		False, simple
	Controlled oral hygiene, oral toilet	
The initial stage of established periodontitis —up to 5·5 mm pockets	subgingival curettage or gingivectomy	True, simple
Loss of supporting tissues in excess of 5·5 mm but less than 8·5 nm	Controlled oral hygiene, oral toilet, gingivectomy in relation to simple pockets, flap surgery in relation to compound pockets	True, simple or compound
Loss of supporting tissues in excess of 8.5 mm		

Diagnostic bacteriology

ASSESSMENT OF PATIENT TREATMENT
NEEDS

There is at present no acceptable reproducible
method of assessing patient treatment need from
individual to individual, or of defining the treatment requirements of a particular patient.

Epidemiological criteria which give a measure
of supragingival plaque or gingival inflammation
have not been directly related to rate of tissue
destruction within the individual or from one
individual to another. Similarly, measurement of
pocket depth and radiographic interpretation of
various degrees of tissue destruction only provide information about prior disease experience
and are poor indicators of an individual's
'current periodontal disease status'. To depend
upon such assessments alone for either initial
diagnosis or subsequent monitoring of therapeutic programmes and their results are clearly
inadequate. Keyes *et al.* [12] have outlined a
diagnostic and therapeutic regimen based on
bacteriological monitoring which requires
further testing and evaluation. He has
postulated:

(1) That certain bacterial complexes firmly
or loosely attached to the radicular surfaces
of teeth are not compatible with periodontal health. (This includes a variety of motile
micro-organisms such as Gram-negative bacilli
and spirochaetes which are substantially non-
attached populations.)

(2) The motile bacteria and white blood cells
(WBC) residing in the sulcus/pocket spaces can
be sampled and readily examined at the chairside
by phase contrast microscopy.

(3) The prevalence of certain bacterial populations can be used to predict potentially
periodontopathic conditions and assess the probable degree of progressive tissue destruction.

(4) The microbiological population in question can be prevented from accumulating or can
be suppressed by appropriate therapy.

(5) When microbiological populations are
controlled, progressive destruction of periodontal tissues abates.

Such principles can be evaluated by the use
of dark ground illumination microscopy [13].

It has been proposed that two easily performed

procedures provide diagnostic information in relation to the current disease status of the
periodontium [12]:

(1) A microscopic assessment of the motile
microorganisms and WBCs obtained from the
sulcus/pocket areas;

(2) A determination of gingival sulcus
bleeding points.

A small curette or periodontal file is used to
remove samples of accumulated bacteria from
several representative root surfaces and pockets.
Any existing supragingival plaque should be removed from the area and a particular effort
made to obtain samples from deeper subgingival
spaces, that are difficult for the patient to clean.
Where phase contrast microscopy is used, the
scrapings are immediately immersed in a drop of
tap water on a standard microscope slide and
dislodged from the curette by an explorer. A
cover slip is quickly placed over the wet preparation and gently compressed to spread and
thin the sample prior to viewing. Two or three
different samples from different sites can be prepared on a single slide. Notations based on
microscopic findings may be recorded so that
initial and subsequent observations can be prepared on a form similar to that shown in fig.
12.23. This permits one to follow microbial
population changes over a period of time and
relate them to the patient performance and
treatment provided.

In patients having excellent periodontal health
where there is no evidence of gingival inflammation, sulcus bleeding or pocket formation the
accumulation of plaque is so scanty that it is
difficult to sample. Accumulations from such
individuals contain only an occasional WBC
and few of the larger motile rods and spirochaetes. Healthy individuals only demonstrate
very small motile cocci which spin around in
erratic circles or tiny darting rods. Such a
description is also typical of patients brought
under control through personal and professional therapy. In contrast, lesions not
under control will continue to harbour larger
motile rods, spirochaetes and numerous WBCs
[12].

The second diagnostic procedure aids in
assessing current tissue condition and is accomplished by gently passing a periodontal probe

Name: .... No. ....
Address: ....
....

	18	17	16	15	14	13	12	11	21	22	23	24	25	26	27	28
SOT	☐	☐	☐	☐	☐	☐	☐	☐	☐	☐	☐	☐	☐	☐	☐	☐
POT	☐	☐	☐	☐	☐	☐	☐	☐	☐	☐	☐	☐	☐	☐	☐	☐
>5·5	☐	☐	☐	☐	☐	☐	☐	☐	☐	☐	☐	☐	☐	☐	☐	☐
>3·5<5·5	☐	☐	☐	☐	☐	☐	☐	☐	☐	☐	☐	☐	☐	☐	☐	☐

	48	47	46	45	44	43	42	41	31	32	33	34	35	36	37	38
SOT	☐	☐	☐	☐	☐	☐	☐	☐	☐	☐	☐	☐	☐	☐	☐	☐
POT	☐	☐	☐	☐	☐	☐	☐	☐	☐	☐	☐	☐	☐	☐	☐	☐
>5·5	☐	☐	☐	☐	☐	☐	☐	☐	☐	☐	☐	☐	☐	☐	☐	☐
>3·5<5·5	☐	☐	☐	☐	☐	☐	☐	☐	☐	☐	☐	☐	☐	☐	☐	☐

Treatment code

Curettage	Gingivectomy	Flap	Chlorhexidine	Occlusal adjustment		Sex	Age
☐	☐	☐	☐	☐		☐	☐

FIG. 12.23. Treatment planning form. SOT, secondary occlusal trauma; POT, primary occlusal trauma.

around the root in sulcus/pocket spaces. If this procedure induces gingival bleeding there is presumptive evidence of capillary fragility associated with erythemogenic bacterial biproducts and/or ulceration within the gingival sulcus or pockets.

Other clinical criteria which have been employed to estimate tissue conditions and rate of destruction are recording of pocket depths, tooth mobility, radiographs and oral photographs. In common with plaque and inflammation scores, measurements of gingival exudate and other periodontal disease indices have at best provided doubtful criteria of an individual's progressive disease status at any particular time.

Listgarten [14] noted that a distinct microbial flora was associated with tooth surfaces of extracted teeth, grouped according to their periodontal status prior to extraction.

Teeth with a clinically healthy periodontium exhibited accumulations of predominantly coccoid cells in a supragingival location. With the electron microscope these bacteria had cell wall features characteristic of Gram-positive as well as Gram-negative organisms, the former being the more common.

Teeth with gingivitis had a supragingival flora of predominantly filamentous cells and a scanty but distinct subgingival flora.

Teeth with periodontitis had well-established periodontal pockets along the surfaces sampled and a well-developed subgingival flora containing many flagellated cells and spirochaetes. The majority of bacteria in pockets had cell wall structures characteristic of Gram-negative microorganisms. The supragingival flora of these teeth was predominantly filamentous and indistinguishable from the supragingival flora of teeth with gingivitis. These observations on extracted teeth were based on time-consuming preparatory techniques and involved transmission electron microscopic examination of many samples per tooth. While the results are informative, the methodology is not suited to the clinician interested in examining the periodontal flora of individual patients. For these reasons a clinically orientated technique has been proposed [14].

When no detectable supragingival microbial accumulations were present bacterial samples were obtained by introducing a clean periodontal curette through the sulcus or pocket orifice as far apically as possible and the bacterial contents removed. If necessary, the process was repeated several times to obtain enough bacteria. If a pocket contained a relatively large volume of bacteria, only a portion of the contents was removed. If the crown was covered with a substantial accumulation of bacterial debris, the latter was first scraped from the tooth surface coronal to the sulcus or pocket orifice prior to sampling.

The sample was suspended in a sterile 0·85 per cent sodium chloride solution containing 1 per cent gelatine. By vigorously agitating the tip of the instrument in the solution, generally 0·1–0·3 ml of solution contained in a small screw top vial was adequate for dispersing bacterial samples from single surfaces. In order to minimise clumping and loss of bacterial motility, samples were prepared and the examination completed within one hour of their collection. The bacterial suspension was dispersed just prior to the examination by aspirating and expelling the fluid three times through a disposable tuberculin syringe equipped with a 23 gauge needle. One drop of the suspension was applied to the microscope slide and the cover slip placed in position. Excess fluid was removed by inverting the slide over an absorbent surface and applying moderate pressure. The slide was examined by dark field microscopy at a magnification of 1200×. If the preparation was too dense the sample was diluted with additional saline and a new slide prepared. Generally from 100–200 bacteria from a field selected at random were classified into nine morphological categories as follows [14]:

(1) *Coccoid cells.* Cells approximately 0·5–1·0 μm in diameter showing a bright outline with a dark centre. In this category were also included coccobacillary forms the length of which was up to, but not more than, twice the width of the cell. Dividing cells were counted as one, unless the daughter cells appeared as distinct, fully formed cocci still attached to one another, in which case each cell was counted separately.

(2) *Straight rods.* Non-flagellated cells with a bright outline and a dark interior, approximately 0·5–1·5 μm in width, with a width to length ratio between 1:2 and 1:6, and blunt or rounded cell ends. Branching cells were excluded.

(3) *Filaments.* Cells with a bright outline and a dark interior, approximately 0·5–1·5 μm in with, with a width to length ratio greater than 1:6. These cells often had an irregular contour and on rare occasions exhibited branching or septa. Shorter cells exhibiting branching were also included in this category.

(4) *Fusiforms.* Cells approximately 0·3 to 1·0 μm in diameter, with a bright outline but not always a dark interior. Cell length was approximately 10 μm or less and cells ends were pointed.

(5) *Curved rods.* Similar to straight rods except for a definite crescent shape. No evidence of flagella. These probably represent dead motile cells in which the flagella could not be detected or had been lost.

(6) *Small spirochaetes.* Helicoidal cells, approximately 0·2–0·3 μm in width and up to 10 μm in length, with a single-contoured outline and relatively tight coils.

(7) *Intermediate spirochaetes.* Helicoidal cells, approximately 0·3–0·4 μm in width and up to 15 μm in length. The cell outline was single-contoured in the darkfield and the coiling not as tight as for small spirochaetes.

(8) *Large spirochaetes.* Helicoidal cells 0·5 μm or wider and up to 20 μm in length. The cells had a wavy rather than a coiled appearance in

FIG. 12.24. All the illustrations are micrographs of sulcular or pocket microorganisms photographed by darkfield ▶ microscopy. For photographic purposes, the microorganisms suspended in Karnovsky fixative (Karnovsky M.J., *J. Cell. Biol.* **27**, 137A, 1965) were smeared on a slide, dried and the preparation coverslipped with glycerin. (Courtesy Dr. M. A. Listgarten.)

a. Coccus (C), fusiform (Fu) and filament (F). × 1000.
b. Cocci (C) and straight rod (R). × 1000.
c. Straight rods (R) and long filament (F). × 1000.
d. Fusiform (Fu), small spirochaete (SS), medium-size spirochaete (MS), coccus (C) and short filament (F). If the latter were at all shorter it would fall into the category of straight rods (compare with rod in (C)). × 1000.
e. Curved rod with distinct flagellum. This cell would be classified as a motile rod because of the presence of a distinguishable flagellum, even in the absence of actual motility. × 2000.
f. Similar cell type as in (e) showing incomplete division. This would be counted as a single cell. × 1500.
g. Medium-size spirochaete (MS), small spirochaete (SS), large spirochaete (LS). × 1000.
h. Relative sizes of spirochaetes of the small (SS), medium-size (MS) and large (LS) variety. The double-contour of the large spirochaetes is not well reproduced photographically. × 1500.

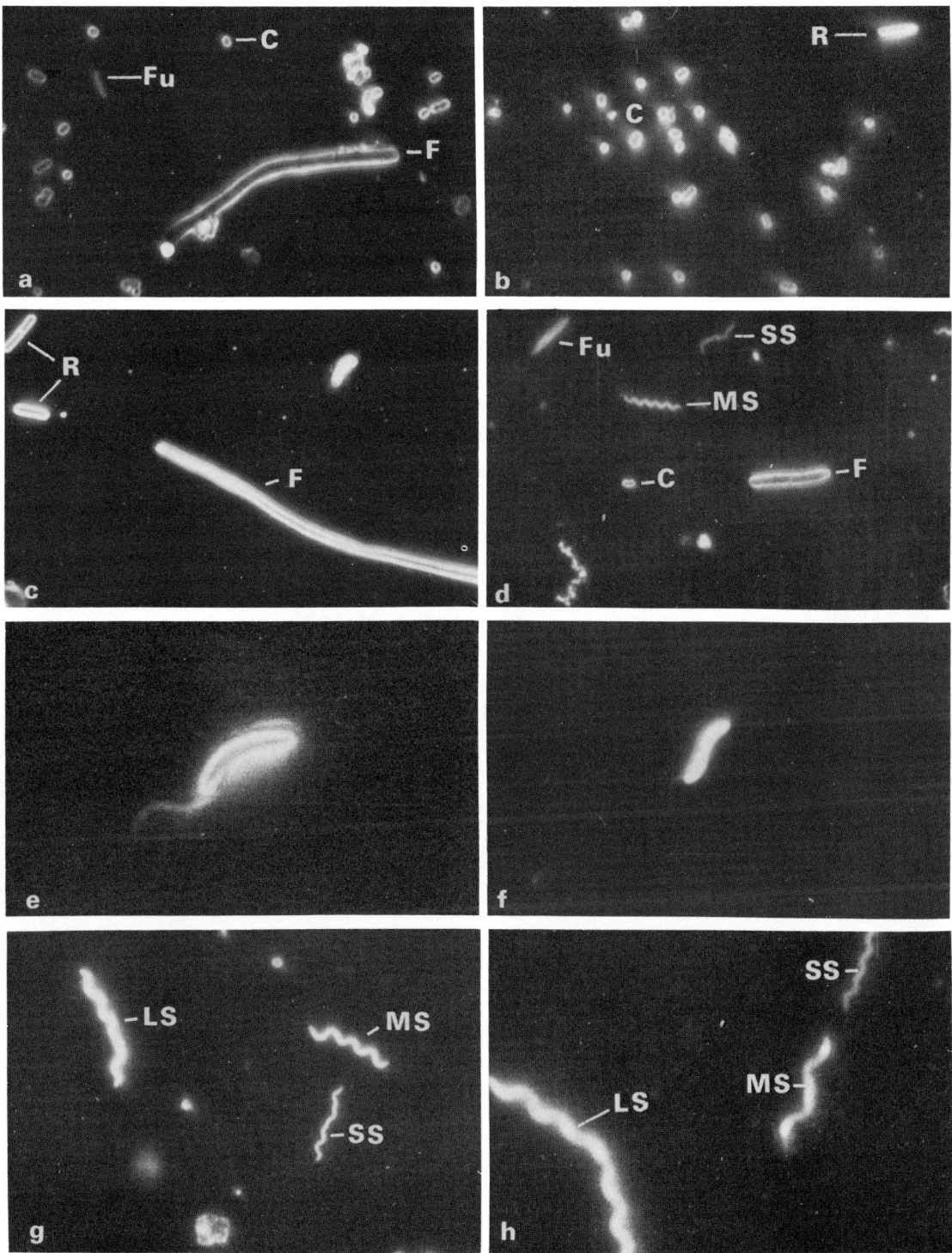

the darkfield and showed a distinct double-contoured outline. This group probably included some chains of spiral organisms such as *Selenomonas* which resemble large spirochaetes.

In distinguishing among spirochaetes, cell width, including presence or absence of a double contour, was more useful than length which varied considerably.

(9) *Motile rods*. This category included all cell types, other than spirochaetes, which exhibited motility in the darkfield. These generally comprised either straight or curved rods and on occasion fusiform and coccoid cells.

Attempts to establish a correlation between certain species of microorganisms and periodontal disease, using data from cultural studies of plaque samples, have indicated that a number of microorganisms, including *Bacteroides melaninogenicus*, vibrio (*Campylobacter sputorum*) and *Fusobacterium nucleatum* [15] and certain as yet unidentified Gram-negative rods [16 & 17] appear to be related to the disease process.

Morphological techniques have repeatedly indicated an association of certain microorganisms with periodontal disease. Kritchevsky and Seguin [18] demonstrated the association of spirochaetes with periodontal disease and were able to distinguish three different types of spirochaetes in smears of bacteria from untreated pockets. Data was presented to show that antisyphilitic therapy had a concomitant beneficial influence on the periodontal status of the patients. More recently, microscopic studies of the undisturbed microbial flora associated with the surfaces of healthy and periodontally diseased teeth showed that the flora at healthy sites consisted predominantly of Gram-positive coccoid bacteria, while Gram-negative and filamentous forms increased in gingivitis. Spirochaetes and Gram-negative flagellated bacteria were primarily a feature of advanced periodontal disease [13].

The proportional increase of the number of spirochaetes in samples from diseased sites demonstrated by Listgarten and Helldén [14] appears highly significant for each category of spirochaete, as well as for spirochaetes taken as a a group. The mean increase for individual categories varies from approximately a factor of 11 for small spirochaetes to a factor of 37 for medium sized spirochaetes and 34 for large spirochaetes. The overall 21-fold increase from 1·8 to 37·7 per cent of spirochaetes as a group is noteworthy not only because of its magnitude but also because an increase was consistently observed in each subject although the magnitude of the increase varied from subject to subject.

Although inherently crude, the technique of classifying the periodontal flora on a proportional basis according to morphological criteria as presented here is simple, relatively rapid, cheap and provides a less distorted overall view of plaque composition than current cultural techniques. There is presently a cumulative error in cultural techniques as applied particularly to organisms of endogenous origin so that what emerges at the end of a complex cultural procedure bears little relationship to the organism as it existed in its own environment, the plaque microcosm of interdependent groups of organisms. Spirochaetes which may account for over a third of the subgingival flora in a severely diseased site are not even detected by cultural methods in current use for assaying the composition of the oral flora.

In studies by Listgarten, Lindhe and Helldén [19] 12 adult patients with severe chronic periodontitis were examined prior to treatment, and after 8 and 25 weeks following the start of treatment. Six subjects received tetracycline during weeks 1 and 2 and weeks 7 and 8, while the other six did not. All subjects were instructed in oral hygiene and received a series of scaling and root planing treatment on one side only of their dentition. The contralateral side received no scalings at any time. The experiment was designed to provide clinical and microbial data at the 0–8 and 25-week intervals for at least six sites in each of four groups: untreated sites (T_0S_0); sites which were scaled only (T_0S_1); sites which received tetracycline only (T_1S_0); and sites which were scaled and were exposed to tetracycline (T_1S_1). In addition biopsies of initially diseased sites which had been treated or left untreated were evaluated by light and electron microscopy at all time intervals.

The results indicated that (T_0S_0) sites remained more or less unchanged with respect to all parameters during the 25-week period, with the exception of a decrease in PlI scores due to improved oral hygiene. T_0S_1 sites showed a marked clinical improvement between time 0 and 8 weeks, i.e. reduced PlI and GI scores and reduced probing depth; the microbial flora showed an increase in the population of coccoid cells with a concomitant decrease in motile rods and spirochaetes; the plasma cell dominated infiltrated connective tissue (ICT) showed a significant decrease in the proportion of plasma cells with a corresponding increase in lymphocytes; evidence of collagen deposition was also observed histologically. This 8-week status persisted after 25 weeks but in addition the tissues showed an increase in the proportion of fibroblasts and a decrease in the proportion of lymphoblasts. T_1S_0 sites showed a similar improvement in the clinical and microbial parameters at 8 weeks, but the ICT showed only a moderate reduction in the proportion of dead and unidentified cells.

After 25 weeks, the clinical parameters remained unchanged from the 8-week interval, but the microbial composition and the tissue characteristics showed a significant rebound toward the values observed at baseline. T_1S_1 sites showed essentially similar changes in the clinical microbial and tissue characteristics as the T_0S_1 sites for all time intervals. However, in the presence of the antibiotic the 8-week proportions of coccoid cells were higher and those for motile rods and spirochaetes lower. Evaluation of all biopsied sites revealed a positive correlation between the proportion of plasma cells in the ICT and the proportion of spirochaetes in the associated microflora.

The results suggest that the microflora of healthy and periodontally diseased sites differ and that some of these differences are associated with detectable differences in the composition of the ICT. Mechanical debridement and/or treatment with tetracycline cause changes in the clinical microbiological and histological parameters. Discontinuation of treatment with tetracycline leads to a return of the microbial and histological parameters toward values observed prior to treatment. These changes appear prior to detectable clinical changes.

Oral hygiene alone did not affect significantly either the GI score or the probing measurement of the untreated control sites.

The changes in the relative proportions of some members of the microbial flora were particularly noteworthy. The results indicated that the proportion of coccoid cells, motile rods and spirochaetes changed significantly during the course of this experiment with the proportion of coccoid cells varying inversely to those of motile rods and spirochaetes. The proportion of coccoid cells increased as a result of scaling and/or tetracycline therapy with the results achieved at eight weeks being maintained throughout the 25-week experimental period for the scaled only group but with a return towards baseline values in the patients who had received tetracycline. This seemed to be due in part to the extremely high proportion of coccal cells which resulted from tetracycline therapy, the latter having just ended at the time of the eight-week examination. It is apparent that such high levels of coccoid cells could not be achieved or maintained by scaling alone or following discontinuation of antibiotic administration.

An identical but reverse pattern was detected with respect to changes in the proportion of motile rods and spirochaetes, the proportions of which were markedly reduced by scaling and/or antibiotic therapy. However the return to baseline values for spirochaetes between the 8- and 25-week examinations seemed to be limited to the tetracycline only group. In the scaled plus tetracycline group, scaling seemed to be able to keep the proportion of spirochaetes reduced to a level close to that observed in the no tetracycline scaled group at the 8- and 25-week examination. It is obvious that scaling and/or tetracycline were able to significantly suppress spirochaetes between the baseline and the eight-week examination. While scaling alone was able to keep the proportion of spirochaetes throughout the experimental period at a level not significantly different from that achieved in eight weeks, discontinuation of the tetracycline, in the absence of scaling, resulted in a significant rebound towards baseline levels between the 8- and 25-week examinations. It is not possible to state on the basis of this 25-week experiment whether the treatments would have been adequate for the long term maintenance of probe-able pockets following an initial series of scalings.

It is worth noting, nevertheless, that there were no detectable changes in the clinical parameters between 8- and 25-weeks in any of the treatment groups following the initial improvement from baseline values. Yet while the clinical parameters remained stable over this time, the composition of the microbial flora which had changed significantly as a result of the initial therapy began to shift back in the direction of baseline values. This was particularly noticeable with respect to the relative proportions of coccoid cells, motile rods and spirochaetes, and most evident in the tetracycline/no scaling treatment group [19].

The results suggest that a microbial flora typical of that observed at a periodontally diseased site [14] can be altered, by treatment, to one more typical of the flora observed at a healthy site. While an effect on the flora is not unexpected following the use of a broad spectrum antibiotic, it is noteworthy that a similar effect can be produced by mechanical debridement. Furthermore, this effect is detectable for at least two weeks following scaling in most patients and most sites. The results of this study are significant since they show definite change in the proportions of certain bacterial forms in response to both mechanical and chemical treatment. It is equally significant that in the absence of mechanical debridement tetracycline therapy merely adds a transient effect.

The improvement in probing measurement over baseline values observed at treated sites after 8- and 25-weeks was probably due largely to the histologically detectable increase in new collagen fibre deposition and the concomitant decrease in the size of the inflammatory infiltrate in the connective tissue.

The reason for the marked increase in the proportion of dead cells in the infiltrate at the eight-week interval was not clear. It was suggested that plasma cells may be produced in response to antigenic stimulus by certain members of the periodontal flora. Tetracycline therapy may produce a more specific and complete reduction of certain microorganisms than mechanical debridement and thereby markedly alter the nature of the antigenic stimulus due to the microbial flora. Since the life span of plasma cells may be as short as two to four days, any alteration in the antigenic stimulus may be followed by a rapid change in the cellular composition of the inflamed connective tissue infiltrate. A clear association seemed to exist between the nature of the connective tissue infiltrate and the presence of spirochaetes in the bacterial sample. Plasma cells tended to dominate in those tissues which were associated with a microbial flora containing 5 per cent or larger proportions of spirochaetes. Infiltrates dominated by lymphocytes tended to come from biopsies associated with microbial floras containing 5 per cent or fewer spirochaetes. All areas in which fibroblasts were the dominant cells, that is in areas which few if any inflammatory cells were observed, were obtained from tissue samples associated with microbial floras in which spirochaetes were absent or constituted less than 5 per cent of the microbial flora.

The inflammatory infiltrate of the initially diseased sites was dominated by plasma cells, which constituted close to 50 per cent of all cells present. However the character of the lesion was markedly changed as the result of scaling. After 8- and 25-weeks of treatment the lesion was reduced in size and the cellular composition of the infiltrate was significantly altered. After treatment, lymphoid cells accounted for approximately 50 per cent of the cells in the infiltrate with plasma cells only present occasionally. In that particular study this shift was accompanied by a pronounced deposition of new collagen in the tissues.

A FOUR VISIT PROFESSIONAL TOOTH CLEANING PROGRAMME

It seems generally agreed that pocket formation is a result of long standing progressive gingival inflammation. Once formed, the periodontal pocket may provide a 'primary ecologic niche' for pathogenic microbial colonies which may cause further connective tissue destruction. Pockets 3·5 mm or more in depth may be regarded as being in need of periodontal treatment.

Present evidence further suggests that oblation of an existing pocket by surgical means is not necessarily the ideal treatment as has been previously widely assumed. The creation of a long epithelial attachment by more conservative means, such as a hygiene phase associated with chemotherapeutic control of subgingival plaque, deep scaling and/or subgingival curettage may produce a comparably acceptable long term result.

The custom in one of our clinics is to admit patients to an initial hygiene and assessment phase which may extend to four visits over a period of approximately eight weeks. The initial objective of this phase is chemotherapeutic control of subgingival plaque and scaling or curettage to create a long epithelial attachment which, if sustainable, will obviate the need for surgical elimination of pockets.

Patients are categorized into three treatment streams, according to a variation of the treatment need index described in the WHO Technical Report Series 621 (see p. 299). In the examination procedure, a blunt periodontal probe is inserted gently into the pocket or sulcus of the designated tooth unit. The probe has two principal gradations, one at 3·5 mm and one at 5·5 mm. Pocket depths may thus be classified as being less than 3·5 mm, more than 3·5 mm, less than 5·5 mm, or greater than 5·5 mm. The only deviation from the WHO recommendation is that for treatment planning purposes all teeth are examined rather than the selected

teeth proposed for epidemiological treatment need surveys. Pocket depth measurement within the limits defined are entered onto a computer data sheet type form as illustrated in fig. 12.23. The time required to complete such an examination is very short. The form is completed at the beginning and at the end of the hygiene phase professional tooth cleaning period.

Chemotherapeutic control of subgingival plaque

The principles of chemotherapeutic control of plaque infection have been well reviewed by Loeshe [20]. While there are certain general indications as to the groups of organisms which may be involved in the various phases of periodontal disease, the information is not as yet precise enough to allow a particular choice of therapeutic agent, and for this reason antiseptics such as chlorhexidene, cetyl pyridinium chloride, or broad spectrum antibiotics such as tetracycline are usually employed.

A variation of the basic therapeutic programme suggested by Keyes [12] is in current use in one of our clinics during the four visit eight-week introductory oral hygiene programme (table 12.2). Patients are instructed in

TABLE 12.2. Routine treatment programme

1.	<3·5	Routine OH programme Cavitron + Chlorhexidine flush		Within limits of self care		1–2 visits—6 months recall interval.
2.	>3·5<5·5	One or more pockets in this category	→	4 visits—routine OH and 'salt out' and chlorhexidine programme over 8 weeks. Cavitron +	→	Curettage or modified Widman Flap any pocket remaining patent.
3.	>5·5	One or more pockets in this category	→	4 visits—routine OH and 'salt out' and chlorhexidine programme over eight weeks. Cavitron −	→	Surgical ablation any pocket remaining patent under antibiotic or metronidazole cover if bacteriology positive.

All patients charted at 1. admission
                    2. after 8 weeks
                    3. following surgery
Treatment programmes in 2 and 3 to be phase contrast monitored.
Occlusal therapy, when required, will always precede surgery.

routine oral hygiene methods of toothbrushing and flossing as usual. At each individual visit they are given a 'salt out' programme in the surgery. A thick mix of baking soda slightly moistened with a few drops of water and 3 per cent hydrogen peroxide is used as a dentifrice and worked between teeth with the toothbrush, dental floss or toothpicks. Teeth are brushed with the mix which is left in place for one minute. Table salt may also be used. Epsom salts (magnesium sulphate) should be used by patients on a low sodium diet. Patients with pockets in excess of 5·5 mm in particular, are advised to use a water pik. As a matter of routine each mouth is irrigated by such a device following the 'salt out' programme to ensure that no residual 'salt out' material is left in the sulcus. Finally, at the end of each visit, each pocket of a depth in excess of 3·5 mm is flushed at four points round the circumference of the tooth with a solution of 2 per cent chlorhexidene delivered from a 10 ml syringe through a 23 gauge needle. Under this system of treatment planning, patients are categorized into one of three treatment streams as shown in table 12.2. Patients with sulci of less than 3·5 mm depth throughout the mouth have a routine oral hygiene programme, the mouth scaled either by hand or with the cavitron and a chlorhexidine flush. Such sulci are considered to be broadly within the limits of patient self care and such a programme should extend through, at most, one to two visits followed by six month recall intervals.

Patients with one or more pockets in the category of greater than 3·5 mm but less than 5·5 mm are placed on the four visit eight-week routine oral hygiene 'salt out' and chlorhexidine programme. The cavitron is still regarded as an effective instrument at this level of pocket depth. Any pocket in this category remaining patent at the end of the eight-week programme is then eliminated by either subgingival curettage or the modified Widman flap procedure (see chapter 15).

A patient with one or more pockets greater than 5·5 mm in depth is placed on the same four visit, eight week oral hygiene 'salt out' and chlorhexidene programme. The cavitron is not regarded as an effective instrument for control of deep tortuous pockets of this depth, which should be scaled by hand. Any pocket in this category which remains patent at the end of the eight-week programme is oblated by the appropriate surgical technique under antibiotic or metronidazole cover if the bacteriological picture is still positive.

The basic rules of the programme are that all patients are charted at admission, after eight weeks, and after any surgery. Patients are monitored by phase contrast or dark ground illumination microscopy during the eight-week programme. Occlusal therapy, when required, always precedes surgery. Antibiotic or metronidazole therapy is only used when spirochaetes in particular and large motile organisms remain persistently present throughout the hygiene phase. The function of systemic therapy is to reduce the levels of such organisms when the pocket is oblated to allow Gram-positive flora to become established during the period of healing.

REFERENCES

[1] GOTTLIEB B. (1920) Etiology and therapy of alveolar pyorrhea. Z. Stomat. **18**, 59.

[2] GOTTLIEB B. (1946) The new concept of periodontoclasia. J. Periodont. **17**, 7.

[3] ORBAN B. & WEINMANN J.P. (1942) Diffuse atrophy of the alveolar bone. (Periodontosis). J. Periodont. **13**, 31–45.

[4] INGLE J.I. (1959) Papillon–Lefèvre syndrome: precocious periodontosis with associated epidermal lesions. J. Periodont. **30**, 230–237.

[5] BASU M.K. (1964) Scleroderma—a rare disease. Edin. dent. Hosp. Gaz. **5**, 9–14.

[6] BRANDTZAEG P. & KRAUS F.W. (1965) Autoimmunity and periodontal disease. Odont. T. **73**, 281–393.

[7] Oral Hygiene in adults, United States 1960–1962. (1966) Washington: U.S. Department of Health Education and Welfare.

[8] CARVEL R.I., HALPERN V. & WALLACE J.H. (1973) Immunological studies in chronic severe alveolar resorptive disease: A report of two young female patients. J. Periodont. **44**, 25–34.

[9] RAMFJORD S.P., KERR D.H. & ASH M. (eds) (1966) World Workshop in Periodontics, p. 192. Michigan: University of Michigan Press.

[10] MacPhee I.T. (1967) Periodontal scoring: A simple method of periodontal scoring as a basis for treatment planning in teaching hospitals and general practice. *Dent. Practit. dent. Rec.* **17**, 269–273.

[11] Massler M. & Schour I. (1949) The P.M.A. Index of gingivitis. *J. dent. Res.* **28**, 634.

[12] Keyes P.H., Wright W.E. & Howard S.A. (1978) The use of phase contrast microscopy and chemotherapy in the diagnosis and treatment of periodontal lesions. An initial report. *Quintessence International*, **1**, 1590–1591.

[13] Listgarten M.A. (1976) Structure of the microbial flora associated with periodontal health and disease in man. *J. Periodont.* **47**, 1–18.

[15] Listgarten M.A. & Hellden L. (1978) Relative distribution of bacteria at clinically healthy and periodontally diseased sites in humans. *J. Clin. Periodont.* **5**, 115–132.

[15] van Palenstein Helderman W.H. (1975) Total viable count and differential count of vibrio (*Campylobacter*) *sputorum. Fusobacterium nucleatum, Selenomonas sputigena, Bacteroides achraceus* and *Veillonella* in the inflamed and noninflamed human gingival crevice. *Journal of Periodontal Research*, **10**, 294–305.

[16] Slots J. (1977) The predominant cultivable microflora of advanced periodontitis. *Scand. J. Dent. Res.* **85**, 114–121.

[17] Newman M.G. & Socransky S.S. (1977) Predominant cultivable microbiota in periodontitis. *J. Periodont. Res.* **12**, 120–128.

[18] Kritchevsky B. & Seguin P. (1918) The pathogenesis of pyorrhea alveolaris. *Dental Cosmos*, **60**, 781–784.

[19] Listgarten M.A., Lindhe J. & Hellden L. (1978) Effect of tetracycline and/or scaling on human periodontal disease. Clinical, microbial and histological observations. *J. Clin. Periodontol.* **5**, 246–271.

[20] Loeshe W.J. (1976) Chemotherapy of dental plaque infections. *Oral Sci. Rev.* **9**, 65.

CHAPTER 13

Systemic conditions which may influence the host–parasite relationship in the mouth

Periodontitis is a complex process involving a wide range of interaction between the commensal population of the mouth and the host tissues. Tissue metabolism is controlled by heredity, age, sex, endocrine secretion, psychosomatic factors and nutrition. Host resistance to the commensal population of the mouth is dependent on these factors.

The common response to reduction in tissue resistance is an increase in nonspecific gingival inflammation, and widely differing pathological processes tend to produce indistinguishable clinical appearances. Some of the factors which may condition the response of the host tissues to bacterial products have been discussed in chaps. 4–7. Such conditioning may occur at any stage in the progress of gingivitis or periodontitis (chap. 12). The use of the term gingivitis to describe the tissue changes associated with pregnancy, puberty or the presence of a blood dyscrasia does not necessarily imply that the lesion is gingivally contained. The term has been used to indicate that clinical change may be most apparent in the superficial gingival tissues. The main conditions which are thought to have the potential to produce tissue alteration or cellular damage in the periodontium sufficient to exacerbate tissue reaction to the noxious products of plaque organisms are:

(1) nutritional deficiencies,
(2) endocrine disturbances,
(3) diseases of blood,
(4) psychosomatic disturbance,
(5) factors producing tissue intoxication.

A clear distinction must be drawn between central factors which are known to be of importance in clinical practice, and those which have only been shown to produce exacerbation of inflammation under experimental conditions. Epidemiological surveys have confirmed that serious metabolic disease and ageing are directly related to the degree of severity of periodontal disease but do not explain the prevalence [1]. Nutritional deprivation states, particularly protein and ascorbic acid deficiency have tended to be associated with increased severity of periodontitis but have never been demonstrated to be initiating factors [2]. Similar conclusions may be reached by reviewing the data on presence of particular systemic diseases such as diabetes [3], leukaemia [4] and the hormonal shifts encountered in puberty, pregnancy and menstruation [5, 6 & 7]. Reduction of host resistance to plaque may result from metabolic change at the cellular level not demonstrable by assay of circulating nutritional or hormonal factors in blood. Numerous surveys have confirmed that homeostatic mechanisms are such that estimation of plasma levels of particular factors such as albumen or total protein bear no direct relationship to whether or not a particular tissue is deprived [8].

NUTRITIONAL DEFICIENCIES

There are several ways in which nutritional deficiencies may disturb the periodontium in theory, or in animal experiment, and these include:

(1) vitamins which have a specific action on cells, deficiency of which may reduce resistance of tissues to irritation and infection, i.e. vitamins A, B complex and C,

(2) deficiency of vitamins which cause change

in the permeability of blood vessels, or in the blood clotting mechanism, i.e. vitamin K,

(3) deficiency of vitamin D which causes a decreased rate of formation of bone and cementum and a decrease in the degree of mineralization,

(4) protein deficiency,

(5) calcium deficiency which can lead to osteopaenia. Experiments in dogs [9] have shown, however, that although osteopaenia of alveolar bone can be induced by feeding a calcium deficient, phosphorus-rich diet, gingivitis and pocketing did not develop, in the absence of plaque. Neither was increased tooth mobility observed. In areas where bacterial deposits were allowed to accumulate, pathologic pockets gradually developed in both test and control animals, but the degree of attachment lost was the same in both groups.

In animal experiment, deficiency of vitamin A has been shown to affect normal development and function of epithelial cells and to predispose to inflammation, hyperkeratosis and pocket formation in the presence of local irritants. Deficiency also interferes with the production of lysozyme, an antibacterial agent in saliva, which is important in control of the oral flora.

Vitamin C has a role in the synthesis of collagen in connective tissues, and prolonged and severe deficiency may result in scurvy, with widespread destruction of the periodontium and loosening of the teeth. It has proved difficult to produce periodontal lesions in experimental animals having severe avitaminosis A or C in the absence of local irritation, bacterial or otherwise, and epidemiological survey has not confirmed the importance of vitamin C deficiency in the prevalence of periodontitis.

Following a survey of the nutritional state of 700 men who underwent complete medical examination, including biochemical analysis of blood [10], the following points were noted.

(1) Periodontal disease in individuals with a clear deficiency of one or more nutritional components showed no difference from periodontitis in males with no diagnosed deficiency.

(2) Eighteen men who had no demonstrable level of vitamin C in their serum showed the same gingival condition as others in the main group. Fifteen men with less than 0·1 mg/ml vitamin C in their serum had a better gingival condition than the average for their age group.

(3) Of 33 vitamin C deficient men, nine had no periodontal disease at all.

The evidence further suggests that deficiency of vitamin A or the B complex vitamins has no direct bearing on the development or existence of periodontal disease throughout the population. Similar conclusions have been drawn with regard to the effect of protein deficiency, even in the presence of experimental occlusal trauma [11].

It has been fully substantiated that periodontal conditions in undernourished individuals or population groups are not essentially different from those on an adequate diet [12 & 13]. Although it is commonly believed that mild vitamin deficiencies contribute to the ease of damage to the periodontium by irritant factors from plaque organisms, it is certain that such a nutritional mechanism produces no specific change except in extreme deficiency. There is no acceptable evidence to support the use of dietary adjustment in the treatment of periodontal disease. It is possible that the established relationship of available sucrose to plaque formation [14] may provide a method of dietary control in the future by replacing dietary sucrose with some other sugar (chap. 4).

ENDOCRINE DISTURBANCES

The ability of sex hormones to affect the degree of aggregation of ground substance of connective tissue, rendering it more fluid, has been discussed in chap. 5. The changes in the endocrine balance which are associated with pregnancy and puberty may be reflected in the mouth, and they may cause a lowering of tissue resistance relative to the commensal microbial population.

Pregnancy gingivitis

An increased level of inflammation has been reported to occur in the mouth during pregnancy in between 30 and 100 per cent of the patients examined [15]. Pregnancy gingivitis has been said to occur in both a specific and a nonspecific form [16], the distinction between the two being based on the tendency of the lesion to heal spontaneously postpartum. Clinical and histological studies support the view that the gingivitis of pregnancy is an inflammatory condition, which in principle does not differ from that which may be found in nonpregnant patients [6]. Following a survey of 121 pregnant and 61 postpartum women for the occurrence and severity of periodontal disease [15], the following conclusions were reached.

(1) 100 per cent of the pregnant women showed signs of gingival inflammation.

(2) The prevalence and severity of gingival disease in pregnant women was significantly higher than in postpartum women.

(3) The increase in the level of inflammation was noticeable from the second month of gestation and reached a maximum in the eighth month. During the last month of gestation a definite decrease occurred.

(4) After parturition the state of the gingivae was similar to that of the second month of pregnancy.

(5) The depth of gingival pockets was significantly increased during pregnancy. The decrease in pocket depth after parturition indicates that deepening was probably caused by enlargement of the gingivae (false pocketing), rather than by apical movement of the crevicular epithelium.

This study failed to support the view that the increased prevalence and severity of gingival inflammation during pregnancy causes lasting injury to the periodontium.

The correlation between oral hygiene status and periodontal condition in this group of patients showed that there was no significant difference in the quantity of deposits on the teeth of pregnant as compared with postpartum patients, and that the character and distribution of the deposits showed no significant difference between the two groups. The general trend of the distribution of both soft and hard deposits on the various surfaces of the teeth during pregnancy did not differ from that in nonpregnant patients. The index of gingival inflammation was significantly higher in pregnant than in postpartum patients [17], but a similar difference could not be found for the plaque index. This suggests that in pregnancy some other factor is present, which together with bacterial plaque may be responsible for the accentuated inflammatory changes in the gingivae. This would support the view that increase in the permeability of ground substance [18], associated with change in the level of circulating sex hormones during pregnancy, may lead to exacerbation of pre-existing inflammation in the presence of dental plaque.

CLINICAL FEATURES

Pregnancy gingivitis may occur as a generalized (fig. 13.1a) or a localized (fig. 13.1b) condition. The gingival tissue is inflamed, oedematous and varies in colour from bright red to bluish red. The change in colour results from a marked increase in the vascularity of the tissues; there is also an increased tendency towards gingival haemorrhage. In the localized form the inflamed papilla is markedly enlarged and forms a discrete tumour-like mass, frequently misdescribed as a pregnancy tumour (fig. 13.1b). The term tumour should be reserved for neoplasms to avoid misunderstanding. The localized lesion occurs in less than 1 per cent of patients with pregnancy gingivitis [5, 6 & 15].

HISTOPATHOLOGY

The microscopic appearance of tissue from a pregnancy gingivitis is that of a nonspecific, proliferative, highly vascular, inflammatory reaction (fig. 13.1c). There is marked infiltration of lymphocytes and plasma cells, characteristic of chronic inflammation. The epithelium may show a marked degree of hyperplasia, downgrowth of the rete pegs and a variable degree of intra- and extracellular oedema. The appearance on the whole is characteristic of nonspecific inflammatory change.

TREATMENT

The basic principle in the treatment of pregnancy gingivitis is reduction of inflammation and control of plaque deposition by means of hygiene phase therapy (chap. 10). Where inflammation remains at a persistently unacceptable level, further reduction may be achieved by the use of

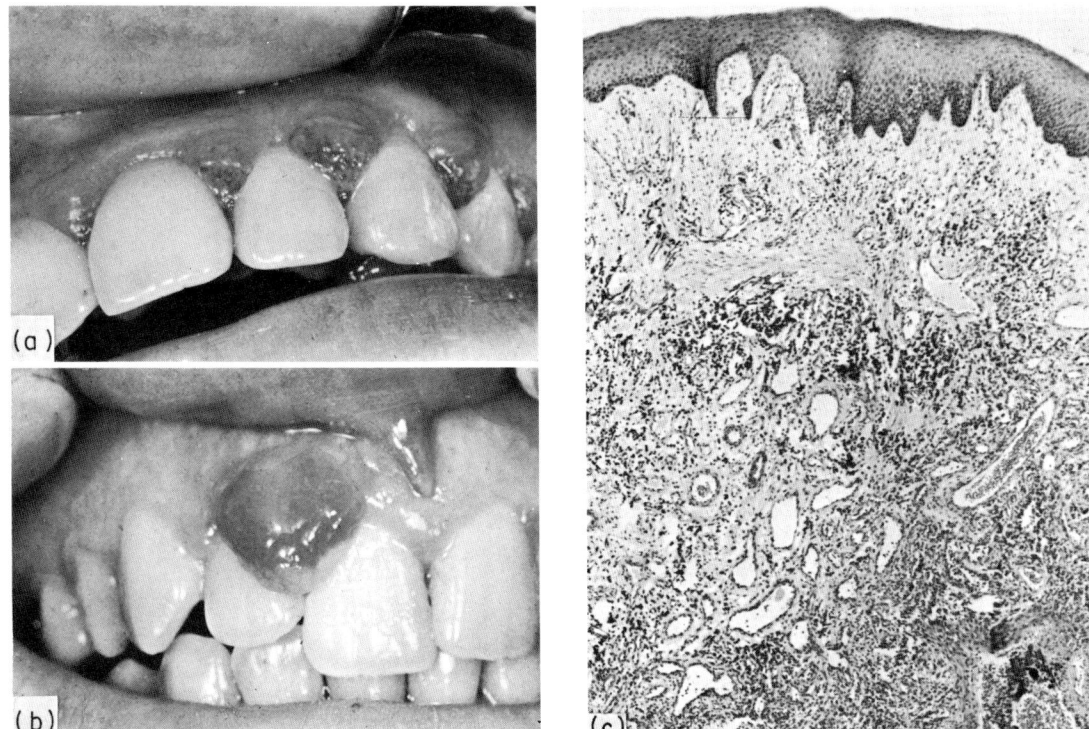

FIG. 13.1. (a) Generalized pregnancy gingivitis characterized by highly vascularized enlarged interdental papillae. (b) Localized pregnancy gingivitis. (c) Histology of (b). A nonspecific proliferative highly vascular inflammatory reaction, with marked infiltration of lymphocytes and plasma cells characteristic of chronic inflammation.

pressure packs. Surgical intervention is directly contraindicated during the course of pregnancy, except when a large localized lesion creats an aesthetic or functional problem. Assessment and treatment planning for routine periodontal therapy should be carried out approximately one month after parturition (chap. 12).

Diabetes and periodontal disease

The ground substance of connective tissue contains a large proportion of high molecular weight carbohydrates in the form of carbohydrate–protein complexes, so that the generalized change in carbohydrate metabolism associated with diabetes may be reflected in the ground substance throughout the body. The diabetic patient is prone to infection as a result of the altered carbohydrate metabolism that produces accumulation of keto acids in the tissues. Local accu-

mulation of lactic acid has a bacteriostatic effect and in inflamed tissue of normal patients lactic acid may concentrate locally to the extent of 200 mg per cent [19]. The lack of the bacteriostatic effect of rising concentration of lactic acid in the diabetic may contribute to an altered host–parasite relationship [20].

Whatever the mechanism, the resulting inflammation of gingival tissues is nonspecific, and diabetics show periodontal changes which are qualitatively no different from those of non-diabetics suffering from a similar degree of periodontal disease [21] (fig. 13.2). Diabetics as a group, however, suffer from an increased prevalence of advanced periodontal disease compared to a normal population [22].

Addison's disease

Addison's disease occurs as a result of adrenocortical insufficiency, most commonly found secondary to bilateral tuberculosis of the adrenal glands [23]. On occasion it may arise secondary to other diffuse cortical necrotizing disorders, such as syphilis, sarcoidosis, amyloid disease or metastatic tumours. The clinical features of Addison's disease are weakness, lassitude, weight loss, anorexia, low body temperature, hypotension and pigmentation of skin and mucous membrane.

The most common oral sign of Addison's disease is bluish grey or brownish pigmentation of the mucous membrane of the gingiva, palate, buccal mucosa, lips or tongue (fig. 13.3). The pigmentation is caused by deposition of melanin in the region of the basal layer of epithelial cells. All patients with diffuse hyperpigmented areas of the oral mucous membrane should be investigated to exclude the possibility of Addison's disease.

A specific example of alteration of the balance of the host–parasite system of the mouth secondary to endocrine dysfunction is to be found in relation to the symptom complex, Addison's disease, idiopathic familial juvenile hypoparathyroidism, keratoconjunctivitis and superficial candidiasis. The association of Addison's disease with fungal infections in general has been widely reported [24 & 25]. The particular association of oral candidiasis with familial idiopathic hypoparathyroidism and Addison's disease has been recognized for several years [26 & 27]. It has

been further suggested that hypothyroidism and a coeliac component may be part of the same symptom complex [28]. Immunodeficiencies in lymphocyte functions may account for recurrences in *Herpesvirus* infections and resistance to antifungal treatment in chronic candidiasis. With increasing severity of candidiasis, the immunodeficiencies increase and may involve all cellular and humoral functions [29].

Not all components of the syndrome appear simultaneously. Candidiasis is nearly always the first to appear, and this may present in the mouth in the absence of pigmentation of mucous membrane, or any other signs and symptoms (fig. 13.4). There is commonly a history of a preceding fungal paronychia. The oral candidiasis presents as diffuse firmly attached hyperkeratotic plaques. Biopsy reveals the fungal hyphae within the superficial layers of the epithelium, orientated approximately at right angles to the surface (fig. 13.4).

A few months to many years later, the presenting candidiasis is followed by evidence of hypoparathyroidism and hypoadrenocorticism, most frequently manifest during the 9–12 year age group.

Candida albicans is a normal mouth commensal which may be isolated from approximately 50 per cent of normal mouths [30]. The relationship of the altered host–parasite balance to the endocrine changes which allows the fungal elements to become dominant is not known. At

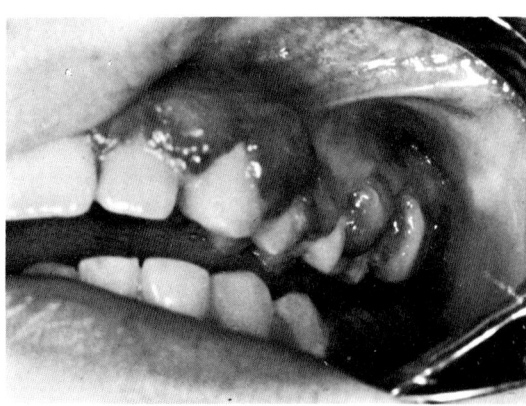

FIG. 13.2. Established periodontitis in an uncontrolled diabetic.

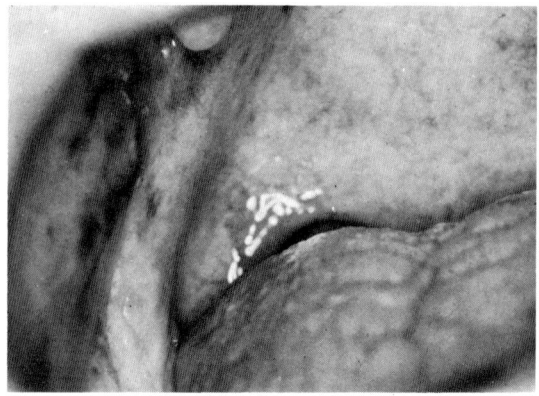

FIG. 13.3. Addison's disease. Melanin deposition in buccal mucosa.

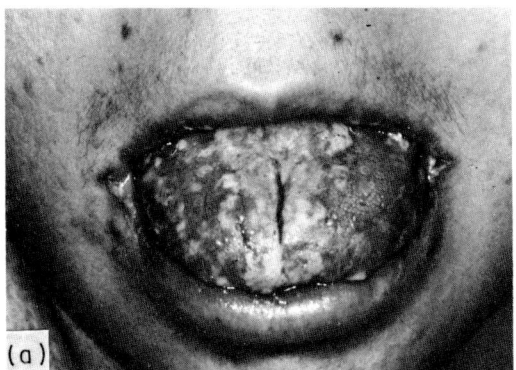

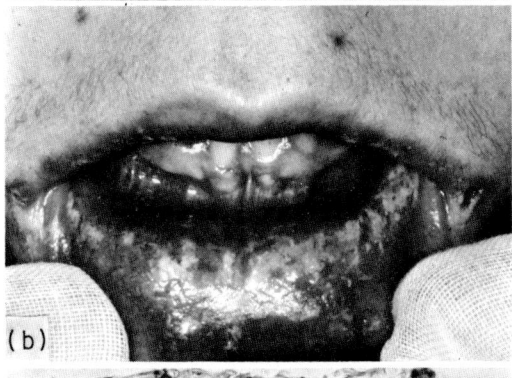

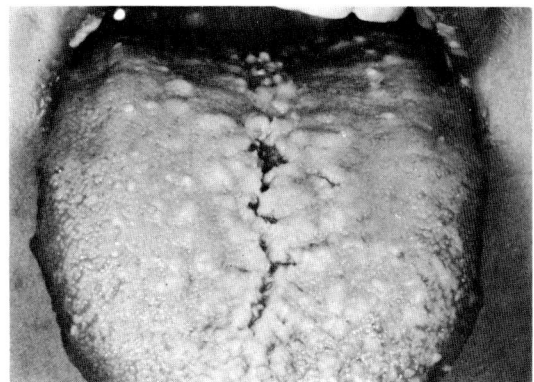

FIG. 13.5. Acute pseudomembranous candidiasis in a debilitated patient. The condition is of sudden onset, and the plaque is easily removed with a napkin to leave a raw bleeding surface.

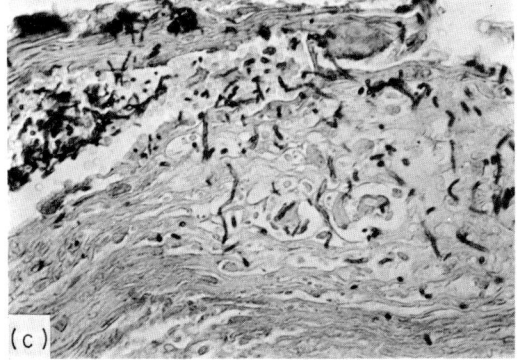

FIG. 13.4. (a & b) Chronic candidiasis in a child with familial hypoparathyroidism, hypoadrenocorticism and chronic candidiasis. (c) Biopsy of (a & b). Fungal hyphae within the superficial layers of the epithelium orientated approximately at right angles to the surface layers.

autopsy there is no evidence of mycotic involvement of the endocrine glands. There is no evidence of advanced periodontitis relative to age in this syndrome.

While oral candidiasis occurs fairly com-

monly in debilitated patients (fig. 13.5), or secondary to drug therapy, any young patient who does not respond to treatment with nystatin or amphotericin should be investigated for possible endocrine dysfunction.

DISEASES OF THE BLOOD

Alteration in the host–parasite relationship of the mouth, most commonly expressed as non-specific inflammatory change of the gingival tissues, may result from the presence of a blood dyscrasia. These conditions may give rise to a large variety of signs and symptoms in the mouth involving the gingival tissues, the lips, cheeks or tongue. In relation to the gingival tissues, the most consistent signs of a haematological disorder are an increase in the level of nonspecific inflammation which is present and an increased tendency towards gingival haemorrhage. The change in the gingival tissues is a direct response to the presence of local irritants resulting from the modification in host resistance which may accompany the blood disorder. In the absence of oral irritants, a blood dyscrasia may show no local signs at all. The most common signs and symptoms in relation to the lips, cheeks and tongue are ulceration, atrophic change, cheilitis (fig. 13.6), glossitis and paraesthesia of the tongue. These signs may be evident in any condition where there is aberration in either the mechanical or biochemical aspects of the control

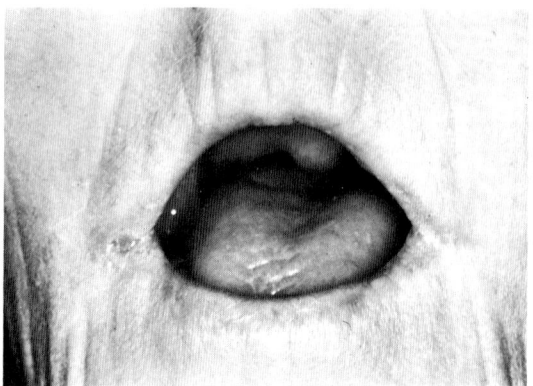

FIG. 13.6. Cheilitis in elderly patient with anaemia and vitamin deficiency, courtesy of Professor John Boyes.

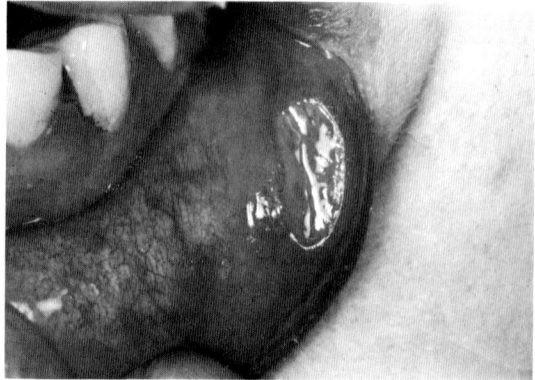

FIG. 13.7. Recurrent ulceration of mouth in patient with no abnormal systemic findings. Periadenitis mucosa necrotica recurrens type ulcer. Ulceration of the oral mucosa is a presenting symptom of acute leukaemia only in a small percentage of cases (6–12 per cent).

of haemorrhage, where there is reduction in the adequacy of the inflammatory response resulting from a deficiency of mature white cells, or in presence of anaemia (table 13.1). When an increased level of gingival inflammation occurs in association with a blood dyscrasia, such inflammation is clinically nonspecific and not diagnostic of the presence of the blood condition. Similarly recurrent ulceration of the mouth (fig. 13.7) has a prevalence of more than 50 per cent in the selected populations which have been examined [31 & 32], and is not particularly

TABLE 13.1. Haematological disorders which may be reflected in the mouth.

Conditions associated with change in the mechanical or biochemical aspects of the control of haemorrhage:
  (1) Thrombocytopaenic purpura,
  (2) Haemophilia,
  (3) Christmas disease,
  (4) Hereditary haemorrhagic telangiectasia,
  (5) von Willebrand's disease,
  (6) Polycythaemia.

Conditions associated with modification of the inflammatory response:
  (1) Leukaemia,
  (2) Agranulocytosis,
  (3) Infectious mononucleosis.

The anaemias:
  (1) Pernicious anaemia,
  (2) Microcytic hypochromic anaemia,
  (3) Aplastic anaemia.

associated with the presence of blood dyscrasias. While these symptoms may occur in patients with blood dyscrasias, there may be no mouth symptoms at all. The blood condition most likely to be associated with oral signs and symptoms is acute leukaemia. Following a survey of 580 patients with acute leukaemia, only 13 per cent presented with an initial complaint of oropharyngeal lesions, and on examination only 20 per cent were found to have mouth lesions [33]. In a further survey of 172 patients with acute leukaemia, mouth sores were an initial complaint in only 6 per cent of cases. On examination gingival enlargement was found in 10 per cent of cases and oral ulceration in 12 per cent [34].

Conditions associated with change in the mechanical or biochemical aspects of the control of haemorrhage

THROMBOCYTOPAENIC PURPURA

Thrombocytopaenic states are a large variety of conditions which are characterized by a decreased number of platelets in the circulating blood. The low platelet count results in prolonged clot retraction and bleeding time, and in a normal or slightly prolonged clotting time. Petechiae and ecchymoses occur in the mouth, particularly in relation to the palate and buccal mucosa (fig. 13.8). The gingivae may be swollen, soft and bleed spontaneously. The condition may arise from primary bone marrow failure, or invasion of bone marrow by metastatic carcinoma or leukaemic cells. Thrombocytopaenia may be induced by drugs such as gold, benzol or arsenicals, which act directly on the bone marrow and cause a decrease in the number of megakaryocytes. Drugs such as sedormid and quinine may induce an allergic response, with formation of an antigen antibody complex, which destroys the platelets in the peripheral circulation. The gingival changes are directly related to the presence of plaque and other local irritants, and marked improvement follows hygiene phase control.

HAEMOPHILIA

Haemophilia is a disease transmitted by a sex linked recessive gene. The affected male exhibits the disease, while females transmit it to the next generation. The affected male does not transmit the disease to his male offspring. The condition arises as a result of deficiency in the production of antihaemophilic globulin (factor 8), which results in haemorrhage of all degrees of severity. There is spontaneous bleeding into joints and into skin, but rarely if ever from mucous surfaces. The condition is reflected in the mouth by severely prolonged clotting time following injury or incision. In the presence of an estab-

lished periodontitis, periodontal treatment should be limited to routine hygiene phase therapy (chap. 10), and conservation of the teeth which can be carried out on an out-patient basis, and which rarely if ever leads to problems of control of haemorrhage. Surgical corrective phase therapy should never be attempted.

CHRISTMAS DISEASE

Christmas disease is an inherited sex linked recessive condition which mimics haemophilia so closely that no distinction is possible without examination of thromboplastin production in blood. It results from the deficiency of plasma thromboplastic component (PTC factor 9), without which there is abnormality in the production of plasma thromboplastins. The same restrictions on treatment apply to patients with Christmas disease as with haemophilia.

HEREDITARY HAEMORRHAGIC TELANGIECTASIA

This is a comparatively rare condition sometimes known as Rendu–Osler–Weber's disease. It is characterized by multiple angiomata of capillaries and venules in the skin and mucous membrane (fig. 13.9), with a resulting tendency towards haemorrhage. The most common sites of involvement are nasal mucosa, tongue, palate, lips and mucocutaneous junction, and gingivae. Lesions may occur, however, anywhere on the skin and mucous membranes of the body. Although the condition may be present in childhood, the lesions increase in number with

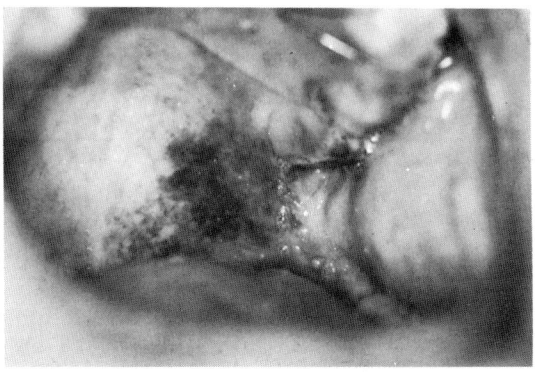

FIG. 13.8. Petechiae and ecchymosis of palate and alveolar mucosa of patient with thrombocytopaenic purpura.

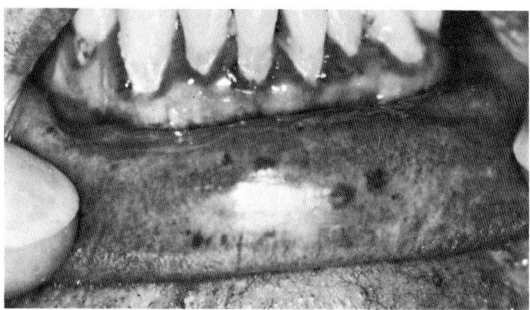

FIG. 13.9. Hereditary haemorrhagic telangiectasia. Similar angiomata occur on the gingival tissue.

advancing age. The blood vessels do not attain their maximal size until about the age of 35 years, by which time the telangiectases appear as bright red violaceous or purple spots. If the gingivae are involved, periodontal treatment should be restricted to hygiene phase therapy and conservation of the teeth.

VON WILLEBRAND'S DISEASE

Von Willebrand's disease is a haemorrhagic condition which has been frequently referred to as pseudohaemophilia. It is a non sex linked dominant inherited condition, in which both males and females are affected. In general the symptoms are less severe than those of haemophilia, but the condition may be manifested by ease of bruising, epistaxis, haematuria and gingival bleeding. Tooth extraction is still a serious hazard. It has been suggested that the condition is associated with an alteration in permeability of the blood vessel walls and with the lack of a labile factor in plasma, the Von Willebrand's factor. Periodontal therapy should be restricted to hygiene phase control and conservation of the teeth. Surgical corrective phase therapy should not be attempted.

POLYCYTHAEMIA

Polycythaemia is a condition in which the quantity of red cells is raised in unit volume of blood in the presence of an increased total blood volume. The condition may occur as an idiopathic phenomenon, or secondary to the presence of anoxic anoxia, cyanotic heart disease, hypernephroma, hydronephrosis or polycystic disease of the kidneys. The clinical features of the condition are those of intense venous engorgement which may be evidenced as congestion of gingival tissues. There is a tendency towards excessive haemorrhage following minor injury, for which there is no satisfactory explanation. Treatment should be confined to hygiene phase therapy.

Conditions associated with modification of the inflammatory response

LEUKAEMIA

Leukaemia is a neoplastic disease characterized by uncontrolled excessive production of any of the white blood cell series, and the appearance in most cases of large numbers of these cells, and their immature precursors in the circulating blood [35]. Those unusual cases in which excessive or abnormal white cells are not found in the peripheral blood are referred to as aleukaemic leukaemia.

Leukaemias are normally classified according to the cell type predominantly involved, e.g. as myelogenous, lymphocytic or monocytic. Mouth symptoms occur in association with leukaemia in about 20 per cent of acute cases, with the greatest frequency in relation to acute and subacute monocytic leukaemia, less frequently in acute and subacute lymphatic and myelogenous leukaemia, and seldom in chronic leukaemia [36]. In all forms of leukaemia the precipitating factor is the presence of local irritants, and in the absence of these there may be no oral signs (fig. 13.11). In the presence of local irritants, clinical changes which may occur include a diffuse cyanotic bluish red discoloration of the gingival tissues and occasionally ulceration, necrosis and pseudomembrane formation of the papillary and marginal tissues. The most frequently occurring change has been said to be a diffuse oedematous hyperplasia, sometimes so severe as to cover the teeth completely [23]. In such cases the gingivae are soft, boggy, violaceous in colour and tend to bleed spontaneously (fig. 13.10). Blood smears made from the gingival tissues may show the presence of large num-

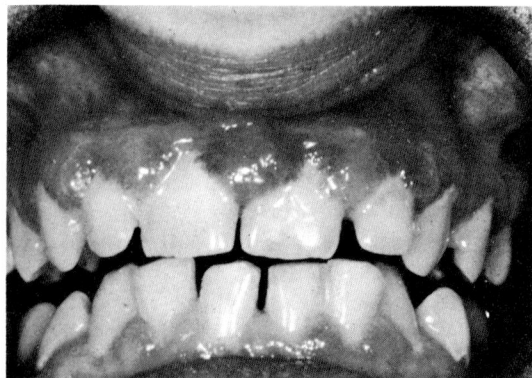

FIG. 13.10. Nonspecific gingival enlargement in patient with acute monocytic leukaemia.

bers of immature white cells. Gingival changes are a direct response to reduction in host resistance, relative to the presence of plaque or other local irritants in the mouth. A marked improvement follows the establishment of adequate patient self-care and routine hygiene phase therapy.

Severe ulceration and abscess formation, which is resistant to treatment and tends to spread rapidly, may follow minor trauma of the oral mucosa.

Occasionally in acute leukaemia, localized nodules of pure leucoblastic tissue occur, generally growing from fascia or from periosteum. The lesions are composed of masses of immature blast cells held together by reticulin, which are capable of eroding and destroying neighbouring tissues. Such localized leukaemic deposits are described as 'chloroma' and may occur in the mouth as firm bluish grey nodules. Chloroma is not a common sign of acute leukaemia but may occur in the mouth in the absence of any other oral signs (fig. 13.11), particularly in children and young adults.

AGRANULOCYTOSIS

Agranulocytosis is characterized by an abnormal decrease in the number of circulating white cells of the granulocyte series. It may be idiopathic, or result from idiosyncrasy to drugs such as amidopyrine, sulphonamides, thiouracil or chloramphenicol. Agranulocytosis may follow irradition, or occur secondary to aplastic anaemia or acute lymphocytic or monocytic leukaemia. The disease may result in ulceration of the mouth and pharynx (fig. 13.12), or severe gingivitis secondary to the presence of local irritants. In common with leukaemia, the acute gingivitis shows marked improvement following hygiene phase therapy.

Agranulocytosis generally occurs as an acute disease but may occur in cyclical episodes as cyclical neutropenia.

INFECTIOUS MONONUCLEOSIS

Infectious mononucleosis is a benign disease associated with infection by the Epstein Barr virus which most commonly occurs in children or young adults of either sex. The condition may be associated with the presence of acute gingivitis, fever, malaise, headache, sore throat and ulceration of the tonsils and buccal mucous membrane. There is marked lymphadenopathy of the cervical lymph nodes and this generally spreads to involve additional groups of nodes. Patients with this condition exhibit a marked leucocytosis. The predominant cell is usually the lymphocyte, and the lymphocyte differential count ranges between 70 and 90 per cent [23]. Many of the lymphocytes are abnormally large and are characterized by an indented nucleus and foamy cytoplasm. A high percentage of patients with this condition have increased levels of agglutinins in the peripheral

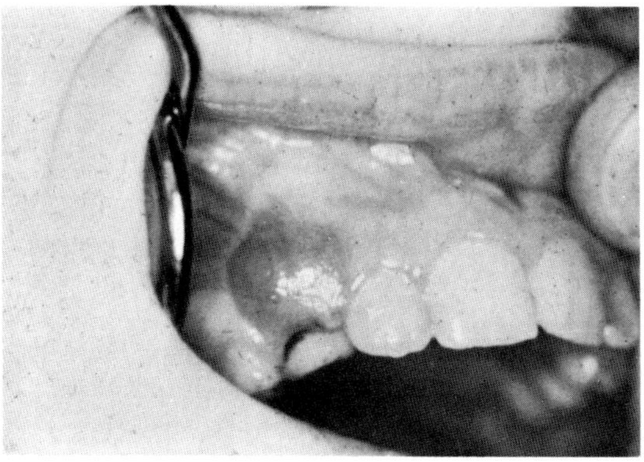

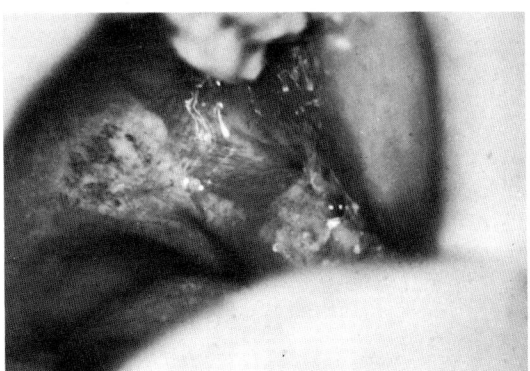

FIG. 13.11. Chloroma in child in terminal stages of acute leukaemia, note clinically normal gingivae in other areas.

FIG. 13.12. Ulceration of buccal mucosa and pharynx associated with nonspecific gingivitis in a patient with agranulocytosis.

blood which are absorbed on ox red cells but not guinea pig kidney cells (Paul Bunnel test). The serum titre rises after the 4th day and may persist for months. The level of the titre is not proportional to the severity of the disease, and an antibody titre of more than 1:56 is diagnostic [37].

The condition is normally self-limiting and runs an average course of 10–21 days. The acute gingivitis is nonspecific and directly related to the presence of local irritants. A marked improvement follows hygiene phase control. Patients with this condition show an increased tendency to develop secondary infections of the mouth. Episodes of acute ulceromembranous gingivitis, herpetic gingivitis and aphthous type stomatitis are especially common.

The anaemias

Anaemia may be defined as a condition in which there is a fall in the quantity of red cells, or haemoglobin, in a unit volume of blood, in presence of a low or normal total blood volume. The most common signs and symptoms in the mouth which may occur secondary to the presence of an anaemia are glossitis, stomatitis and cheilitis.

PERNICIOUS ANAEMIA

Pernicious anaemia is a disease of adults seldom occurring before the age of 30 years, which arises secondary to a deficiency of vitamin B12. The condition occurs most frequently in the over 40 year age group and is characterized by numbness and tingling of the extremities, malaise and weakness, and a sore tongue in about 75 per cent of cases. Some patients with this condition may show evidence of central nervous system damage. Patients with pernicious anaemia exhibit an atrophic gastritis, have a histamine fast achlorhydria, and do not secrete the intrinsic factor from gastric mucosa, which is necessary for the absorption of vitamin B12. The blood changes include a fall in the red call count, often to a level of 1 million cells or less per mm^3, and a small reduction in the haemoglobin level. Variation in size and shape of the

red cells described as anisocytosis and poikylocytosis is commonly seen on blood smears. The platelet count is reduced and there may be a marked neutropenia.

The oral symptoms associated with pernicious anaemia may be extremely severe, and the most common complaint is a burning sensation of the tongue. The tongue appears beefy red, smooth and shiny (fig. 13.13), as a result of atrophy of the fungiform and filiform papillae. The mucosa and lips may be pale and yellowish in colour and susceptible to ulceration following minor trauma. There may be a nonspecific gingivitis which is directly related to the presence of local irritants, and which responds dramatically to hygiene phase control. The course of the other symptoms is dependent on the treatment, which is administration of vitamin B12.

MICROCYTIC HYPOCHROMIC ANAEMIA

Microcytic hypochromic anaemia occurs most commonly secondary to chronic blood loss, nutritional deficiency, inadequate absorption of iron and hookworm infection. There is a moderate fall in the red cell count and a marked reduction in the haemoglobin level. The red cells are microcytic and hypochromic and may show a moderate degree of anisocytosis and poikylocytosis. The white cell and platelet counts are usually normal.

Oral signs which are commonly associated with this condition are a pale mucosa, erythema

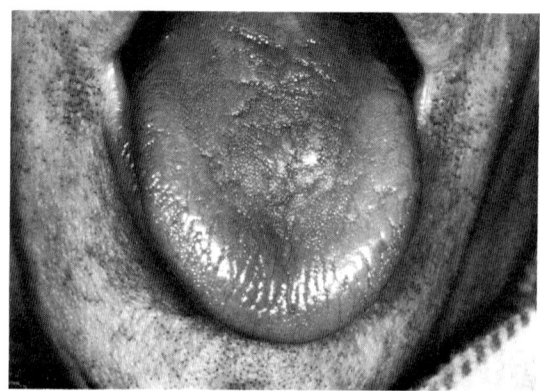

FIG. 13.13. Beefy red, smooth, shiny tongue of patient with pernicious anaemia.

of the lateral border of the tongue, glossitis and a nonspecific gingivitis related to the presence of local irritants. The same general oral signs and symptoms may occur in relation to normochromic normocytic anaemia and sickle cell anaemia.

Iron deficiency anaemia associated with the presence of a smooth tongue, ulceration of oral mucosa, angular cheilitis and dysphagia is generally described as Plummer Vinson syndrome. The significance of this symptom complex lies in the fact that the tissue changes act as a predisposing factor in the subsequent development of carcinoma of the upper alimentary tract. According to Ahlbon, approximately one half of all women with carcinoma of upper oesophagus seen at a clinic in Stockholm had Plummer Vinson syndrome [38].

APLASTIC ANAEMIA

Depression of formation of blood cells in the bone marrow may be idiopathic, secondary to the presence of diseases such as miliary tuberculosis, hypopituitarism and myxoedema, or may follow drug therapy. The condition has been recorded as following administration of chloramphenicol, arsphenamine, sulphonamides, trinitrotoluene, gold salts and mesantoin. In general the oral signs and symptoms are similar to those which have been described in relation to acute leukaemia. Where an uncontrolled gingi-

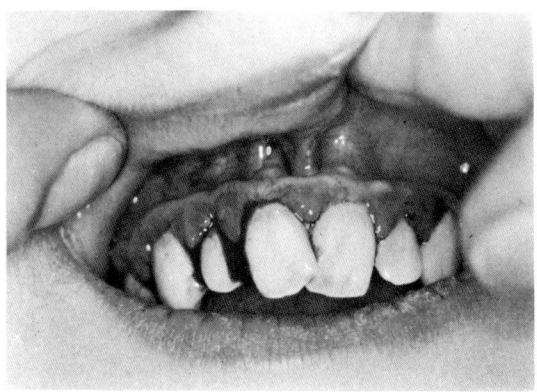

FIG. 13.14. Haemorrhage from uncontrolled nonspecific gingivitis following transfusion of patient with aplastic anaemia.

vitis is present, considerable haemorrhage from the gingival tissues may follow the transfusion of fresh blood (fig. 13.14).

OTHER ANAEMIAS

Many other types of anaemia exist, notably those which are associated with excessive destruction of blood cells, but since specific lesions of the soft tissues in the mouth are not commonly associated with these conditions they have not been considered here. Excessive destruction of blood cells in the peripheral circulation, such as is associated with Rhesus incompatibility (Erythroblastosis foetalis), may give rise to deposits of blood pigment in enamel and dentine. These conditions are not commonly associated with lesions of the gingival tissues beyond the occurrence of nonspecific gingivitis associated with local irritants.

PSYCHOSOMATIC FACTORS

Selye introduced the concept of stress as a determining factor in the causation of disease [39]. The elaboration and action of adrenocorticotrophic hormone, somatotrophic hormone, mineral and glucocorticoids, and adrenaline and noradrenaline under stress has an influence on general metabolism, and this may be reflected in the mouth as a result of alteration in host resistance relative to the commensal population. Selye has described the General Adaptation Syndrome which includes: 'the sum of all those nonspecific systemic reactions of the body which ensue upon long-continued exposure to stress'. It includes a number of morphological and functional changes in the endocrine glands, especially in the adrenal cortex. The presence of these endocrine substances in the bloodstream causes vascular changes, altered respiration and temperature changes of tissue surfaces. There is evidence to suggest that in persons under mental stress, blood calcium and phosphorus levels decline, low sugar tolerance and glycosuria occur and white cell counts are reduced [40].

A multitude of factors have been implicated in the aetiology of ulceromembranous gingivitis. Prominent amongst them have been the emotional effects which may elicit an endocrine response, detectable by change in steroid metabolism. Stress can be measured by determining the level of 17 hydroxycorticoids in blood. It has been shown that patients with ulceromembranous gingivitis have higher than normal 17 hydroxycorticoid blood levels [41], and that the levels decline as the clinical picture improves.

Clinical studies undertaken to investigate the relationship of personality and periodontal disease confirmed a statistically significant relationship between periodontal pathology, age, marital adjustment, broken home, somatization, the Minnesota Multiphasic Personality Index hysteria scale and a number of other variables [42]. The results of such surveys suggest that even in the presence of adequate dental care and good oral hygiene, periodontal disease can occur with increased frequency amongst individuals with anxiety states. Such studies have not established definitely that there is an important relationship between general personality adjustment and periodontal disease, which is a significant factor in the prevalence of periodontitis throughout the population. They have, however, established that psychosomatic factors may influence at least some periodontitis.

FACTORS PRODUCING TISSUE INTOXICATION

A wide spectrum of drugs may give rise to oral signs and symptoms as a result of direct tissue intoxication, alteration in the metabolism of host tissues, allergy or a combination of these effects.

Metallic intoxication

The therapeutic use of heavy metals has been largely discontinued, but local reaction in the mouth may result from filling materials misplaced in the gingival tissues during restorative procedures (fig. 13.15), from industrial contact or from the use of contaminated water supplies.

In the extreme, mercury intoxication may result

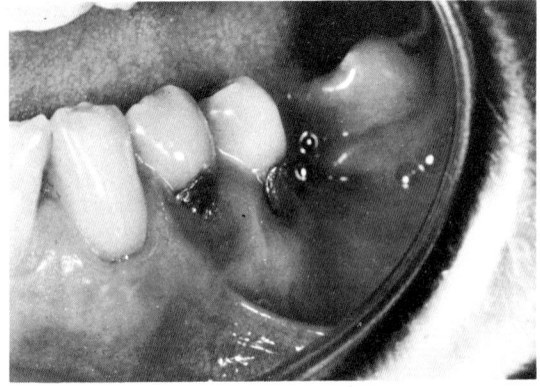

Fig. 13.15. Blue staining of tissue buccal to $\overline{/4}$ due to inadequate control of amalgam while packing a class V cavity.

in headache, insomnia, ptyalism and pigmentation following deposition of mercuric sulphide in the gingivae. A local reaction without the general symptoms may be associated with the presence of amalgam misplaced within the soft tissues (fig. 13.15). Heavy metal ions result in a modification of host resistance, reflected as exacerbation of pre-existing inflammation, which may lead to ulceration of the gingival tissue and adjacent mucosa and resorption of underlying bone.

BISMUTH

Bismuth intoxication is much less common either as a general or a local reaction but may result from industrial contact. The general symptoms of chronic bismuth intoxication are gastrointestinal disturbance, nausea, vomiting and jaundice. It may be accompanied by an ulcerative gingivitis and a narrow blue black discoloration of the gingival margin in areas of pre-existing gingival inflammation. Such pigmentation results from deposition of particles of bismuth sulphide in tissues, following exudation from blood vessels in areas of gingival inflammation. The deposition may occur in the absence of general symptoms of metallic intoxication.

LEAD

Lead intoxication may arise as a result of in-

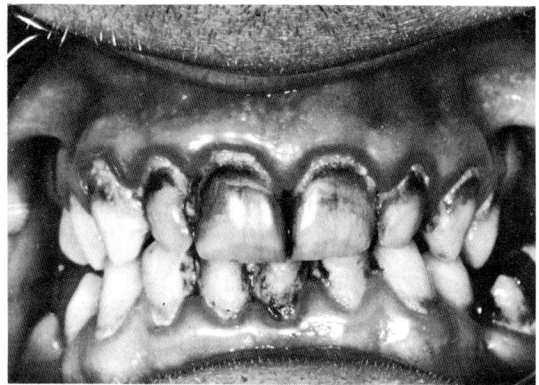

FIG. 13.16. Steel grey deposit in marginal gingivae of plumber under treatment for lead poisoning.

dustrial contact or the use of a contaminated water supply. It may be associated with pallor of the face and lips, nausea and vomiting, abdominal colic and peripheral neuritis. The most common oral signs are increased salivation and a steel grey deposit at the gingival margin in inflamed areas (fig. 13.16). The oral signs may occur in the absence of general toxic symptoms.

OTHER

Even more rarely other chemicals such as phosphorus, arsenic, chromium and benzene may give rise to acute inflammation, necrosis of alveolar bone and loosening and exfoliation of the teeth.

DRUG-INDUCED ALTERATION IN METABOLISM OF HOST TISSUES

The classic example of drug-induced alteration of host tissue metabolism is the gingival hyperplasia which may follow administration of the anticonvulsant drug dilantin sodium (sodium diphenylhydantoinate). Hyperplastic enlargement of the gingival tissues does not occur in all patients who are taking the drug, and there are no reliable figures as to the percentage of patients affected. In selected populations the incidence has been reported as varying from 0 to 84 per cent [43]. The mechanism whereby the hyperplasia is produced is not completely understood.

Animal experiment has shown that the enlargement of gingivae originates in the connective tissue of the marginal and interproximal gingivae as a proliferation of fibroblasts and capillaries in a meshwork of collagen strands [44]. Evidence from tissue culture experiments on cells from human gingival tissues has suggested that an increased rate of emmigration of 'fibroblastoid' cells [45] follows administration of the drug.

Hyperplasia can occur in the mouth in the absence of clinically obvious inflammation (fig. 13.17). The distortion of gingival form which results from the drug-induced hyperplasia gives rise to food stagnation and an increased rate of accumulation of plaque. In a high percentage of cases inflammation of local factor origin supervenes. In the same way a percentage of patients on anticonvulsant therapy, who do not show the drug-induced hyperplasia, may acquire a purely inflammatory hyperplasia which is in no way related to the drug therapy. Gingival hyperplasia occurring in patients taking dilantin sodium has been classified as [36]:

(1) noninflammatory hyperplasia directly caused by dilantin (fig. 13.17a),

(2) chronic inflammatory enlargement entirely unrelated to dilantin (fig. 13.17b),

(3) combined enlargement consisting of hyperplasia caused by dilantin, and inflammatory hyperplasia caused by local irritants; this is the type of enlargement most commonly found in patients receiving dilantin therapy (fig. 13.17c).

Drug-induced noninflammatory hyperplastic gingivitis may exist for a considerable period of time as a limited lesion without being associated with the destruction of deeper supporting tissues. Treatment in these circumstances is restricted to hygiene phase control and surgical excision of the hyperplastic tissue for aesthetic reasons. Such tissue may be removed by gingivectomy (chap. 15). Chronic inflammatory enlargement unrelated to dilantin, and combined hyperplasia, may occur at any stage in the progression of periodontitis, and may be associated with considerable destruction of the deeper supporting tissues and the presence of compound pockets. Treatment consists of hygiene phase control and elimination of all sources of local irritation, followed by surgical excision of the hyperplastic tissue by a technique appropriate to the stage of periodontitis (chaps 12 & 15).

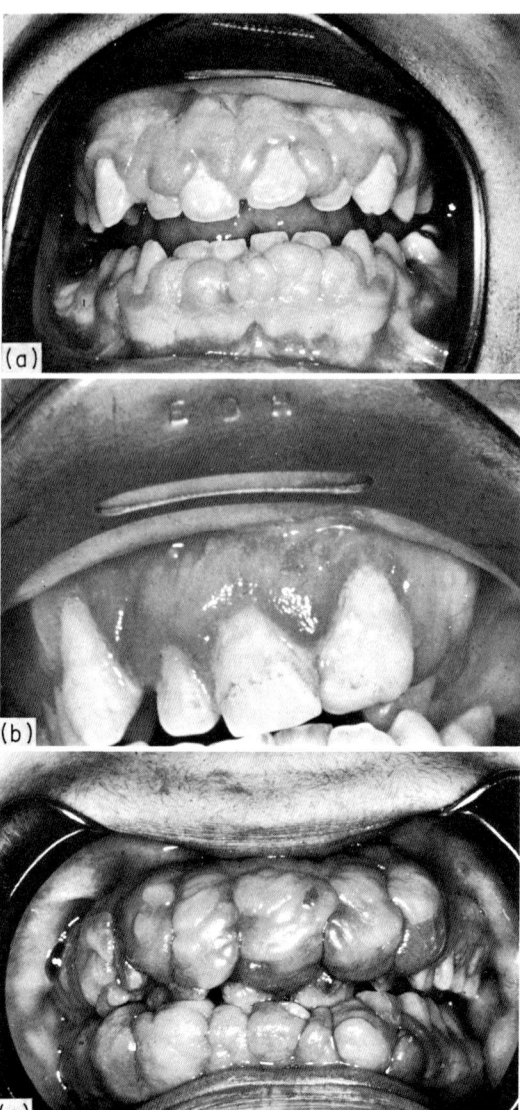

FIG. 13.17. (a) Noninflammatory hyperplasia directly caused by dilantin. (b) Chronic inflammatory hyperplasia occurring in a patient taking dilantin. Since some 40 per cent of patients taking dilantin do not show gingival hyperplasia at all, it is assumed that chronic inflammatory hyperplasia occurs in some patients taking dilantin which is entirely unrelated to administration of the drug. (c) Combined inflammatory and drug-induced gingival hyperplasia.

ALLERGY

The probability that allergic reactions to bacterial antigens from the commensal population of the mouth are associated with the aetiology of periodontitis has been discussed in chap. 6. Several groups of commensal organisms may produce allergic responses in humans, and the eosinophilia which is associated with some cases of periodontitis suggests that allergic mechanisms may play a part in the disease process. The most common response in the mouth to either commensal or exogenous antigens is increase in the level of nonspecific inflammation which is present. The gingival tissues may be highly vascularized, oedematous and may vary in colour from bluish red to purple. On occasion this change may be associated with a variable degree of hyperplasia (fig. 13.18). A wide range of ulcerative lesions of the oral mucosa are considered to be of allergic origin. These are typified by erythema multiforme.

ERYTHEMA MULTIFORME

Erythema multiforme is an acute inflammatory process which may involve skin, occular, genital and oral mucous membranes. Occasionally the mouth lesions may occur in the absence of involvement of other areas, and the condition presents as a symptom complex characterized by eruptive lesions of oral mucous membrane, particularly in children and young adults [46].

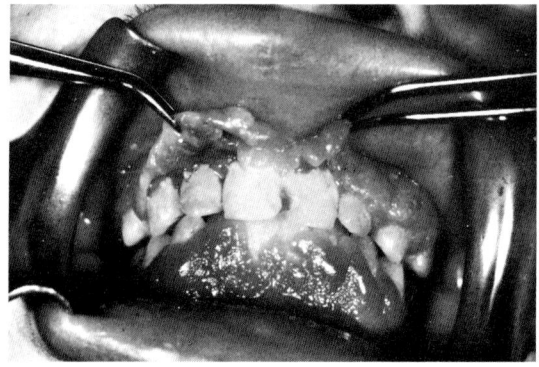

FIG. 13.18. Gross gingival hyperplasia of allergic origin occurring in paint sprayer. Raised eosinophil count in peripheral blood and blood directly from gingival tissues.

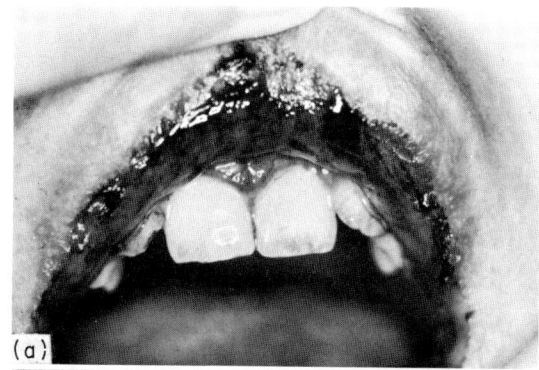

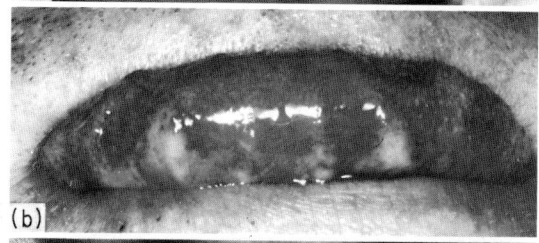

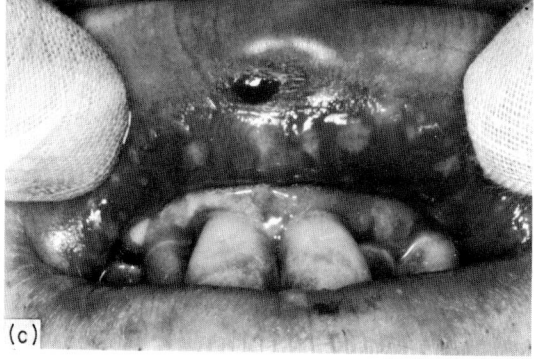

FIG. 13.19. Erythema multiforme, ulceration and crusting of lips, (b) ulceration of tongue, (c) acute gingivitis.

The lesions of the mouth are initially vesicles and bullae which tend to rupture more easily than similar lesions on skin, giving rise to extensive ulcerations of varying depth and size. The periphery of each ulcer presents a zone of erythema, and large areas of the oral mucosa may be markedly reddened. The lips, tongue and gingivae are usually severely involved, with erosion of bullae and extensive ulceration (fig. 13.19). The skin lesions are characterized by central vesicles or bullae surrounded by an urticarial zone. Approximately 50 per cent of the patients with skin involvement present oral lesions.

The aetiology of erythema multiforme is unknown. It is, however, widely regarded as an allergic condition in which the vascular bed acts as the shock tissue. It has been suggested that the condition should be regarded as a symptom complex rather than a specific disease entity [46], and that Behcet's, Stevens–Johnston's and Reiter's syndromes are variations of erythema multiforme which do not justify individual description [47].

Infections (e.g. typhoid fever, tuberculosis, measles, diphtheria and streptococcal infection), drugs (e.g. bromides, antipyretics, barbiturates, phenolphthalein, sulfonanides and penicillin) and various foods have been implicated as causal allergens [48]. Urbach observed that erythema multiforme occurs frequently about 8 days after an attack of herpes labialis [49] and suggested that the condition might be an allergic response to the herpes simplex virus. This view has been supported by the work of Forrester and Scott [50] and Smidt [51], and by the fact that a few reports on small endemics of erythema multiforme suggest a contagious aspect.

The pathogenesis of erythema multiforme may be sensitization of small cutaneous and mucosal blood vessels of certain individuals to any one of a variety of allergens, such as drugs, viruses, bacteria and microbial products [48].

Newman reported one case in which the condition markedly regressed following removal of all the patient's teeth because of 'pyorrhea alveolaris' [52], which suggests that commensal organisms may act as allergens.

REFERENCES

[1] Löe H. (1963) Epidemiology of periodontal disease. *Odont. T.* **71**, 479.

[2] Stahl S.S. *et al.* (1970) Autoradiographic evaluation of gingival response to injury. 1. Surgical trauma in young rats. *Arch. oral Biol.* **13**, 71.

[3] Ray H.G. & Orban B. (1950) Gingival structures in diabetes mellitus. *J. Periodont.* **21**, 85.

[4] Glickman I. (1958) *Clinical Periodontology*, 2nd Edition, p. 409. Philadelphia: Saunders.

[5] Ziskin D.E. & Nesse G.J. (1946) Pregnancy Gingivitis, history, classification aetiology. *Amer. J. Orthodont.* **32**, Sec. Oral Surg. 390–432.

[6] Maier A.W. & Orban B. (1949) Gingivitis in pregnancy. *Oral Surg.* **2**, 334–373.

[7] Larato D.C. *et al.* (1960) The effect of a prescribed method of toothbrushing on the fluctuation of marginal gingivitis. *J. Periodont.* **40**, 142.

[8] MacPhee I.T. (1973) Host resistance to dental plaque, in *Host Resistance to Commensal Bacteria*, Ed. MacPhee I.T., p. 1. Edinburgh: Churchill Livingstone.

[9] Svanberg G., Lindhe J. & Hugoson A. (1973) Effect of nutritional hyperparathyroidism on experimental periodontitis in the dog. *Scand. J. dent. Res.* **81**, 155–162.

[10] Russell A.L., Consalazio F. & White C.L. (1961) Periodontal Disease and Nutrition in Eskimo Scouts of the Alaska National Guard. *J. dent. Res.* **40**, 604–613.

[11] Stahl S.S., Miller S.C. & Goldsmith E.D. (1957) Effects of vertical occlusal trauma on the periodontium of protein deprived young adult rats. *J. Periodont.* **28**, 87–97.

[12] Green J.C. (1960) Periodontal disease in India: report of an epidemiological study. *J. dent. Res.* **39**, 302–312.

[13] Ramfjord S.P. (1961) Periodontal status of boys 11 to 17 years old in Bombay, India. *J. Periodont.* **32**, 237–248.

[14] Carlson J. & Egelberg J. (1965) Effect of diet on early plaque formation in man. *Odont. Revy.* **16**, 112–125.

[15] Löe H.E. & Silness J. (1963) Periodontal disease in pregnancy: 1. Prevalence and severity. *Acta Odont. scand.* **21**, 532–551.

[16] Hilming F. (1950) Gingivitis gravidarum. Dissertation, University of Copenhagen.

[17] Löe H. & Silness J. (1964) Periodontal disease in pregnancy: 2. Correlation between oral hygiene and periodontal condition. *Acta. Odont. scand.* **22**, 121–135.

[18] Gersh I. & Catchpole H.R. (1949) The organisation of ground substance and basement membrane and its significance in tissue injury, disease and growth. *Amer. J. Anat.* **85**, 457–521.

[19] Burnett G.W. & Scherp H.W. (1962) *Oral Microbiology and Infectious Disease*. Baltimore: Williams and Wilkins.

[20] Dubois R.J. (1954) *Biochemical Determinants of Microbial Diseases*. Cambridge, Mass.: Harvard Univ. Press.

[21] Glickman I. (1946) Periodontal structures in experimental diabetes. *N.Y. St. dent. J.* **16**, 226–251.

[22] Sandler H.C. & Stahl S.S. (1960) Prevalence of periodontal disease in a hospitalised population. *J. dent. Res.* **39**, 439–449.

[23] Tiecke R.W. (1955) *Oral Pathology*, p. 478. New York: McGraw-Hill.

[24] Gorlin R.J. & Pindborg J.J. (1964) *Syndromes of the Head and Neck*, p. 27. New York: McGraw Hill.

[25] Del-Negro G., Wajchenberg B.L., Pereira V.G., Shnaider J., Cintra A.B., Assis L.M. de & Sampaio S.A. (1961) Addison's disease associated with South American blastomycosis. *Ann. intern. Med.* **54**, 189–197.

[26] Whitaker J., Landing B.H., Esselborn V.M. & Williams R.R. (1956) Syndrome of familial juvenile hypoadrenocorticism, hypoparathyroidism and superficial maniliasis. *J. clin. Endocr.* **16**, 1374–1387.

[27] Lehner T. (1964) Chronic Candidiosis. *Brit. dent. J.* **116**, 539–545.

[28] Collins-Williams C. (1950) Idiopathic hypoparathyroidism with papilledema in a boy of six years of age: Report of a case associated with moniliasis and celiac Syndrome and a brief review of the literature. *Pediatrics*, **5**, 998–1007.

[29] Lehner T., Wilton J.M.A. & Ivanyi L. (1972) Immunodeficiencies in chronic muco-cutaneous candidosis. *Immunology*, **22**, 775.

[30] Young G., Resca H.G. & Sullivan M.T. (1951) Yeasts of the normal mouth and their relation to salivary activity. *J. dent. Res.* **30**, 426–430.

[31] Ship I.I., Morris A.L., Durrocher R.T. & Burkett L.W. (1960) Recurrent aphthous ulcerations and recurrent herpes labialis in a professional school population. *Oral Surg.* **13**, 1191–1202.

[32] Ship I.I., Brightman V.J. & Laster L.L. (1967) The patient with recurrent aphthous ulcers and the patient with recurrent herpes labialis: A study of two population samples. *J. Amer. dent. Ass.* **75**, 645–654.

[33] Roath S., Israels M.C. & Wilkinson J.F. (1964) The acute leukemias: A study of 580 patients. *Quart. J. Med.* **33**, 256.

[34] Southam C.M., Craver L.F., Dargean H.W. & Burchenal J.H. (1951) Study of the natural history of acute leukaemia with special reference to duration of disease and occurrence of remissions. *Cancer*, **4**, 39–59.

[35] Anderson W.A.D. (1957) *Synopsis of Pathology*, 4th Edition, p. 498. London: Kimpton.

[36] Glickman I. (1964) *Clinical Periodontology*, 3rd Edition. Philadelphia: Saunders.

[37] Eastham R.D. & Pollard B.R. (1964) *A Laboratory Guide to a Clinical Diagnosis*, p. 10. Bristol: Wright.

[38] Ahlbom H.E. (1936) Simple achlorhydric anaemia, Plummer Vinson Syndrome, and carcinoma of the mouth, pharynx and esophagus in women: Observations at Radium–Hemmett Stockholm. *Brit. med. J.* **ii**, 331–333.

[39] Selye H. (1951) *First Annual Report on Stress*. Montreal: Acta Inc.

[40] Henry G.W. & Ebeling W.W. (1926) Blood calcium and phosphorus in personality disorders. *Archs. Neurol. Psychiat. (Chic.)*. **16**, 48–54.

[41] LOVING R.H., WEBER T.B. & MAZERELLA M.A. (1960) Blood serum total 17 hydroxycorticoids levels in necrotising ulcerative gingivitis. *J. dent. Res.* **39**, 663.

[42] BAKER E.G., CROOK G.H. & SCHWABACHER E.D. (1961) Personality correlates of periodontal disease. *J. dent. Res.* **40**, 396–403.

[43] ANGELOPOULOS A.P. & GOAZ P.W. (1972) Incidence of diphenylhydantoin gingival hyperplasia. *Oral surg. oral med. oral path.* **34**, 898–906.

[44] ISHIKAWA J. & GLICKMAN I. (1961) Gingival response to the systemic administration of sodium diphenyl hydantoin (Dilantin) in cats. *J. Periodont.* **32**, 149–157.

[45] NEASE W.J. (1965) The effect of sodium diphenyl-hydantoinate on tissue cultures of human gingivae. *J. Periodont.* **36**, 22–23.

[46] SKLAR G. & McCARTHY P.L. (1966) Oral manifestations of erythema multiforme in children. *Oral Surg.* **21**, 713–723.

[47] ROBINSON H.M. & McCRUMB F.R. (1950) Comparative analysis of the muco cutaneous-ocular syndromes: Report of eleven cases and review of the literature. *Archs. Derm. Syph. (Chic.).* **61**, 339–560.

[48] BRANDTZAEG P. (1964) Erythema multiforme exudativum: A review of the literature with special reference to oral manifestations. *Odont. T.* **72**, 363–390.

[49] URBACH E. (1945) Erythema multiforme. *Arch. Dermat. Syph. (Chic.).* **51**, 228. Cited by Brandtzaeg [48].

[50] FORRESTER D.W. & SCOTT L.V. (1958) Isolation of herpes simplex virus from a patient with erythema multiforme exudativum (Stevens–Johnson syndrome). *New Eng. J. Med.* **259**, 473–475. Cited by Brandtzaeg [48].

[51] SCHMIDT H. (1961) Isolation of herpes simplex virus from blisters of a patient. (Stevens–Johnson syndrome). *Acta. derm.-venerol. (Stockh.).* **41**, 53–55. Cited by Brandtzaeg [48].

[52] NEWMAN C.W. (1956) Electron microscope study of erythema multiforme. *Oral Surg.* **9**, 962–969.

CHAPTER 14

Corrective phase therapy

CORRECTION OF TOOTH RELATIONSHIPS

Corrective phase therapy may be divided into two parts. Firstly, correction of tooth relationships, and secondly, surgical correction of soft tissue and bone architecture.

On completion of hygiene phase therapy, inflammation may persist in some areas of the mouth in association with obvious local factors, such as malpositioned teeth, lack of contact points or marginal ridges, poorly designed prostheses or appliances which lead to food stagnation and the accumulation of plaque. The initial objective of corrective phase therapy is correction of such factors. Elimination of local factors may lead to resolution and healing in the area, particularly in the presence of a limited oedematous gingivitis. Where subsequent surgical elimination of pockets is required, it is necessary to create an environment in which the wound may be expected to heal, by the prior elimination of local causative factors. As a generalization, consideration of correction of individual tooth relationships and the relationships of restorations and appliances to the teeth should precede any attempt at the surgical elimination of pockets.

On occasion it may be necessary to correct soft tissue architecture prior to preparing restorations or taking impressions for dentures, particularly where the cervical margins of restorations or dentures are directly associated with the gingival tissues. If there is significant delay in placing the finished restorations subsequent to gingival surgery, plaque accumulation around temporary restorations may lead to inflammation and further distortion of gingival form. In the extreme it may prove necessary to repeat the surgery after the restorations or dentures have been finally placed. Correction of tooth relationships and surgical correction of soft tissue and bone architecture should never be considered in isolation from each other.

Factors which may be responsible for the presence of persistent localized inflammation despite an adequate standard of oral hygiene are:

(1) malpositioned teeth,

(2) inadequately designed or positioned restorations,

(3) poorly designed dentures,

(4) interocclusal factors:

    (a) hyperfunction,

    (b) hypofunction,

    (c) parafunction,

(5) functionally poor soft tissue or bone architecture (see chap. 15).

MALPOSITIONED TEETH

The presence of stagnation areas, resulting from malpositioning of teeth, has long been considered a contributory factor in the establishment of periodontal disease [1, 2 & 3]. One study using objective criteria in a group of young patients with a high standard of oral hygiene failed to confirm this view. In this group there was no apparent association between disease and axial inclination or displacement of posterior teeth [4]. Malpositioning may produce poor functional self-cleansing of teeth by lips, cheeks or tongue, and lead to the exacerbation of pre-existing inflammation in the periodontitis susceptible patient. Ideally, a malpositioned tooth should be repositioned in the arch prior to any surgical attempt to eliminate pockets associated with the tooth. Loss of functional tooth–tissue relationships (chap. 2) due to palatal inclination or displacement of maxillary central or lateral incisors may frequently be associated with inflammation, fibrosis and pocket formation on the buccal side of the displaced tooth (fig. 14.1). In the young patient in particular, the arch form may be restored by orthodontic realignment of teeth, although sufficient space may not be available without serial extraction. In a small percentage of older patients, where space allows, it is possible to push a tooth through the bite prior to surgical elimination of any pockets (fig. 14.2). In the majority of older patients, where major orthodontic therapy would be required to restore a tooth to a functional position, it is necessary to accept that corrective phase elimination of an existing pocket is not necessarily permanent, and that over the long-term the condition may recur.

The proper treatment for periodontal problems associated with malpositioned teeth is interceptive orthodontics at the appropriate stage of growth and development. Orthodontic tooth movement, when necessary, usually takes precedence over any other occlusal therapy short of emergency procedures.

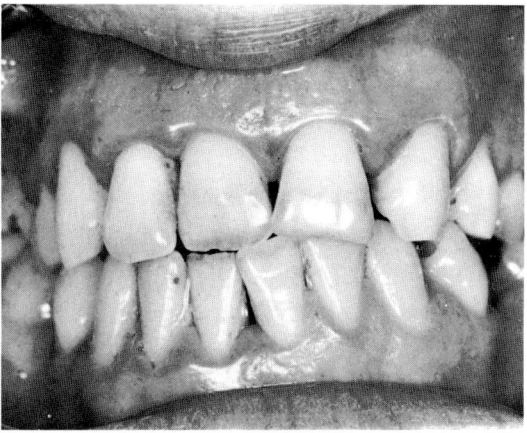

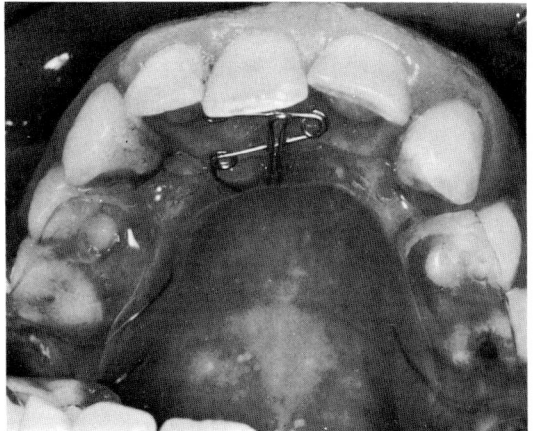

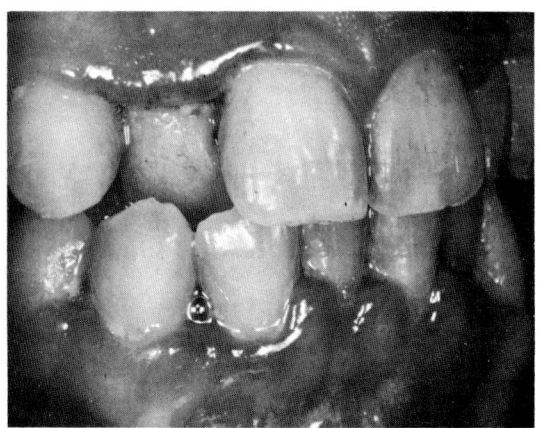

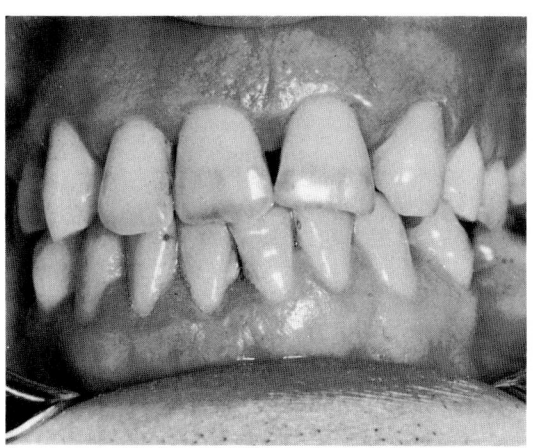

FIG. 14.1. Inflammation and pocket formation associated with palatal displacement of 2 /.

FIG. 14.2. Orthodontic realignment of 1 / prior to surgical treatment of pockets, 30-year-old man.

INADEQUATELY DESIGNED OR POSITIONED RESTORATIONS

The importance of correct tissue relationships at the contact area has been stressed in chapter 2, as has the cleansing action of lips, cheeks and tongue in minimizing plaque formation. Where necessary, deficient restorations should be re-designed with particular regard to:

(1) design of the contact area,

(2) contour and position of the cervical margins of the restoration relative to the adjacent gingival tissues,

(3) surface smoothness, particularly of the cervical margin area,

(4) morphology of the occlusal surface,

(5) functional movements of the dentition as a whole.

Design of the contact area

In the natural dentition of the young patient, adjacent teeth meet in a narrow contact area approximately halfway between the level of the marginal ridges of the occlusal surface and the gingival tissues, in the interdental region. Where a restoration is placed such that the contact area approximates to the occlusal surface, this may result in flattening of the marginal ridges, and may predispose to trapping of food interproximally. The interdental col has been found to vary in size in different areas of the mouth [5], and the creation of a broad buccolingual contact rather than a narrow contact area may cause a change in the anatomy of the tissues of the col, which may lead to the persistence of local inflammatory change. The saddle shaped area of the normal col (fig. 14.3a) becomes broadened (fig. 14.3b) in proportion to the width of the contact area. Plaque may accumulate against the increased area of thin col epithelium, and the area in which incipient periodontal disease may develop is markedly increased [6]. When amalgam restorations are placed, it is impossible to achieve an adequate marginal ridge/contact area/tissues of the col relationship, unless the filling is placed by means of a wedged matrix (fig. 14.4). Rubber dam may also be used to advantage [6].

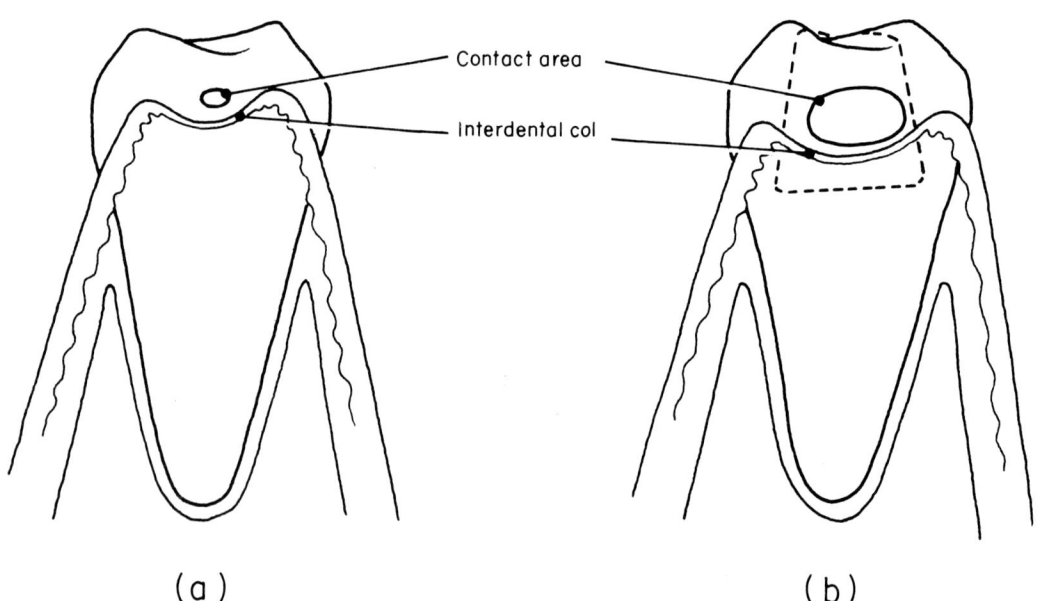

Contact area

Interdental col

(a)　　　　　　　　(b)

FIG. 14.3. (a) Narrow col associated with narrow contact area. (b) Buccolingually broadened col as a result of poorly designed broad contact area.

USE OF THE AMALGAM SPLINT FOR EMBRASURE PROTECTION

The amalgam splint was initially proposed as a permanent fixed splint for use in a mouth with mobile teeth and gross destruction of the supporting tissues [7]. The technique is also applicable where it is impossible to place adjacent restorations with an adequate marginal ridge or contact area because of excessive crowding, excessive separation or lateral displacement of adjacent teeth.

TECHNIQUE

MOD amalgam cavities are prepared in the teeth to be splinted. A rubber-base impression is taken of these cavities and a cast poured in stone. Wax is inserted into the cavity preparations on the models and physiologic interproximal contours carved. The entire stone cast is then coated with a separating medium, and plasticine is placed on the lingual side to fill one half of the interproximal space from lingual to buccal. Cold cure acrylic resin is placed on the buccal side and as far into the interproximal region as the physiologically carved wax and the plasticine will allow. The buccal flange of the matrix is allowed to set and then removed from the model. The plasticine is removed from the lingual side, and the lingual side of the model and the interproximal area recoated with a separating medium. The interstitial part of the buccal acrylic flange is coated with separating medium and replaced on the buccal side. Cold cure acrylic resin is placed on the lingual side and packed through the interproximal region as far as the physiologically carved wax and the buccal flange will allow. The two halves of the matrix are removed from the model, and a small hole is drilled in each flange with a rose-head burr. After the removal of the temporary dressings the

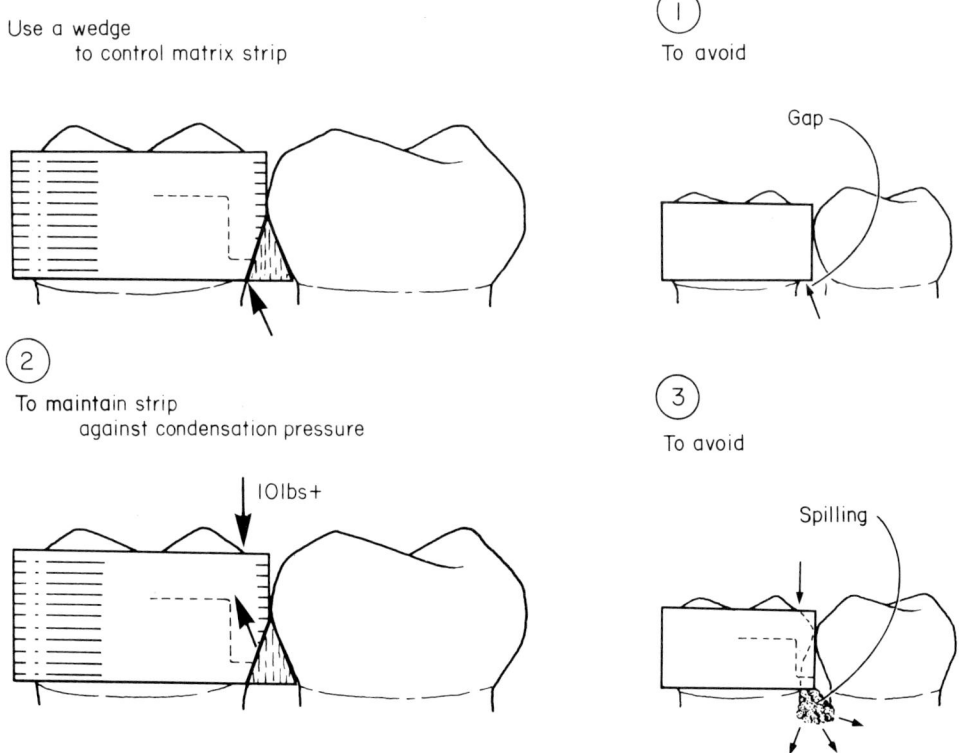

FIG. 14.4. The use of a wedge to control embrasure design of restoration, courtesy of Professor G. S. Beagrie.

acrylic matrix is inserted into the patient's mouth and fixed in position by means of an Ivory's matrix clamp (fig. 14.5b). By condensing amalgam into the entire cavity preparation a one-piece periodontal splint is formed with a bridge of amalgam crossing at an occlusal level, and with amalgam accurately positioned at the cervical margins of the restorations (fig. 14.5c). When the initial set has taken place the matrix is removed, and the fillings are contoured and carved. The acrylic matrix will have governed the design of the interproximal area as dictated by the wax on the model and have prevented the formation of overhanging edges. Final finishing may be carried out by means of linen and sandpaper strips. The occlusal bridge of amalgam fulfils the protective function of the marginal ridges and contact area and allows the tissues of the embrasure to assume a close approximation to a physiological contour. The space apical to the bridge of amalgam may be maintained by routine oral hygiene measures, the use of wood points and/or an interspace brush (fig. 14.6).

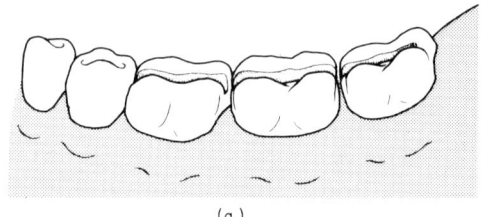

(a)

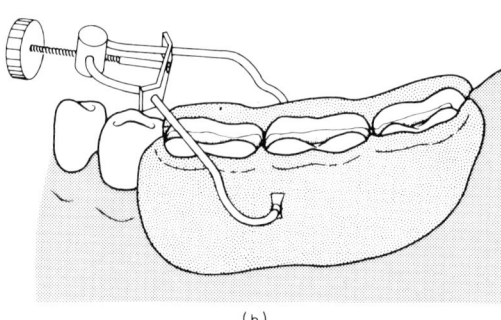

(b)

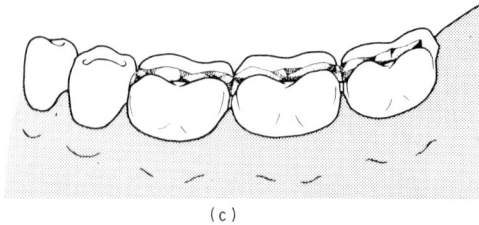

(c)

FIG. 14.5. (a) Poor fillings, inadequate contact points, mobile teeth. (b) Cavities prepared, acrylic matrix in position. (c) Completed amalgam splint.

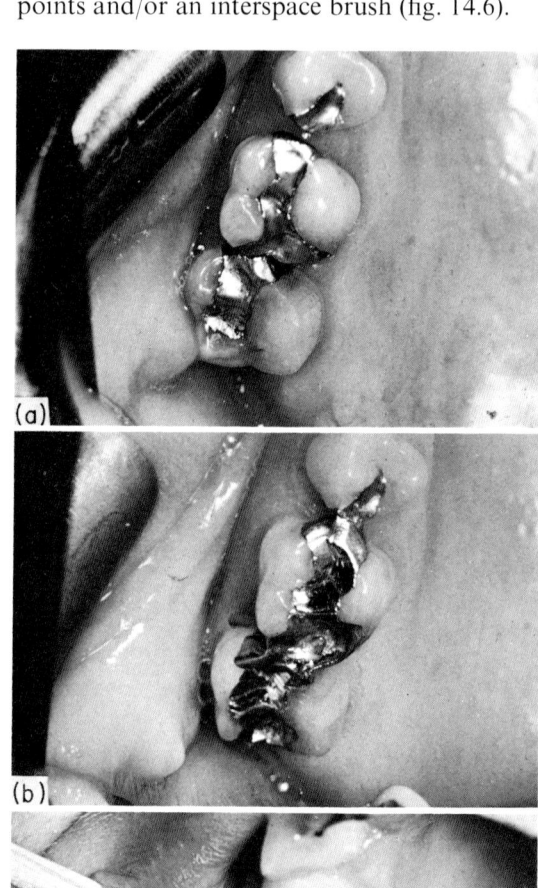

(a)

(b)

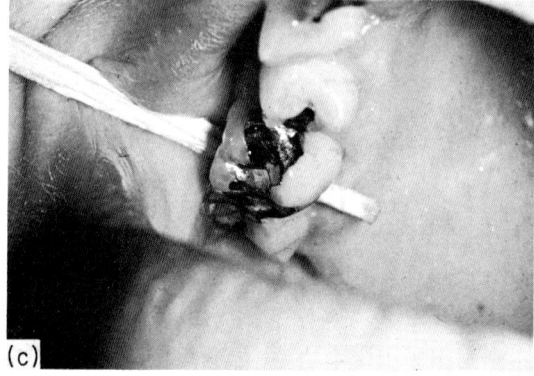

(c)

FIG. 14.6. (a) Contact point problem due to buccal displacement of ⌐7⌐. (b) Amalgam splint in position. (c) Use of wood stick apical to amalgam bridge.

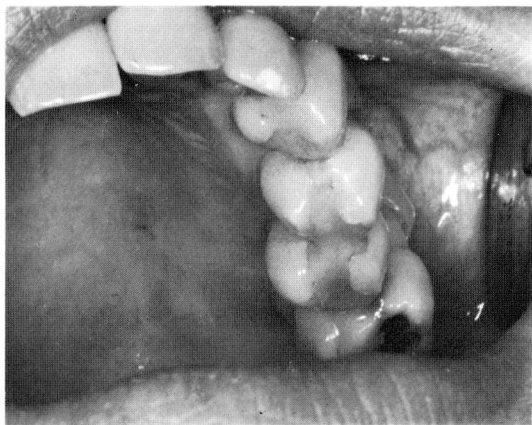

FIG. 14.7. Fixed acrylic splint.

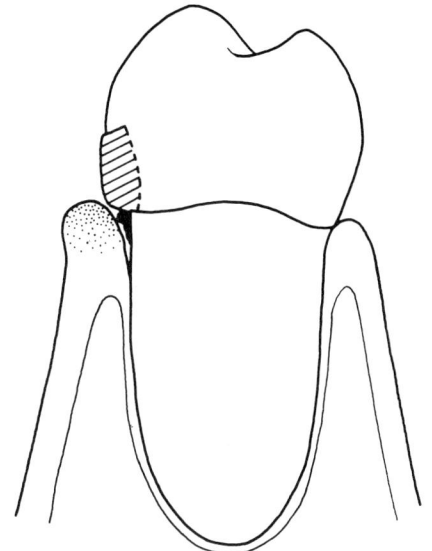

FIG. 14.8. Plaque formation in deadspace beneath over contoured restoration.

A similar result may be obtained by placing a cold cure acrylic splint [8] directly in the mouth without the intermediate use of a model, and without prefabricating a matrix. MOD retentive cavities are prepared in the mouth as before. Soft bite wax is placed interstitially and laterally to act as a matrix contoured to a physiological form, clear of the cervical edges. The cavities are lined, and cold cure acrylic resin flowed into position and allowed to set. The bite wax matrix is removed, and the fillings polished and contoured with burrs and polishing strips. Materials such as Adaptic, Concise, and Nuvafil may be similarly employed. Secondary caries is commoner around acrylic splints than around amalgam splints, but these may be expected to function adequately for periods up to, and in excess of, 5 years (fig. 14.7).

Contour and position of cervical margin of restorations relative to gingival tissues

BUCCAL AND LINGUAL CONTOURS OF RESTORATIONS

It has been widely held that buccal and lingual contours of restorations should protect the gingival crevice from food impaction. The suggestion has been made that this should be accomplished by selectively placing a bulge in the filling at the cervical margin which serves to: 'deflect the food over the crevice and on to the kera-tinized surface of the attached gingival tissues' [9].

The contour of the natural crown is not of itself adequate protection against food impaction in the crevice [10]. The maximum bulge is not more than 0·5 mm [11 & 12]. The main self-cleansing mechanism at the gingival margin is movement of lips, cheeks and tongue constantly passing over the gingival margin, massaging and cleansing. The role of saliva in such a cleansing mechanism has been discussed in chapter 2. Over-contouring and exaggeration of the buccal and the lingual margins of a restoration can promote the accumulation of plaque (fig. 14.8), and exaggerate rather than prevent inflammation. Restorations should be shaped to follow the natural contour of the tooth, or where in doubt narrowed buccolingually to reduce the deadspace at the cervical margin.

POSITION OF CERVICAL MARGIN RELATIVE TO THE GINGIVAL MARGIN

Traditionally, it has been variously held that the cervical margin of restorations should be placed 'at the gingival crest', 'slightly below the gingival crest', 'slightly above the crest'. Such generalizations have led to conflicting statements such as: 'the margins of a crown placed beneath the crest of the gum tissue 20–25 years ago, maintain the same healthy relationship today' [13], and: 'The periodontal health is maintained more easily when the buccal (and lingual) margins of the restoration are well above the gingival tissue' [14]. Apart from aesthetics on anterior teeth, wherever possible margins should be placed above the gingiva where they can be adequately finished by the dentist and cleaned easily by the patient. Factors which are of importance in deciding the location of the cervical margin of a restoration are:

(1) degree of susceptibility to periodontitis,
(2) caries rate of the patient,
(3) type of filling material used,
(4) degree of marginal adaptation, and smoothness of the restoration,
(5) aesthetics,
(6) standard of oral hygiene.

DEGREE OF SUSCEPTIBILITY TO PERIODONTITIS AND CARIES

Subgingival placement of the cervical margin of a restoration may cause gingival irritation. There may be no alternative if extensive caries is present. Initial caries does not develop below the gingival margin, and it has been suggested that the margin of an interproximal cavity preparation should be extended subgingivally to prevent secondary caries developing at the cervical edge of the filling [15 & 16].

Waerhaug has shown experimentally, in dogs and monkeys, that subgingival rough surfaces or overhanging edges of restorations do not mechanically irritate the gingival tissues with which they lie in contact [17 & 18]. Such factors, however, favour retention of bacterial plaque, and the severe gingival inflammation associated with such restorations is primarily the result of bacterial rather than mechanical irritation [19].

In a patient with a high caries rate and a low susceptibility to periodontitis, deliberate extension of the cavity below the gingival margin may occasionally be justified. In such a patient diet control, topical fluoride application and improved oral hygiene measures should be utilized to reduce the caries attack rate. It is undesirable

to extend the restoration below the gingival margin in a patient with a high susceptibility to periodontitis. When such extension is unavoidable, particular attention must be paid to:

(1) type of filling material to be used,
(2) marginal adaptation and polish of the restoration,
(3) instruction in patient self-care.

TYPE OF FILLING MATERIAL TO BE USED

The most commonly used filling materials, amalgam, composite and silicate, are less well tolerated by the gingivae than gold or porcelain and give rise to an inflammatory reaction which is more severe with silicate than with amalgam [20 & 21]. Pure gold and inlay gold are chemically inert in oral fluids and produce no chemical irritation [22]. High fusing porcelain is probably inert, but Waerhaug believes that low fusing porcelain may have a slightly irritant effect because of its slight solubility [19].

From animal experiments, Waerhaug has concluded that heat-cured acrylic resins are non-irritating since they become covered with epithelium which adheres to the acrylic and, histologically, they cause little or no inflammation [19]. Self-curing acrylic resins are very irritating during and shortly after polymerization because of chemical irritation by the monomer, but later they produce little or no irritation [23] except that which is associated with thermal expansion.

Where subgingival extension is obligatory in a periodontitis susceptible patient, gold and porcelain are the materials of choice.

DEGREE OF MARGINAL ADAPTATION AND SMOOTHNESS OF THE RESTORATION

Poor marginal adaptation of a restoration, whether the result of inadequate gingival retraction or resection before filling, of poor filling technique, or of setting or thermal dimensional changes in the filling material, allows bacterial plaque to form in the marginal defects, thus resulting in gingival irritation [24]. The poor marginal adaptation of acrylic resins, associated to some extent with thermal expansion, make these materials unsuitable for use in the periodontitis prone patient (fig. 14.9).

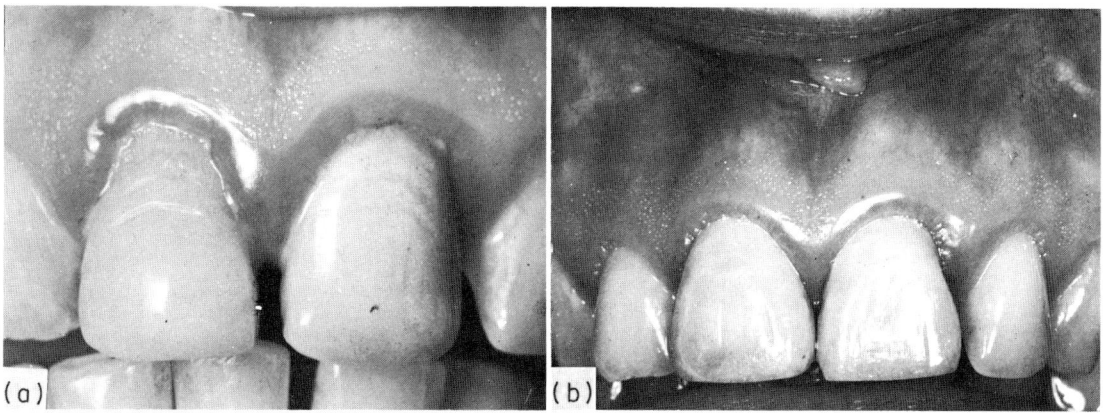

FIG. 14.9. (a) Marginal inflammation resulting from thermal expansion of acrylic crowns. (b) Following replacement of acrylic crowns by porcelain crowns, courtesy of Professor G. S. Beagrie.

However suitable the filling material, the degree of adaptation and finish of the resulting restoration at the cervical margin is critical in preventing the accumulation of dental plaque.

STANDARD OF ORAL HYGIENE OF THE PATIENT

Where possible, the margins of restorations should be situated where they can readily be kept clean. Planning the surgical correction of an existing periodontitis should, where necessary, include designing margins of restorations such that they can be easily maintained postoperatively. Surgery may precede or follow placing of restorations. The patient should be formally instructed in the use of aids to oral hygiene, with as much stress on maintenance of restorations as on maintaining gingival health. In the control of periodontitis these factors are inseparable.

ANATOMY OF THE OCCLUSAL SURFACE OF THE RESTORATION IN FUNCTION

The importance of design of the occlusal surface of a restoration from the point of view of food shedding and embrasure protection has previously been stressed (fig. 14.10). The occlusal surface must be shaped in such a way that the

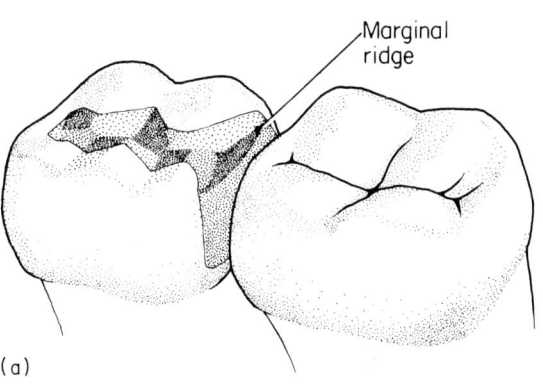

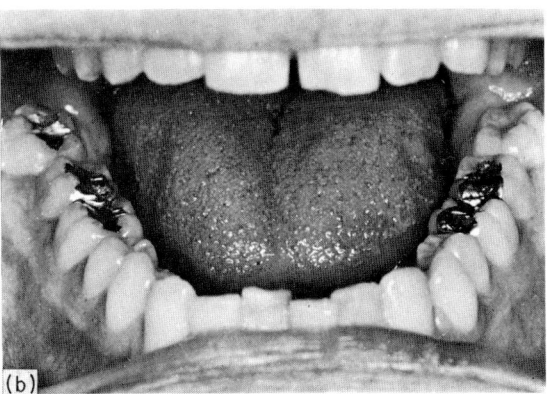

FIG. 14.10. (a) Anatomically carved restoration with functional marginal ridge and narrow contact area. (b) Clinical photograph of functional restorations.

restoration functions in harmony with the movements of the dentition as a whole. An occlusal surface which is too low may lead to over-eruption or tipping of the restored tooth or its opponent. A high filling may lead to undesirable compensatory adjustment in the position of the restored tooth or of the neuromuscular mechanisms which control mandibular movement.

POORLY DESIGNED DENTURES

During hygiene phase therapy, persistent inflammation is frequently found in association with the presence of an ill-fitting denture. The denture should be taken from the patient and the correction of any poor tooth relationships undertaken. The design of restorations should be considered with a view to providing a new denture.

The restorations and the denture must be designed to meet the biologic requirements of the periodontium as a whole. A toothborne fixed or removable prosthesis is best tolerated by the supporting tissues and should be used wherever possible (fig. 14.11).

Where compromise is necessary, a tooth and tissue borne partial denture must be designed with the maximum of respect to the potentially damaging effect of such appliances on the periodontium. The principles of design have been well described by Liddelow [25].

Several reports have shown that gingival inflammation, mobility and bone destruction increase drastically in teeth adjacent to partial dentures. This is another warning against using partial dentures and removable splints in periodontal therapy. The question may even be raised whether partial dentures in many cases do not cause more harm then good, and it may be that partial dentures should only be made when the patient, for aesthetic or functional reasons, cannot be without them [26].

Poorly designed dentures cause damage to:

(1) mucous membrane,
(2) gingival margins specifically, leading in time to severe damage to the supporting structures of the teeth,
(3) alveolar bone,
(4) teeth.

Damage to the mucous membrane can be caused by failing to cover sufficient area, thus overloading the area which is covered. A loose denture causes frictional damage by movement. A proportion of patients with such dentures develop a denture stomatitis associated with infection by *Candida albicans* (fig. 14.12a & b). In many such mouths, the inflammation will not resolve completely following removal of the denture and hygiene phase therapy alone. Resolution may be expedited by use of Amphotericin B (10 mg) lozenges, 2 per cent Nystatin cream, or Nystatin (500 000 units) lozenges allowed to

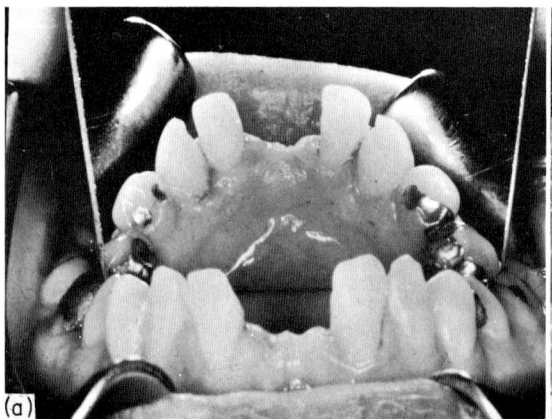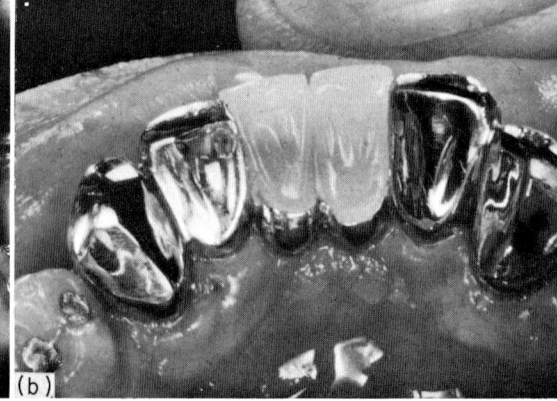

FIG. 14.11. Fixed bridge replacing 1 / 1, courtesy of Professor G. S. Beagrie.

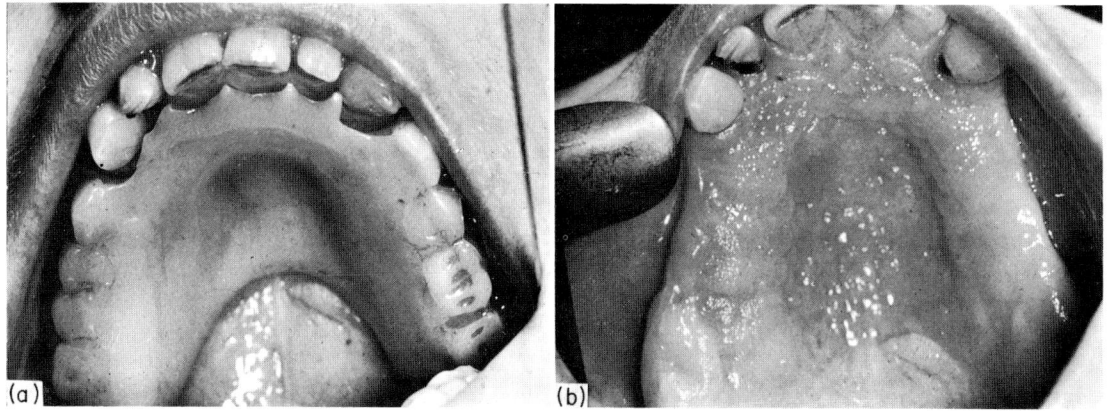

FIG. 14.12. (a) Poorly designed tissue borne acrylic denture. (b) Denture sore mouth.

dissolve in the mouth, three times daily, for 7–10 days. Occasionally supportive drug therapy may be required for much longer periods to eliminate infection and prevent recurrence.

Damage to mucous membrane may also be caused by fitting a denture which opens the bite so that the weight of chewing is transmitted by the denture entirely to the mucous membrane and not the standing teeth, or by fitting a denture so that there is gross cuspal interference or locking during functional movements of the mandible. The maintenance of a healthy periodontium is aided by insisting that dentures are not worn during the night and that they are cleaned and placed in water.

Relationship of the denture to the cervical region of the teeth

If a tissue borne partial denture is made to fit the gingival margins of the teeth accurately, its every movement will press or drag on the margins, causing traumatic injury to the gingival tissues. A degree of settlement of a tissue borne denture is inevitable and this will tend to cause the fitting part of the denture to compress the gingival tissue, stripping the tissue away from the tooth. Conversely, failure to fit the denture accurately around a standing tooth will leave a space down which food will be forced directly onto the gingival margin (fig. 14.13b). The correct relationship of the denture to the tooth is shown in fig. 14.13d. The denture should fit in close con-

tact with the tooth just on or above its most bulbous part, free of the cervical margin of the tooth and directing food away from the embrasure and not between the denture and the tooth. Such a result cannot be achieved by arbitrary grinding at the time of fitting; the denture must be made on a surveyed model. The denture must not finish gingivally to the survey line (fig. 14.13c), or sufficiently far occlusally to displace the teeth (fig. 14.13a).

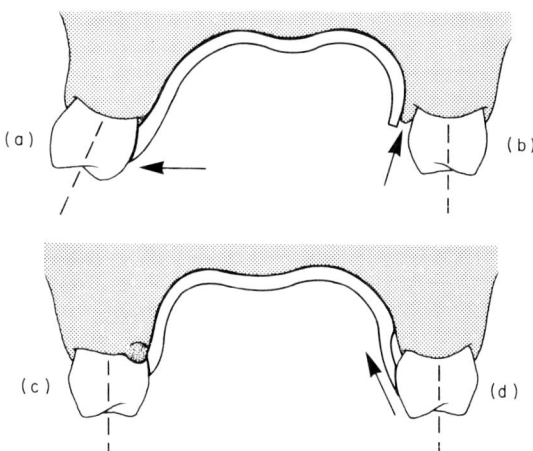

FIG. 14.13. (b) Denture cut short of tooth leading to food packing. (d) Denture in close contact with tooth on or above its most bulbous part relieved from the cervical margin, i.e. correct design. (c) Denture fitting gingivally at cervical margin causing stripping of gingivae from tooth. (a) Denture fitting occlusal to survey line causing lateral displacement of tooth.

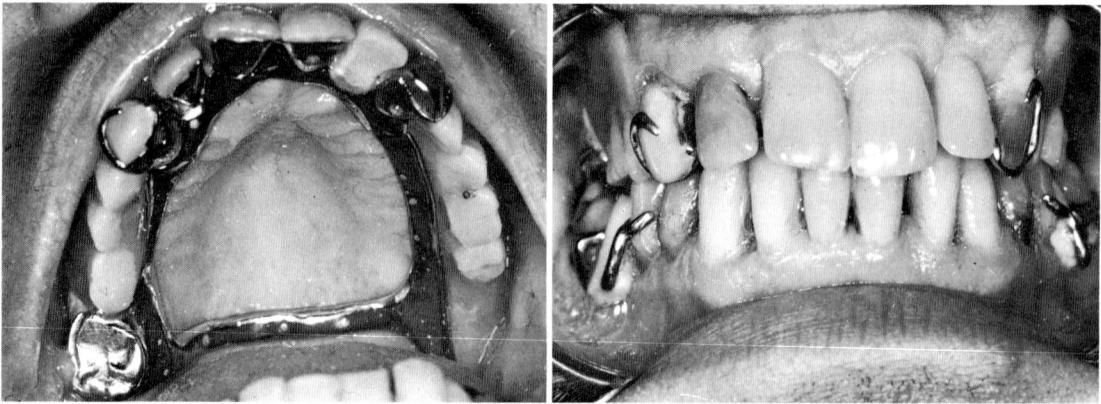

FIG. 14.14. Tooth and tissue borne partial denture, courtesy of Mr K. W. Tyson.

Tooth and tissue borne acrylic dentures, adequately designed, may be acceptable where there is a well supported dentition. Tooth borne, or tooth and tissue borne metal dentures are preferable from the point of view of gingival health and may be obligatory as part of the treatment of advanced periodontitis (fig. 14.14).

INTEROCCLUSAL FACTORS

The dynamic concept of occlusion

The extent to which the health of the tissues of the mouth is dependent upon good functional anatomical relationships of individual tissues has been discussed on pages 22–24. The teeth and their supporting structures, the bone of maxilla and mandible, the temporo-mandibular joint, the investing sheath of the masticatory muscles and the oral mucosa act as a single functional unit whose individual tissues are mutually interdependent (fig. 2.3). If teeth are removed, the remaining teeth are free to move through the supporting bone in response to the resultant of the total forces to which they are subjected. They will continue to move until they reach a position of functional stability relative to these forces. Changes in position of the teeth may produce changes in the pattern of movement of the temporomandibular joint. They can also change the relationship of the gingival tissues to the tooth and lead to plaque accumulation and disease.

The masticatory apparatus is a dynamic system with a considerable total capacity to adapt through a wide range of functional requirements. The individual tissues are in a dynamic relationship to each other, each with a variable individual adaptive capacity to meet alteration in the functional requirements of the apparatus as a whole. There is constant turn-over and adjustment of supporting bone and the connective tissue elements of the perio-dontium to maintain a balanced relationship. Where the total functional adaptive capacity of the masticatory system is exceeded, breakdown of any of the individual tissues involved may result.

The function of the masticatory apparatus is comminution of food and the clearance of food debris from the oral cavity. Ideally, functional relationships of the tissues should be such that the mouth is largely self-cleansing. In the past, the study of tooth relationships has tended to concentrate on interocclusal relationships, and masticatory efficiency has been considered in terms of ability to comminute food without exceeding the adaptive capacity of the supporting tissues. An increasing weight of evidence suggests that even in the presence of malocclusion, it is unlikely that the adaptive capacity of the system will be exceeded by normal functional demands, and that the self-cleansing capacity of the system is at least as important a factor from the point of view of disease of the mouth [27]. The functional relationships of teeth to each other within an arch merit at least as much consideration as the inter-arch relationship.

The physiology of occlusion

Until recently, two concepts of occlusion have virtually governed the practice of dentistry. The first is the prosthetic concept of balanced occlusion whereby functional stability of full dentures may be increased by creating bilateral, working and balancing cuspal contacts in lateral and protrusive excursions (fig. 14.15). While this concept has obvious merits in full denture construction, there is no evidence that the principle is applicable to the natural dentition. On the contrary, several workers have suggested that nonworking (balancing) contacts in the natural dentition are harmful [2, 28–32].

It has been stated that the nonworking contact in the natural dentition is unnecessary and that interferences on this side should be eliminated [33]. In a study of 413 teeth in the mouths of fifty-four periodontally involved patients, it was found that 53 per cent of the molar teeth had nonworking contacts, and that mobility, bone loss and pocket depths were significantly greater in relation to these teeth [34].

On the evidence available, it appears that nonworking contacts may contribute to the aetiology and progression of periodontitis, and it is clear that there is no evidence to justify applying the prosthetic concept of balanced occlusion to the natural dentition as a therapeutic procedure.

The second concept which has greatly influenced the practice of dentistry is the orthodontic attitude that defines normal occlusion in terms of static cusp and fossa relationships which are considered acceptable. An occlusion that does not conform to these relationships is classified as a malocclusion. Until recently, consideration of the natural occlusion has been based on these two concepts and large numbers of patients have received extensive bite rehabilitation for no reason other than that their occlusion did not conform to these standards.

A wider concept of dynamic individual occlusion has recently emerged, whereby the requirement for alteration of tooth relationships is assessed on the broader basis of the health and function of each individual masticatory system, without respect to the restrictions imposed by formal prosthetic and orthodontic concepts of ideal occlusion [35].

NEUROMUSCULAR CONTROL OF MANDIBULAR MOVEMENT

Some simple movements of the masticatory muscles are thought to be caused by innate reflexes [36 & 37]. With growth and development, conditioned reflexes are acquired which modify these primitive reflexes. The nerve endings in the periodontal membrane and oral mucosa, the tension receptors of the muscles of mastication and the receptors in the temporomandibular joints are the sources of reflex control of the movements of the mandible [37 & 38].

The postural position of the mandible

This is the position which is maintained by just enough muscle contraction to overcome gravity [39]. The pull of gravity causes a constant shower of asynchronous motor discharges to the mandibular muscles, resulting in a slight degree of contraction at all times. When the mandible is held in a balanced position against gravity symmetrically opposed to the cranium, it is said to be in the postural position. This has been called the 'physiologic rest position', but the muscles are

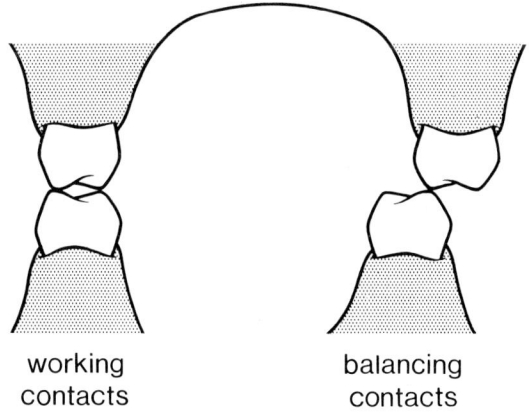

working
contacts

balancing
contacts

FIG. 14.15. Working and balancing contacts, courtesy of Miss Jenny Mitchell.

not at rest and it is no more physiologic than any other position [39].

Centric relation

The postural position of the mandible is the only mandibular position which is consistently observed before eruption of the teeth. With growth and development, modification of innate reflexes by acquired conditioned reflexes should result in a position of occlusion that provides a maximum of occlusal cuspal contact, with a minimum of lateral strain on the teeth. This is the ideal occlusal position. In centric relation, the mandible is held above the postural position and greater neuromuscular activity is required. Moyers has defined centric relation as the position of the mandible determined by the neuromuscular reflex first learned for controlling mandibular position when the primary teeth were in occlusion [40]. At first, centric occlusion is simply the relationship of the teeth when the mandible is in centric relation. Since centric relation is a neurologic concept, partly governed by acquired conditioned reflexes, growth and development must change the centric relation; centric relation and centric occlusion may not then coincide. Centric relation has also been defined as the first point of contact between opposing teeth in the path of closure from the postural position towards centric occlusion. The implication of this latter definition is that when centric relation does not coincide with centric occlusion (the point of maximum cuspal interdigitation), the patient has disharmonies and a slide into centric occlusion occurs. It has been suggested that such disharmony predisposes to periodontal disease and to temporomandibular joint problems.

The majority of studies suggest that centric relation and centric occlusion are two separate positions [41]. In a study of 200 patients said to be free from periodontal disease, only nine patients were seen in whom centric relation and centric occlusion were identical [42].

While it is desirable that the path of closure to centric occlusion should be without lateral or anteroposterior slides resulting from cuspal interference the absence of such a situation does not necessarily lead directly to disease. Adjust-

ment of tooth position occurs throughout life, in response to changes in occlusal forces resulting from wear, pathologic changes in the supporting tissues, changes in muscle tonicity, or following the provision of fillings or dentures. Within the adaptive capacity of the masticatory system, a balance of force is maintained such that the dentition as a whole is in equilibrium with its environment [43].

ADAPTIVE CHANGES IN THE PERIODONTAL TISSUES TO PHYSIOLOGIC FORCES

Alveolar bone

Alveolar bone, like bone anywhere in the body, is in a constant state of reorganization, primarily in response to functional stimuli but also to some extent influenced by intrinsic metabolic factors. When a tooth is moved by forces within physiological limits, intermittent resorption and repair occurs in the alveolar bone on the side to which the tooth is moving (the pressure side). The areas of active bone resorption constitute only a small part of the total surface of alveolar bone related to the tooth on the pressure side [44], so that the total support of the tooth is not much reduced at any particular time. More bone is resorbed from the pressure side than would be needed to reconstitute the normal width of periodontal membrane. This results in a series of concavities in the pressure surface of the alveolar bone where the periodontal membrane and bone are gradually replaced, initially, by granulation tissue. Repair and regeneration in the granulation tissue results in reorganization of the periodontium, while further resorption may be initiated in an adjacent region. Throughout this dynamic process, all stages of replacement by granulation tissue, repair and regeneration are evident until the tooth reaches a position of stability relative to its environment.

On the tension side, the side from which the tooth is moving, the alveolar bone adjacent to the tooth is lamellated, indicating that new bone is being laid down on the periodontal membrane side of the cribriform plate. On the marrow side there is evidence of resorption, and the lamina dura and periodontal membrane are thus maintained at their normal width.

If teeth are moved a limited distance labially by physiologic forces, bone is resorbed on the periodontal membrane side of the alveolus and new bone is deposited on the labial aspect of the alveolar process. If the rate of the new bone formation does not match the rate of resorption on the periodontal membrane side, the tooth may move through the labial bone plate, causing fenestration or dehiscence (chap. 15 & fig. 15.19).

Cementum

Cementum formation is probably a continuous process throughout the life of the tooth; the lamellated structure is presumably due to intermittent deposition. The lamellation may be related to changes in the direction of the forces acting on the teeth, resulting in reorientation of the Sharpey's fibres [45]. As has been stated previously, functional adjustment of tooth position takes place mainly by alteration in alveolar bone, rather than cementum, which is a stable tissue in comparison to supporting bone. Functional hyperplasia of cementum may occasionally occur in the apical region when a tooth has been exposed to heavy function.

Changes in collagen structure of the periodontal membrane

The periodontal membrane is on average about 0·2 mm thick and acts as a buffer layer between bone and tooth. It consists of collagen fibres which support the tooth, with a fluid or gel-like interfibrous phase (ground substance) which behaves like a fibrostatic cushion [46]. A change in orientation of the fibres occurs when eruption brings the tooth into occlusion [47]. The supracrestal fibres of the marginal ligament (chap. 2) are arranged in an intricate pattern which contributes to the stability of the tooth and promotes the self-cleansing action of the gingival sulcus during normal function. The degree of organization and structure of the collagen fibres of the periodontium is governed by the direction and magnitude of occlusal stress and, to some extent, by the systemic status of the individual. The turnover of mature collagen is slow, and such fibres are not generally sensitive to systemic changes,

unless trauma or other forms of injury establish a need for reparative processes [47].

If the forces applied to the tooth are mainly vertical (in the long axis), the periodontal fibres assume an oblique pattern, in some instances almost parallel to the long axis of the root of the tooth. If the stress is largely horizontal, there are well developed groups of alveolar fibres with a horizontal arrangement in the region of the alveolar crest (alveolar crestal fibres) and around the apex of the tooth. There is very little evidence of a functional arrangement of fibres in the region of the mid portion of the root [47]. Lateral stress on the tooth within physiologic limits is desirable, since it stimulates development of the marginal ligament. This may limit the spread of gingival inflammation more effectively than would a loose, nonfunctionally arranged connective tissue structure [47]. In general the width of the periodontal membrane will increase with increase in functional demand [48].

Changes in the vascular system

The vascularity of the periodontal tissues decreases with increase in functional demands, and an increase in the proportion of functionally orientated collagen fibres occurs. It has been suggested that hydraulic principles are applicable to the periodontal membrane and that blood and tissue fluids absorb at least part of the initial impact of occlusal forces [49, 50 & 51]. The main factors in resistance to compressive forces are fibres of the periodontal membrane, the bone walls of the socket, the degree of aggregation of the ground substance of connective tissue, and the vascularity of the periodontal tissues. Experiments on monkeys have shown that many venules pass through the cribriform plate apertures in the lower two thirds of the socket wall, which connect two reservoirs of low pressure blood, one in the venous network of the periodontal membrane, and one in the bone marrow [46]. Local areas of high pressure in the periodontal vascular bed occasioned by tooth movement may thus be reduced by flow towards the marrow reservoir. Teeth respond differently to different types of forces, but the evidence suggests that vascular continuity between the periodontal membrane and bone reservoir is at least a factor in resistance to compressive forces.

Hyperfunction

RELATIONSHIP OF OCCLUSAL
DISHARMONY TO PERIODONTAL
DISEASE

Occlusal stress as an aetiological factor in periodontal disease was first suggested by Karolyi in 1901 [52], and since then hyperfunction has been widely considered to play a major role in the aetiology of periodontal disease. Occlusal forces in excess of physiologic limits produce specific changes in the periodontal membrane, supporting bone and cementum. Changes are produced such as necrosis, haemorrhage, thrombosis, undermining resorption and endosteal and periosteal bone formation [53]. The tissue changes associated with occlusal trauma often have the character of functional adaptation, and it is difficult to assess at what point the trauma assumes pathological significance. The weight of opinion is that in the absence of additional complicating factors, these changes are largely reversible, and that the supporting tissues will repair and reorganize around the tooth in its new position, when the provoking force is removed, or when the tooth has moved to a stable position relative to its environment [27, 54–59].

Muhleman and his co-workers have established that normal occlusal stress causes changes in tooth mobility [60]. According to the same author, in the normal mouth, the diagnosis of occlusal trauma is permitted only if increased tooth mobility decreases after elimination of suspected traumatogenic factors.

The adaptive capacity of the supporting tissues varies between individuals and, to some extent, in the same individual from time to time.

Tooth mobility is a function of:

(1) the degree and duration of the applied stress either in normal or abnormal function,

(2) the total amount of supporting tissue which is present and the length of root which is supported by the alveolus (fig. 14.16),

(3) the position of the axis of rotation of the intra alveolar root portion (fig. 14.16),

(4) the 'biological quality' of the supporting tissues.

In experimental animals, severe nutritional disturbance has led to reduction in the func-

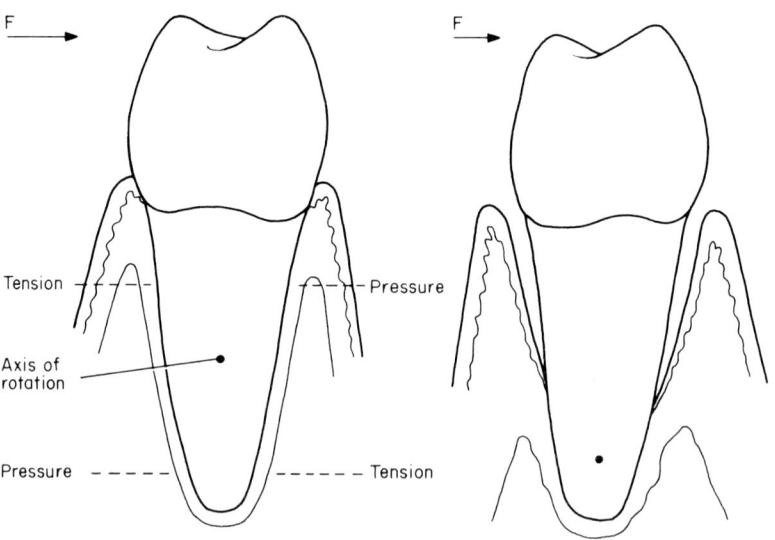

FIG. 14.16. Tooth mobility is related to quantity and quality of tooth support and to the position of the axis of rotation of the intra alveolar part of the root.

tional capacity of the periodontal tissues [61], but as has been stated previously, in general, the turnover of mature collagen in the periodontal membrane is slow and the tissue is not sensitive to changes of systemic origin, unless trauma or injury increases the need for reparative processes. The degree of aggregation of connective tissue is, however, altered by hormonal changes as in pregnancy gingivitis [62, 63 & 64], and by the presence of gingival inflammation [65] (chap. 7). Such changes in the degree of polymerization of the ground substance of connective tissue are reflected as increased tooth mobility. Forces which are within physiologic limits for the healthy periodontium may be hyperfunctional if tissue resistance is reduced in the presence of inflammation of the supporting tissues. Such forces may contribute to further breakdown of the supporting tissues [66 & 67].

In the natural dentition, the concept of occlusal imbalance cannot be regarded in terms of the mechanical ideal, of working and balancing cuspal contacts. It is now widely held that it is acceptable for teeth to have harmonious group function in the working segments only [2 & 68]. It is further accepted that although the adaptive capacity of the neuromuscular system makes it possible for the mandible to adapt its movements to the presence of prematurities or changes in interocclusal relationships [38, 68–71], where it is at all possible cuspal relationships should always allow smooth gliding movements [2]. This principle is of particular importance in the mouth with established periodontal disease, and particularly where there has been gross disorganization and loss of the supporting tissues.

With the multitude of factors involved it is impossible to define precisely at what stage in the progression of periodontal disease occlusal trauma becomes a significant factor [72].

DEFINITION OF OCCLUSAL TRAUMA

Common usage of the term 'occlusal trauma' is inclusive of forces which are capable of causing the microscopic changes described as adaptive changes to physiologic forces. The term 'occlusal trauma' should refer only to a lesion or injury

to the periodontal tissues which is due to abnormal, but not necessarily excessive, occlusal stress. It is convenient to distinguish two forms:

(1) abnormal occlusal stress with anatomically normal supporting tissues—primary occlusal trauma,

(2) normal or abnormal stress in presence of pre-existing gingivitis or periodontitis—secondary occlusal trauma.

Primary occlusal trauma

Studies on experimental animals [56, 73–76] and on humans [59, 77–80] confirm that primary occlusal trauma does not initiate gingival inflammation and pocket formation.

Secondary occlusal trauma

In presence of inflammation of the connective tissues and reduced alveolar support, small forces may assume pathological significance [81].

RELATIONSHIP OF OCCLUSAL TRAUMA TO THE SPREAD OF GINGIVAL INFLAMMATION

Goldman has stated that pocket formation cannot occur without destruction of the supracrestal gingival fibre group [82]. Trauma does not destroy the supracrestal fibres of the marginal ligament, since they are coronal to the alveolar crest and while these are intact, the cuff epithelium cannot proliferate apically along the root surface. In the normal mouth, the effects of primary occlusal trauma are limited to those areas of the periodontium which lie apical to the alveolar crest. Primary occlusal trauma can, by itself, cause migration and transient or permanent loosening of teeth, but it cannot produce gingivitis, pocket formation, apical migration of the epithelial cuff or gingival hyperplasia. As has been previously stated, if teeth are moved a limited distance labially or buccally by physiologic forces, bone is resorbed on the periodontal membrane side of the alveolus, and new bone is deposited on the labial aspect of the alveolar process. If the rate of new bone formation does not match the rate of resorption on the periodontal membrane side, the tooth may move through the labial bone plate causing fenestration or dehiscence (see fig. 15.19). Primary occlusal trauma may lead to dehiscence at the cervical margin, and inflammation may supervene (secondary occlusal trauma) (fig. 14.17).

Where occlusal trauma occurs in presence of pre-existing periodontal disease (secondary occlusal trauma), it may facilitate the deeper spread of the inflammatory process. In 1941, Weineman reported that gingival inflammation follows the course of the blood vessels, directly into the interdental septum of alveolar bone, and labially and lingually to the periosteal side [83]. Only occasionally was inflammation found to extend directly into the periodontal membrane. Later experiments demonstrated that excessive pressure and tension may produce damage to the periodontal tissues, which permits the inflammation to extend directly into the periodontal membrane [84]. These findings have been supported by Glickman and Smulow [67].

The role of occlusal trauma in initiation and subsequent progression of periodontitis has been a matter of dispute for many years. A number of essentially clinical studies have suggested that occlusal trauma is an important factor in causation of pocket formation [81, 85–91]. Other authors have claimed occlusal trauma to be an aggravating factor in existing periodontal disease [27, 57, 67, 84, 92 & 93], and some have been unable to demonstrate any relationship at all [94–97]. Further studies have investigated the effects of experimental occlusal trauma, essentially in the form of tissue reactions, to unilateral forces against individual teeth or groups of teeth in various animals [57, 73, 75, 79, 98–106].

There is general agreement from such studies that unilaterally applied forces like these cause 'temporary pressure areas' characterized by transient vascular thrombosis, disorganization of cells and fibres, resorption of alveolar bone and cementum and loosening of the tooth. After a variable period the tooth moves to a position of stability relative to the resultant of the forces to which it is being subjected and a phase of repair leads to complete re-organization of the supporting tissues around the tooth in its new position.

A lesser number of experiments have studied the effect of reciprocating forces such as occur in the mouth [58 & 105]. As the experimental teeth in these studies were unable to migrate away from the applied force they became permanently hypermobile. The consequent cone-shaped widening of the marginal periodontal space of the side exposed to pressure was considered the main indication of occlusal trauma [93].

It is clearly the consensus of such studies that hyperfunction does not damage the supracrestal tissues, and that the density of the collagen structure of the marginal ligament may be related to the degree of function to which the tooth is subjected.

While it seems equally clear that occlusal forces will not cause irreversible tissue damage in the subcrestal areas of non-inflamed periodontium, the evidence with regard to the role of hyperfunction in dissemination of existing inflammation throughout connective tissue has been conflicting. Data from human autopsy material [67, 92 & 107] and experiments in rats [84] suggest that trauma enhances the spread of gingival inflammation to the deeper tissues. However, occlusal trauma failed to accelerate deepening of the gingival pockets in short-term experiments in monkeys and rats with chronic gingival inflammation [106]. Experiments have been designed [108 & 109] specifically to investigate the effects of induction and mainten-

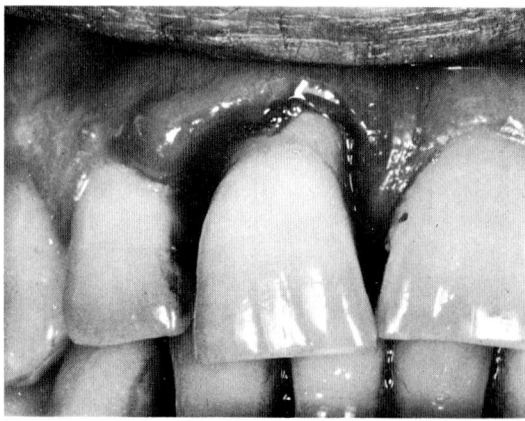

FIG. 14.17. Dehiscence resulting from secondary occlusal trauma.

ance of increased mobility of a single tooth in dogs over a prolonged period of time in the absence and in the presence of gingival inflammation and true pocket formation.

During the pre-experimental period the teeth of all dogs were scaled and polished with a rubber cap and pumice so that at the beginning of the experiment none of the animals had chronic gingivitis as judged from gingival exudate measurements [110]. An occlusal shearing force was applied by means of an onlay which caused premature contact on closing. Forces were also produced by a spring attached to a mandibular lingual bar to act on one lower premolar alternately in a mesial and distal direction. The spring device in the lower jaw prevented the test tooth from moving out of premature occlusion. Radiographs from the 60, 90, and 180 day experiments in this study consistently revealed a cone-shaped widening of the marginal periodontal membrane on the pressure side of the test teeth. Svanberg and Lindhe [108] concluded from this work that '. . . These findings closely resemble the infrabony pockets or angular destructions of the alveolar bone described by Glickman and Smulow [67, 92 & 105] and related to trauma from occlusion. This means that long-term tooth "jiggling" in the dog will result in roentgenologically distinguishable alterations similar to those defined as cardinal signs of traumatizing occlusion'. Pockets were not, however, detected clinically.

The study was extended to investigate the effect of 'jiggling' forces applied by the same apparatus in the presence of surgically induced periodontitis [109]. Pathological pocket formation was induced in beagle dogs by surgical creation of a local osseous defect, prevention of initial reattachment by means of a copper band and promotion of gross plaque formation by application of a non-elastic rubber band around the tooth at the level of the cemento-enamel junction. Radiographs of test tooth regions obtained at necropsy after 6 months of 'jiggling' and continued plaque formation displayed not only advanced horizontal bone loss but also angular or crater-like osseous defects. The bony defects were most pronounced in the pressure areas. The defects in the bone resembled the

lesion frequently described by Glickman and collaborators as the result of trauma from occlusion [111].

Though the plaque index scores and the degree of gingival inflammation of test and control teeth were similar throughout the experimental period, the test teeth showed an apical shift in pocket epithelium which was three times that of the controls [109]. It was concluded from these studies [108 & 109] that any effect of occlusal trauma on the attachment level requires the presence of a plaque induced inflammatory cell lesion in the supra-alveolar connective tissue. Trauma from occlusion appears to accelerate progression of experimental periodontitis in dogs.

This supports the view that hygiene phase control of inflammation should precede occlusal adjustment and reconstruction, since it can be assumed that a traumatized tooth may not be in its normal position [112]. The weight of evidence suggests that secondary occlusal trauma in the presence of pre-existing periodontal disease accelerates the destructive process [41].

Secondary occlusal trauma may be a cause of vertical bone resorption and compound pocket formation [67] (fig. 14.18).

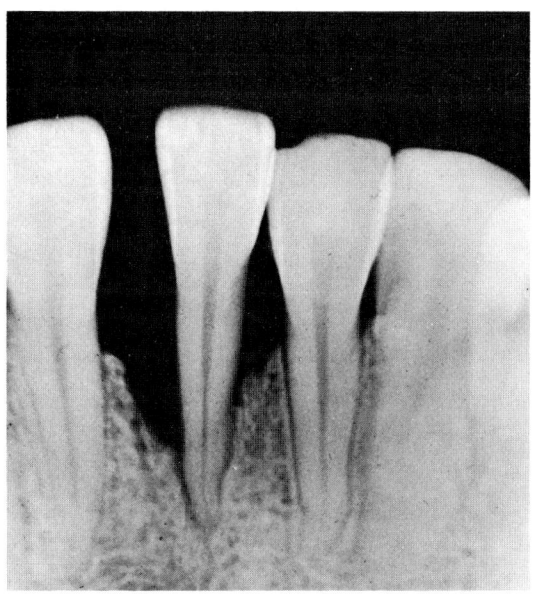

FIG. 14.18. Compound pocket formation associated with occlusal trauma.

Altered occlusal forces leading to periodontal injury do not initiate gingival inflammation, but may change the pathway of inflammation from the gingivae to the supporting periodontal tissues, aggravating the tissue destruction and altering the morphology of the pockets and the pattern of bone destruction [26].

Hypofunction

There is constant reorganization and adaptive change of the periodontal tissues in response to forces applied to the teeth during normal and hyperfunction. Reports in the literature have suggested that when such functional stimulation is reduced, or absent, the periodontal tissues undergo degenerative change (disuse atrophy). Studies have been carried out on both animals [113–117] and humans [107, 118–121]. On the basis of a review of this literature, Anneroth and Ericsson [116] have stated that the present generally accepted view on the changes associated with hypofunction was formulated by Goldman *et al.* [122]:

'If function is greatly decreased over a long period of time, as around teeth having lost their antagonists, the supporting cancellous bone of the alveolar process undergoes atrophy of disuse. Thus one may find only the thin alveolar wall proper, and this may be broken and less compact than normal. The supporting bone may be entirely missing so that only fatty marrow is present. The periodontal ligament is thin and consists principally of indifferent fibres, most of the principal fibres having been lost.'

It has been further stated that in long term hypofunction, there is reduced osteoblastic and cementoblastic activity [47], and that the cribriform plate of the socket is reduced in width. Kronfield, however, reported hyperplasia of cementum of human teeth which had been non-functional for a lengthy period [119]. This was supported by the work of Gottlieb and Orban in man [120], and Anneroth and Ericsson in monkeys [116].

Where the cribriform plate is completely missing, bone marrow may extend into an area previously occupied by periodontal membrane. Even in such areas of replacement of periodontal membrane by bone marrow, the surface of the root is always covered by fibrous connective tissue, and ankylosis does not occur [47]. Henry and Weinmann reported that collagen fibres were relatively few in number and loosely arranged in the periodontal membrane of hypofunctional teeth [121]. Reduction of functionally oriented periodontal membrane fibres, as a result of hypofunction, develops slowly in adults. It has been reported that gingival and alveolar crest fibres of anterior teeth maintain a functional orientation for at least 6 months following loss of opposing teeth [44].

Clinical experience and animal experiment suggest that although disuse atrophy may occur, the tissue response to hypofunction is essentially an adaptive change of the tissues of the periodontium to altered functional need [116 & 123]. It is common clinical experience that over-erupted teeth do not always show increase in the length of the clinical crown which is commensurate with the degree of over-eruption. Studies of hypofunctional teeth in monkeys up to a maximum period of 720 days have demonstrated that the gingival cuff seemed to follow the tooth during over-eruption [116]. There was no evidence of apical proliferation of crevicular epithelium and compensatory formation of new alveolar bone and cementum occurred to support the tooth in its new position.

These findings led Anneroth and Ericsson to conclude: 'The results of the present study indicate a physiological adaptation of the periodontal tissue to the new position and functional conditions of the erupted tooth. No evidence was found that the status of the tooth might decisively be impaired' [116].

Similar studies in rats over a maximum period of 6 months demonstrated compensatory growth of gingival tissue and alveolar bone in association with over-eruption of unopposed molar teeth [123] (fig. 14.19). Such studies confirm the potential for physiologic adaptation of the periodontal tissues to the new tooth position and new functional conditions.

The importance of hypofunctional changes in the supporting tissues is the reduced ability of such tissues to withstand the reapplication of stress if the tooth is restored to function. Although hypofunctional teeth may appear firm, traumatic occlusion will readily develop if such

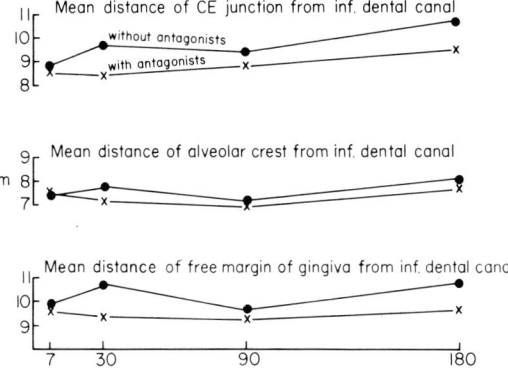

FIG. 14.19. Compensatory growth of gingival tissue and alveolar bone during a period of 6 months, measured in mm on an expanded scale, courtesy of M.K. Basu.

teeth are abruptly restored to function by conservative or prosthetic means. In the absence of pre-existing gingivitis, abrupt restoration of the tooth to function will result in changes in the supporting tissues which have been described as primary occlusal trauma (see above). Such tissue changes are reversible and, over the long term, adaptive change will increase the functional capacity of the hypofunctional tissues, and the tooth may become successfully restored to function within a few months. Where there is a pre-existing gingivitis, this will be exacerbated by restoration of the hypofunctional tooth to normal function and the irreversible tissue changes associated with secondary occlusal trauma may result. Plaque and calculus tend to accumulate around hypofunctional teeth [124], partly as a result of the lack of frictional cleansing whilst chewing food with a particular group of teeth, and partly because the tooth may be tilted or over-erupted so that areas of its surface are isolated from the cleansing action of the lips, cheeks and tongue. Gingivitis in association with hypofunctional teeth is fairly common and tends to be exacerbated if the tooth is abruptly restored to function. Studies by Muhleman have shown that tooth mobility values are higher in areas which have been hypofunctional for many years [125]. This has led to the suggestion that hypofunction may be more detrimental to the periodontal tissues than is hyperfunction.

Parafunction

The interdependence of the individual tissues of the masticatory system has been described in chapter 2. Functional disturbance of the system may result in injury to the periodontium, to the temporomandibular joint or in spasm of the masticatory muscles. Parafunctional habits may condition the rate of progression of periodontitis. Such habits may be performed at a subconscious reflex level and the patient may be unaware of their existence. Habits of significance have been classified by Sorrin into three main groups [126]:

(1) neuroses
(2) Occupational habits
(3) Miscellaneous habits

NEUROSES

Neuroses such as cheek biting and lip biting are quite common and may lead to parafunctional positioning of the mandible. Tongue thrusting and abnormal swallowing habits may lead to anterior open bite or tilting of anterior teeth. The biting of pencils, pens or finger nails may also lead to dysfunction and occlusal trauma. Bruxism, the repetitive or continuous clenching or grinding of the teeth during the night or day is probably the most important habit (see below).

Bruxism

Bruxism has been described as a gnashing or grinding of the teeth for nonfunctional purposes, and more fully as a nonfunctional or involuntary mandibular movement which may occur by day or night, manifested by periodic grinding, crunching or clicking of the teeth [127]. The general tendency to gnash and grind the teeth in association with anger or aggression has been recognized and described for both humans and animals [128]. Comparisons of bruxist and non-bruxist groups of patients have demonstrated that bruxists tend to exhibit a higher level of anxiety as measured by the Cornell Medical Index [129].

Karolyi recognized the role of occlusal interference in addition to psychic factors in the development of bruxism [52]. Occlusal interferences such as a sharp cusp were thought to receive undue attention from neurotic individuals, and to act as trigger areas for grinding habits.

Nonfunctional crunching, grinding or gnashing may occur in centric occlusion or in eccentric positions of the mandible. Bruxism does not necessarily occur in the intercuspal or the retruded position, during sleep it may happen in some eccentric contact position, often an extreme one which the patient can take up only with difficulty when awake. Under these circumstances, many possibilities exist for tooth loading, including loading of a single pair of teeth [130]. It has been proposed that centric bruxism is associated with a prematurity in the region of centric acting as a trigger area, and that eccentric bruxism is associated with a prematurity in eccentric excursions [47].

While greater emphasis has always been placed on the importance of the psychic components [131], it has been shown experimentally, and observed clinically, that occlusal interference may precipitate bruxism. Following a combined clinical and electromyographic study of bruxism in thirty-four adults, Ramfjord concluded that any type of occlusal interference may, when combined with nervous tension, initiate bruxism, and that such bruxism may be eliminated by occlusal adjustment [132]. A large variety of local factors other than occlusal interference may contribute to hypertonicity of the masticatory muscles and initiate abnormal jaw movements. Such conditions are said to be local infection, pericoronitis, periodontal disease, surface irregularities of lips, cheeks and tongue and pain and discomfort in the temporomandibular joint or masticatory muscles. Bruxism may be performed on a subconscious reflex control level, and in the majority of instances, may be unrecognized by the patient unless specifically called to his attention. For this reason, there are no figures as to the prevalence or incidence of bruxism throughout the general population. Boyens found the condition in seventy-eight out of 100 patients and Leof [133] reporting on 171 instances, found 81 per cent of his periodontal patients were so involved [134]. In an extensive electromyographic study of 167 patients, Kraft reported that about half the patients were gnashing their teeth during sleep,

and the others were biting or pressing them together [135]. The forces measured during bruxism do not seem to be excessive and do not seem to differ extremely from the forces applied during mastication [130].

Relationship of bruxism to periodontitis. In the absence of periodontal disease, any of the microscopic tissue changes which have been described in relation to normal function or hyperfunction may be associated with the presence of bruxism. As with other forms of primary hyperfunction, the tissue changes are confined to the tissues apical to the alveolar crest, and it is accepted that bruxism does not initiate gingivitis or pocket formation. The most frequent results of bruxism in a normal mouth are compensatory hypertrophy of the periodontal structures and increase in width of the periodontal membrane.

Where there is pre-existing gingival inflammation, and particularly where there is some loss of tooth support, the weight of evidence suggests that bruxism probably accelerates the destructive process as does any other form of secondary occlusal trauma (see p. 235). The principles of treatment of bruxism are based on the use of flat plane bite splints to redistribute stress, and to prevent any cuspal interference which may act as a trigger area, followed by selective grinding of the dentition to eliminate any occlusal interference.

OCCUPATIONAL HABITS

Thread biting by tailors, hair clip opening by hairdressers (fig. 14.20), and the holding of nails by cobblers and carpenters may all, on occasion, cause damage to the teeth or tissues of the periodontium.

MISCELLANEOUS HABITS

Incorrect teeth cleaning habits, thumb sucking and pipe smoking are all habits which may lead to damage of periodontal tissues.

Occlusal disharmony

THE RESULTS OF TOOTH LOSS

The extraction of a tooth or teeth at any stage

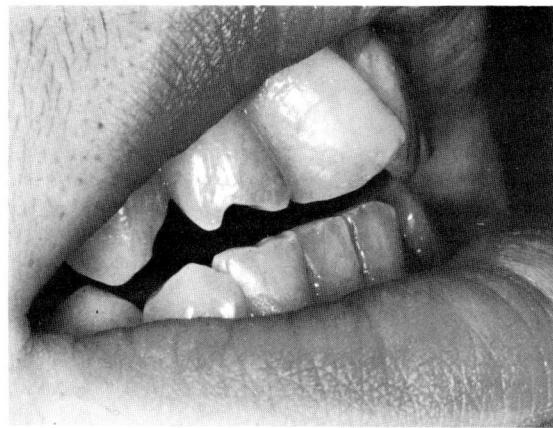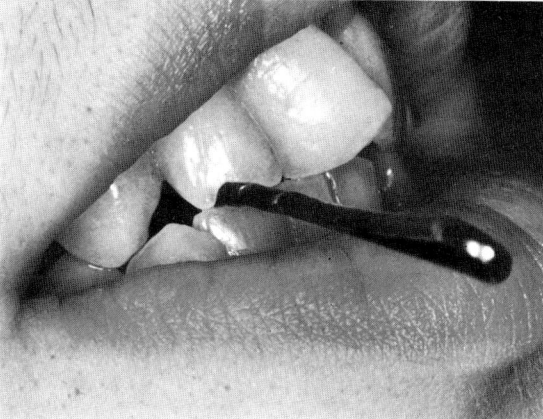

FIG. 14.20. Trauma due to kirby grip biting, courtesy of Dr J.W. Galloway.

during growth and development or thereafter is followed by change in functional relationships of the masticatory system as a whole. The supporting tissues are constantly in a state of dynamic readjustment according to the resultants of the forces applied to the teeth. The position of individual teeth is, in part, determined by the confining influence of adjacent teeth, by occlusal forces and by forces exerted by movement of lips, cheeks and tongue. Following loss of a tooth, there is a period of readjustment during which teeth adjacent to the site of extraction may move, in an attempt to reach a position of stability, relative to the change in environment resulting from the extraction. Such large scale readjustment of tooth relationships commonly follows extraction of deciduous teeth without the subsequent use of space maintaining appliances, or extraction of permanent teeth without replacement by bridges or dentures. In the course of time, these changes may be reflected in areas of the mouth distant from the site of the extraction. The readjustment of functional relationships is not always complete and occlusal disharmony frequently results from casual extraction of teeth. For example, the changes which commonly follow the loss of mandibular first molars are as follows [47 & 136]:

(1) Lingual and mesial tipping of the mandibular second and third molars (fig. 14.21). This may result in the formation of a stagnation area and gingivitis on the lingual and mesial side of

the tipped tooth and, as a result of the excessive mesial leverage on the tooth, a compound pocket may form. The elevated distal cusps of the tilted molars may assume a plunger relationship in the embrasures between the opposing maxillary teeth.

(2) Over-eruption of the unopposed maxillary first molars (fig. 14.22).

(3) Protrusion of the anterior segments of the maxillary arch, with opening of contacts between the mandibular first and second premolars and, possibly, rotation of these teeth.

It is likely that these changes are the result of

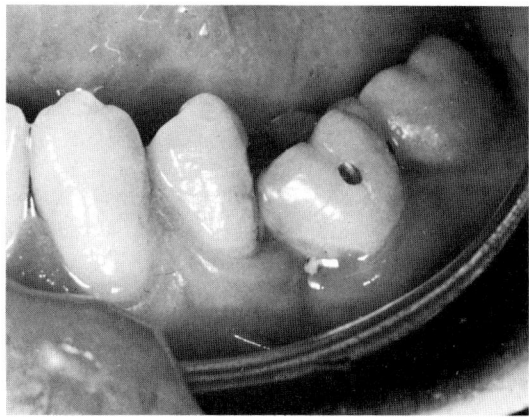

FIG. 14.21. Lingual and mesial tipping of mandibular second and third molars following extraction of first molar.

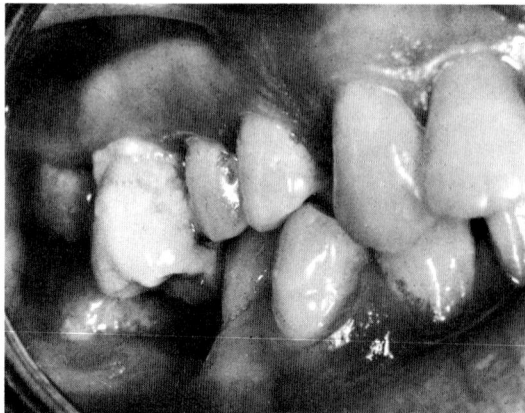

FIG. 14.22. Over-eruption of unopposed maxillary first molar.

a considerable number of factors [47], prominent among which are:

(1) Cuspal deviation in the path of closure between centric relation and centric occlusion, which follows tipping of the posterior teeth. This may result in an increased posteroanterior slide into centric, causing the mandibular incisors to impact on the palatal surface of the maxillary incisors, forcing the incisors forward.

(2) The adjustment of the neuromuscular mechanism which follows the presence of such prematurities in the path of closure may induce a change in masticatory habits, or muscle tonicity, which alters the balance of forces on teeth distant from the site of extraction. Tipping of the mandibular molars may also cause cuspal interference between the disto-buccal cusps of the mandibular molars, and the lingual cusps of the opposing maxillary molars on the non-working side.

The effects of tooth loss are not restricted to areas adjacent to the extraction, change may result in other areas of the mouth. This principle has been emphasized by Thielemann [137].

THIELEMANN'S DIAGONAL LAW

'If an interference such as a hypererupted or tipped tooth, third molar, gum flap, etc, restricts the functional gliding movement of the mandible, elongation of the anterior teeth and often periodontal disease will develop in the anterior region diagonally opposite to the interference.'

'Extrusion of the maxillary anterior teeth will occur only if these teeth do not have a well-defined cingulum or worn-in centric stop on the lingual aspect' [138].

In general, extrusion of anterior teeth is probably caused by the restricted masticatory pattern caused by molar interference. In a proportion of cases, readjustment of tooth relationships following extraction may balance the occlusion such that these changes do not occur. After a period of adjustment during which there is an increased requirement for repair of the supporting tissues, the dentition may again achieve a position of stability relative to the forces to which it is subjected. It is likely that a pre-existing periodontitis would be exacerbated during the period of readjustment, as a result of the increased requirement for repair.

CORRECTION OF OCCLUSAL DISHARMONY

Selective grinding

'Occlusal adjustment of the natural teeth is one of the more common therapeutic measures in dentistry. By the same token, it has been approached with so many variations that confusion and controversy are all too often in evidence. Most investigators concur that pathology is necessary before any occlusal adjustment is performed' [139].

'Assessment of traumatic articulation meets with severe difficulties as there is no agreement as to the criteria of trauma. Stillman's clefts, McCall's festoons (fig. 14.23), increased mobility, various types of bone resorption, increased width of periodontal space, increased thickness of lamina dura, premature contacts have all, in one or the other combination, been taken as criteria of traumatic articulation. However, these clinical manifestations are all, at the same time, symptoms of periodontal disease of bacterial aetiology' [140].

It has been stated that the primary objective of occlusal adjustment is improvement of the functional relationships of the dentition, such that the teeth and the periodontium receive uniform functional stimulation, and the occlusal

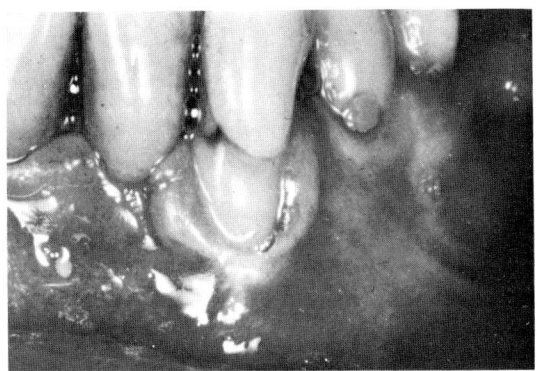

FIG. 14.23. McCall's festoon.

surfaces of the teeth are exposed to even physiologic wear. Unrestricted multidirectional occlusal function is thought to increase the rate of clearance of food from the mouth, and to reduce plaque accumulation and subsequent gingivitis.

Ramfjord has grouped the main indications for occlusal adjustment into the following categories [132]:

(1) the improvement of functional relations and the inducement of physiologic stimulation of the entire masticatory system;

(2) the elimination of traumatic occlusion;

(3) the elimination of abnormal muscle function, bruxism and associated discomfort or pain;

(4) the elimination of dysfunctional temporomandibular joint discomfort or pain;

(5) the establishment of an optimal occlusal pattern prior to extensive restorative procedures;

(6) the re-shaping and contouring of teeth for masticatory efficiency and gingival protection;

(7) the stabilization of orthodontic results;

(8) the reconditioning of some abnormal swallowing habits.

It has been shown that occlusal adjustment may induce multidirectional functional pathways, if the adjustment results in equally convenient and efficient functional relations in the various directions [2]. At the present time, there is considerable variation of opinion as to how this result should be achieved. While the majority of studies suggest that centric relation and centric occlusion are two separate points [41],

it is widely accepted as desirable that the path of closure of the mandible should be such that the translation from centric relation to centric occlusion is made without lateral or anteroposterior slides resulting from cuspal interference, particularly where there is evidence of traumatic occlusion, bruxism, muscle spasm or temporomandibular joint dysfunction.

There is considerable variation in opinion as to the technique of recording centric relation as the starting point for occlusal analysis. The majority of recording devices which have been proposed attempt to relate the mandible to the maxilla in the terminal hinge position, using intra- or extra-oral gothic arch tracings, check bites or plaster registrations [141–146].

Such registrations precede mounting of the related models on an articulator for subsequent analysis. Registration and mounting of models on an articulator by such techniques is a demanding and time consuming procedure, with a large potential error during bite registration and subsequent mounting [147].

'The profession is plagued with hundreds of articulators and the battle waged over these instruments creates confusion and tends to delay progress in occlusal reconstruction ... An articulator, any one, must be considered only as a device that will facilitate the construction of the restorations at the bench in the laboratory. It is not practical to depend primarily upon a particular articulator to determine the patient's mandibular movements.'

'The mouth should have the last word in what is correct and comfortable for the mouth. The operator who, by using the hinge axis recording and time consuming devices, obtains good results in occlusal rehabilitation, should be complimented. By the same token, we should not condemn the operator who obtains equally good results by using less intricate techniques' [148].

While there is no unequivocal evidence in favour of any particular approach, experience suggests that occlusal adjustment is best performed as a clinical procedure, by recording jaw relationships directly via the teeth, and marking initial tooth contact with wax or articulating paper. The presence of models mounted on an articulator may, however, be a valuable supplement to the clinical examination of the dentition.

Recording centric relation

Centric relation may be considered to be the first point of contact between opposing teeth during the terminal hinge phase of the path of closure of the mandible. Taking centric relation as the starting point of occlusal analysis, the initial objective of selective grinding is to achieve a translation from centric relation to centric occlusion, which is a hinge movement, devoid of lateral or antero-posterior slides resulting from cuspal interference. The first essential of accurate recording of centric relation is to obtain the maximum degree of relaxation of the masticatory muscles. This problem is exacerbated where there is muscle spasm present and, according to Ramfjord and Ash, three factors which may induce abnormal muscle tension must be controlled [47]. These factors are psychic or emotional tension, pain in the temporomandibular joints or other parts of the masticatory system, and 'muscle memory' or protective reflex action caused by faulty occlusal contacts [149]. Where the degree of muscle spasm present is marked, it is necessary to use a flat plane bite splint (vide infra) for a short period to free the cuspal guidance and eliminate the muscle spasm. This should be done before any other attempt is made to record centric relation. Ramfjord and Ash have proposed a step by step procedure for recording centric relation which takes these factors into consideration [149].

(1) Seat the patient comfortably in the dental chair with the back rest reclined to about 60–70°, and place the headrest under the occipital ridge so that there is no tension in the neck muscles when the patient rests his head.

(2) Ask the patient to relax his arms and feet.

(3) Have the patient focus his eyes on an object in the line of straight forward vision between 12 and 15 inches away, and have him breathe slowly through his nose.

(4) Ask the patient to open his mouth as far as possible and to hold it open for about 30–60 sec.

(5) Place the right thumb on the patient's mandibular central incisors and the forefinger under the patient's chin. Hold the thumb high enough on the teeth to prevent contact of opposing teeth in case the patient should try to bite together or to swallow.

(6) Speak to the patient in a soft monotonous voice during the entire procedure. Repeat over and over that he should relax his arms and feet and breathe slowly through his nose.

(7) Tell the patient also that you will guide and move his jaw, and reassure him that he is doing very well (regardless of how tense his jaw muscles may be at the time). It is very important that the operator should not cause pain when he starts to move the patient's jaw towards closure. The room should be as quiet as possible and the operator should concentrate all his efforts towards establishing rapport with the patient. This approach obviously includes features of hypnotic induction or relaxation technique.

(8) Guide the patient's jaw first from maximum opening, until the jaw seats back into the most open stationary hinge position. Opening and closing the jaw slightly often helps in obtaining the posterior hinge position. It is important to approach recording of centric relation from wide opening, because muscle orientation and protective reflexes associated with faulty contacts are much less active when the teeth are far apart, than when they come close together.

(9) As soon as the jaw has been placed in the open hinge position, the operator should move the jaw up and down on the arc of stationary hinge closure, gradually bringing the teeth closer together, until the operator's thumbnail strikes the maxillary anterior teeth. If, during these exercises, the patient starts to use his tongue to orient his jaw position by touching both the maxillary and mandibular teeth, he should be told either to place the tongue in the floor of the mouth or against the anterior or middle aspect of the hard palate. Do not have the patient roll the tongue back in the pharynx since this will strain some of the jaw muscles and will have a tendency to bring the condyle down and back from the normal seat in the glenoid fossa.

(10) The operator should gradually move the thumb down on the mandibular incisors while moving the mandible up and down on the path of the stationary hinge axis, or centric relation, until initial contact is established between

mandibular and maxillary teeth. This can easily be felt, and heard, and establishes the patient's initial occlusal contact in centric relation. Once this initial contact has been established correctly, it is much easier to guide the patient back to it in subsequent manipulations.

The most reliable method of marking the initial tooth contact in centric relation is by use of thin sheets of soft bite wax. Strips of wax are heated and placed on the mandibular posterior teeth on both sides. The premature contacts will penetrate the wax as the patient's jaw is manipulated, the wax can then be removed from the mouth, and inspected against a light source. Any perforation in the wax will indicate areas of premature contact.

To examine for a slide into centric occlusion, tap the patient's teeth together in centric relation to the point of initial cusp contact and ask him to complete the act of closure. Where a slide is present, observe the direction of the slide carefully, since a straight forward slide is of less significance than a lateral shift. The teeth that make contact during the slide can usually be marked by carbon paper or traced by wax. The traumatic impact of a slide in centric tends to be much greater upon the teeth engaged at the end of the slide, than on the teeth that provide the pathway for the slide. Protrusion of maxillary anterior teeth may result from an anteroposterior slide into centric, guided on posterior teeth which remain unaffected by the action of the slide.

Examination for occlusal interference in lateral and protrusive excursions

Examination for cuspal interference in lateral and protrusive excursions should be carried out on the basis of bilateral sweeping movements of the mandible, starting from centric occlusion, guided by the operator's hand. If the patient is allowed to freely perform such movements, there is a tendency to follow the acquired path of closure, and the major interference may be avoided. It is desirable to achieve maximum cuspal contact on the working side, and no balancing contacts on the nonworking side. A considerable proportion of patients will show anterior cuspal contact only on the working side

and no effort should be made to increase the area of posterior contact by excessive reduction of anterior teeth. It is further necessary to be sure that grinding of cusps on the working side does not result in the creation of further balancing contacts on the nonworking side.

With regard to protrusive function, it should be accepted that in the great majority of cases, the anterior teeth disengage posterior teeth.

Technique of occlusal adjustment

Grinding teeth to create harmonious functional relationships and simultaneous group contact may be divided into two phases [68]. Firstly, preliminary grinding, which consists of reshaping the teeth and establishing an occlusal plane, and secondly, grinding for the establishment of group function.

PRELIMINARY GRINDING: Reshaping of teeth and establishment of an occlusal plane

(1) reshape malposed, extruded, tilted or rotated teeth,
(2) eliminate any plunger cusps,
(3) establish adequate interdental contact areas,
(4) provide physiologic embrasures,
(5) reshape worn teeth to re-create marginal ridges and assist food shedding,
(6) reduce over-erupted teeth to plane of occlusion,
(7) adjust the length of the clinical crowns of teeth for favourable crown:root ratio.

Grinding to establish centric relation with group contact of teeth

Numerous techniques have been advocated to determine centric relation, such as placing the tongue to the roof of the mouth, or asking the patient to keep his mouth open for a minute or more thus causing the muscles to become tired. Many other methods, including muscle relaxants, have been proposed.

Some clinicians advocate the use of a bite-freeing appliance with a flat occlusal surface for a week or two, to prevent cuspal contact and reduce any tendency for the patient to use an acquired path of closure during occlusal adjustment.

Location of premature contacts in centric relation

As previously described, mandibular closure from rest position to centric relation should not be left to the patient but should be guided by the operator, since proprioceptive signals from the teeth may change during the various stages of occlusal adjustment. Articulating paper, or preferably thin bite registration wax, may be used to determine where premature occlusal contacts occur, and where interfering sliding contacts are located.

Adjustment of centric

The aim of occlusal adjustment for a slide into centric is to eliminate premature contacts, and to stabilize the occlusion by fitting the buccal cusps of the mandibular teeth into the central fossae of the maxillary teeth, and the lingual cusps of the maxillary teeth into the central fossae of the mandibular teeth. This is achieved by grinding any offending cusp inclines such that a seat is ground for the cusps in the central fossae of opposing teeth. Such grinding provides a flat

area of contact between centric relation and centric occlusion. This flat area provides a so-called 'long centric' [150].

Premature contact may prevent occlusal harmony without producing a slide when the patient bites. Such 'high-spots' should be eliminated according to Schuyler's well established principle for adjustment of premature contacts in centric [151].

> *If a cusp is making premature contact in centric and does not make contact in the lateral excursions, the fossa opposite the high cusps should be deepened. Only when the cusp is making a premature contact both in centric and lateral excursions should the cusp height be reduced* (fig. 14.24).

The aim should be group function of the canine, pre-molar and molar teeth. On the balancing side, any contacts must be removed by grinding. An important rule for adjustment of centric is never to leave the impact of the occlusal forces in centric relation or centric occlusion on inclines that may induce tooth

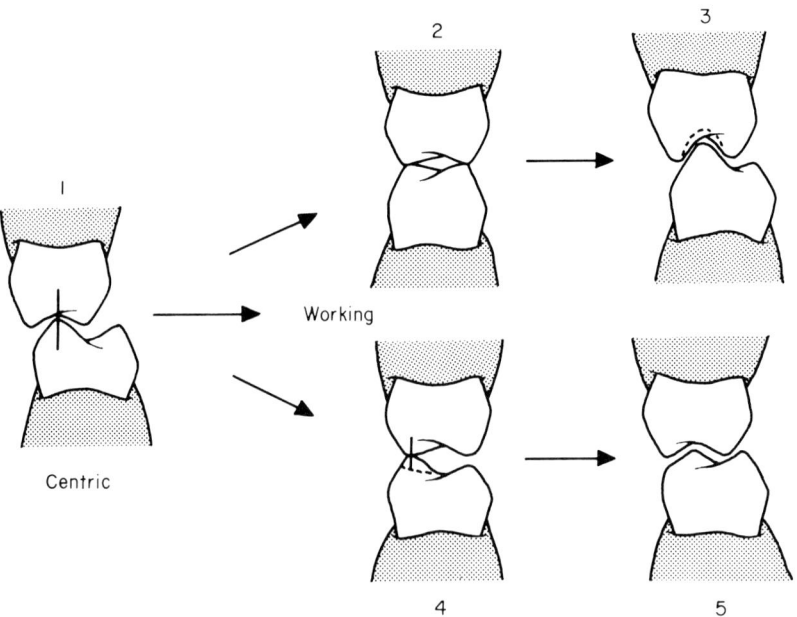

FIG. 14.24. When there is a premature contact (1) in centric check the working bite. If the prematurity is not evident in the working bite (2) grind the fossa opposite the cusp (3). If the prematurity is evident in the working bite (4) reduce the cusp height (5).

movement. If this cannot be achieved, consideration should be given to stabilization of the occlusion by occlusal and marginal restorations, especially in patients with temporomandibular joint dysfunction or bruxism [47].

Adjustment of working side and protrusive interference

The elimination of occlusal interference on the working side during lateral excursion should be done according to Schuyler's 'bull' rule (buccal of upper, lingual of lower). This means grinding the lingual inclines of the buccal cusps of maxillary teeth, and the buccal inclines of the lingual cusps of the mandibular teeth (fig. 14.25). This method of grinding maintains centric contacts, leaves occlusal stability undisturbed, and provides maximal functional contact around centric occlusion. The buccal aspect of the buccal mandibular cusps and lingual aspect of the maxillary lingual cusps should never be ground since such grinding may jeopardize occlusal stability and function in an area where functional contacts are most important.

Interference between the maxillary and mandibular anterior teeth either in lateral or protrusive excursions should be corrected where necessary, by grinding on the lingual aspect of the maxillary anterior teeth along the path of the interference. The grinding should be extended incisally from the point of initial contact in lateral or protrusive excursion, leaving this point itself undisturbed (fig. 14.26). On occasion, there is no functional contact between the maxillary and mandibular anterior teeth. The position of the teeth is then thought to be maintained by tongue or lip habits. If the incisal edges of the mandibular incisors or canines are ground out of contact with the maxillary anterior teeth, these teeth usually erupt back to their previous incisal relationship. No attempt should be made to establish heavy contacts in the posterior regions during protrusive excursions. There is no evidence to suggest that posterior contacts are desirable during protrusion in the natural dentition.

Removal of balancing side contacts

The presence or absence of balancing side contacts can be established by techniques similar to those used for the detection of centric and working side interferences. Balancing side interferences are those which occur between maxillary and mandibular supporting cusps and their occlusal inclines. Since these cusps maintain the position of the teeth, grinding to remove interferences has to be done with care. After centric, lateral and protrusive excursions have been adjusted, the entire field of occlusal function should be examined by letting the patient

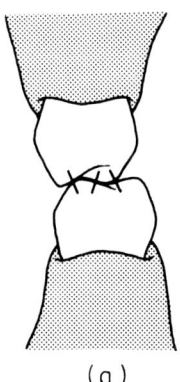 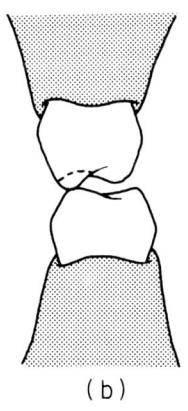 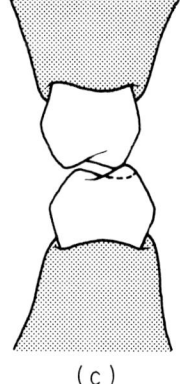

(a)   (b)   (c)

FIG. 14.25. Adjustment of prematurities present in working excursion (bull rule). (a) Ideal centric contact between cusps and opposing inclines of molar teeth. (b) Working excursion prematurity between two buccal cusps. Grind the lingual incline of the maxillary buccal cusp. (c) Working excursion prematurity between two lingual cusps. Grind the buccal incline of the mandibular lingual cusp.

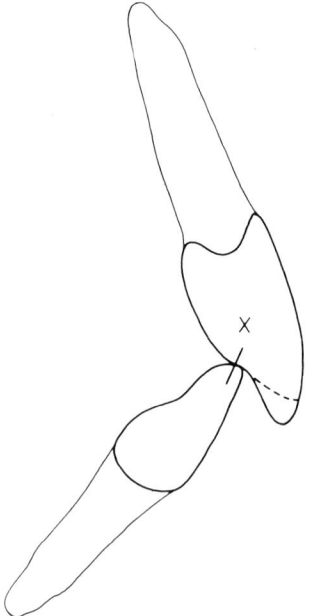

FIG. 14.26. Incisor grinding to correct interference in lateral or protrusive excursion, retaining centric stop (x).

perform occlusal contact movements in various directions. While this is done, the operator should hold his hand on the patient's chin to feel whether all movements are smooth and unstricted. Following the elimination of all premature contacts and occlusal interferences, occlusal surfaces, incisal edges and cusps should be reshaped for optimal functional efficiency and aesthetics. The occlusal anatomy of fillings and teeth can usually be sharpened without loss of centric stops or contacts to protect against food impaction.

After grinding has been completed, it is important to polish all the ground surfaces thoroughly, since any roughness may act as a trigger for bruxism, and it will be more difficult for the patient to keep these areas clean. Such polishing is accomplished by the use of stones, sand paper discs and finally by the use of pumice and fine polishing paste with a rubber cup.

SPLINTS

There is probably no area in dentistry in which treatment procedures are more empirical than when splinting is used for therapeutic purposes [152]. As yet, no research has defined when a splint should be used, the relative efficacy of the different types of splint, or even if a splint is of benefit to the patient [153]. The extreme view is that occlusal trauma neither initiates periodontal disease nor contributes to the further progress of existing periodontal disease [59]. It is more generally held that while the basic treatment of periodontitis is prevention of bacterial deposits, optimal function assists resolution of inflammation of supporting tissues. A large proportion of patients referred for periodontal treatment are those with mutilated occlusions, and advanced periodontal disease, and here it is desirable to bring the teeth under as favourable functional conditions as possible, as a basic principle of treatment.

The theoretical basis for splinting has been described as:

(1) to rest the supporting tissues in accord with the general principle that rest promotes resolution of inflammation;

(2) to redistribute stress to a group of teeth, so that forces act mainly in an axial direction and the force on any single tooth does not exceed the adaptive capacity of its supporting tissues;

(3) to prevent tipping, migration, or over-eruption of teeth following extraction, and to stabilize proximal contacts of mobile teeth and reduce food impaction into the embrasures.

Splints can be classified as either 'temporary' or 'permanent' and as either 'removable' or 'fixed'.

Temporary splints are employed for a limited period of time to aid healing by limiting the mobility of a tooth or teeth and therefore assisting in healing. Temporary splints may also be used as a diagnostic measure to assist in the determination of prognosis of questionable teeth. Ramfjord and Ash have classified splints into (1) 'temporary' (2) 'diagnostic' and (3) 'permanent' [47]. Such splints have also been grouped as either external or internal to the circumference of the tooth.

External splints are placed outside the crown of the teeth, e.g. wire ligature splints; internal splints are fitted or attached inside the circumference of the teeth, e.g. amalgam splints, p. 224, or parallel gold inlay splints.

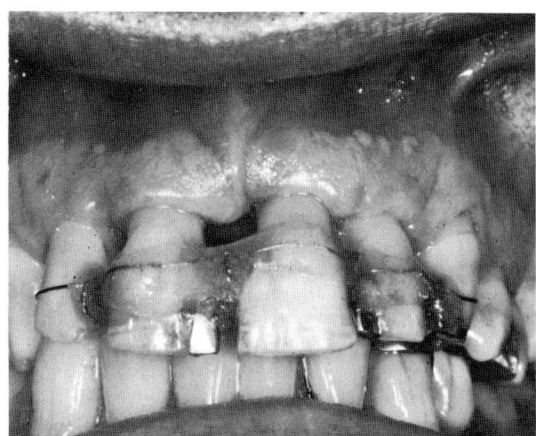

FIG. 14.27. Wire and acrylic splint used to stabilize teeth during periodontal surgery.

Temporary splints

These are usually used over a period of from 1–6 months. The most frequently used temporary splint is a brass or stainless steel wire ligature splint (chap. 8), stabilized with cold curing acrylic resin (fig. 14.27). This is an excellent splint for anterior teeth and provides a high degree of stability. It is acceptable from the aesthetic viewpoint and, if properly constructed, the embrasures are protected from food impaction. This type of splint has largely replaced welded orthodontic bands and wire ligature splints without acrylic, which were commonly used in the past. Direct bonding of composite material after acid etching is now gradually replacing wire and acrylic splints due to ease of fabrication, improved aesthetics and access for cleaning.

Practically all removable temporary splints are modifications of acrylic bite plates used as bite-freeing appliances (fig. 14.28). Splinting action is gained by carrying the acrylic over onto either the labial surface of anterior teeth or the buccal aspect of posterior teeth.

Indications for the use of temporary splints or bite-freeing appliances

(1) Following loosening of teeth by trauma.
(2) To prevent cuspal contact and interlocking in bruxists or patients with temporomandibular joint pain-dysfunction syndrome.

(3) To stabilize teeth during surgical corrective phase therapy of advanced periodontitis.
(4) For stabilization of teeth during comprehensive occlusal reconstruction.

Permanent splints

Permanent splints are constructed to provide stability for teeth that have lost so much support that normal forces act as hyperfunctional forces. Permanent splints are also used for retention of teeth following orthodontic procedures.

All fixed and removable appliances should be designed to increase the stability and function of the dentition as a whole. There are a number of principles to be considered when fixed splints are to be made:
(1) All gingival irritation by the splint must be avoided.
(2) Fixed splints must allow adequate access for oral hygiene.
(3) Abutment teeth must be chosen carefully to provide adequate support and retention for the fixed restoration.

For technical, aesthetic and economic reasons, the minimal number of teeth are usually included to provide the support needed for the splint. This does not always lead to the most desirable type of splint and the decision as to the number of teeth to be included is often based on poorly defined clinical factors. Whenever feasible, pin-ledge preparations or three-quarter crowns should be used for fixed splints (fig. 14.29). The complete coverage type of preparation with subgingival extension is the last choice from the view point of biological acceptability. Full coverage crowns should only be used when unavoidable. Precision attachment connections between various parts of a splint come next to fixed rigid splints in providing stability and controlling the distribution of stress in a dentition. Present day techniques frequently combine splinting with occlusal reconstruction. Fixed retainers are preferable to removable appliances with clasps. The use of the precision attachment brings the forces closer to the axial centre of the tooth when a removable partial denture is necessary.

In two clinical trials, the effect of removable splints (fig. 14.30), on mobility was investigated.

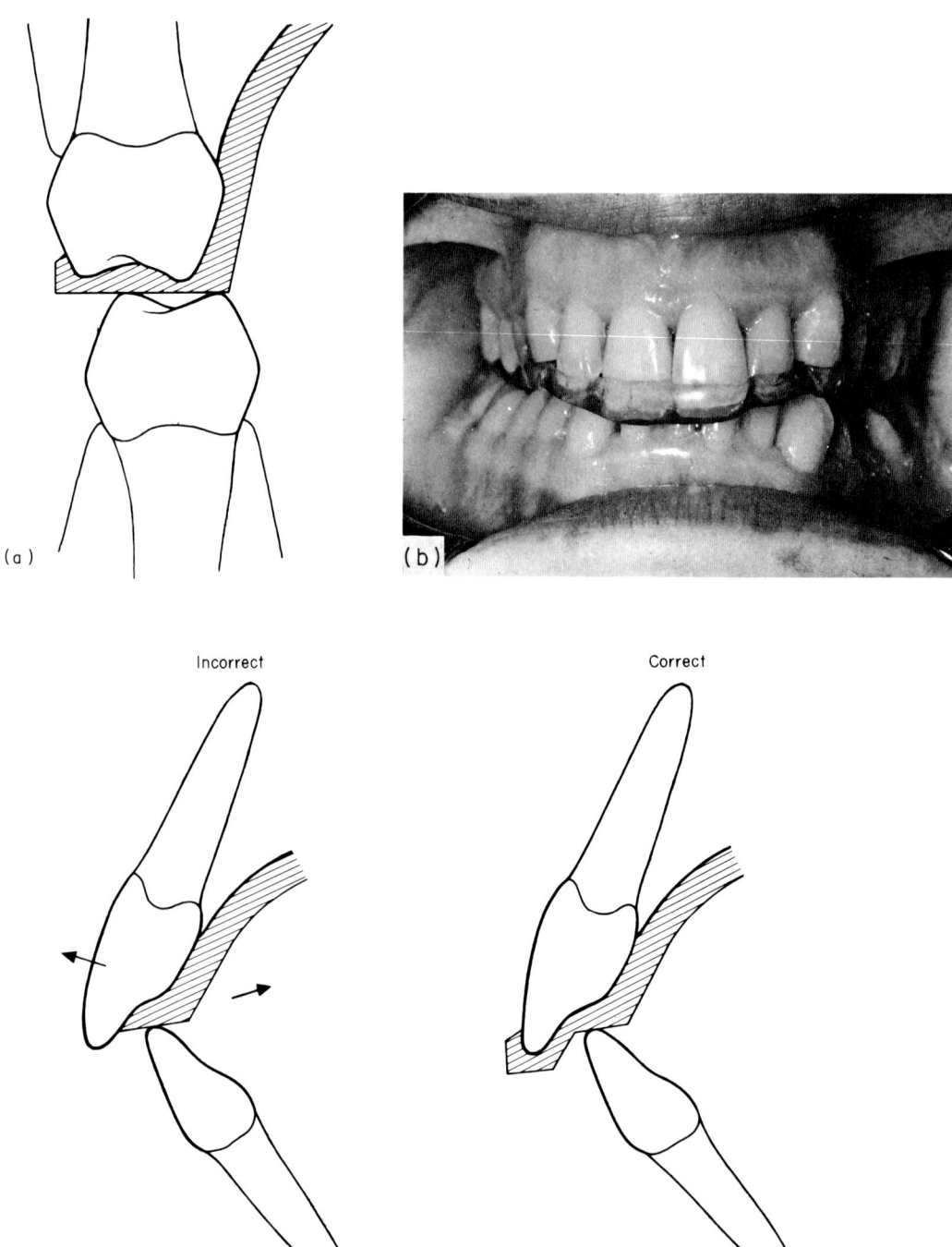

FIG. 14.28. (a) Flat plane splint. (b) With incisor edge cover. (c) Sved splint. Correct and incorrect design. Incisor edge cover prevents displacement of appliance of teeth.

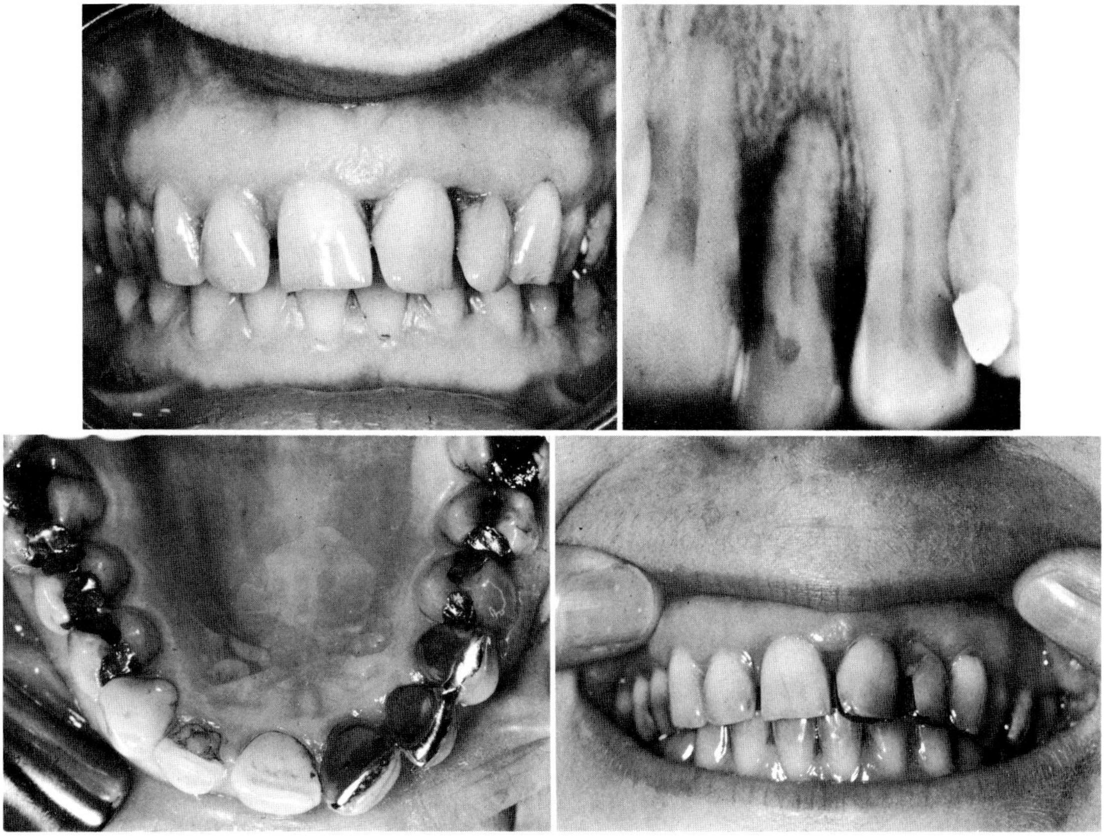

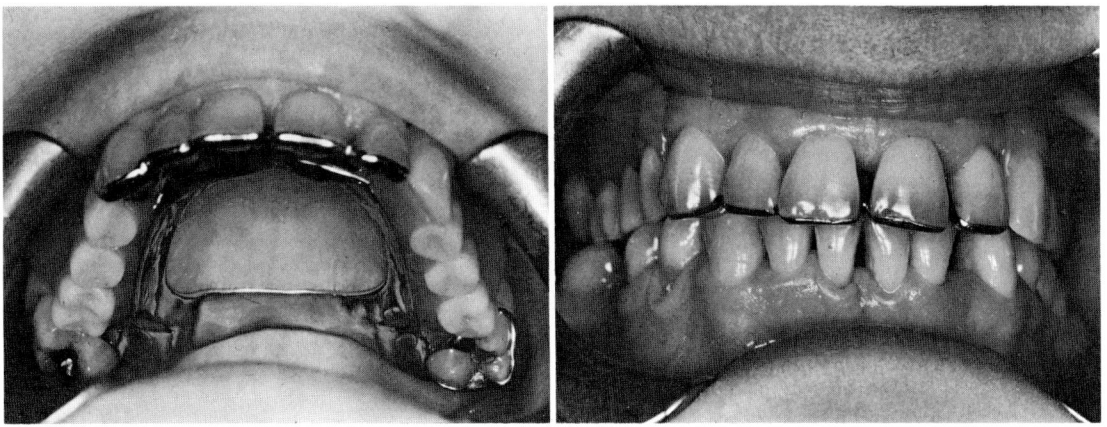

FIG. 14.29. Lateral incisor splinted by parallel three quarter crowns prior to surgery, courtesy of Professor G.S. Beagrie.

FIG. 14.30. Chrome cobalt removable periodontal splint with incisor edge cover.

Instead of reducing mobility, splinting led to increased mobility as compared with patients who received ordinary local hygiene treatment [154 & 155]. The results of such studies indicate that removable splints can cause an increased mobility of about 15 per cent during long term use.

Disadvantages of splinting teeth

The disadvantages of splinting may be broadly grouped as hygienic, biological or mechanical. All splints have a tendency to interfere with patient self-care, and the self-cleansing action of teeth and gingival tissues. Whenever splints contact the gingivae, it is almost impossible to avoid irritation of a mechanical nature. If bacterial deposits also form, persistent inflammation is likely to ensue. This is of great importance in a patient with a high susceptibility to periodontitis; unfortunately it is this type of patient whose need is greatest for periodontal splinting.

A study by Glickman, Stein and Smulow reported the influences of increased occlusal forces on the periodontium of monkeys both when the teeth were splinted and when they were not [156]. The authors stressed that the study did not allow definite conclusions to be drawn regarding the benefits or shortcomings of fixed splints, but suggested that the inclusion of a tooth in a fixed splint does not necessarily shield it from the risk of injury by occlusal forces. Even splinted teeth which were not in occlusal contact did not escape injury, when only one member of the splint was traumatized. When one of the teeth in a splint is subjected to excessive occlusal force, the remaining teeth share the load.

Nabers has reported that night-guard appliances can open interproximal contacts between teeth [157], and Saturen has reported that wire ligatures are an undesirable form of temporary splinting because they induce active forces on the ligated teeth, causing them to be moved into new positions [158].

Extensive caries may develop under loose abutments and gross sepsis may follow with minimal symptoms. It is therefore imperative that all splints be inspected regularly.

Since splints have many disadvantages accompanying their obvious stabilizing advantages, splinting of teeth should be restricted to the minimum needed to achieve occlusal stability and adequate masticatory function. Splints should never be used as a substitute for accuracy and exactness in occlusal therapy of the individual teeth [47].

REFERENCES

[1] HELLGREN A. (1954) On the relationship between some occlusal characteristics and periodontal disease. *Europ. orthodont. Soc. Trans.* 221–234.

[2] BEYRON H.L. (1954) Characteristics of functionally optimal occlusion and principles of occlusal rehabilitation. *J. Amer. dent. Ass.* **45**, 648–656.

[3] CROSS W.G. (1958) Co-report: local etiological factors in periodontal diseases. *Int. dent. J.* **8**, 333–335.

[4] BEAGRIE G.S. & JAMES G.A. (1962) The association of posterior tooth irregularity and periodontal disease. *Brit. dent. J.* **113**, 239–242.

[5] KOHL J.T. & ZANDER H.A. (1961) Morphology of interdental gingival tissues. *Oral Surg.* **14**, 287–295.

[6] HAZEN S.P. & OSBORNE J.W. (1967) Relationship of operative dentistry to periodontal health. *Dent. Clin. N. Amer.* **March**, 245–254.

[7] LLOYD R.S. & BAER P.N. (1959) Permanent fixed amalgam splint. *J. Periodont.* **30**, 163–165.

[8] OBIN J.N. & ARVINS A.N. (1951) The use of self-curing resin splints for the temporary stabilization of mobile teeth due to periodontal involvement. *J. Amer. dent. Assn.* **42**, 320–322.

[9] AMSTERDAM M. & FOX L. (1959) Provisional splinting principles and techniques. *Dent. Clin. N. Amer.* **March**, 73–99.

[10] HERLANDS R.E., LUCCA J.J. & MORRIS M.L. (1962) Full coverage in occlusal reconstruction. *Dent. Clin. N. Amer.* **March**, 147–162.

[11] WHEELER R.C. (1958) *A Textbook of Dental Anatomy and Physiology*, 3rd Edition. Philadelphia: Saunders.

[12] WHEELER R.C. (1961) Complete crown form and the periodontium. *J. prosth. Dent.* **11**, 722–734.

[13] TYLMA S.D. (1960) *Theory and Practice of Crown and Bridge Prosthodontics*, 4th Edition, p. 124. St. Louis, Mosby.

[14] KAHN A.E. (1960) Partial versus full coverage. *J. prosth. Dent.* **10**, 167–178.

[15] DAVIS W.C. (1945) *Operative Dentistry*, 4th Edition, p. 61. London: Kimpton.

[16] McGEHEE W.H.O. (1948) *A Textbook of Operative Dentistry*, 2nd Edition. London: Churchill.

[17] WAERHAUG J. (1956) Effect of rough surfaces upon gingival tissue. *J. dent. Res.* **35**, 323–325.

[18] WAERHAUG J. (1956) Effect of zinc phosphate cement fillings on gingival tissues. *J. periodont.* **27**, 284–290.

[19] WAERHAUG J. (1960) Histologic considerations which govern where the margins of restorations should be located in relation to the gingiva. *Dent. Clin. N. Amer.* **March**, 161–176.

[20] ZANDER H. (1957) Effect of silicate cement and amalgam on the gingiva. *J. Amer. dent. Ass.* **55**, 11–15.

[21] ZANDER H. (1958) Tissue reaction to dental calculus and to filling materials. *J. dent. Med.* **13**, 101–104.

[22] WAERHAUG J. (1956) Observations on replanted teeth plated with gold foil. *Oral Surg.* **9**, 780–791.

[23] WAERHAUG J. & LOE H. (1958) Tissue reaction to self-curing acrylic resin implants. *Dent. practit. dent. Rec.* **8**, 234–240.

[24] WAERHAUG J. & ZANDER H. (1957) Reaction of gingival tissues to self-curing acrylic restoration. *J. Amer. dent. Ass.* **54**, 760–768.

[25] LIDDELOW K.P. (1956) The simple all-acrylic partial denture. *Brit. dent. J.* **101**, 411–428.

[26] RAMFJORD S.P., KERR D.A. & ASH M. (eds) (1966) *World Workshop in Periodontics*. Ann Arbor: Michigan.

[27] POSSELT U. & EMSLIE R.D. (1959) Occlusal disharmonies and their effect on periodontal disease. *Int. dent. J.* **9**, 367–381.

[28] AHLGREN J. & POSSELT U. (1963) Need of functional analysis and selective grinding in orthodontics. A clinical and electromyographic study. *Acta odont. scand.* **21**, 187–226.

[29] LAURITZEN A.G. (1951) Function, prime object of restorative dentistry, a definite procedure to obtain it. *J. Amer. dent. Ass.* **42**, 523–534.

[30] PARFITT G.I. (1960) Occlusal adjustment during periodontal therapy. Is it always necessary to equilibrate the teeth during periodontal treatment? *Dent. Clin. N. Amer.* **Nov.** 687–692.

[31] POSSELT U. (1962) *The Physiology of Occlusion and Rehabilitation*, Oxford: Blackwell Scientific Publications.

[32] SCHUYLER C.H. (1961) Factors contributing to traumatic occlusion. *J. prosth. Dent.* **11**, 708–715.

[33] GRANT D., STERN I.B. & EVERETT F.G. (eds.) (1963) *Orban's Periodontics*, 2nd Edition, St. Louis: Mosby.

[34] YUODELIS R.A. & MANN W.V. (1965) The prevalence and possible role of non-working contacts in periodontal disease. *Periodontics* **3**, 219–223.

[35] RAMFJORD S.P. & ASH M. Jr. (1966) *Occlusion*, 1st Edition, p. 62. Philadelphia: Saunders.

[36] BALLARD C.F. (1955) Consideration of the physiological background of mandibular posture and movement. *Dent. practit. dent. Rec.* **6**, 80–89.

[37] ORBAN B. & WENTZ F.M. (1954) Operative dentistry and the supporting dental structures. *Illinois dent. J.* **23**, 717–721.

[38] BRILL N. (1957) Reflexes, registration and prosthetic therapy. *J. prosth. Dent.* **7**, 341–360.

[39] PRITCHARD J.F. (1965) *Advanced Periodontal Disease: Surgical and Prosthetic Management*. Philadelphia: Saunders.

[40] MOYERS R.E. (1963) *Handbook of Orthodontics*, 2nd Edition. Chicago: Year Book Medical Publishers.

[41] BHASKER S.N. & FRISCH J. (1967) Occlusion and periodontal disease. *Int. dent. J.* **17**, 251–266.

[42] FRISCH J. Unpublished work cited in BHASKER S.N. & FRISCH J. (1967) Occlusion and periodontal disease. *Int. dent. J.* **17**, 251–266.

[43] RAMFJORD S.P. & ASH M. Jr. (1966) *Occlusion*. 1st Edition, p. 83. Philadelphia: Saunders.

[44] RAMFJORD S.P. & KOHLER C.A. (1959) Periodontal reaction to functional ecclusal stress. *J. Periodont.* **30**, 95–112.

[45] GUSTAFSON A.G. & PERSSON P. (1957) The relationship between the direction of Sharpey's fibres and the deposition of cementum. *Odont. T.* **65**, 457–463.

[46] CASTELLI W.A. & DEMPSTER W.T. (1965) The periodontal vasculature and its responses to experimental pressures. *J. Amer. dent. Ass.* **70**, 890–905.

[47] RAMFJORD S.P. & ASH M. (1966) *Occlusion*, 1st Edition. Philadelphia: Saunders.

[48] COOLIDGE E.D.J. (1937) The thickness of the human periodontal membrane. *Amer. dent. Ass. J. & Dent. Cosmos*, **24**, 1260–1270.

[49] BOYLE P.E. (1938) Tooth suspension: A comparative study—paradental tissues of men and of the guinea pig. *J. dent. Res.* **17**, 37–45.

[50] BOYLE P.E. (1955) *Kronfields Histopathology of Teeth*, 4th Edition. Philadelphia: Lea & Febiger.

[51] PARFITT G.J. (1967) The physical analysis of the tooth-supporting structures, in *The Mechanisms of Tooth Support*, A symposium, pp. 154–156. Bristol: Wright.

[52] KAROLYI M. (1901) Beobachtungen über pyorrhea alveolaris. *Öst. Vjschr. Zahnheilk.* **17**, 279.

[53] GRUPE H.E. (1964) Consideration of secondary occlusal trauma in the use of periodontally involved teeth in partial denture prosthesis. *Dent. Clin. N. Amer.* **March**, 175–181.

[54] BHASKAR S.N. & ORBAN B. (1955) Experimental occlusal trauma. *J. Periodont.* **26**, 270–284.

[55] GLICKMAN I. & WEISS L. (1955) Role of trauma from occlusion in initiation of periodontal pocket formation in experimental animals. *J. Periodont.* **26**, 14–20.

[56] STAHL S.S., MILLER S.C. & GOLDSMITH E.D. (1957) Effects of vertical occlusal trauma on the periodontium of protein deprived young adult rats. *J. Periodont.* **28**, 87–97.

[57] WAERHAUG J. (1955) Pathogenesis of pocket formation in traumatic occlusion. *J. Periodont.* **26**, 107–118.

[58] WENTZ F.M., JARABAK J. & ORBAN B. (1958) Experimental occlusal trauma initiating cuspal interferences. *J. Periodont.* **29**, 117–127.

[59] LOVDAL A., SCHEIL O., WAERHAUG J. & ARNO A. (1959) Tooth mobility and alveolar bone resorption as a function of occlusal stress and oral hygiene. *Acta. odont. scand.* **17**, 61–77.

[60] MÜHLEMAN H.R., HIRT H. & HERZOG H. (1955) Tooth mobility—bruxism selective grinding. *Transactions of the 14th A.R.P.A. Congress*, Venice.

[61] WAERHAUG J. (1958) Effect of C-avitaminosis on the supporting structures of the teeth. *J. Periodont.* **29**, 87–97.

[62] LÖE H. & SILNESS J. (1963) Periodontal disease in pregnancy: 1. Prevalence and Severity. *Acta. odont. scand.* **21**, 532–551.

[63] LÖE H. & SILNESS J. (1964) Periodontal disease in pregnancy ii. Correlation between oral hygiene and periodontal condition. *Acta odont. scand.* **22**, 121–135.

[64] MÜHLEMAN H.R. (1951) Periodontometry, a method for measuring tooth mobility. *Oral Surg.* **4**, 1220–1233.

[65] GERSH I. & CATCHPOLE H.R. (1960) The nature of ground substance of connective tissue. *Perspect. Biol. Med.* **3**, 282–319.

[66] GLICKMAN I. (1963) Inflammation and trauma from occlusion, co-destructive factors in chronic periodontal disease. *J. Periodont.* **34**, 5–10.

[67] GLICKMAN I. & SMULOW J.B. (1962) Alterations in the pathway of gingival inflammation into the underlying tissues induced by excessive occlusal forces. *J. Periodont.* **33**, 7–13.

[68] GOLDMAN H.M., SCHLUGER S., COHEN D.W., CHAIKIN B.S. & FOX L. (Eds.) (1966) *An Introduction to Periodontia*, 3rd Edition. St. Louis: Mosby.

[69] WALSH J.P. (1951) Neurophysiological aspects of mastication. *Aust. dent. J.* **23**, 49–62.

[70] SICHER H. (1956) The biologic significance of hinge axis determination. *J. prosth. Dent.* **6**, 616–620.

[71] PERRY H.T. (1957) Muscular changes associated with temporomandibular joint dysfunction. *J. Amer. dent. Ass.* **54**, 644–653.

[72] MÜHLEMAN H.R., HERZOG H. & VOGEL A. (1956) Occlusal trauma and tooth mobility. *Schweiz. Mschr. Zahnheilk.* **66**, 527.

[73] BHASKAR S.N. & ORBAN B. (1955) Experimental occlusal trauma. *J. Periodont.* **26**, 270–284.

[74] WAERHAUG J. (1955) Pathogenesis of pocket formation in traumatic occlusion. *J. Periodont.* **26**, 107–118.

[75] GLICKMAN I. & WEISS L.A. (1955) Role of trauma from occlusion in initiation of periodontal pocket formation in experimental animals. *J. Periodont.* **26**, 14–20.

[76] STAHL S.S., JOLY O. & GOLDSMITH E.D. (1961) Adaptation of periodontal tissues to combined insults. *Dent. Progr.* **1**, 121–125.

[77] ORBAN B. (1928) Tissue changes in traumatic occlusion. *J. Amer. dent. Ass.* **15**, 2090.

[78] ORBAN B. & WEINMANN J.P. (1933) Signs of traumatic occlusion in average human jaws. *J. dent. Res.* **13**, 216.

[79] MÜHLEMAN H.R. & HERZOG H. (1961) Tooth mobility and microscopic tissue changes produced by experimental occlusal trauma. *Helv. odont. Acta.* **5**, 33–39.

[80] PRITCHARD J., SIMON P. & LORIMER J.W. (1958) Periodontal prosthesis in occlusal trauma. *J. Periodont.* **29**, 131–136.

[81] BOX H.K. (1928) *Treatment of the Periodontal Pocket*. Toronto: University of Toronto Press.

[82] GOLDMAN H.M. (1944) The relation of the epithelial attachment to the adjacent fibres of the periodontal membrane. *J. dent. Res.* **23**, 177–180.

[83] WEINMAN J.P. (1941) Progress of gingival inflammation into the supporting structures of the teeth. *J. Periodont.* **12**, 71–81.

[84] MACAPANPAN I.C. & WEINMAN J.P. (1954) Influence of injury to the periodontal membrane on the spread of gingival inflammation. *J. dent. Res.* **33**, 263–272.

[85] STONES H.H. (1938) An experimental investigation into the association of traumatic occlusion with parodontal disease. *Proc. Roy. Soc. Med.* **31**, 179.

[86] McCALL J.O. (1939) Traumatic occlusion. *J. Amer. dent. Ass.* **26**, 519.

[87] McLEAN D.W. (1939) Diagnosis and correction of occlusal deformities prior to restorative procedures. *J. Amer. dent. Ass.* **26**, 928.

[88] LEONARD J.J. (1943) Occlusal factor in periodontal disease. *J. Periodont.* **14**, 12.

[89] GRATZINGER M. (1948) Dynamic irritation as a cause of periodontal disease. *J. Amer. dent. Ass.* **37**, 294.

[90] McCALLUM B.B. (1950) In our opinion. *J. Amer. dent. Ass.* **21**, 116.

[91] WAUGHAM O.B. (1951) Functional analysis of occlusion as it relates to periodontal conditions. *North W. Univ. Bull dent. Res.* **52**, 18.

[92] GLICKMAN I. & SMULOW J.B. (1965) Effect of excessive occlusal forces upon the pathway of gingival inflammation in humans. *J. Periodont.* **36**, 141.

[93] GLICKMAN I. (1965) Clinical significance of trauma from occlusion. *J. Amer. dent. Ass.* **70**, 607.

[94] LOVDAL A. *et al.* (1959) Tooth mobility and alveolar bone resorption as a function of occlusal stress and oral hygiene. *Acta odont. scand.* **17**, 61.

[95] BELTING C.M. & GUPTA O.P. (1961) The influence of psychiatric disturbances on the severity of periodontal disease. *J. Periodont.* **32**, 219.

[96] BAER P. *et al.* (1963) Alveolar bone loss and occlusal wear. *Periodontics.* **1**, 91.

[97] KNOWLES J.W. (1967) Occlusal interferences and loss of periodontal attachment. *I.A.D.R. Abstract No. 517,* 45th meeting, 1967.

[98] BOX H.K. (1935) Experimental traumatogenic occlusion in sheep. *Oral Health* **25**, 9.

[99] HAUPL K. & PSANSKY R. (1938) Histologische Untersuchungen der Wirkungsweise der in der Funktions Kiefer-Orthopaedie verwendeten Apparate. *Dtsch. Zahn-, Mund-u, Kieferheilk.*, **5**, 214.

[100] OPPENHEIM A. (1942) Human tissue response to orthodontic intervention of short and long duration. *Amer. J. Orht. & Oral Surg.* **28**, 263.

[101] REITAN K. (1951) The initial tissue reaction incident to orthodontic tooth movement as related to the influence of function. *Acta odont. scand.* **9**, Suppl. 6.

[102] ZANDER H.A. & MUHLEMANN H.R. (1956) The effect of stresses on periodontal structures. *Oral Surg.* **9**, 380.

[103] RAMFJORD S.P. & KOHLER D.A. (1959) Periodontal reaction to functional occlusal stress. **30**, 95.

[104] EWEN S.J. & STAHL S.S. (1962) The response of the periodontium to chronic gingival irritation and long-term tilting forces in adult dogs. *Oral Surg.* **15**, 1426.

[105] GLICKMAN I. & SMULOW J.B. (1968) Adaptive alterations in the periodontium of the Rhesus monkey in

chronic trauma from occlusion. *J. Periodont.* **39**, 101.

[106] COMAR M.D. *et al.* (1969) Local irritation and occlusal trauma as co-factors in the periodontal disease process. *J. Periodont.* **40**, 193.

[107] REICHBORN-KJENNERUD I. (1948) *Marginale Paradentitter.* Groteborg: Elanders Boktryckeri.

[108] SVANBERG G. & LINDHE J. (1973) Experimental tooth hypermobility in the dog. A methodological study. *Odont. Rev.* **24**, 269.

[109] LINDHE J. & SVANBERG G. (1974) Influence of trauma from occlusion in progression of experimental periodontitis in the beagle dog. *J. clin. Periodont.* **1**, 3–14.

[110] LÖE H. & HOLM-PEDERSEN R. (1965) Absence and presence of fluid from normal and inflamed gingiva. *Periodontics* **3**, 171.

[111] GLICKMAN I. (1967) Occlusion and the periodontium. *J. dent. Res. Suppl.* **1**, 53.

[112] COCKLER L.G. & LAINEY W.R. (1963) *Partial Dentures*, 3rd Edition. St. Louis: Mosby.

[113] PREISSECKER O. (1931) Beeinflussung des periodontiums durch experimentelle Enttastung. *Z. Stomat.* **29**, 442.

[114] ANDERSON B.G., SMITH A.H., ARNHIM S.S. & ORTEN A.U. (1936) Changes in molar teeth and their support-structures of rats following extraction of the upper right first and second molars. *Yale J. Biol. Med.* **9**, 189.

[115] GLICKMAN I. (1945) The effect of acute starvation upon the apposition of alveolar bone associated with the extraction of functional antagonists. *J. dent. Res.* **24**, 155–160.

[116] ANNEROTH G. & ERICSSON S.G. (1967) An experimental histological study of monkey teeth without antagonist. *Odont. Revy.* **18**, 345–359.

[117] COHN S.A. (1965) Disuse atrophy of the periodontium in mice. *Archs. Biol.* **10**, 909.

[118] REICHBORN-KJENNERUD I. (1936) Om cementdannelse under fysiologiske og patologiske fonhold. *Den Norske Tand Tidende*, **8**, 341.

[119] KRONFIELD R. (1938) The biology of Cementum. *J. Amer. dent. Ass.* **25**, 1451–1461.

[120] GOTTLIEB B. & ORBAN B. (1936) *Zahnfleischentzündung und Zahnlockerung.* Berlin: Berlinische Verlagsanstalt.

[121] HENRY J.L. & WEINMANN J.P. (1951) The pattern of resorption and repair of human cementum. *J. Amer. dent. Ass.* **42**, 270–290.

[122] GOLDMAN H.M., SCHLUGER S., FOX L. & COHEN D.W. (1964) *Periodontal Therapy*, 3rd Edition, p. 158. St. Louis: Mosby.

[123] BASU M.K. (1968) Personal Communication.

[124] EAER P.N. & WHITE C.L. (1966) Studies on experimental calculus formation in the rat—Effect of function. *J. Periodont.* **37**, 34–35.

[125] MUHLEMAN H.R., HERZOG H. & RATEITSCHAK K.H. (1957) Quantitative evaluation of the therapeutic effect of selective grinding. *J. Periodont.* **28**, 11–16.

[126] SORRIN S. (1935) Habit: An etiologic factor in periodontal disease. *Dent. Dig.* **41**, 290–297.

[127] NADLER S.C. (1966) The effects of bruxism. *J. Periodont.* **37**, 311–319.

[128] NADLER S.C. (1957) Bruxism: a classification, a critical review. *J. Amer. dent. Ass.* **54**, 615–622.

[129] THALLER J.L., ROSEN G. & SALTZMAN S. (1967) Study of the relationship of frustration and anxiety to bruxism. *J. Periodont.* **38**, 193–197.

[130] RAMFJORD S.P., KERR D.A. & ASH M. (eds) (1966) *World Workshop in Periodontics*, p. 234. Ann Arbor: Michigan.

[131] LANDER J.F. (1956) Psychosomatics in relation to periodontus. *J. Periodont.* **27**, 209–215.

[132] RAMFJORD S.P. (1961) Bruxism, a clinical and electromyographic study. *J. Amer. dent. Ass.* **62**, 21–44.

[133] BOYENS P.J. (1940) Value of autosuggestion in the therapy of 'bruxism' and other biting habits. *J. Amer. Dent. Ass.* **27**, 1173–1777.

[134] LEOF M. (1944) Clamping and grinding habits, their relation to periodontal disease. *J. Amer. Dent. Ass.* **31**, 184–194.

[135] KRAFT E. (1960) Cited in *Occlusion*, p. 103. Eds. RAMFJORD S.P. & ASH M. (1966) Philadelphia: Saunders.

[136] HIRSCHFELD I. (1937) The individual missing tooth: a factor in dental and periodontal disease. *J. Amer. Dent. Ass.* **24**, 67–82.

[137] THIELEMANN K. (1938) *Biomechanik der Paradentose.* Leipzig: Herman Meusser.

[138] RAMFJORD S.P. & ASH M. (1966) *Occlusion*, 1st Edition, p. 119. Philadelphia: Saunders.

[139] RAMFJORD S.P., KERR D.A. & ASH M. (eds) (1966) *World Workshop in Periodontics*, p. 361. Ann Arbor: Michigan.

[140] RAMFJORD S.P., KERR D.A. & ASH M. (eds) (1966) *World Workshop in Periodontics*, p. 199. Ann Arbor: Michigan.

[141] YURKSTAS A. & KAPUR K.K. (1957) Evaluation of centric relation records obtained by various techniques. *J. Prosth. Dent.* **7**, 770–786.

[142] KURTH L.E. (1938) Occlusion in dentistry. *J. Amer. dent. Ass.* **25**, 1067–1070.

[143] LAURITZEN A.G. (1951) Function, prime object of restorative dentistry; a definite procedure to obtain it. *J. Amer. Dent. Ass.* **42**, 523–534.

[144] POSSELT U. & ADDIEGO B.J. (1958) A gnatho-thesiometric study of various mandibular positions in individuals with normal and abnormal function of the temporomandibular joints. *Odont. Revy.* **9**, 1–9.

[145] BOOS R.H. (1940) Intermaxillary relation established by biting power. *J. Amer. Dent. Ass.* **27**, 1192–1199.

[146] STEWART C. & STALLARD H. (1957) Diagnosis in treatment of occlusal relations of the teeth. *Texas dent. J.* **75**, 430.

[148] BRECKER S.C. (1962) A clinical approach to occlusion. *Dent. Clin. N. Amer.* **March**, 163–182.

[149] RAMFJORD S.P. & ASH M. (1966) *Occlusion*, 1st Edition, p. 186. Philadelphia: Saunders.

[150] MANN A.W. & PANKY L.D. (1963) Concepts of occlusion: The P.M. philosophy of occlusal rehabilitation. *Dent. Clin. N. Amer.* **Nov.**

[151] SCHUYLER C.H. (1935) Fundamental principles in the correction of occlusal disharmony, natural and artificial. *J. Amer. Dent. Ass.* **22**, 1193.

[152] RAMFJORD S.P., KERR D.A. & ASH M. (eds) (1966) *World Workshop in Periodontics*, p. 373. Ann Arbor: Michigan.

[153] RAMFJORD S.P., KERR D.A. & ASH M. (eds) (1966) *World Workshop in Periodontics*, p. 370. Ann Arbor: Michigan.

[154] WÜST B., RATEITSCHAK J.H. & MÜHLEMANN H.R. (1960) Der Einfluss der lokalen paradontal Behandlung auf die Zahnlockerung und den Entzundungsgrad des Zahnfleisches. *Helv. odont. Acta.* **4**, 58.

[155] RATEITSCHAK K.H. (1963) The therapeutic effect of local treatment on periodontal disease assessed on evaluation of different diagnostic criteria. Changes in tooth mobility. *J. Periodont.* **34**, 540–544.

[156] GLICKMAN I., STEIN S. & SMULOW J. (1961) The effect of increased functional forces upon the periodontium of splinted and non-splinted teeth. *J. Periodont.* **32**, 290–300.

[157] NABERS C.L. (1963) Open contacts caused by night guard appliance. Case report. *J. Periodont.* **34**, 436–437.

[158] SATUREN B. (1960) Wire ligature: an undesirable form of temporary splinting. *J. Periodont.* **31**, 37–39.

CHAPTER 15

Corrective phase therapy

SURGICAL CORRECTION OF SOFT TISSUE AND BONE ARCHITECTURE

There has been considerable development in the field of periodontal surgery, and a wide and confusing choice of techniques has been proposed. The fundamental aim of periodontal surgery, and of all periodontal therapy, is tissue health that the patient can maintain. Five year longitudinal studies have demonstrated that with effective plaque control and pocket elimination, even substantially reduced periodontal units can be controlled and further tissue loss prevented [1 & 2]. Present opinion, however, holds that the need for surgery is much less than has previously been considered necessary, largely as a result of improved means of control of the ecology of subgingival plaque. Where surgery is used the simplest technique appropriate to the particular problem should be utilized.

Simple pocket

A simple pocket may be defined as a pocket where all the peripheral walls are formed by soft tissue. In the case of an early periodontitis the base of the pocket is formed by granulation tissue overlying the resorbed alveolar crest. Generally the pattern of resorption is initially horizontal and for practical purposes the whole of the pocket is coronal to the alveolar crest (chap. 12). Such a pocket is not characterized by marked differences in pocket depth around the involved tooth, and tends to be shallow and broad rather than narrow and tortuous.

Compound pocket

A compound pocket is defined as a pocket which has one or more bone walls. Such a pocket is frequently narrow and tortuous, resulting in marked variation of pocket depth around a single tooth (chap. 12). The incidence of compound pocket formation is greatest in the presence of advanced bone destruction.

There is no generally accepted classification of periodontal surgery, although at least three partial classifications [3, 4 & 5] and one complete classification [6] have been proposed. Complete classification of all existing techniques is necessarily complex, and it is convenient to classify the methods most commonly used into three groups, and to relate these groups to the stages described in table 15.1.

It should be appreciated that problems in mucogingival relationships, such as high muscle attachments, a shallow vestibule or a functionally inadequate width of attached gingivae, may also arise in the normal mouth which is not periodontally involved. It is essential to recognize such potentially damaging situations and to employ such surgical techniques as are necessary to achieve a functionally adequate state of periodontal health. In the past many techniques have been developed and used in an attempt to achieve results which were either functionally unnecessary or not maintainable by the patient. Many of these methods were complicated, slow to heal, and over the long term tended to relapse. The most difficult situations arise where problems in mucogingival relationships exist in association with the presence of compound pockets (fig. 15.1b).

TABLE 15.1. The progression of periodontitis and appropriate treatment.

Stage in progression of periodontitis	Range of therapy	Type of pocket
Limited oedematous gingivitis	Controlled oral hygiene, oral toilet	False, simple
Limited fibrous gingivitis	Controlled oral hygiene, oral toilet	False, simple
The initial stage of established periodontitis	Indirect curettage or gingivectomy	True, simple
Loss of supporting tissues greater than the initial stage but less than half the length of the root of the tooth	Controlled oral hygiene, oral toilet, gingivectomy in relation to simple pockets, flap surgery in relation to compound pockets	True, simple or compound
Loss of supporting tissues in excess of half the length of the root of the tooth		

PRINCIPLES OF PERIODONTAL SURGERY

Selection of patients

Periodontal surgery should be carried out only on patients who have demonstrated a high level of self-care. If this rule is not strictly followed, the probability of achieving consistently good surgical results is small, and much time and effort is wasted by both patient and operator. There are two groups of patients in whom periodontal surgery is contraindicated.

There is short term contraindication in patients who have acute oral infections, or have not reached a sufficiently high standard of self-care during the hygiene phase of treatment. Similarly, periodontal surgery is contraindicated during pregnancy, and occasionally in adolescents with severe puberty gingivitis.

No patient should undergo surgery unless the operator is completely aware of the full medical history. There may be a further short term contraindication in patients taking drugs which they cannot immediately identify, and such patients should be treated only following consultation with a physician. Particular care must be taken with patients taking anticoagulants, steroids or monoamine oxidase inhibitors, and the dosage may require adjustment for a period before and following surgery. Patients who have a history of rheumatic fever, open heart surgery or recurrent kidney infections require scaling

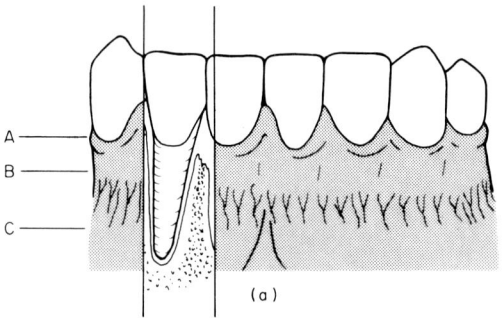

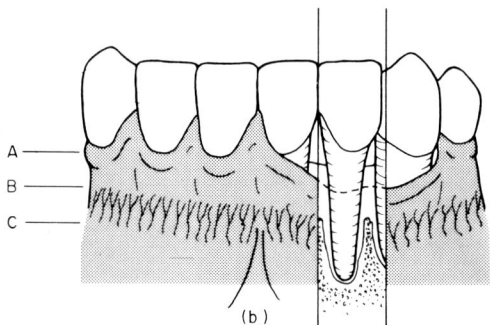

FIG. 15.1. A, free gingivae; B, attached gingivae; C, alveolar mucosa. (a) Compound pocket in presence of an adequate width of attached gingivae and an adequate sulcus depth. The base of the pocket is coronal to the mucogingival line. Such a pocket may be treated in presence of an inadequate width of attached gingivae. The base of the pocket is apical to the mucogingival line. Treatment involves alteration of mucogingival relationships. The techniques applicable are listed in group 3.

and any subsequent surgery to be carried out under antibiotic cover. An antibiotic such as penicillin or erythromycin should be administered 1 M, 30 mins preoperatively [7] and maintained at an adequate dose level for 48 hours postoperatively. Antibiotics administered 24 hours or more preoperatively will increase the risk of heart damage by strains of mouth organisms resistant to the particular antibiotic used.

There may be a permanent contraindication for periodontal surgery in handicapped patients incapable of carrying out adequate self-care, or in those with severe debilitating disease, such as uncontrolled diabetes, Addison's disease or haemorrhagic diathesis (chap. 13).

Anaesthesia for periodontal surgery

PREMEDICATION

Apprehension prior to surgery is common to most patients. In most cases reassurance and a considerate attitude on the part of the operator are all that is required. In a few cases, a sedative or tranquillizer may be necessary. This can be given by the dental surgeon or may be arranged through the patient's physician. The latter course has the advantage that the complete medical history is known to the physician, who is well placed to select the premedication of choice.

There is no ideal drug for sedation of the ambulatory patient. Barbiturates act as sedatives in small doses and as hypnotics in large doses. It has been stated that pentobarbitone (Nembutal) given in small doses (dose range 100–200 mg) approximates to being the ideal drug for premedication [8], and that for a single administration of a sedative or hypnotic there is no reason to prefer anything to quinalbarbitone, (Seconal) (dose range 50–200 mg) or amylobarbitone (Dorminal) (dose range 100–300 mg) [9]. Diazepam may also be used with minimal tendency towards inducing sleepiness. Patients for whom such premedication is prescribed should always be accompanied to the surgery and must be warned not to drive a motor vehicle.

LOCAL ANAESTHESIA

It is customary to perform most periodontal surgery under infiltration anaesthesia, where the local anaesthetic solution is injected directly into the site in which the wound will be developed. The drug of choice is Xylocaine containing noradrenaline 1:80000. The noradrenaline causes minimal cardiac side effects, and has sufficient vasoconstrictor activity to delay circulatory clearance of the anaesthetic solution from the injected tissues. Studies of blood loss during gingival surgery to some extent support the traditional concept that injection of a vasoconstrictor containing anaesthetic solution directly into the wound site reduces the extent of haemorrhage at operation [10 & 11].

Regional block anaesthesia is used most commonly where flap operations involving extensive bone surgery are proposed. Following a block it is the custom of some operators to infiltrate the proposed wound site to reduce haemorrhage.

Prior to inserting the needle, the site of injection should be sterilized with merthiolate or topical anaesthetic applied on a pledget of cotton wool or via a spray. One of the sprays containing an antiseptic can be used, although with present-day presterilized, disposable needles, the incidence of puncture wound infections is extremely low, and the value of topical anaesthetic preparations is debatable.

For infiltration, anaesthetic solution is deposited in the submucosal connective tissue at

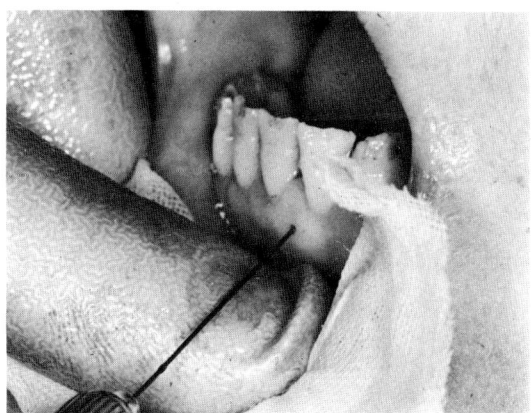

FIG. 15.2. Blanching of tissue following infiltration of local anaesthetic.

the base of the sulcus, and further injections are placed painlessly at the base of each papilla. Care must be taken not to pass the needle through the tissue and inject directly into the pocket. Blanching of the tissues indicates that sufficient solution has been injected (fig. 15.2). If an excess of solution is injected into the base of the sulcus when mucogingival surgery is planned, distortion of the soft tissues makes it difficult to judge where incisions for frenectomy or vestibular deepening should be placed.

GENERAL ANAESTHESIA

General anaesthesia is occasionally used for periodontal surgery. Where an aspirator and facilities for washed field techniques are available, haemorrhage is no problem, but some operators prefer to infiltrate local anaesthetic to reduce haemorrhage and improve visibility.

Control of haemorrhage

If the patient has no bleeding disorder, excessive bleeding during periodontal surgery is not common. In order to reduce bleeding to a minimum, a number of rules should be observed.

(1) Reduce gingival inflammation to a minimum by oral hygiene control prior to surgery. No patient should come to surgery who has not fulfilled the standards of the hygiene phase (chap. 10).

(2) Use a local anaesthetic containing a vasoconstrictor and inject into the proposed wound site.

(3) Always attempt to cut soft tissue cleanly and handle it gently.

(4) Where possible, suture the tissues back in position, preferably using an atraumatic needle.

Occasionally, in spite of these precautions, excessive bleeding occurs which must be controlled before placing a surgical dressing. Where an obvious vessel can be found this should be tied off. More commonly, however, the operator is faced with persistent oozing from a raw surface. Irrigation of the wound with warm saline, followed by gentle pressure from sterile gauze soaked in saline, or, if necessary, 1:100 adrenaline, usually controls bleeding. The patient should be observed for 30 min. before leaving

the surgery. He should be instructed how to apply pressure should the wound start to bleed after leaving the premises, and be advised to avoid violent exercise or excess of alcohol for 24 hours.

Suturing

Accurate apposition of tissue edges reduces the size of a wound, keeps the blood clot to a minimum, aids in haemostasis and rapidity of healing and reduces postoperative discomfort. Suturing plays an important part in surgical procedures where flaps are employed. It is generally agreed that interdental ligation is the most useful type of suturing [12] producing the firmest adaptation of soft tissues to underlying bone and teeth.

When wound edges are kept in close approximation, healing may occur by primary intention, which is much more rapid than healing of a bed of exposed granulation tissue. Poor apposition of tissues results in a space filling clot which heals by granulation, a much slower process.

In the mouth space restriction necessitates the use of a curved needle. The authors' preference is for fine braided silk ophthalmic sutures with attached eyeless reverse cutting needles (fig. 15.3a). These atraumatic needles can be passed through the tissues with minimum trauma, and eliminate the possibility of clamping the needle holders on the eye of the needle which may result in fracture and difficulty in locating the small pieces of metal from the broken needle.

The needle is usually passed through the palatal tissue first (fig. 15.3), as it is difficult to engage the palatal tissue from the buccal side. The needle is passed through the embrasure below the contact area to pierce the buccal flap. The free end of the suture is passed apical to contact area (fig. 15.3), and the knot tied on the buccal side. The ends of the tied suture are covered with gauze before applying a dressing. If the ends of the suture are not covered they become embedded in the dressing and are torn through the soft tissues during pack removal. This is uncomfortable for the patient and damages the healing wound.

It is important that the suture should pass through the tissue at a point where it will not tear through during tying. Sutures should not be

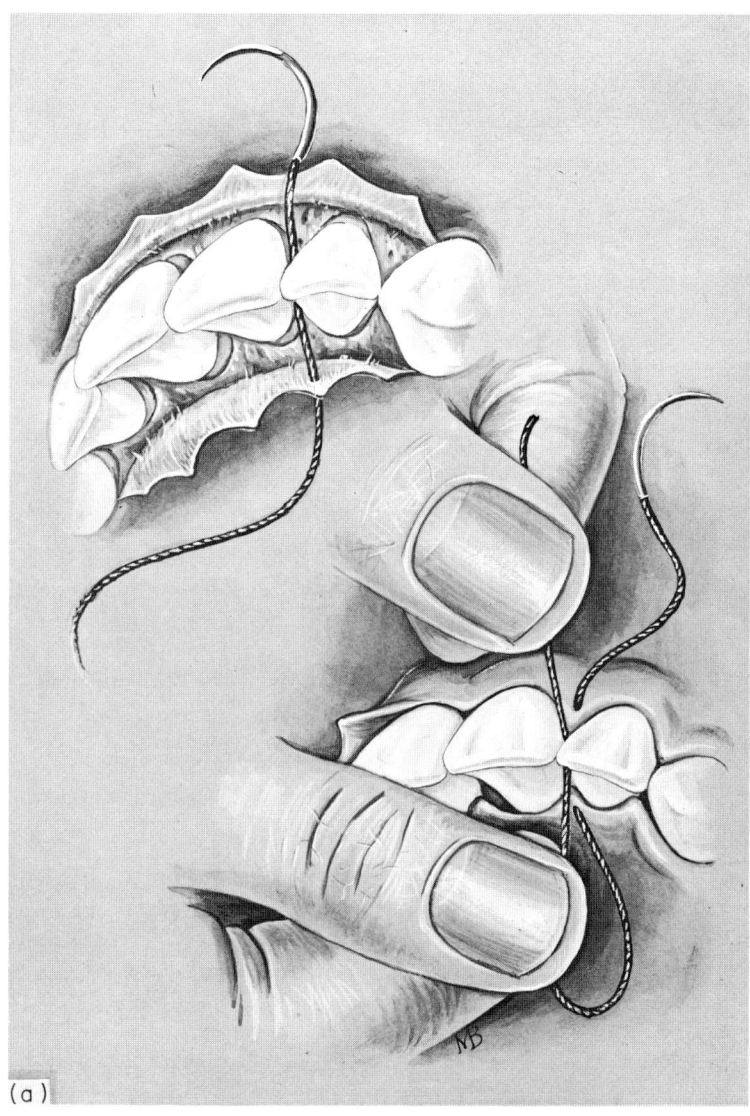

(a)

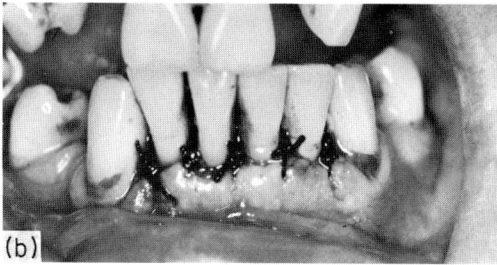

(b)

FIG. 15.3. (a) Technique of placing interdental sutures. Note reverse cutting needle with cutting edge on convexity of curve. (b) Replaced flap stabilized by interdental sutures.

tied excessively tightly, but tension must be enough to ensure good tissue apposition. The distance of the suture from the edge of the tissues depends on the type of tissue being sutured. Thin friable tissues require a greater margin than firm, mature tissue. In most instances 1·5–2 mm from the wound edge will be found satisfactory. In general, interrupted sutures are preferable to continuous, as they are easier to place accurately, and they do not have the disadvantage that the full length of the wound may become displaced should one loop of the suture tear through the tissues.

Temporary splints and surgical dressings

As a general rule abnormalities of interocclusal relationships should be corrected before periodontal surgery is undertaken. Occasionally following surgery a tooth or teeth increase in mobility to an extent where movement during the postoperative period is likely to retard healing. In this situation a temporary splint should be used until healing is well advanced when it can normally be discarded.

Consideration should be given to the correct type of splint during the preoperative planning stage (chaps 10 & 14). Splinting forms a definite part of the overall treatment plan rather than an emergency that arises during or following an operative procedure. A splint placed prior to surgery may make suturing more difficult and time consuming.

The wound should carefully be inspected to check the adequacy of suturing and that there are no soft tissue tags. Any pack must cover the wound without penetrating between wound and tooth (thus re-forming the pocket), and without encroaching on muscle attachments. The dressing prevents food impaction against the healing tissues and helps to keep the soft tissues in close contact with the underlying bone and teeth. The modified zinc oxide eugenol pack described in chap. 10 serves as an excellent dressing, and it can be applied directly to the wound except where bone is to be left exposed (fig. 15.4).

Where bone is to be left exposed the pack should be applied over a strip of gauze dipped in Friar's balsam. Alternatively, one of the proprietary packs can be used (Coe Pack), or ortho-

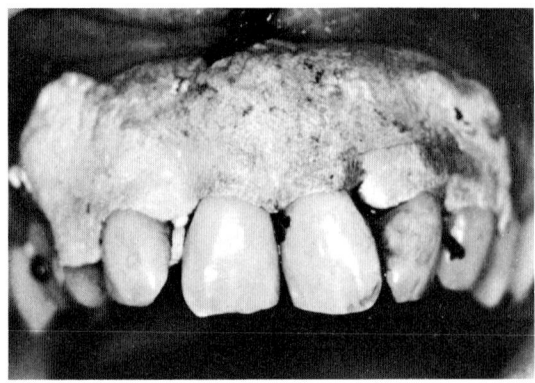

Fig. 15.4. Pack in position following frenectomy and replaced flap surgery, see also figs 15.28 & 15.32.

dontic weight dry foil may be placed over the wound.

The dressing and sutures are routinely removed after 1 week and careful debridement carried out. Depending upon the stage of wound healing, the wound may be left uncovered or may be redressed for a further week. It should rarely be necessary to protect wounds for longer than 2 weeks. Increasingly chlorhexidine (0·05–1·0%) as a mouthwash night and morning is used to obviate the need for surgical pack placement. Patients should be advised only to use toothpaste when cleaning gently with a brush in the middle of the day, as the abrasives in some toothpastes complex with and thus reduce the effectiveness of the chlorhexidine.

POSTOPERATIVE PERIOD

The patient must be carefully instructed in the care of his mouth during the immediate postoperative period. Written instructions should be given. The general principles are:

(1) Avoid excess of exercise or alcohol for the first 24 hours following the operation.

(2) Whilst taking care not to disturb any dressing, clean all undressed teeth after meals.

(3) Postoperative pain is rare following periodontal surgery, but in the event of severe discomfort take codeine (single adult therapeutic dose 10–60 mg), or DF.118 (dihydrocodeine single adult therapeutic dose 10–30 mg) as instructed. If discomfort persists contact the dentist.

(4) In the event of any pack becoming dislodged, bleeding or facial swelling, contact the dentist immediately.

(5) Bring your toothbrush at the time of your next appointment.

In the initial weeks after surgery oral hygiene control is the vital part of treatment. It is essential to check and, if necessary, reinforce oral hygiene instruction at the pack removal stage with a simple explanation about the nature of the wound and the absolute necessity for keeping it free from bacterial deposits. The patient's mouth is readily available for demonstration purposes and should be used to demonstrate oral hygiene techniques. Following such instruction the patient should repeat the techniques to the satisfaction of the operator, preferably using his own brush which should be brought to the surgery at the time of the pack removal appointment.

PROCEDURES FOR SIMPLE POCKETS

Procedures which are designed for the treatment of simple pockets include:
(1) Subgingival curettage,
(2) Gingivoplasty,
(3) Gingivectomy.

Subgingival curettage

The term curettage is descriptive of scraping and debridement of a surface tissue or the lining of a body cavity. Subgingival curettage involves scraping and debridement of the tooth surface and the soft tissue walls of a periodontal pocket. Periodontal curettes and hoes are used to remove bacterial deposits and dead cementum from the tooth surface and diseased soft tissue from the lateral walls of the pocket.

Subgingival curettage is an extension of the scaling procedure and is predominantly of value in resolving a persistent gingivitis, occasionally in reducing slight gingival fibrosis or in eliminating a shallow suprabony periodontal pocket. Following administration of a local anaesthetic the instruments gain access to the lesion through the opening of the gingival pocket (fig. 15.5). Instrumentation of both tooth and

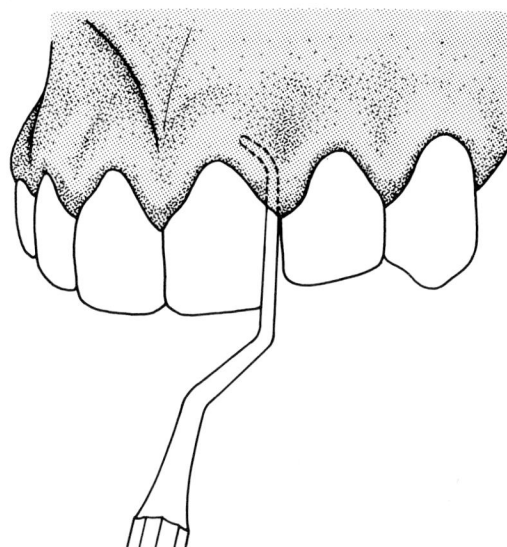

FIG. 15.5. Subgingival curettage. Root planing with McCall's curette.

crevicular soft tissue surfaces is aimed at reducing pocket depth, and improving the functional anatomical form of the papillae and marginal gingivae.

OBJECTIVES

There are three principal aims of subgingival curettage.

(1) The removal of all deposits from the tooth surface, and preparation of the root surface within the pocket to receive the exposed connective tissue, following the removal of the epithelial lining of the pocket (fig. 15.5).

(2) Removal of the epithelial lining of the pocket and underlying inflamed connective tissue (fig. 15.6a & b).

(3) Some reduction in bulk of the connective tissue of the margins and papillae is made (fig. 15.6b & c). It is, however, not possible to produce significant reduction of fibrotic gingivae by this approach.

INSTRUMENTS

Suitable instruments for subgingival curettage are a set of four tungsten carbide tipped periodontal hoes (Ash TC 210, 211, 212, 213) (chap. 10 & fig. 10.19) and two tungsten carbide tipped McCall's curettes (Ash TC. 2L, 2R). A Cross calculus probe (fig. 10.11) can be used to check that deposits are removed and that the root surface is smooth. It is desirable to have a duplicate set of curettes reserved solely for soft tissue curettage, so that the cutting edges remain sharp. The ultrasonic scaling apparatus (p. 152) is suitable for subgingival curettage if this equipment is available.

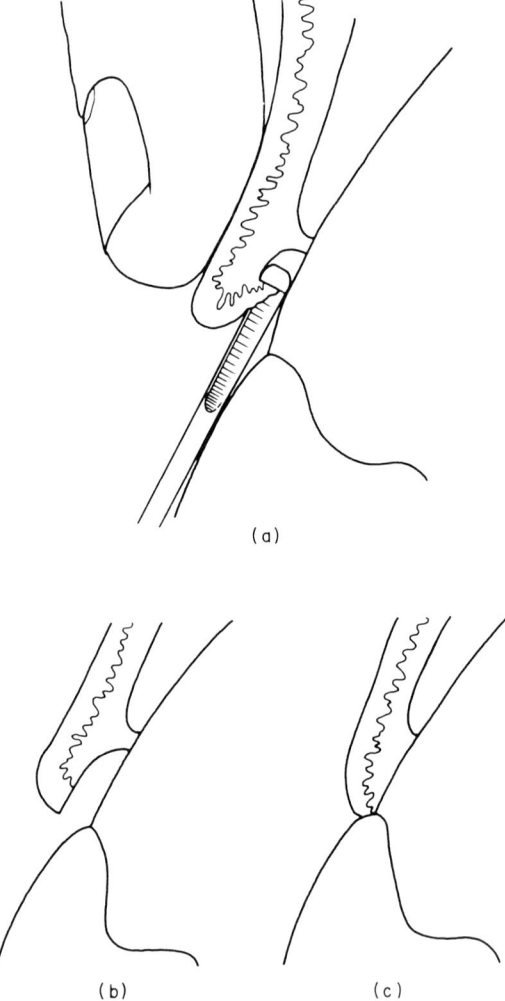

FIG. 15.6. (a & b) Removal of hyperplastic epithelium from the lateral wall of the pocket using a McCall's curette. (c) Exposed connective tissue collapsed against prepared root surface.

OPERATIVE PROCEDURE

Following administration of a local anaesthetic the morphology of the pockets in the area of the mouth to be curetted should be examined by probing. Curettage of each individual pocket is carried out round the complete circumference of each tooth. A periodontal hoe is inserted into the full depth of the pocket, such that the working edge of the instrument is adjacent to the tooth surface within the pocket. The shank of the instrument should be approximately parallel to the long axis of the tooth to avoid gouging. The hoe is then rhythmically withdrawn cervically until the root surface is planed free of all deposits and dead cementum, always withdrawing the instrument along the long axis of the tooth rather than obliquely, which would create a rough surface. The same procedure is then followed using McCall's curettes (fig. 15.5) until the operator is confident that all deposits are removed and that the root surface is planed smooth.

A curette should then be placed in the pocket so that the working edge is adjacent to the lateral wall of the pocket (fig. 15.6a). A finger is pressed against the labial tissues to force the lateral wall of the pocket against the edge of the instrument, which is then rhythmically rotated cervically against finger pressure, stripping the epithelium from the lateral wall of the pocket. The same procedure is repeated until the operator is confident that the epithelial lining of the pocket has been excised, and that such small reduction in the bulk of connective tissue of the pocket wall has been achieved as desired.

When curettage is complete the exposed connective tissue of the pocket wall is pressed against the prepared root surface (fig. 15.6c) and held in position by a periodontal pack. Removal of the pack and polishing of the teeth should be carried out from 4 to 7 days later (fig. 15.7).

It has been suggested that the degree to which the reorganizing connective tissue of the pocket wall differentiates into collagen, which becomes attached to the prepared root surface, is partly governed by the speed at which the crevicular epithelium becomes re-established along the root surface [13 & 14]. Downgrowth of epithelium apical to the amelocemental junction before the connective tissues have fully differen-

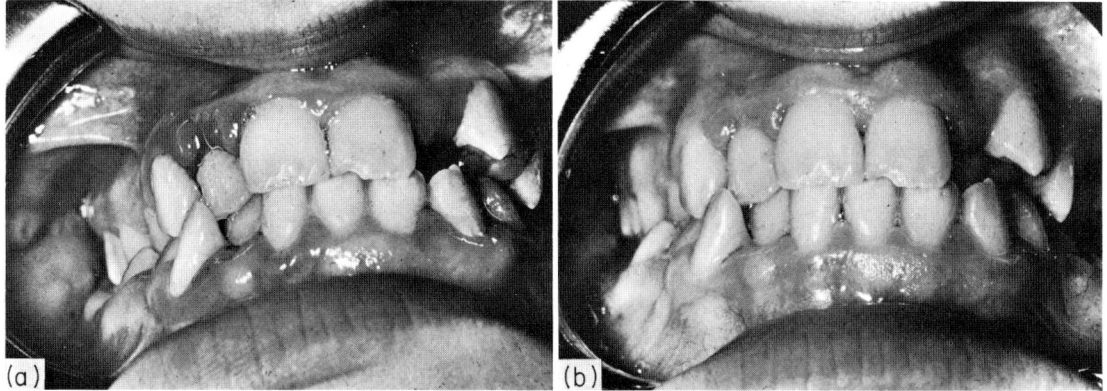

FIG. 15.7. (a) Before subgingival curettage. (b) Following removal of the pack, 4 days postoperative.

tiated may limit the degree of attachment of connective tissue which is obtained. The extent of reattachment of connective tissue to the root surface which is obtained during the process of healing has been described as the result of a race between epithelial downgrowth and connective tissue differentiation. Delay in the epithelium becoming re-established has been said to increase the probability of reattachment of connective tissue to the prepared root surface. For this reason it has been suggested that indirect curettage should be accompanied by the removal of 1–1·5 mm of tissue by means of an external gingivectomy incision, regardless of the pocket depth [15]. The objective is to place the epithelial margin at a distance from the reorganizing connective tissue, and thereby to increase the probability of re-attachment of connective tissue to the root surface.

The metabolism of epithelium and connective tissue is to some extent interdependent (chap. 7), and it is doubtful to what extent connective tissue can reorganize and reattach to root surface in the absence of epithelium from the area. Without some degree of epithelial covering overlying the connective tissue, toxic factors from the mouth provoke inflammatory change which interferes with repair of connective tissue [16].

It has been concluded that the new gingival sulcus following such operative procedures may be the result of either epithelium growing down into the crevice made between the tooth and soft tissue during root planing, or connective tissue proliferation building up a new free gingivae [17]. Healing is a combination of these two mechanisms. Studies have shown that in most instances cemental curettage is followed by downgrowth of new cuff epithelium instead of connective tissue reattachment [17].

It has been further suggested that regeneration of the supporting structures may occur without the removal of the pocket epithelium, and formation and organization of a blood clot. The epithelium may move 'crown wise' as well as 'root wise' depending on what has occurred in the underlying tissues following therapy [18]. There is thus no clear indication for gingivectomy to be performed as part of the subgingival curettage procedure.

The majority of reports indicate that gingival tissue surgically detached is capable of reattaching to the newly exposed root [18–21]. The consensus is that new soft tissue attachment is achieved by longer epithelial adhesion to the tooth rather than by a more coronal connective tissue attachment [22].

INDICATIONS

(1) To reduce a persistent oedematous gingivitis.

(2) To reduce a hyperplastic gingivitis, where the bulk of connective tissue is not sufficient to require complete excision.

(3) To eliminate early periodontitis in the presence of simple pockets where the peripheral walls are soft tissue.

(4) As a palliative operation in an advanced periodontitis to reduce the inflammation.

(1) Where thin atrophic marginal tissue makes soft tissue curettage difficult, increasing the probability of leaving a ragged wound, gingivoplasty would be preferable.

(2) In the presence of well-established suprabony pockets where gingivectomy is indicated (vide infra).

Gingivoplasty

Gingivoplasty, or surgical reshaping of the gingival tissues to a functional form, is designed to treat slight hyperplasia which cannot be reduced sufficiently by curettage.

Gingivoplasty is a limited form of gingivectomy suitable for treatment of false pockets and minor gingival deformity whereas gingivectomy may be the treatment for a true pocket.

Correction of gingival form is carried out by means of an incision made at an angle of 45° to the long axis of the tooth (fig. (15.8a). It has been widely proposed that such minor contouring of gingivae can be performed using cone shaped or round coarse bonded diamond stones rotating under a water or saline spray (fig. 15.8b), or by means of a diathermy unit. The wound base should be thoroughly curetted as described for subgingival curettage (fig. 15.9). Uneventful wound healing follows a clean incision of tissue made with a knife, and overheating of tissue during the use of rotating stones or a diathermy unit tends to result in slower healing and postoperative discomfort.

The wound should be carefully examined to make sure that no tags of tissue are left, the patient's lips are covered with petroleum jelly, and a pack is applied and left in place for 1 week. After removing the pack, any exuberant granulations should be removed with a curette and the teeth polished to remove any deposits or remnants of pack. Trichloracetic acid should never be used to control exuberant granulation as this will result in delayed healing. Finally, the patient should receive instructions as to the care of the wound as defined previously.

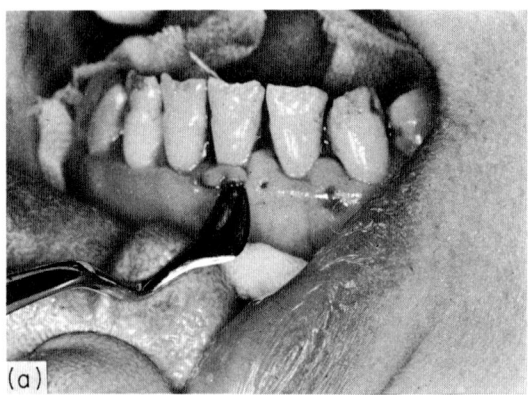

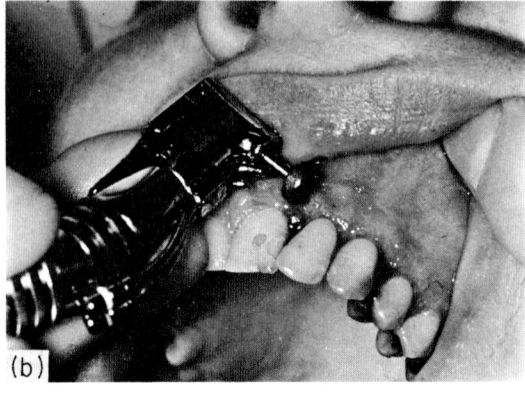

FIG. 15.8. (a) Gingivoplasty incision at 45° to long axis of tooth made with a Kirkland knife. Such fixed blade knives require constant sharpening and removable blade knives such as a Blake knife (fig. 15.12) are more convenient. (b) Gingivoplasty with a coarse bonded diamond stone.

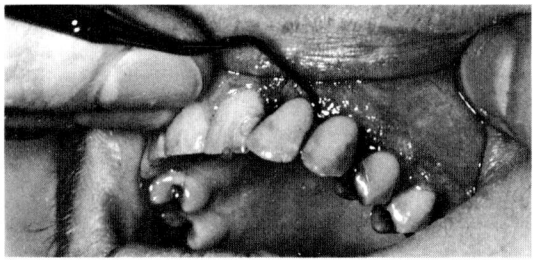

FIG. 15.9. Curettage with McCall's curette following gingivoplasty.

INDICATIONS FOR GINGIVOPLASTY

To eliminate a slight degree of gingival hyperplasia.

CONTRAINDICATIONS

Gingivoplasty must not be undertaken when the alteration of tissue form is associated with deformity of the underlying bone contour. Its use is limited to treatment of the gingivally contained lesion (fig. 15.10).

GINGIVECTOMY

Gingivectomy is a limited soft tissue operation designed to eliminate simple pockets. The objective is complete excision of a pocket which is superficial to the underlying bone contour if the bone has retained an acceptable anatomical form.

Gingivectomy is the traditional approach to excision of a simple pocket. The pocket should be excised in toto by means of an external incision made buccally and lingually at approximately 45° to the long axis of the tooth (fig. 15.11). It is not possible to excise a compound pocket by this technique.

INSTRUMENTS

Suitable instruments for this technique are (fig. 15.12):

(1) mirror, probe and dressing tweezers,

(2) Swann–Morton scalpel with a No. 12 blade,

(3) right and left Blake knives with No. 11 blades,

(4) an Orban knife or serrated Ward's wax carver made by cutting 0·5 mm deep notches into the standard carver, with $\frac{7}{8}$ in diameter carborundum disc,

(5) Crane–Kaplan pocket markers,

(6) periodontal hoes, Ash TC.2L, 2R (see fig. 10.19),

(7) McCall's curettes, Ash TC.210–213 (see figs. 10.19 , 15.5 & 15.6).

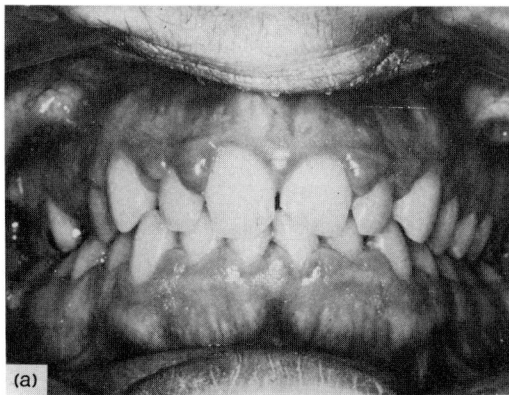

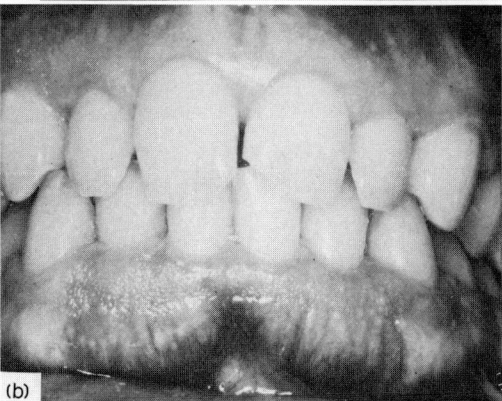

FIG. 15.10. Gingivally contained lesion before (a) and after (b) gingivoplasty.

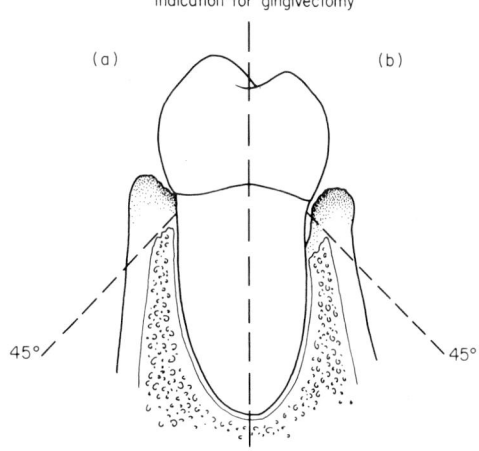

FIG. 15.11. (a) Simple pocket; total excision of pocket by gingivectomy incision. (b) Compound pocket; it is impossible to totally excise a pocket with one or more bone walls by a gingivectomy incision.

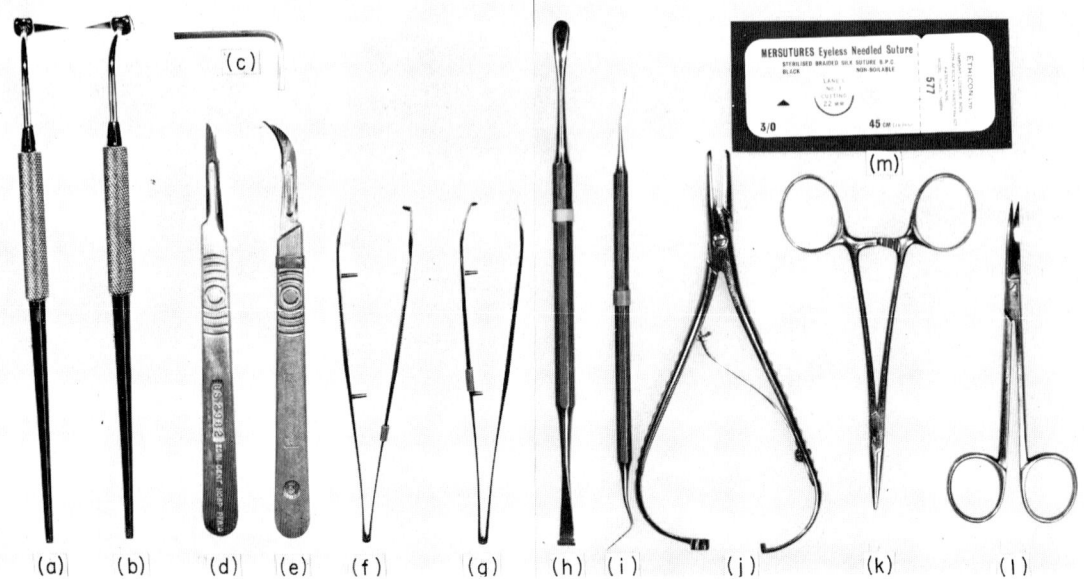

FIG. 15.12. Instruments for periodontal surgery. (a, b & c) Right and left Blake knives and Allan key. The blades are Swann–Morton No. 11 blades locked in position by the Allan key and broken off to size by artery forceps. (d) Scalpel with Swann–Morton No. 15 blade. This broad ended blade is suitable for flap surgery but not for gingivectomy. (e) Scalpel with Swann–Morton No. 12 blade. This curved pointed blade penetrates to the full depth of the embrasure between teeth and is suitable for gingivectomy. (f & g) Right and left Crane–Kaplan pocket markers. (h) Periosteal elevator. (i) Serrated wax carver, Ward's No. 1. (j) Needle holder. (k) Artery forceps. (l) Suture scissors. (m) Sutures.

PLANNING THE INCISION

Factors to be taken into consideration when planning the incision for gingivectomy are:
(1) the depth and morphology of the pocket,
(2) the width of the zone of attached gingivae,
(3) the vestibular depth.

To maintain gingival health there must be an adequate zone of attached gingivae between the cervical margins of the teeth and the line of reflection of alveolar mucosa towards the lips and cheeks (fig. 15.13). Similarly, a shallow vestibule tends to promote food stagnation around the teeth and makes the use of a toothbrush difficult.

A limitation of gingivectomy is that excision of tissue must not reduce the width of attached gingivae and the vestibule depth below a functionally acceptable level. A 'functionally adequate' amount of attached gingiva is not a matter of millimetres but rather a sufficient amount to dissipate the pull of the musculature transmitted through the frenum or the alveolar mucosa that may retract the marginal gingiva or interproximal papilla [23]. If the base of the pocket is sited at or below the junction of the attached gingivae and alveolar mucosa (fig. 15.13), some other technique must be used which will preserve or even increase the width of attached gingivae, and the vestibular depth. One of several flap techniques may be appropriate.

If sufficient attached gingiva is available to perform gingivectomy, it is preferable to plan the line of incision over the whole of the potential wound area, rather than to attempt to excise the walls of each individual pocket separately. Separate incisions for each pocket subsequently connected result in a ragged wound base.

Following administration of local anaesthetic the morphology of the pockets should be confirmed by probing. The incision may be planned with the aid of Crane–Kaplan pocket markers (fig. 15.12). The pocket marking tweezers are inserted into the pocket so that the straight blade is parallel to the long axis of the tooth. The tweezers are closed so that the right angled blade marks the position of the base of the

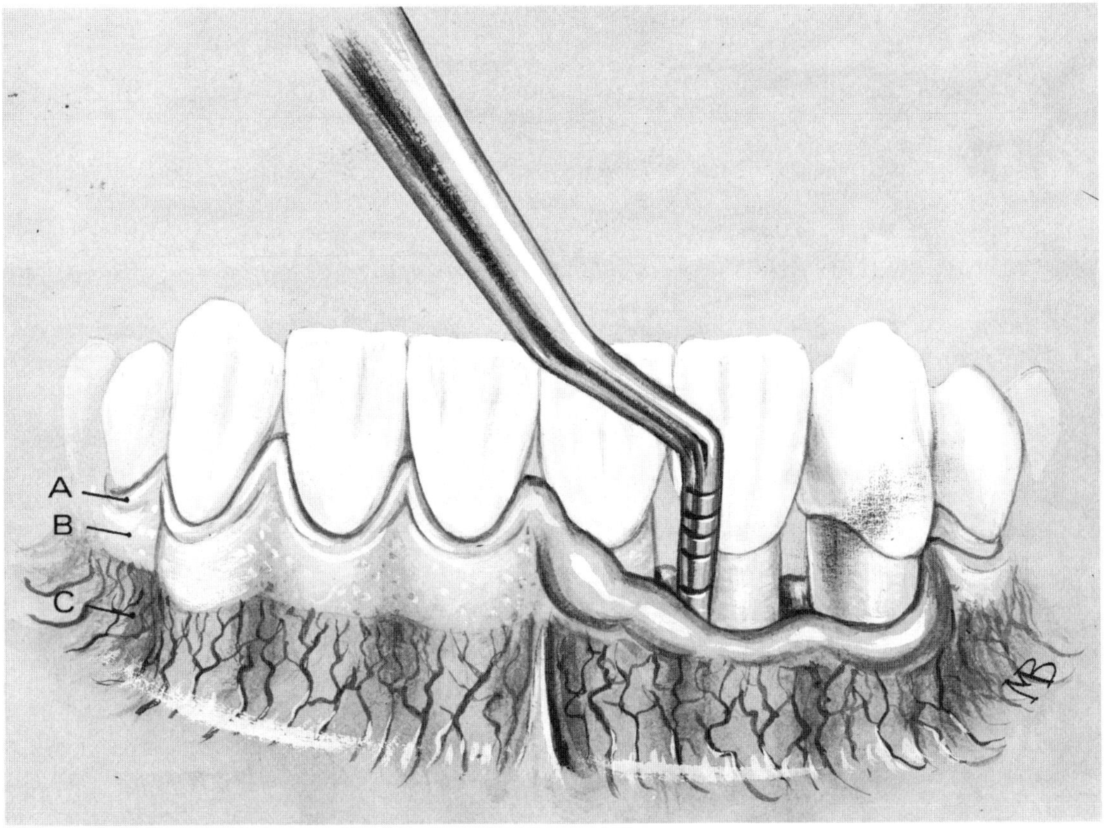

FIG. 15.13. A, free gingivae; B, attached gingivae; C, alveolar mucosa. A limitation of gingivectomy is that excision of tissue must not reduce the width of attached gingivae and vestibular depth below a functionally acceptable level.

pocket by a puncture wound on the surface of the gingivae (fig. 15.14). Crane–Kaplan pocket markers are of limited use in planning the line of incision in the palate as access is restricted. The line of palatal incisions is determined by probing.

The incision should be made at an angle of 45° to the long axis of the tooth, apical to the puncture marks on the gingivae the knife impacts against tooth surface slightly apical to the base of the pocket (fig. 15.15) [24 & 25]. The objectives of the incisions are total excision of the pocket and restoration of gingival architecture to a functional anatomical form. On the buccal side the incision can be made either with a Blake knife (fig. 15.15) or a scalpel (fig. 15.16), but due to restricted access on the palatal or lingual side the use of an angled knife is obligatory. Even with a Blake knife it may be

difficult to achieve an angle of 45° to the long axis of the teeth, palatal to the maxillary teeth, and considerable dexterity may be required. As a matter of convenience, the lingual or palatal

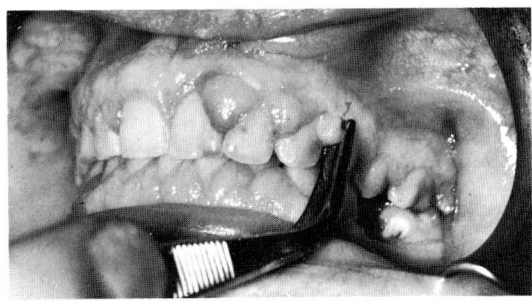

FIG. 15.14. The use of Crane–Kaplan pocket markers, see also fig. 15.12.

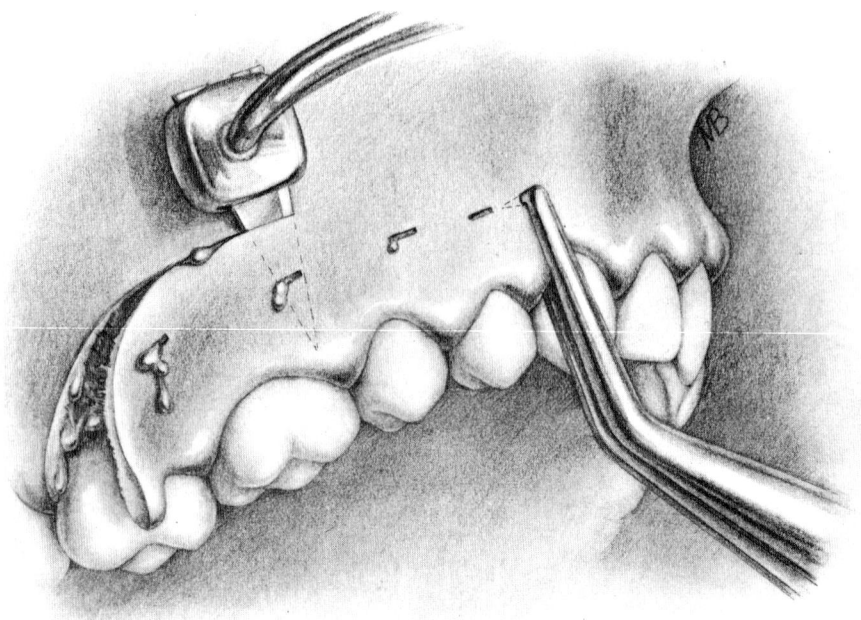

FIG. 15.15. Gingivectomy incision at an angle of 45° to the long axis of the tooth. The incision is made apical to the Crane–Kaplan marks so the blade of the knife impacts against tooth surface slightly apical to the base of the pocket.

incision may be placed prior to the buccal incision. This prevents masking of the more inaccessible areas by blood.

Following placing the incisions, the lateral walls of the pocket should be dissected free using an Orban knife or serrated wax carver.

Where the case has been well selected and the incision well placed, there should be no residual pocket. The wound base should be curetted free from granulation tissue with the aid of the serrated carver and curettes (fig. 15.9), and the exposed tooth substance should be planed as described for subgingival curettage and gingivoplasty. Where necessary, minor adjustment to soft tissues can be made with a coarse bonded diamond stone. This may be necessary where it has proved impossible to place a properly angled incision because of a narrow vaulted palate, but in general the use of rotary instruments should be kept to a minimum. Care should be taken to ensure that the interdental spaces are free from tissue tags and that the soft tissues are restored to a functional form.

An objection to this technique is the creation

of a large external wound which heals by second intention. In certain circumstances such as that following excision of hyperplastic tissue from the palate, the external wound is of considerable area, and the patient may experience marked postoperative discomfort. On occasion an aesthetic problem is created in the anterior region of the mouth when large amounts of tissue are removed.

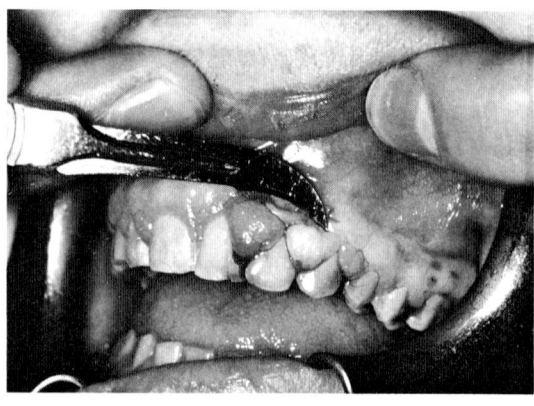

FIG. 15.16. Gingivectomy incision by scalpel with Swann–Morton No. 12 blade.

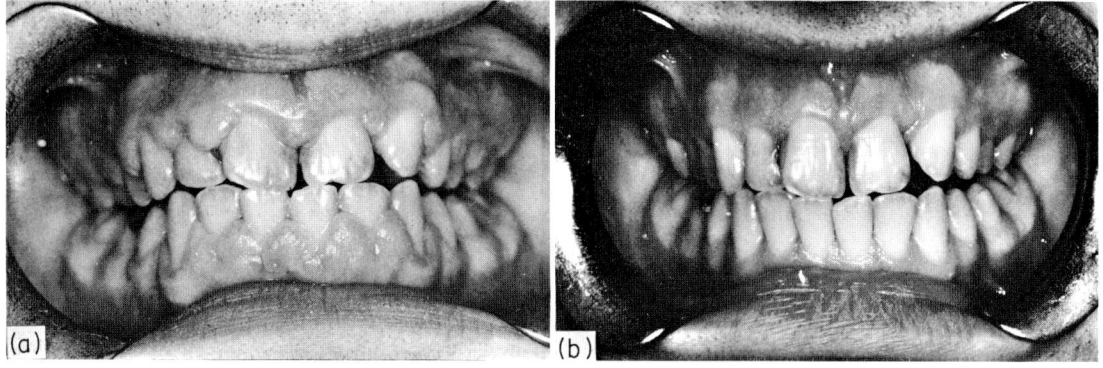

FIG. 15.17. Early periodontitis before (a) and after (b) gingivectomy.

Gingivectomy gives functionally acceptable and aesthetic results, and given an adequate standard of patient self care a predictable result over the long term (fig. 15.17).

WOUND HEALING FOLLOWING GINGIVECTOMY

Few studies have been carried out on wound healing following gingivectomy [26]. McHugh and Persson [27] and Persson [28] concluded that 2 days after operation epithelium begins to regenerate from the basal layers of the old epithelium. Numerous leucocytes are present in a mesh of fibrin covering the wound. By the end of 4 days the deeper aspect of the covering blood clot has been replaced by granulation tissue. Epithelium, without rete ridges, has migrated between the granulation tissue and the superficial aspect of the clot and extends over part of the surface. There is a dense inflammatory cell infiltrate in the underlying connective tissue [29]. By the sixth day the entire wound has been covered by fairly well differentiated stratified squamous epithelium. Some collagen fibres are evident in the granulation tissue with reduction in the level of inflammatory infiltrate.

In dogs it has been shown that a new stratum corneum is evident by 7 days [30]. Following gingivectomy in monkeys, Listgarten [31] has demonstrated that junctional epithelium reforms from the oral epithelium at the wound edge. An epithelial attachment, consisting of a basement lamina and hemidesmosomes was noted between the regenerated junctional epithelium

and the tooth surface as early as 12 days postoperatively [32]. It has also been shown that a new epithelial attachment can form over surgically exposed dentine as well as against enamel or cementum [32]. By the end of 16 days the reformed gingival epithelium appears mature, with new rete ridge reformation. A slight chronic inflammatory cell infiltrate is still present but the connective tissue is much more mature. In a study on human tissue, epithelialization was completed by fourteen days after surgery although active connective tissue repair was still evident after 28 days [33]. Complete healing and restoration of a new gingival sulcus has been reported to occur in monkeys between 3 and 5 weeks postoperatively [34].

Flap surgery

GENERAL INDICATIONS

(1) The presence of compound pockets where changes in the architecture of the alveolar process necessitate surgical intervention (fig. 15.1a).

(2) When the depth of a periodontal pocket extends to or beyond the mucogingival junction (fig. 15.11b & 15.13).

Flaps have been broadly classified into four groups on a geometric basis in an attempt to standardize terminology [35].

(1) Curved: a flap mobilized by means of a single curved incision (fig. 15.18a).

(2) Triangular: a flap mobilized by means of a horizontal incision and one relaxing incision (fig. 15.18b).

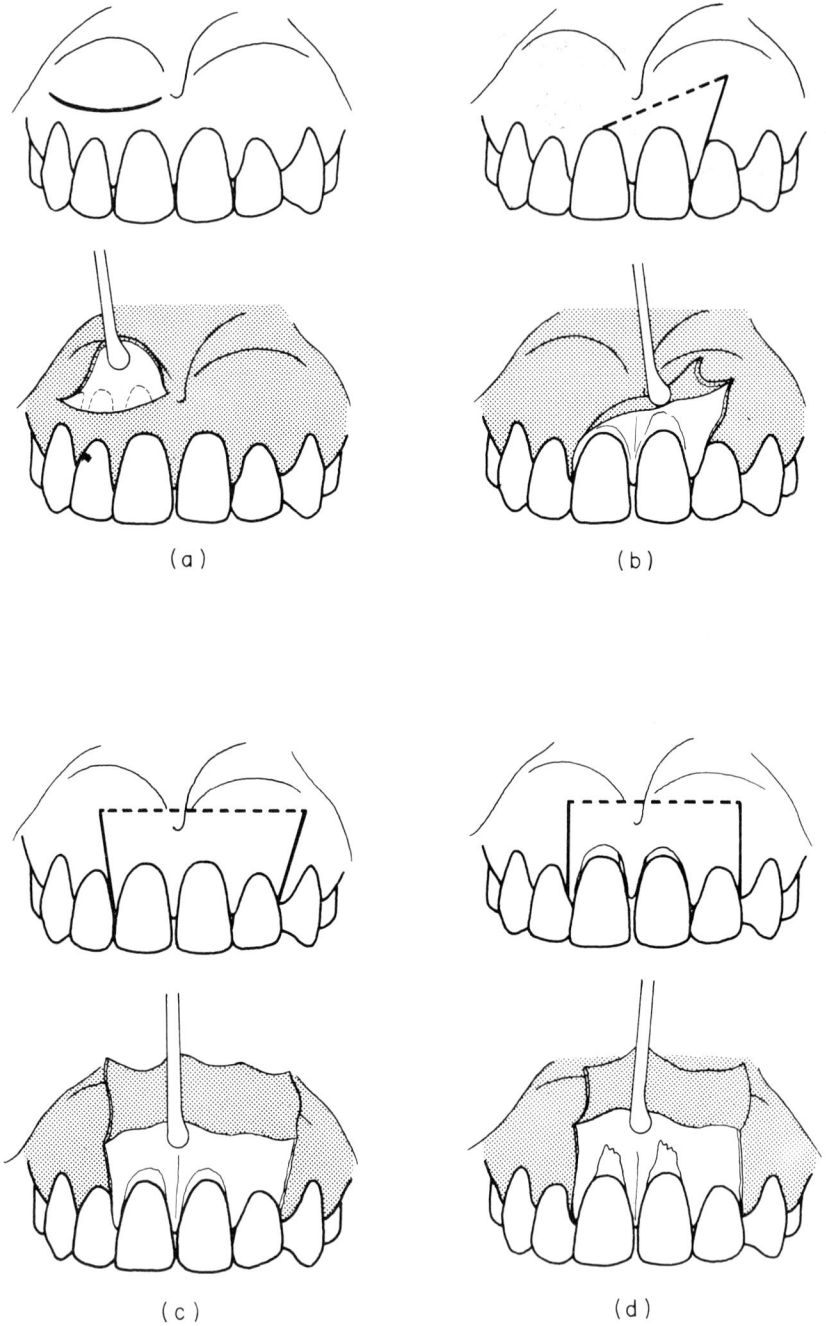

FIG. 15.18. Geometric nomenclature for mucoperiosteal flaps. (a) curved, (b) triangular, (c) trapezoidal, (d) rectangular.

(3) Trapezoidal: a flap mobilized by means of a horizontal incision and two oblique relaxing incisions (fig. 15.18c).

(4) Rectangular: a flap mobilized by means of a horizontal incision and two vertical relaxing incisions (fig. 15.18d).

The general requirements of any well designed flap are as follows [5].

(1) There should be free access to the lesion it is designed to approach. Relaxing incisions should not be directly related to the lesion and the flap should extend peripherally to healthy tissue (fig. 15.19).

(2) There should be an adequate blood supply. As a generalization a flap with two relaxing incisions should be raised on a minimum of three teeth (fig. 15.19).

For periodontal surgery, a flap with two relaxing incisions should be rectangular in design rather than trapezoidal. The relaxing incisions

should be vertical rather than oblique. Oblique incisions cross the thin mucosa overlying the root eminence and may involve a previously unrecognized root fenestration or dehiscence and subsequently fail to heal (fig. 15.19a). Vertical incisions parallel to the long axis of the roots of the teeth are concealed in the thicker mucosa between the root eminences, and are based on sound bone (fig. 15.19b).

Relaxing incisions should join the cervical margin at the junction of a margin and papilla where there is sufficient bulk of tissue to absorb subsequent scar contraction. Incisions joining the margin over the thin mucosa of a root eminence may result in a V shaped notch following scar contraction (fig. 15.20).

In the palate, incisions should follow the line of the cervical margin either directly against the teeth (fig. 15.21A), or displaced towards the vault (fig. 15.21B), dependent on the bulk of soft

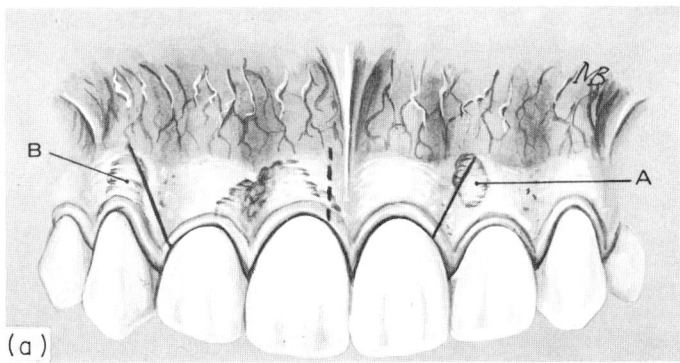

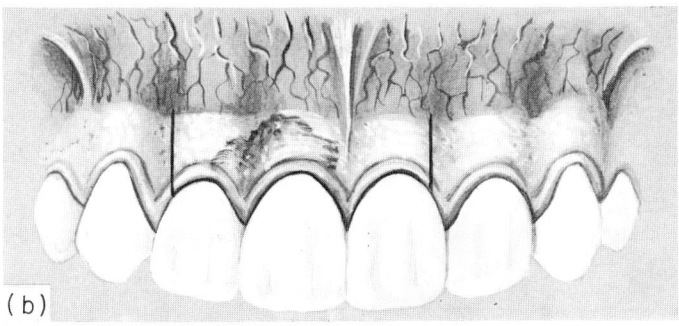

FIG. 19.19. (a) Trapezoidal flap; A, fenestration of bone involved by oblique incision; B, dehiscence of marginal bone involved by oblique incision. Relaxing incisions should not be directly related to the lesion. (b) Rectangular flap. Vertical incisions are concealed in the thicker mucosa between the root eminences and join the margin at the junction of a margin and papilla where this is sufficient bulk of tissue to absorb subsequent scar contraction.

tissue to be removed, and the extent of under-lying bone destruction which subsequently re-quires to be corrected. Relaxing incisions across the line of the blood vessels are rarely, if ever, necessary (fig. 15.21C).

There should be a minimal amount of dead space between the corrected bone contour and the replaced flap following surgery (fig. 15.22). The soft tissues must accord closely with the cor-rected bone architecture. Deadspace invites infection and re-epithelialization of the tooth surface within any residual pocket before the connective tissues are reorganized.

The objectives of flap design may be sum-marized as:

(1) the elimination of pockets and the re-designing of soft tissue and bone architecture to an acceptable anatomical form;

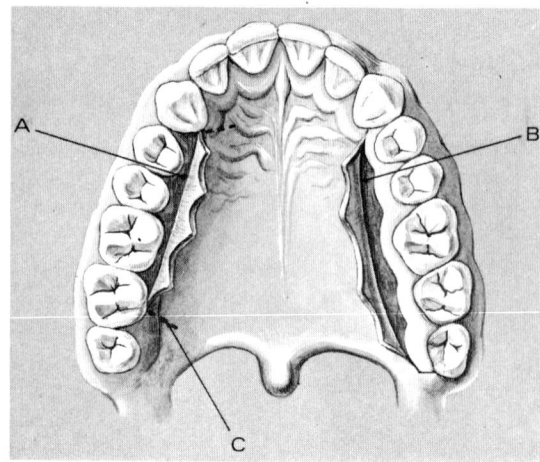

FIG. 15.21. Incisions in the palate. A, incision directly against the teeth; B, incision displaced to-wards the vault of the palate; C, relaxing incisions across the line of the blood vessels are not necessary for access.

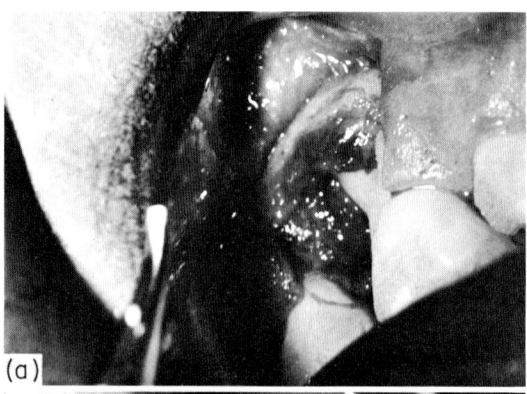

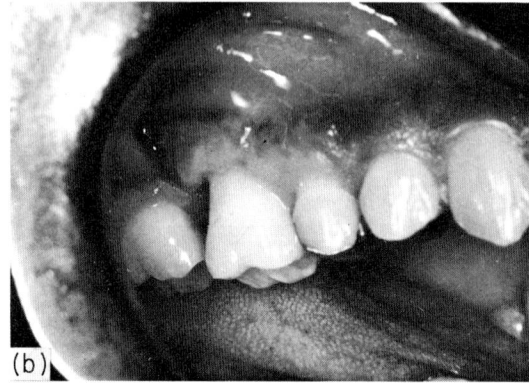

FIG. 15.20. (a) Poorly designed trapezoidal flap. Oblique approach incision directly related to the lesion and to the cervical margin of tooth. Note re-placement of bone by granulation tissue. (b) 'Notch-ing' of cervical margin following scar contraction.

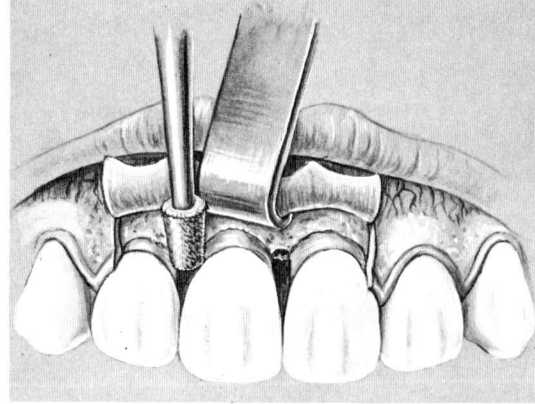

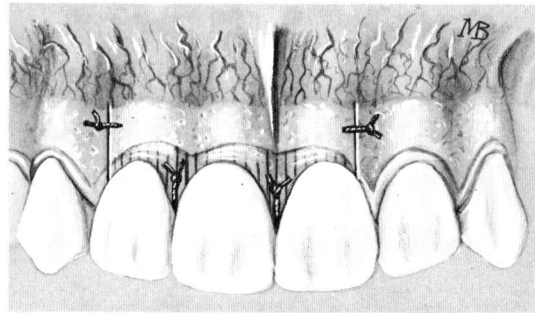

FIG. 15.22. Deadspace. The replaced soft tissues must accord closely with the corrected bone archi-tecture with no deadspace intervening.

(2) the maintenance or, where necessary, the creation of an adequate width of attached gingiva between the cervical margin of the teeth and the line of reflection of the mucosa on to the lips and cheeks;

(3) the maintenance or, where necessary, the creation of an adequate depth of buccal or labial vestibule.

PROCEDURE FOR COMPOUND POCKETS

The procedure which is designed for the treatment of compound pockets which are not related to a problem in mucogingival relationships, i.e. where there is an adequate width of attached gingivae and an adequate vestibular depth (figs 15.1a & 15.13), is flap replacement.

Replaced flaps

A replaced flap may be defined as a flap which is replaced directly onto the original donor site [5]. The limitations of this approach are:

(1) that there must be an adequate width of attached gingiva between the cervical margin and the line of reflection of the mucosa onto the lips or cheeks,

(2) that this existing width of attached gingiva should not be significantly reduced during the course of the operation.

The design of flap is most commonly triangular with one relaxing incision, or rectangular with two relaxing incisions.

The objectives of the procedure are:

(1) the elimination of the soft tissue walls of pockets,

(2) the thinning of any thickened attached gingiva which is to be preserved,

(3) the correction of bone architecture to a functional form,

(4) the replacement of the flap to accord closely with the corrected bone architecture with the minimum of dead space between the two tissues.

The design of choice is based on the principle of the reverse bevel incision [36]. The knife is placed at an oblique angle to the tooth at least 1–2 mm apical to the cervical margin (fig. 15.23). The degree to which the incision is placed apical to the cervical margin is governed by the amount of excess supra-bony soft tissue which must be eliminated. The greater the excess of soft tissues the more apically placed the incision, and the larger the coronal wedge of tissue that will be discarded (fig. 15.23). The incision is made firmly down to the crest of the alveolar bone, extended horizontally, and scalloped at each embrasure. A full thickness mucoperiosteal flap, consisting largely of attached gingiva, is reflected using a periosteal elevator (fig. 15.24). Such an incision thins the attached gingiva, excises the epithelial lining of the pocket from the inside of the flap, and develops a flap which will in the main accord with the corrected bone architecture when allowed to relapse into

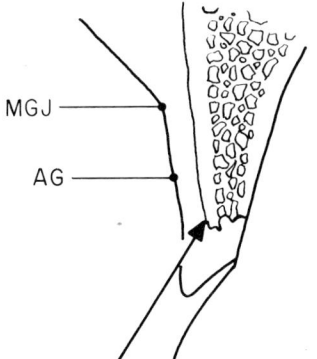
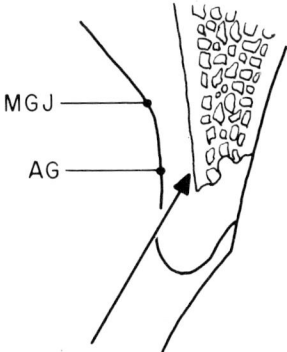

FIG. 15.23. Reverse bevel incision for full thickness flap; MGJ, mucogingival junction; AG, attached gingivae.

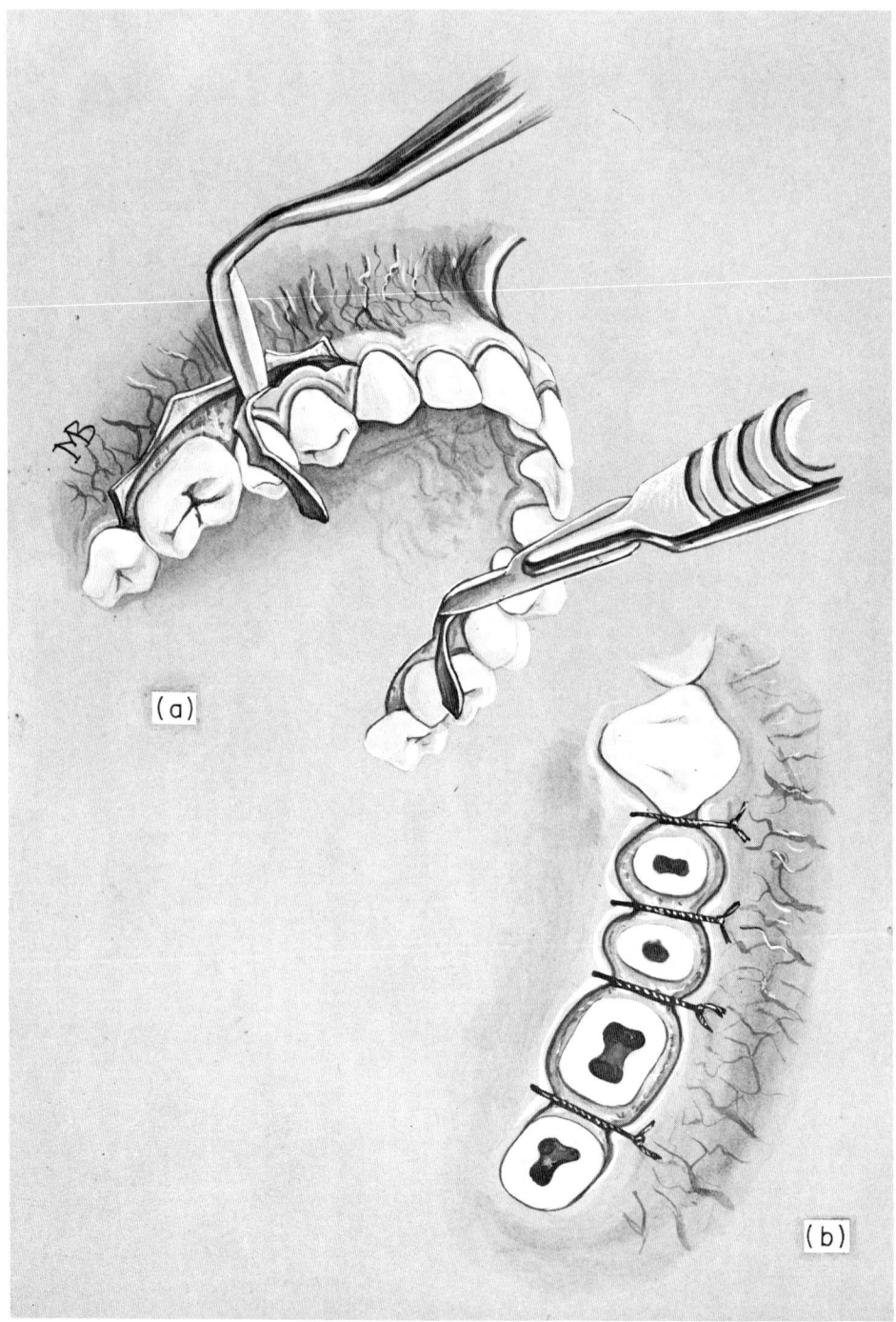

FIG. 15.24. (a) A full thickness mucoperiosteal flap developed by reverse bevel incision. The flap is fully prepared by the initial incision, and in (b) accords with the corrected bone architecture when allowed to relapse into position.

position. The coronal wedge of tissue is dissected free and discarded.

The technique has advantages over the more widely used incision around the cervical margins of the teeth (fig. 15.25). A flap developed by reverse bevel incision requires the minimum of manipulation during the remainder of the operation. The flap has been thinned and prepared to fit the corrected bone form, and the epithelial lining of the pocket has been discarded in the coronal wedge of tissue.

A flap developed from an incision around the cervical margins of the teeth requires to be thinned and cut to size after it has been raised, and the epithelial lining of the pocket which has been raised as part of the flap must be curetted away from the deep surface. It is doubtful if the operator can be sure that all the epithelium has been removed from the deep surface and such unnecessary trauma of tissue which is to be preserved is undesirable.

A modification of the standard flap procedure, the modified Widman flap, has been described by Ramfjord and Nissle [37] and the results of studies using this technique reported following a longitudinal study [38 & 39]. In this procedure initial incisions parallel to the long axis of the teeth are made followed by raising of a mucoperiosteal flap only 2–3 mm from the alveolar crest. Following a crevicular incision around the necks of the involved teeth the resulting collar of tissue is excised and discarded.

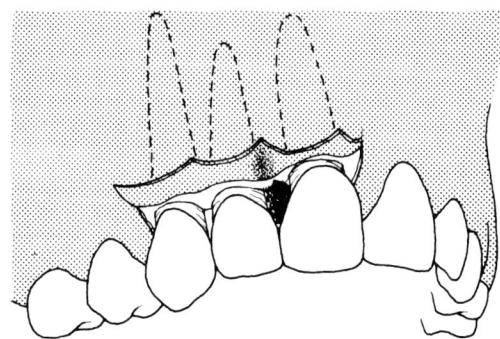

FIG. 15.25. A flap developed by an incision around the cervical margin of the teeth. The epithelial lining of the pocket is raised as part of the flap, and the flap requires to be thinned and cut to size after it has been raised.

Root surfaces are planed and the scalloped wound closed with close adaptation of the interproximal flap edges. In comparing modified Widman flap surgery with curettage and conventional pocket elimination surgery Knowles *et al.* [38] reported that moderate and deep periodontal pockets can be reduced in depth and stay reduced following each of the techniques. They also reported that pocket reduction for moderately deep pockets is greater following the modified Widman procedure or pocket elimination surgery than following curettage.

CORRECTION OF BONE ARCHITECTURE

The shape of alveolar bone in health parallels to a large degree the form of the overlying gingivae.

Deviation from this normal functional form either genetically determined or because of periodontal disease may render the mouth more susceptible to a progressive periodontitis.

Abnormal gingival form resulting from defects in underlying bone form cannot be corrected merely by reshaping the soft tissue. Reshaping of the underlying alveolar bone must also be carried out. Gingival tissue and bone appears to have the characteristic of attempting to retain its original scalloped form. Where this normal tissue pattern is altered as a result of disease, such that the interdental bony crest lies apical to the level of the bone at the buccal or lingual cervical margins of the tooth, surgical correction to reform the scalloped pattern of the soft tissues alone will result in the re-establishment of a pocket in the embrasure region postoperatively. In this situation the basic principle is to correct bone form by creating a gently scalloped pattern of osseous surfaces that the soft tissue can follow.

Removal or recontouring of bone to treat periodontal disease is not a new concept. This was first advocated over fifty years ago [40, 41 & 42]. At that time many favoured bone removal because it was thought to be necrotic and infected although a few, at this time, advocated removal or recontouring of irregular margins [43 & 44]. This latter concept has been revived and expanded since 1949 when Schluger restated the principle of harmonious gingival and osseous architecture to prevent the recurrence of pockets after periodontal surgery [45]. A number of recent reports have suggested technical improvements but the underlying principle remains unchanged [46, 47 & 48].

Although the bone deformity is occasionally due to exostosis of buccal or lingual plates, an overdeveloped zygomatic process or pronounced external oblique line, osseous deformities are most frequently caused by periodontal disease. In the presence of inflammation bone resorption tends to follow the course of the blood vessels [49] (p. 36). This is principally due to blood vessels being supported by loose connective tissue which is the 'stage upon which the drama of inflammation is played' [50]. The pattern of bone loss is dependent upon the original site of the inflammation, the morphology and thickness of the bone adjacent to it, the course of the blood vessels, and the collagen structure in the region. In the interdental region an inflammatory reaction beneath the epithelium of the col will follow the perivascular connective tissue through the transeptal fibres and will extend along the intraseptal vessels. Alternatively, it may extend from the amelocemental junction down between the cementum and the mesial or distal

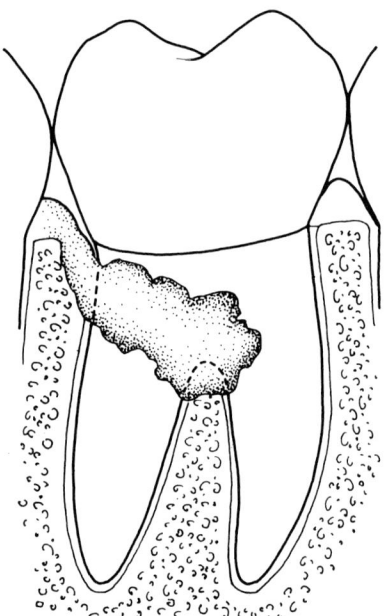

FIG. 15.26. Extension of a pocket to involve the bifurcation of the roots of a mandibular molar.

cortical plate along the line of the vessels of the periodontal membrane. As the cortical plate of the supporting bone is cribriform in nature the zone of resorption may well pass laterally through any of the small openings caused by the joining up of periodontal vessels and the intraseptal vessels. As the bone within the confines of the outer cortical plates and that lining the tooth sockets is cancellous in nature it tends to resorb more easily than the denser cortical bone. In this way irregular patterns of bone resorption occur frequently leaving unsupported cortical bone, and the resultant pockets have a complex topography. Frequently bone at the base of a pocket is apical to the neighbouring bone forming a compound pocket. In multirooted teeth extension of the pocket into the bifurcation or trifurcation is a common problem (fig. 15.26). This complicates elimination of the pocket surgically.

Correction of bone form is carried out using chisels, burs (Nos. 8 and 10 round) or coarse bonded diamond stones (fig. 15.22). Two procedures are described, osteoplasty and osteotomy.

Osteoplasty has been defined as reshaping of bone contour to reduce thickened buccal or lingual plates, to eliminate hollowing of the interdental crest between the plates, and to re-create a functional form [46].

Ostectomy has been described as deliberate excision and sacrifice of bone to restore the scalloped pattern of the supporting tissues [46].

Osteoplasty and ostectomy are most frequently performed in conjunction and are best described by the single term osseous contouring.

Some resorption of bone follows surgical correction of the contour in the immediate postoperative period [51]. These techniques should be applied with reserve and allowance made for the postoperative resorption which may follow.

TREATMENT OF COMPOUND POCKETS

Compound pockets have been classified according to the number of walls in the bone defect, as one wall, two wall, three wall and four wall pockets [52 & 3] (fig. 15.27). Where the number of walls is different in the apical area of the pocket from that in the occlusal area, this has

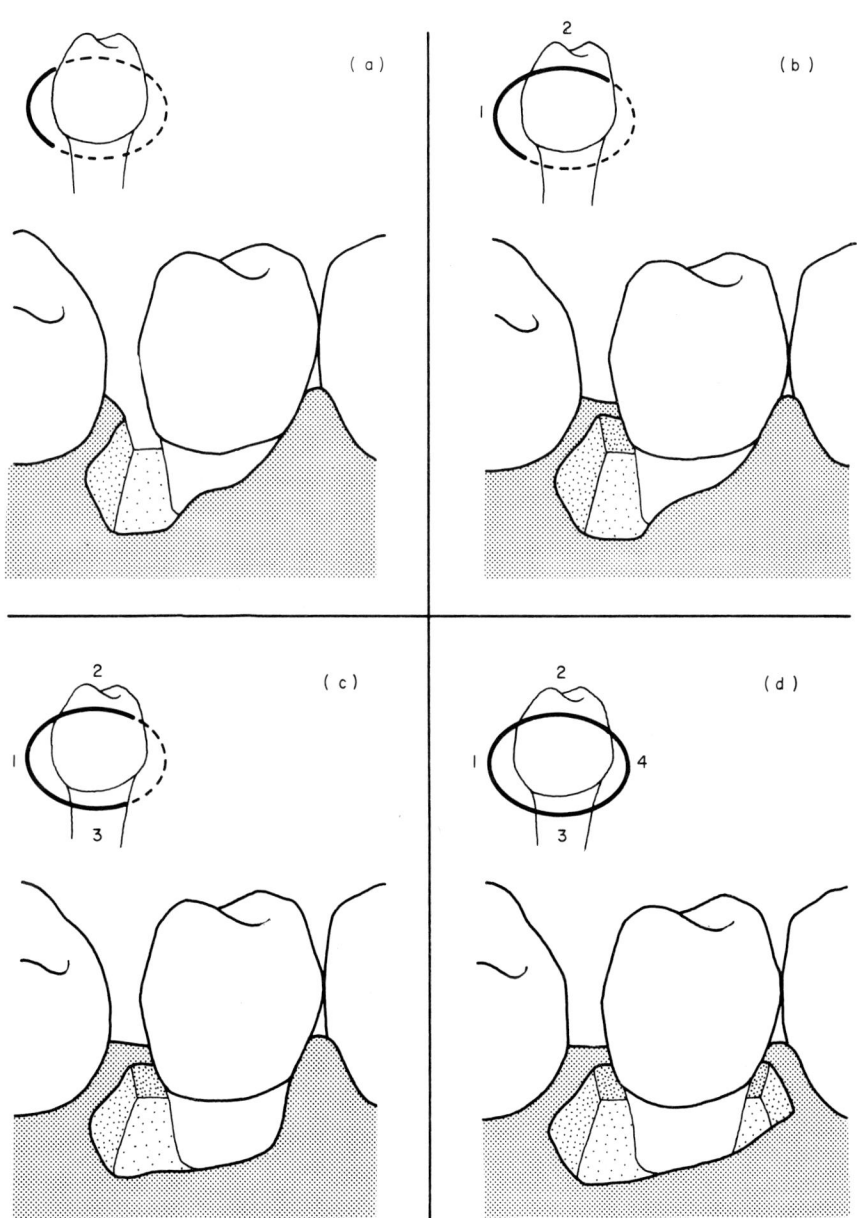

FIG. 15.27. Classification of compound pockets, (a) one wall compound pocket, (b) two wall compound pocket, (c) three wall compound pocket, (d) four wall compound pocket.

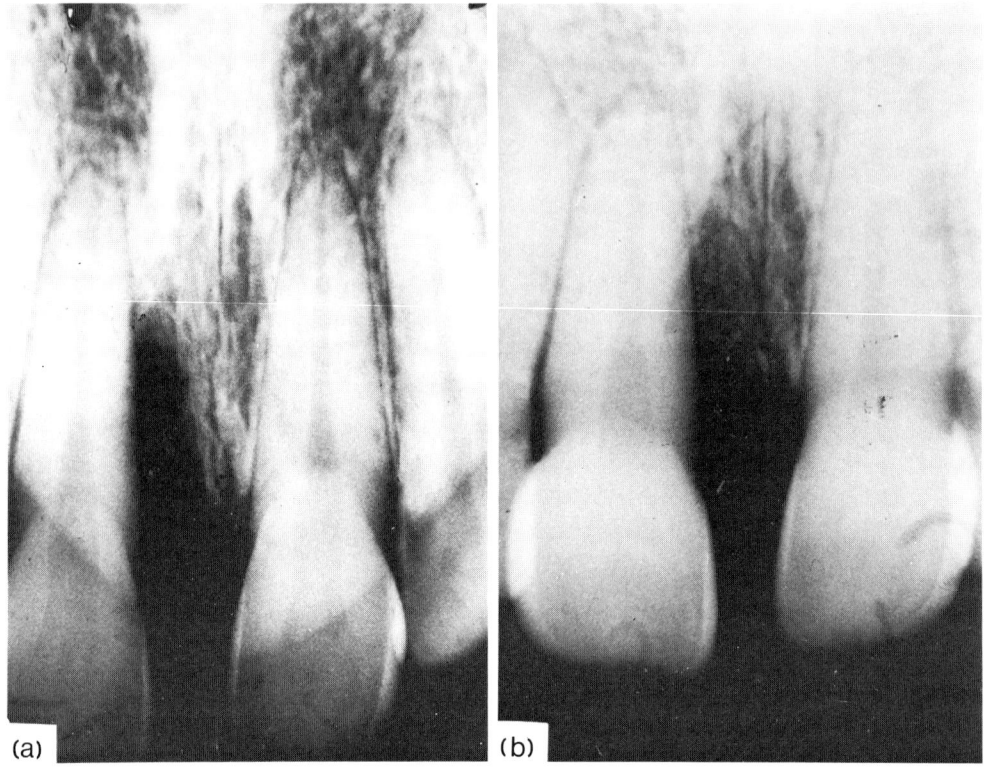

FIG. 15.28. (a) Radiograph of 10 mm infra bony pocket mesial to $\underline{1}$ treated with flap surgery and graft. (b) Repeat radiograph 3 months postoperative showing established graft.

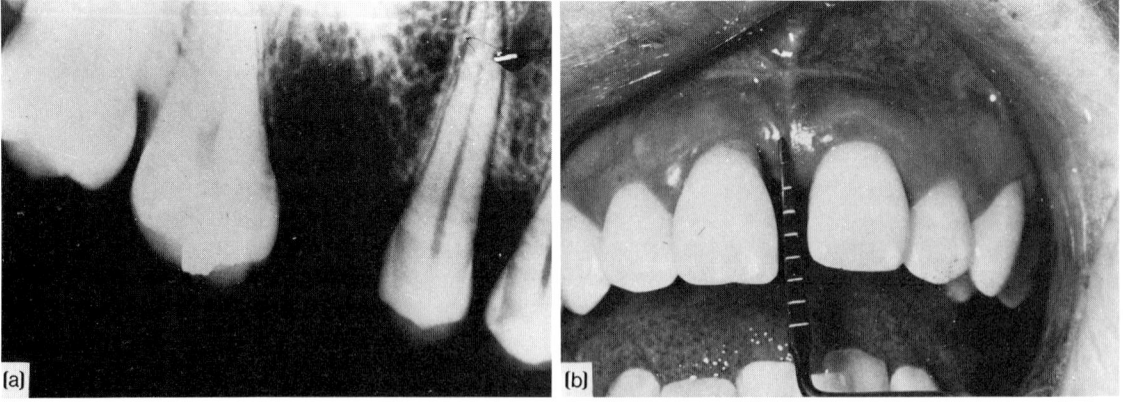

FIG. 15.29. (a) Radiograph of donor site for operative site shown in Fig. 15.28(a). (b) 3 months postoperative, probe can now only penetrate 3 mm.

been described as a combined osseous defect. Postoperative repair is dependent on organization of a clot in the defect, and the population of this clot by mesenchymal cells from the surrounding bone surfaces, which will subsequently induce calcification. The success of treatment is thus related to the number of walls in the osseous defect. It has been stated that at least three osseous walls are mandatory for predictable success [52 & 3]. One and two wall deformities should be reshaped by osseous contouring to eliminate the defect altogether.

When the flap is raised, thorough curettage of the tooth surface, the bone defect and the wound base should be carried out.

In many instances sufficient access may be gained to carry out the correction of bone architecture without the use of relaxing incisions at all (fig. 15.30b).

The use of autogenous and heterogenous bone transplants have been described [53, 54 & 55], but longitudinal studies in humans require to be undertaken before bone grafting of this area is worthy of widespread application (fig. 15.28 & 15.29).

Bone is a delicate tissue and when cut or left uncovered by mucoperiosteum varying amounts become necrotic and sequestrate or are resorbed by osteoclasts which are thought to form from undifferentiated mesenchymal cells in the vicinity. Granulation may also be initiated from cells of the periodontal membrane and adjacent wound margins. The bone becomes covered with a young proliferating connective tissue. Complete postoperative coverage of bone with a mucoperiosteal flap speeds up this process and reduces the amount of resorption which takes place.

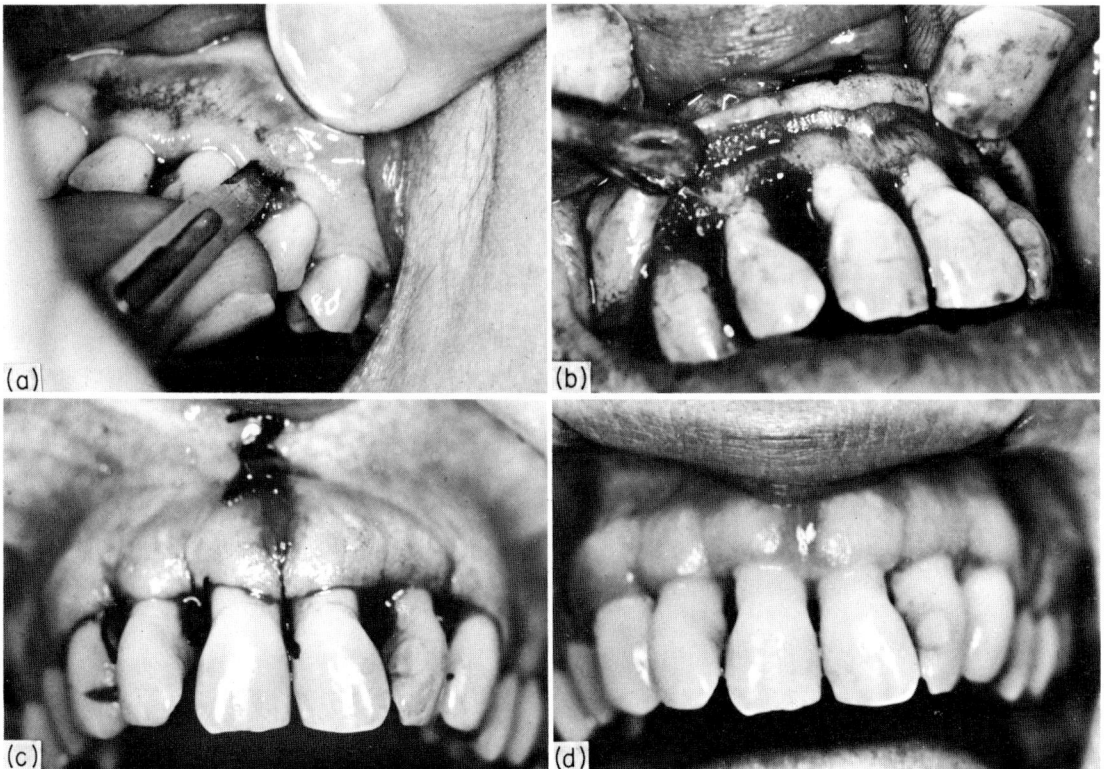

FIG. 15.30. Replaced flap. (a) Reverse bevel incision. (b) Access without vertical relaxing incisions. (c) Flap secured by interdental sutures. (d) 3 weeks postoperative (see also fig. 15.34).

REPLACING THE FLAP

A flap raised by reverse bevel incision should accord closely with the corrected bone form when replaced in position on the donor site. Occasionally it may be necessary to trim the edge of the flap with scissors before suturing to reduce excess tissue but this should not be required if the reverse bevel incision has been well placed. It should be secured in position by interdental sutures with no attempt made to draw the tissues fully across the embrasure region by placing sutures under tension. Suturing is most easily performed by the use of a reverse cutting needle and fine silk (p. 260) (fig. 15.3). The palatal flap is pierced first, the needle passed through the embrasure to pick up the buccal flap, and the free end of the suture pulled through the contact area. The suture may then be tied on the buccal side. If the contact point is too tight to allow passage of the suture, the free end should be threaded onto a large needle and passed beneath the contact area to the buccal side. Sutures are removed after 1 week when the lesion should be well healed (fig. 15.30).

HEALING AFTER FLAP SURGERY

Studies have shown that healing following reverse bevel periodontal flap surgery may be by first, second or third intention depending mainly on the state of flap adaptation to teeth and bone [56]. Good adaptation of the flap to the teeth and complete coverage of bone leads to a much faster and more uncomplicated healing than occurs following apical repositioning of a flap. It was also found that healing was better following a split flap approach than following a full thickness mucoperiosteal flap. Untraumatized bone, covered by well adapted flaps, showed only mild, delayed and very superficial bone resorption, 2–3 weeks after the procedure. Bone that had been traumatized during reshaping by chisels or files showed superficial necrosis followed by resorption, which began as soon as 5 days after surgery. Under a well adapted flap this resorption was transient, superficial and underwent prompt repair. Where bone was left exposed, much more severe inflammation occured, resorption was still present 35 days post-

operatively, and healing was not entirely complete even in the 72 day specimens.

Electron microscopic examination of tissues 4 months after flap surgery in a human patient has demonstrated that connective tissue regeneration can occur with the formation of a new epithelial attachment [57], although the degree of bone regeneration is variable and is dependent on the nature of the osseous lesion and the surgical technique being used.

Histological studies following transplants of cancellous bone and marrow have suggested that the degree of regeneration, in an osseous defect of a given volume and morphology, varies directly with the adequacy of the soft tissue cover and with the surface area of the vascularized bony walls lining the defect. It varies inversely with the root surface area. In a series of 166 transplants in 40 patients, an average coronal bone regeneration of 3·4 mm was obtained using transplants from the maxillary tuberosity or from healing sockets or edentulous areas of the mandible or maxilla [58].

REVERSE BEVEL GINGIVECTOMY

The principle of the reverse bevel incision can be applied in treatment of the early lesion even when the lesion is gingivally contained. Two limitations of external wound gingivectomy are insufficient width of attached gingivae and lack of vestibular depth.

A gingivally contained lesion should be excised by reverse bevel incision when it is necessary to eliminate the lesion while preserving the existing width of attached gingivae and sulcus depth. The position of the coronal edge of the alveolar crest is defined by the method used for the open wound procedure. The knife is placed at a 25° angle to the long axis of the tooth 1–2 mm apical to the cervical margin and the incision made firmly down to the bone edge, as described for a replaced flap. The incision is then extended across the planned wound area, buccally and palatally, and scalloped at each embrasure. The wedge of tissue coronal to the incision is then dissected free. Where the lesion has been gingivally contained there is no need to traumatize the tissues further by reflecting a flap. The wound area is curetted free from residual granulation tissue, and the exposed tooth substance prepared with hoes and curettes as for subgingival curettage. The buccal and palatal tissues are collapsed against the underlying alveolar bone such that the peaks of tissue created by the scalloped incision meet in the centre of the embrasure. The tissues are secured in position by means of interdental sutures, or simply by placing of a pack.

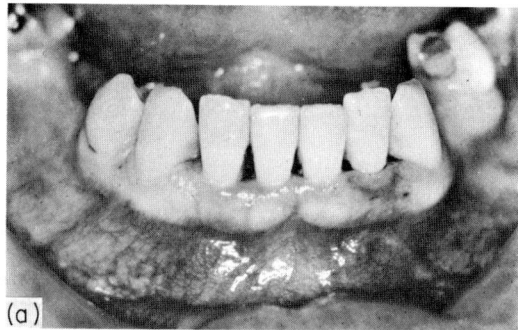

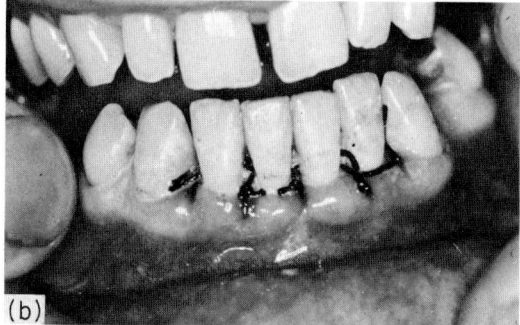

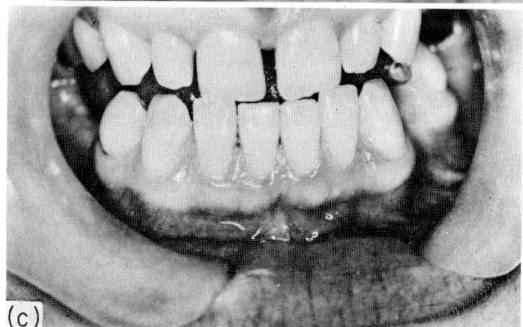

FIG. 15.31. Reverse bevel gingivectomy. (a) Early periodontitis. Simple pockets in presence of shortage in width of attached gingivae. (b) Pockets excised by reverse bevel gingivectomy without developing a flap. Soft tissue collapsed into embrasure and secured by sutures. (c) Pockets eliminated with no reduction in width of attached gingivae.

The advantages of this technique for surgical treatment of the gingivally contained lesion are considerable.

(1) The operation is conducted on the principle of conservation of the maximum amount of healthy tissue whilst still ensuring complete removal of all diseased tissue. The width of the zone of attached gingivae is not significantly reduced.

(2) The reverse bevel incision creates an internal wound which heals to some extent by first intention (fig. 15.31).

Treatment of the gingivally contained lesion by this approach has been described as split difference gingivectomy [6] or gingivectomy with an internal wound.

PROCEDURES INVOLVING ALTERATION OF MUCOGINGIVAL RELATIONSHIPS

Procedures which involve alteration in mucogingival relationships in presence or absence of compound pockets include:

(1) Frenectomy,
(2) Repositioned flaps,
(3) Retracted flaps,
(4) Mucosal flaps,
(5) Gingival grafts.

Alteration of mucogingival relationships may be indicated in the presence of the following.

(1) A frenum attachment high on the papilla such that tension from the lip movement may

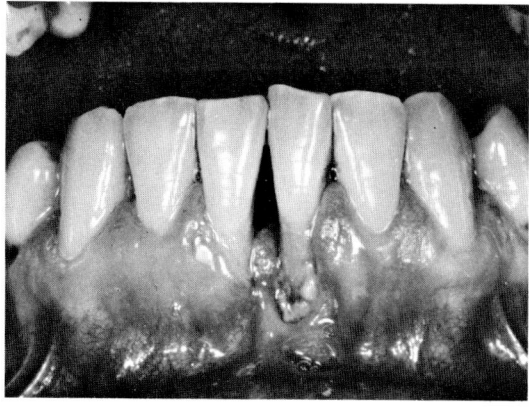

FIG. 15.32. Recession of tissue associated with the presence of a high frenum attachment.

result in detachment of the papilla from the tooth or recession of the tissue away from the tooth (fig. 15.32). This situation may arise as the normal developmental relationship of the tissues in a particular mouth, as a result of tissue loss in the presence of chronic periodontitis, or as the result of any surgical procedure which involves the excision and sacrifice of existing tissue.

(2) A functionally inadequate width of attached gingiva, between the cervical margin and the line of reflection of the mucosa onto the lips or cheeks. This may result in detachment of the gingivae from the tooth as a result of tension transmitted from movement of the lips or cheeks (fig. 15.33).

(3) Pockets which extend apical to the existing width of attached gingiva (fig. 15.33).

(4) An inadequate vestibular depth.

(5) Extreme recession of the soft tissues around a tooth.

Frenectomy

The excision of a frenum is easily achieved by the use of a scalpel with a number 11 blade and one or two pairs of artery forceps [59]. Local anaesthetic is placed in the sulcus on each side of the frenum sufficiently far from the frenum not to distort its preoperative anatomical form. The lip is held under tension and a pair of artery forceps placed parallel to the surface of the lip that the points of the forceps impinge on the

buccal alveolus at what is judged to be the most coronal point to which the frenum should extend postoperatively (fig. 15.34). The vertical angle of the forceps is adjusted so that the beaks extend to the mucolabial fold and the forceps are locked in that position. An incision is made down the lip side of the forceps to where the point impinges on the alveolus, and a second incision made parallel to the surface of the alveolus, from the most coronal point of attachment of the frenum to the point of the forceps. Where a large bulk of tissue has to be excised, a second pair of forceps may be placed parallel to the alveolus so that the points of the two pairs of forceps coincide. The second incision is then made on the alveolar side of the second pair of forceps.

These incisions are made through mucosa and submucous layers only, and result in a diamond shaped wound. Muscle is rarely if ever evident in the superficial tissues although it may be found deep in the wound. The attachment of the fibrous layer of the periosteum in the depth of the wound should be freed by sharp dissection. The lip side of the wound is closed by sutures placed through mucosa only, but no attempt should be made to close the alveolar side of the wound which heals by second intention (fig. 15.34).

Alternatively, frenectomy may be performed by placing the lip under tension and incising down to bone around the alveolar attachment of

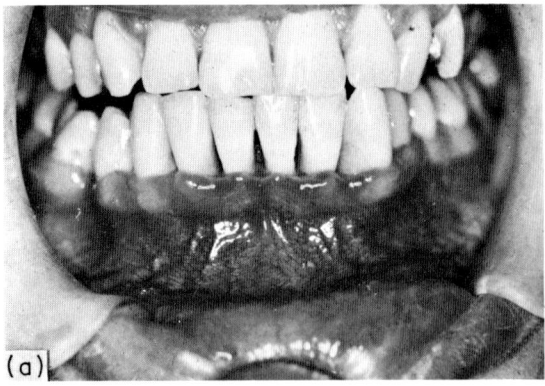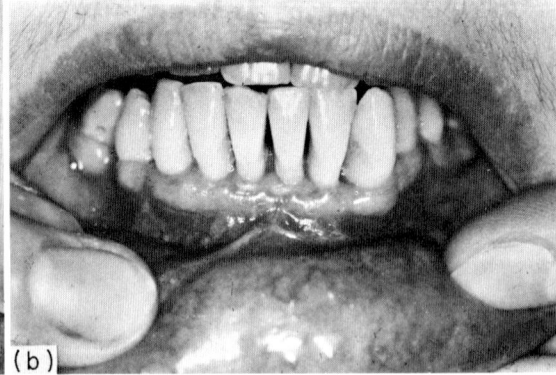

FIG. 15.33. (a) A functionally inadequate width of attached gingivae and pockets extending apical to the mucogingival line. The result of mismanaged recurrent ulceromembranous gingivitis. (b) Following treatment by apically repositioned flap.

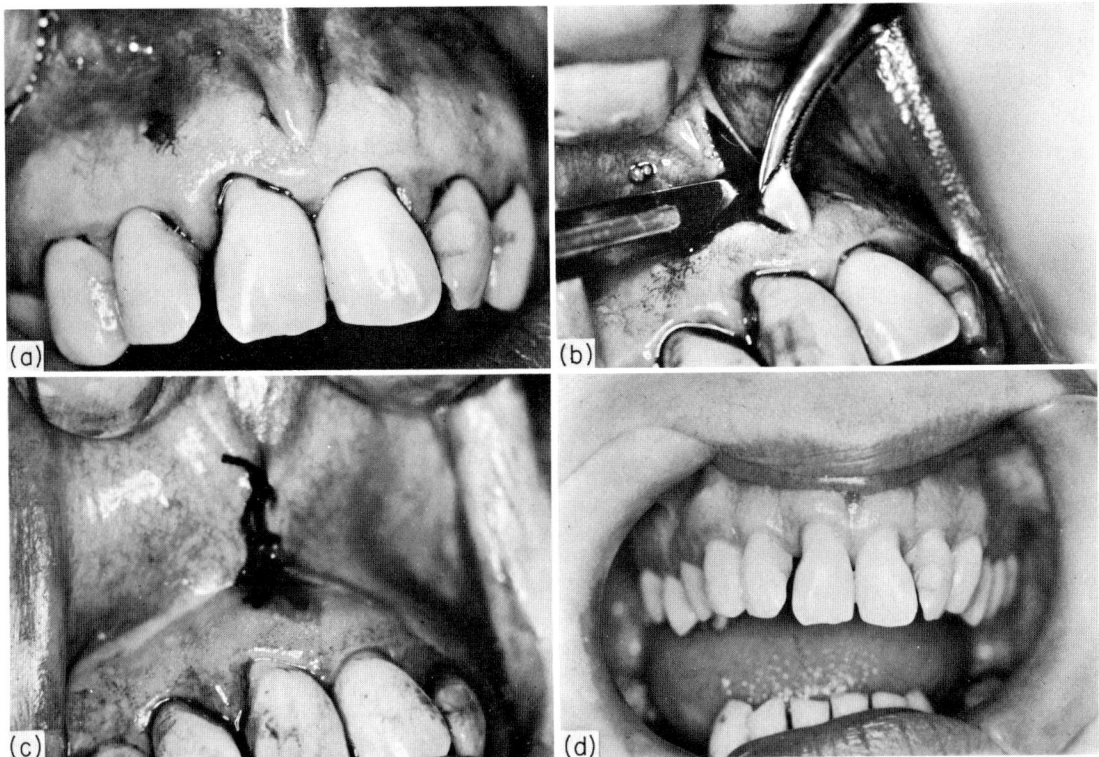

FIG. 15.34. (a) Mouth prior to frenectomy and replaced flap operation. (b) Incision down the lip side of artery forceps. (c) Lip wound sutured. (d) 12 months following frenectomy and replaced flap (see also fig. 15.30).

the frenum. Using a periosteal elevator lift or a mucoperiosteal flap to detach the frenum from alveolar bone, grasp the freed tissue in forceps, hold away from the lip and excise the excess frenal tissue, suture the lip side of the wound.

While the method initially described has been widely criticized as crude by experienced operators, we find that the use of artery forceps to define the position of the incision on the lip side of the wound lends confidence to those less experienced.

Flap procedures

Mucogingival surgery is concerned with the treatment of abnormality of form involving the attached gingiva and its relation to the underlying alveolar support, the alveolar mucosa, and depth of the vestibular sulcus [60].

Goldman described three problems which in-

volved interrelating gingival, mucosal and vestibular surgery [61]:

(1) extension of pocket depth through the attached gingivae into the alveolar mucosa,

(2) extension of the frenum attachment into the marginal gingivae,

(3) a shallow vestibular trough resulting from surgical pocket reduction procedures.

The objectives of mucogingival surgery are the elimination of pockets, the production of a new and wider zone of attached gingivae and increase in depth of the vestibular sulcus.

During the last decade a wide and confusing choice of design of flaps for mucogingival surgery have been proposed. A technique of apical repositioning of attached gingivae was introduced by Nabers in 1954 [62], and the first detailed discussion of the techniques which had emerged was published by Goldman, Schuger and Fox in 1956 [63]. The original extension procedures, the Schluger 'pouch', and Fox 'push back' operation were open wound procedures which involved leaving areas of exposed alveolar bone to heal by second intention. Healing of such wounds tends to be slow and to be associated with considerable postoperative discomfort.

Histological studies have demonstrated that healing following exposure of bone by open wound procedures took place by granulation from the marrow spaces of the underlying bone [51]. The exposed cortical plate was removed either by resorption or sequestration and replaced by a bed of granulation tissue which differentiated into new cortical plate covered by fibrous gingival tissue during a protracted healing period. Cephalometric studies show that postoperative shrinkage of the new attached gingivae could result in loss of up to 87 per cent of the original operative depth increase [64].

The objective of the modifications of technique which have been proposed since that time has been the development of closed wound procedures which are associated to some extent with healing by primary intention and less postoperative discomfort.

There is no standard classification of mucogingival surgical techniques and classification of all the modifications which have been proposed is complex [6 & 65]. In some circumstances the use of open wound procedures is unavoidable although this is undesirable. Flap techniques associated with alteration in mucogingival relationships can be put in one of three groups [5], repositioned, retracted and mucosal flaps.

REPOSITIONED FLAPS

Apically repositioned flap

The apically repositioned flap has wide general application where increase in width of the zone of attached gingivae is the desired result. The concept of apical repositioning was introduced by Nabers in 1954 [62], and has been further developed by Friedman [66] and Bohannan [67].

A flap to be apically repositioned should be developed by reverse bevel incision placed oblique to the bone edge in an attempt to split the mucosa from the underlying periosteum (fig. 15.35). The object of a split flap procedure

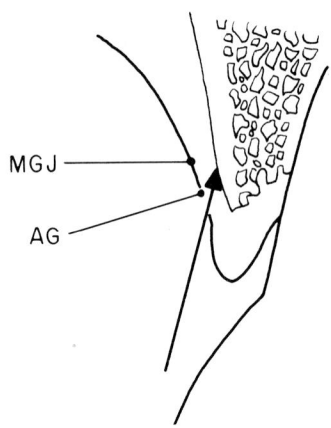

FIG. 15.35. Reverse bevel incision to develop split thickness flap; MGJ, mucogingival junction; AG, attached gingivae. A reverse bevel incision to develop a split flap is placed oblique to the bone edge.

is to produce the minimum exposure of areas of bone which do not require alteration during correction of bone form but which must be transiently exposed to allow repositioning of the flap. With split flap dissection exposed bone should remain covered to the maximum extent by periosteal remnants.

The splitting of mucoperiosteum into its individual layers is easily achieved under reflected mucosa, where the periosteum has a wide fibrous layer; but in the region of the attached gingiva, mucoperiosteum tends to function as an integral unit in which the individual layers are difficult to separate.

A split flap is developed by reverse bevel incision and released by two peripheral relaxing incisions (figs. 15.35 & 15.36). The relaxing incisions should be full thickness through mucoperiosteum down to bone in the area of the attached gingiva, but through mucosa only apical to the mucogingival junction [5]. The flap should be dissected free by sharp dissection leaving the maximum amount of periosteum on the exposed bone surface. Curettage of the wound area and correction of bone architecture should be carried out as previously described.

Such a flap is easily displaced apically, either to accord with the corrected bone edge (fig. 15.36b), or apical to the corrected bone edge (fig. 15.36c) to leave exposed a margin of bone

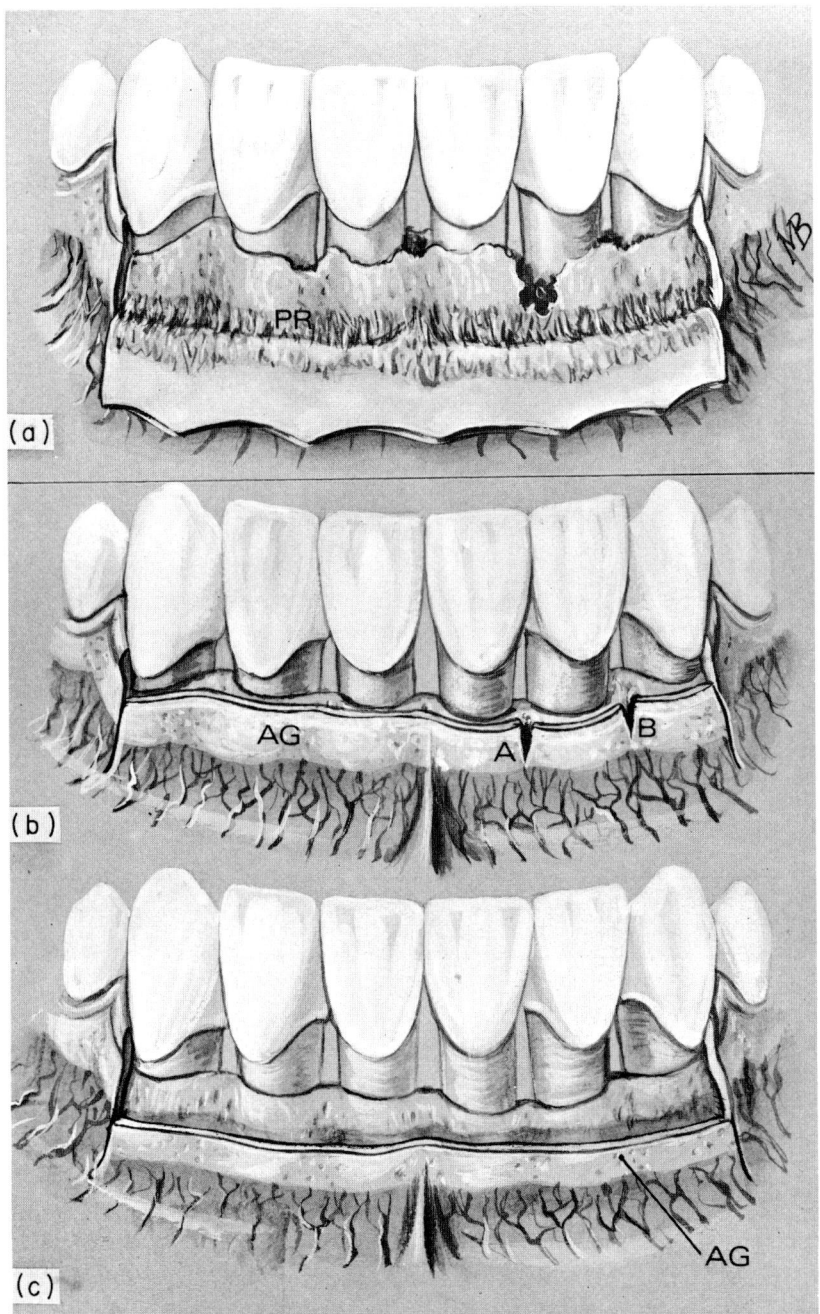

FIG. 15.36. Apical repositioning. (a) Split flap developed by reverse bevel incision, note the periosteal remnants (PR) on bone apical to the mucogingival line. (b) Flap apically repositioned to accord with the corrected bone edge; AG, attached gingivae; A & B, where the flap does not lie closely against the bone edge short vertical relaxing incisions should be placed. (c) Flap repositioned apical to the corrected bone edge. The permanent gain in width of attached gingivae which will be achieved is directly related to the area of denuded bone left exposed.

covered by periosteal remnants which will heal by second intention to form a new area of attached gingiva. No attempt should be made to reposition a flap to a functional knife edge relationship to the teeth. Healing is dependent on the proliferation of connective tissue from the flap edge and from the periodontal membrane.

Where a flap is repositioned to accord with the bone edge the normal relationship of soft tissue to teeth is restored by the formation of 2–3 mm of new gingiva at the coronal edge of flap. This takes place by proliferation of connective tissue elements which are subsequently covered by keratinizing stratified squamous epithelium.

Where a flap is repositioned apical to the corrected bone edge the gain in width of attached gingiva which is achieved will be directly related to the area of bone left exposed [64 & 48].

The repositioned attached gingiva acts as a barrier to creeping return of the mucogingival junction towards the teeth and leads to a permanent gain in width of attached gingiva, and vestibular depth.

Such flaps must be adequately secured against coronal return of the flap from the displaced position and from further apical displacement of the flap during the period of healing. Coronal return is prevented by suturing the base of the flap to the underlying periosteum in the depth of the vestibule and by suturing across the vertical incisions in the displaced position (fig. 15.37b). Further apical movement of flaps displaced to the bone edge may be prevented by a continuous horizontal mattress suture tied without tension (fig. 15.37a). Further displacement of flaps apical to the bone edge is stopped by simple suspensory sutures tied on the lingual side (fig. 15.37b).

The apically repositioned flap is the design of choice to meet problems associated with an inadequate width of attached gingiva, pockets which extend through the existing width of attached gingiva, and an inadequate sulcus depth in that situation. The limitations of this technique are that there must be at least some attached gingiva existing preoperatively, and that it must be possible to place this attached gingiva against bone in the fully displaced position. If there is no pre-existing attached gingiva, or if such attached gingiva as there is will be on the lip side of the wound in the apically displaced

position, this tissue must be excised and discarded, and some other operative procedure used. In a well selected case apical repositioning of attached gingiva gives a predictable and functionally acceptable result (fig. 15.38).

A longitudinal study in humans has been reported where curettage and surgical pocket elimination (gingivectomy or apically repositioned flap) were carried out on 104 patients and observed for periods of up to 10 years. The allocation of surgical procedures was undertaken on a random basis and variations in attachment levels were assessed at yearly intervals [39]. Evaluation of the results indicated that over 1–3 years curettage resulted in a slight gain of attachment, while there was a slight loss following surgical pocket elimination. A statistically significant loss of attachment occurred between 3 and 5 years following completion of the treatment for both experimental procedures. The long term (4–7 years) loss of attachment was not significantly different for the two procedures and pocket reduction was greater, and sustained better, following surgical elimination than following curettage. All cases received regular three-monthly prophylaxis, and during the period of the study, progression of the disease was retarded, indicating that both forms of therapy, in conjunction with regular prophylaxis, were of benefit to the patient. Although the two forms of surgical treatment were shown to give statistically significantly different results, these results were not of such magnitude as to have clinical significance over the period of the study.

Laterally repositioned flap

The most common indication for a laterally repositioned flap [68] is localized recession of the soft tissue around a tooth (fig. 15.40a). The degree of recession may be such that the attached gingiva is either greatly reduced in width or completely absent. Plaque and calculus accumulate at the base of the lesion which becomes self perpetuating as a result of mechanical irritation of lip movement.

Following administration of a local anaesthetic, the edges of the defect should be excised by means of a box shaped incision to remove the

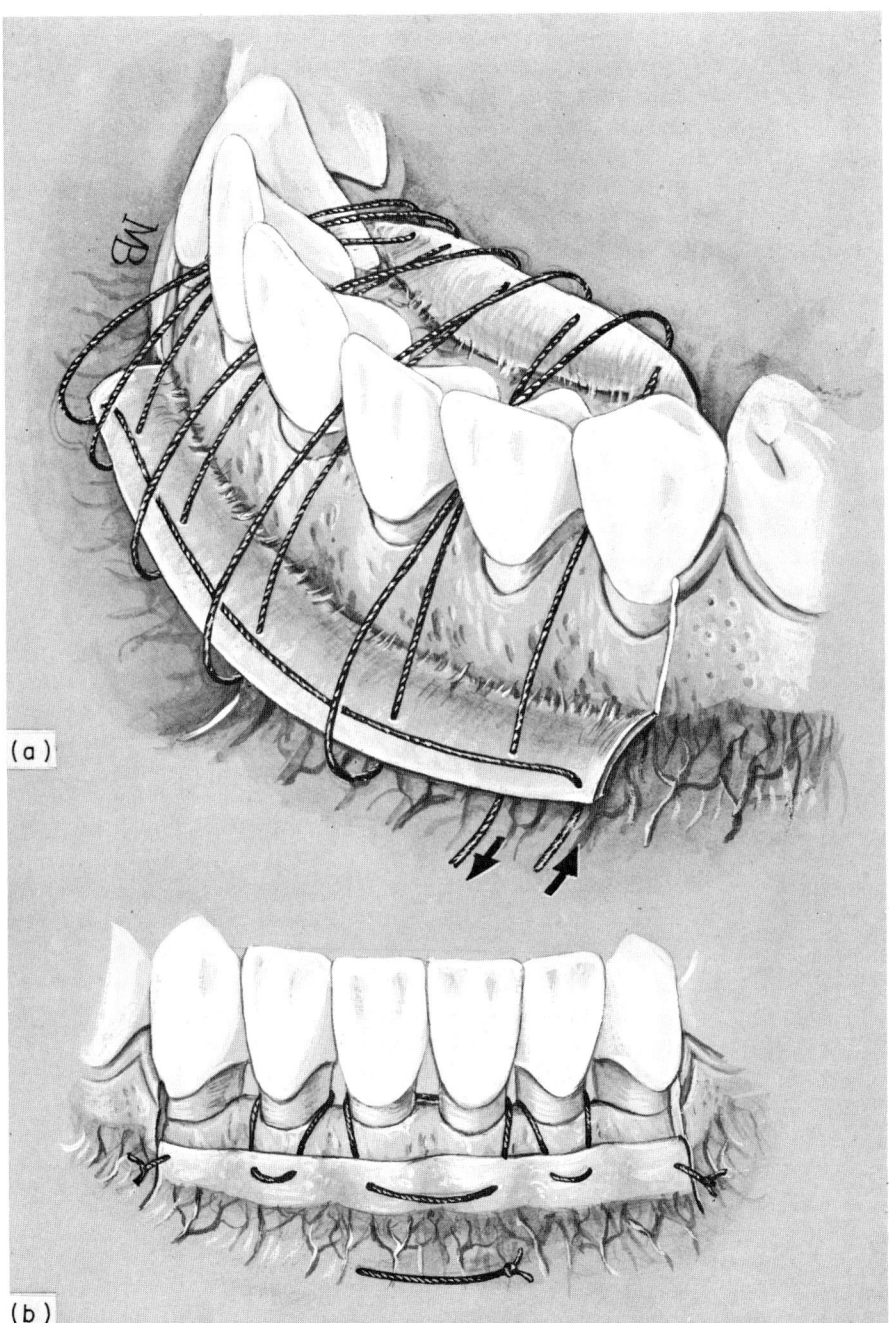

FIG. 15.37. Suturing apically repositioned flaps. Repositioned flaps must be stabilized to prevent further apical displacement during the healing period, or coronal return of the flap from the displaced position. Further apical displacement may be prevented by a continuous horizontal mattress suture (a) or by suspensory sutures tied round the lingual side of the teeth (b). Coronal return of the flap is prevented by a suture at the base of the sulcus through undisturbed periosteum and muscle and suturing the relaxing incisions in the displaced position (b).

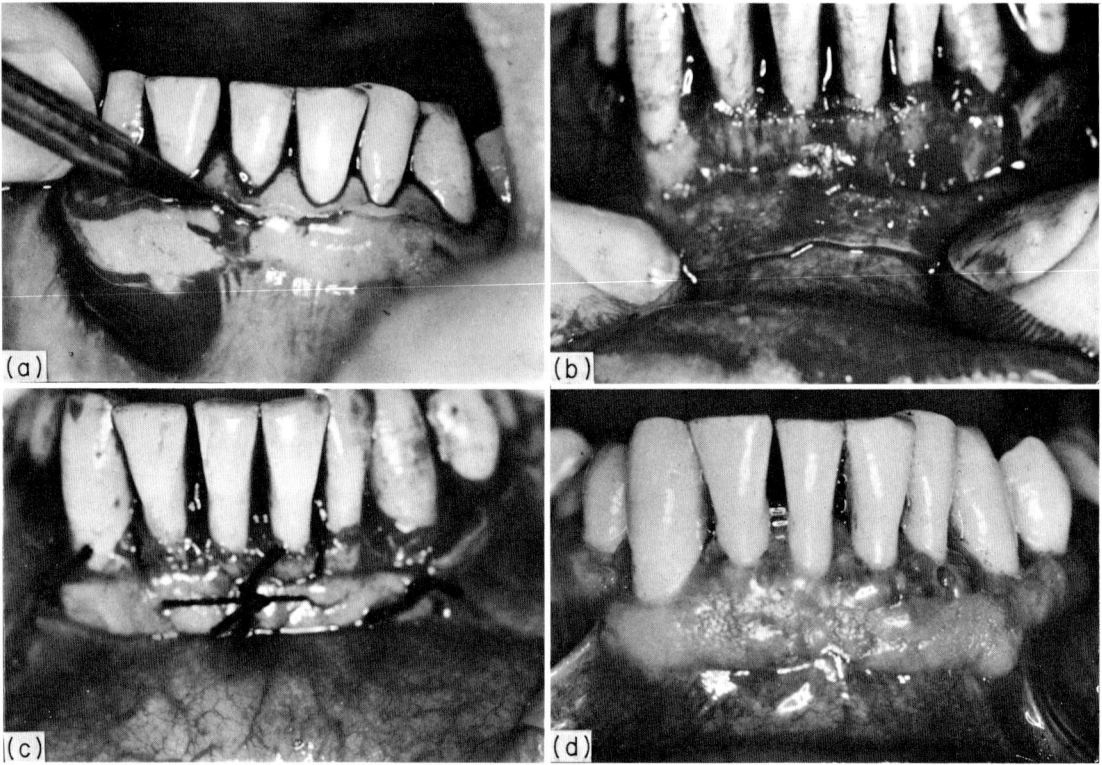

FIG. 15.38. (a) Reverse bevel incision. (b) Split flap developed; note periosteal remnants apical to mucogingival line. (c) Flap sutured in displaced position apical to the corrected bone edge. (d) Healing 4 weeks postoperative. Note the formation of new tissue coronal to edge of the repositioned flap.

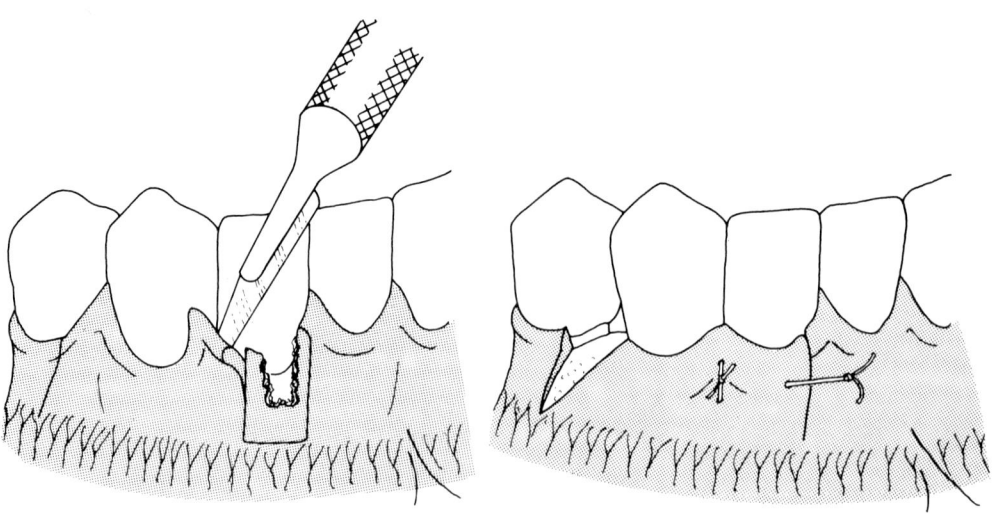

FIG. 15.39. Technique of laterally repositioned flap.

epithelial lining of the crevice and to prepare an exposed connective tissue surface at the edges of the wound (fig. 15.39). The edges of the defect and the exposed root should then be thoroughly prepared by curettage to receive the repositioned flap. A vertical relaxing incision (fig. 15.39) is placed at least $1\frac{1}{2}$ teeth away from the defect. The relaxing incision should be full thickness down to bone through the attached gingiva, but through mucosa only below the mucogingival line. A reverse bevel incision is made on the principles previously described, from where the relaxing incision joins the cervical margin to the edge of the defect. The flap should be mobilized as a full thickness mucoperiosteal flap by blunt dissection through the depth of the existing attached gingiva, and as a split thickness flap by sharp dissection apical to the mucogingival line. Such a flap is readily transferred laterally across the defect and secured in position by interdental sutures (fig. 15.40). The flap should be sutured to the prepared edge of the defect using a fine ophthalmic needle and 000 silk, and the wound covered by surgical dressing. The area of exposed bone in the region of the relaxing incision granulates and heals by second intention. The dressing is removed after 1 week when the area is gently cleansed and, if necessary, the donor site is redressed for a further week.

A refinement of this technique is to attempt a split flap dissection of the attached gingiva in the region of the donor site, so that the bone to be left exposed remains covered by periosteal remnants above the mucogingival line.

The laterally repositioned flap is not a predictable technique in comparision to the results achieved by apical repositioning. The initial cause of the recession is generally not known and the repositioned flap is placed on prepared tooth surface rather than on bone.

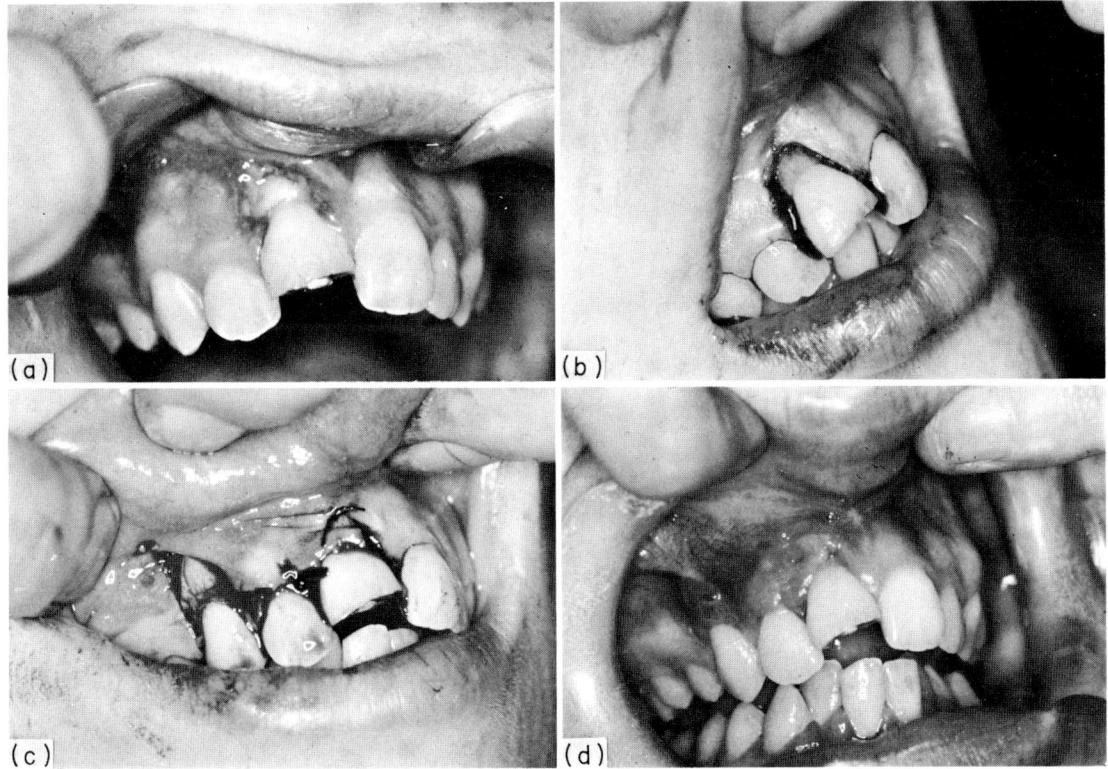

FIG. 15.40. (a) Defect buccal to central incisor. (b) Edges of defect excised following resolution of inflammation. (c) Flap transferred laterally and sutured in position. (d) 6 months postoperative.

A series of twenty-five cases of laterally re-positioned flaps has been reported [69].

The criteria for success have been described:

(1) Selection of the receptor site.

Selection of the operative site is dependent on the amount of tissue destruction present, the ability to eliminate the causative factors and the position, quality and support of the tooth itself. Recession can take place as a result of frenal tension, thin or absent buccal bone, malpositioning of teeth, plaque, calculus, food impaction, or there may be no obvious causative factors at all. All gingival recession does not justify surgical intervention, but progressive denudation of the tooth root or the presence of periodontal pockets does warrant therapy.

(2) Selection of the donor area.

The donor site should be associated with a healthy stable tooth and a site with gingival inflammation or periodontal pockets present should not be utilized.

In the well selected case the procedure gives a satisfactory result (fig. 15.40d).

RETRACTED FLAPS

A retracted flap may be defined as a flap developed following the excision and sacrifice of any existing attached gingivae (fig. 15.41).

The principle of denudation of bone for purposes of increasing the zone of attached gingivae was developed by Fox as the gingival replacement procedure [63]. Gingival replacement means that all the attached gingiva has been removed during surgery and its replacement with a wide new zone of attached gingiva is the therapeutic goal. Gingival replacement was performed only in presence of an adequate vestibular depth, and where increase in vestibular depth was required in addition to increasing the zone of attached gingiva. Schluger developed the vestibular trough extension procedure [63]. The Fox push back (gingival replacement) and the Schluger pouch (vestibular extension) procedures involved denudation of areas of alveolar bone which healed by granulation, and the healing period was frequently associated with considerable postoperative discomfort. These procedures have been refined to retain or create a protective cover of mucosa or periosteum for

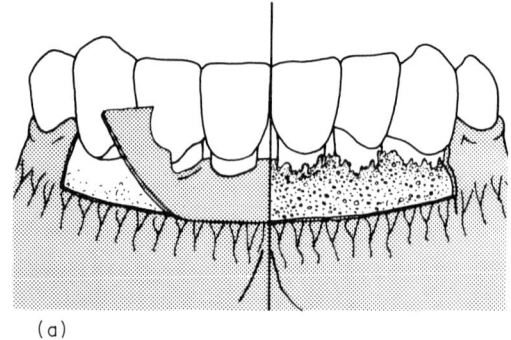

(a)

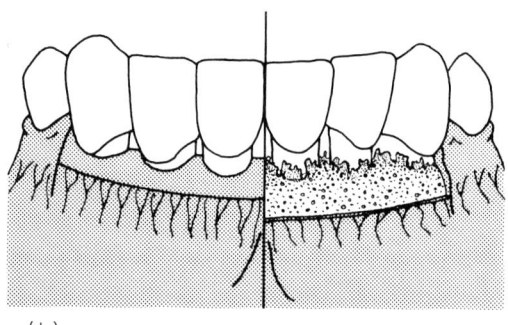

(b)

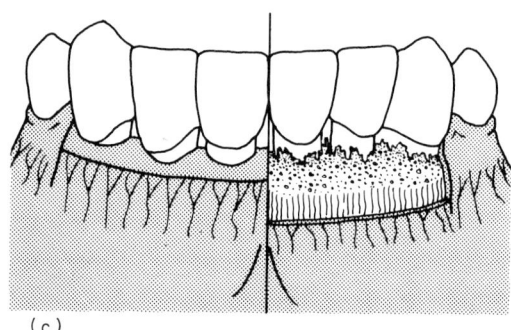

(c)

FIG. 15.41. Technique of retracted flaps. (a) Complete denudation to the depth required. (b) Excision of attached gingivae followed by retraction of full thickness flap which results in complete denudation. (c) Excision of attached gingiva followed by retraction of a split thickness flap leaving periosteal remnants apical to the mucogingival line. The design of choice.

bone which has been exposed at operation [48 & 70].

The need for retracted flaps arises most commonly as a result of shortage of attached gingiva in the mandibular incisor region, as a result of high frenal attachment in the mandibular premolar region, and in the mandibular molar region where the buccal surface of the mandible forms a flat plane covered by reflected mucosa sweeping out towards the external oblique ridge. The limitation of apically repositioning any existing attached gingiva is that it must be possible to place this attached gingiva against bone in the fully displaced position. While apical repositioning is the design of choice to increase the zone of attached gingiva, where any remaining attached gingiva will be on the lip side of the wound in the displaced position this must be excised and discarded and a retracted flap design used.

To develop a retracted flap (fig. 15.41), any remaining attached gingiva should be excised and a flap consisting of alveolar mucosa retracted to the required depth. The area of bone exposed will granulate and heal by second intention to form a new area of attached gingiva.

Three designs have been used.

(1) An incision through the alveolar mucosa at the depth required followed by discarding all tissue coronal to the level of the incision (fig. 15.41a). This results in complete denudation of bone coronal to the incision. The exposed bone becomes necrotic and replaced by a granulation tissue bed which subsequently differentiates into attached gingiva. There is considerable postoperative discomfort, healing is slow and packs may be required for four or five weeks postoperatively. This technique has no place in contemporary practice.

(2) An incision along the mucogingival line followed by discarding of attached gingiva and retraction of alveolar mucosa and periosteum to the required depth (fig. 15.41b). This again results in complete denudation of all exposed bone and has no advantage over the techniques described above.

(3) The design of choice is an incision along the mucogingival junction, discarding the attached gingiva, and thereafter sliding the alveolar mucosa developed as a split flap to the

required depth relative to the periosteum [48] (fig. 15.41c).

The alveolar mucosa should be freed from the underlying periosteum as previously described and retracted to the required depth. The bone remains covered with periosteal remnants apical to the mucogingival line and the area of denuded bone coronal to the mucogingival line is sufficient to establish an adequate width of attached gingiva. The permanent gain in width of attached gingiva which will be achieved is proportional to the area of bone which is denuded. No more bone should be denuded than is necessary to create a functionally adequate width of attached gingiva. Flaps retracted by this double flap procedure give a permanent gain in width of attached gingiva and a predictable result (fig. 15.42).

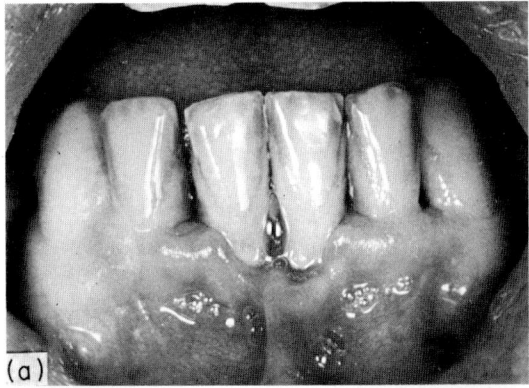
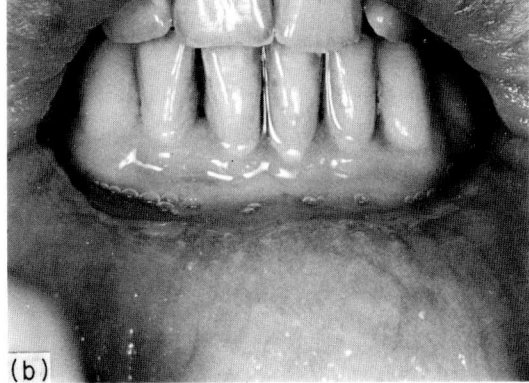

FIG. 15.42. Before (a) and after (b) retracted flap operation. Note how frenum has been removed during retraction.

MUCOSAL FLAPS

The objective of the procedure is to increase the vestibular depth while retaining such attached gingiva as remains (fig. 15.43). At the same time, if necessary, the width of attached gingiva can be increased by grafting, often from a palatal donor

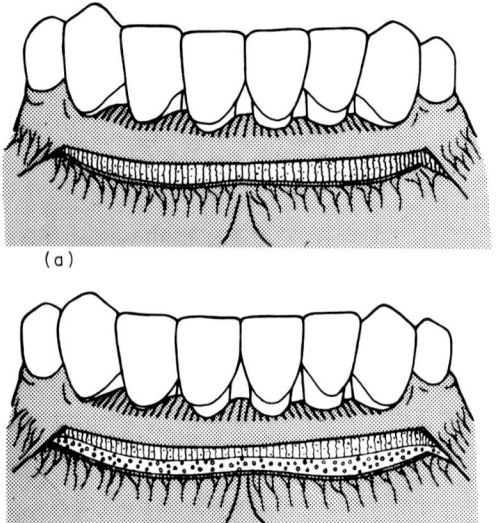

(a)

(b)

FIG. 15.43. (a) Mucosal flap developed without periosteal fenestration at the mucogingival line. This does not lead to a permanent gain in width of attached gingiva and sulcus depth. (b) Mucosal flap with periosteal fenestration. Differentiation of attached gingivae in the area of fenestration prevents creeping return of the mucogingival line towards the teeth.

site, a strip of keratinized tissue, immediately below any existing gingiva.

An incision is made along the mucogingival junction and a flap consisting of alveolar mucosa reflected either as a split flap (fig. 15.43a) or with some degree of periosteal fenestration (fig. 15.43b). Where there is no periosteal fenestration retraction of a split flap will result in increase in sulcus depth, but no permanent increase in width of the zone of attached gingiva. Where there is periosteal fenestration the resulting scar tissue will form an attachment which prevents creeping return of the mucogingival junction toward the teeth [71]. Where necessary, the operation is performed as a combination procedure with deliberate periosteal fenestration with graft insertion sufficient to increase the zone of attached gingiva, and subsequent split flap sharp dissection to increase the vestibule depth.

On this basis the technique gives a permanent and predictable result although scar tissue in the area of periosteal fenestration is occasionally unsightly (fig. 15.44).

The pouch may be dissected to any depth required and may be lined with gingival grafts, split skin grafts (fig. 15.45), or graft of mucosa from the cheeks.

Gingival grafts

Gingival grafts may be used to create a wider zone of attached gingiva or to deepen the vestibule in association with single defects or

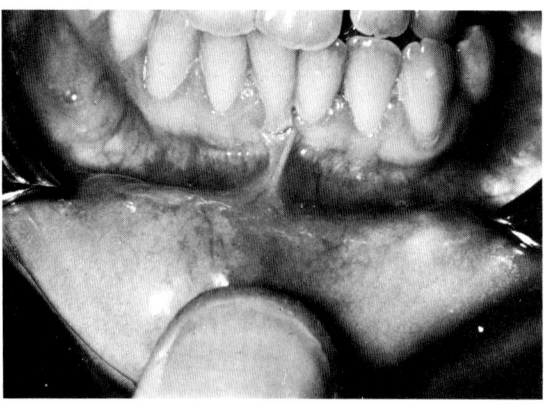
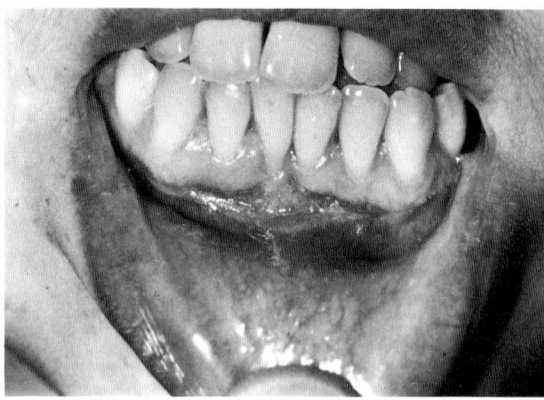

FIG. 15.44. Scar following periosteal fenestration at the mucogingival line.

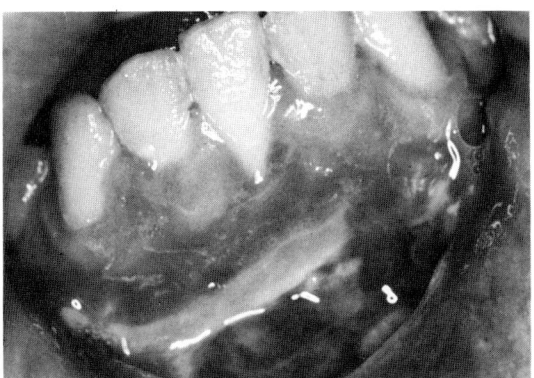

FIG. 15.45. Mucosal flap pouch dissection lined by split skin graft, 3 weeks postoperative.

mucogingival problems in relation to groups of teeth [72]. Using this technique, mature keratinized tissue is removed from the palate, edentulous areas or other donor areas having adequate width of attached gingiva, and the resulting split thickness, free graft transferred to the recipient site (fig. 15.46). In cases of individual defects the recipient site is prepared as previously described for a laterally repositioned flap and where an increased width of attached gingiva is required in association with a shallow vestibule, a mucosal flap is first raised and displaced apically to allow insertion of the graft on the prepared connective tissue bed below the line of incision at the mucogingival junction. Care should be taken when removing the graft from the donor site to ensure that the tissue is large enough to accommodate any

shrinkage which might occur postoperatively, the graft should be as thin as possible and care should be taken to cause minimal trauma. When bleeding at the prepared recipient site has ceased, the graft is carefully sutured into place using atraumatic needles and compressed to the underlying connective tissue for 1–2 minutes to allow adhesion by fibrin to occur. The graft is then covered by sterile gauze and a pack carefully placed. Consideration should also be given to the placement of a dressing over the wound in the donor area. This wound is shallow and although when on the buccal aspect or in an edentulous area they can be packed, palatal wounds are difficult and frequently the dressing causes the patient more problems than simply leaving the wound open. Healing of the donor area is by granulation and is well advanced by 1 week. At that time, the pack and sutures are removed from the recipient area, when healing should also be well advanced. The associated teeth should be carefully polished and the wound cleaned. Where necessary, a pack can be replaced for a further week but in many instances this will not be found necessary. When the pack has been removed, the patient should be encouraged to clean the area gently with a toothbrush, gradually increasing the thoroughness of brushing so that by 1 week after pack removal, cleaning is at preoperative levels. The use of free gingival grafts to cover denuded roots has been discussed [73]. Over a period of 2 years free gingival autografts were used in the treatment of twenty areas of localized gingival recession with root

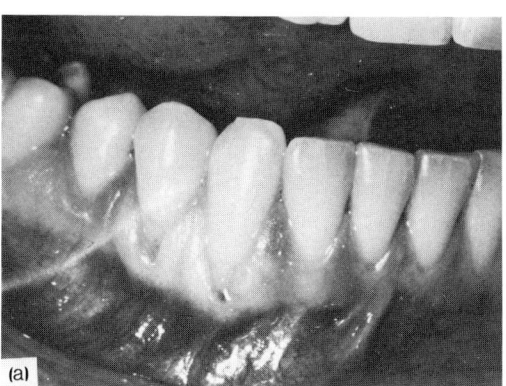

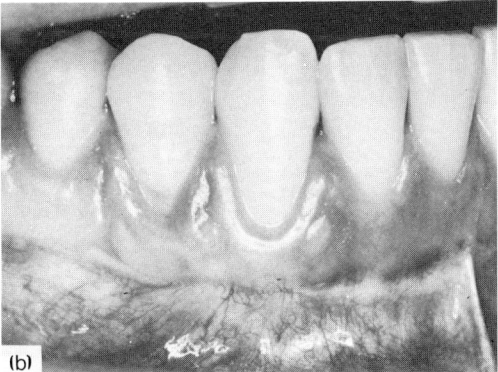

FIG. 15.46. (a) Recession of gingiva leaving inadequate width $\overline{43}$. (b) Postoperative situation 2 years after free gingival graft from palate. Satisfactory width of attached gingiva and depth of vestibule.

exposure. The size of the defect was carefully measured both pre- and postoperatively. Where defects were less than 3 mm in width and depth approximately 70 per cent of the root defect could be covered. Where lesions were of greater width, only 13 per cent of the defect could be covered. Experiments in dogs [74] have shown that revascularization of the graft does not begin until the fifth postoperative day and not until the tenth postoperative day is an effective peripheral vascular plexus re-established. As the graft depends on adjacent tissue for nitrients,

it is clear that large grafts cannot survive when placed over cementum.

Provided the latter reservation is noted, free gingival grafts have a place in periodontal surgery, particularly in cases of recession in relation to anterior teeth where the lifting of a pedicle graft on an adjacent tooth might expose an underlying bony defect.

Completion of corrective phase therapy constitutes control and not cure. All patients must be recalled for regular maintenance at intervals which should not exceed 6 months.

REFERENCES

[1] LINDE J. & NYMAN S. (1975) The effect of plaque control and surgical pocket elimination on the establishment and maintenance of periodontal health. A longitudinal study of periodontal therapy in cases of advanced disease. *Journal of Clinical Periodontology*, **2**, 67–79.

[2] AXELSSON P. & LINDHE J. (1978) Effect of controlled oral hygiene procedures on caries and periodontal disease in adults. *Journal of Clinical Periodontology*, **5**, 133–151.

[3] GOLDMAN H. & COHEN D.W. (1958) The infrabony pocket, classification and treatment. *J. Periodont.* **29**, 272–291.

[4] FRIEDMAN N. & LEVINE L. (1964) Mucogingival surgery current status. *J. Periodont.* **35**, 5–21.

[5] MACPHEE I.T. (1967) The design of flaps for mucogingival surgery. *Edin. Dent. Hosp. Gazette*, **7**, No. 3, 8–15.

[6] KRAMER G.M. & KOHN J.D. (1966) A classification of periodontal surgery. An approach based on tissue coverage. *Periodontics*, **4**, 80–89.

[7] GARROD L.P. & WATERWORTH P.M. (1962) The risks of dental extraction during penicillin treatment. *Brit. Heart J.* **24**, 39–46.

[8] JORGENSON N.B. & HAYDEN J. (1967) *Premedication, Local and General Anaesthesia in Dentistry*, p. 28. London: Kimpton.

[9] JOYCE C.R.B. (1961) Sedatives and analgesics in dental practice. *Dent. Practit. dent. Rec.* **12**, 111–118.

[10] BERDON J.K. (1965) Blood loss during gingival surgery. *J. Periodont.* **36**, 102–107.

[11] McIVOR J. & WENGRAF A. (1966) Blood loss in periodontal surgery. *Dent. Practit. dent. Rec.* **16**, 448–451.

[12] MORRIS M.L. (1965) Suturing techniques in periodontal surgery. *Periodontics*, **3**, 84–89.

[13] GOLDMAN H.M. (1944) The relationship of the epithelial attachment to the adjacent fibres of the periodontal membrane. *J. dent. Res.* **23**, 177–180.

[14] SHAPIRO M. (1953) Reattachment in periodontal disease. *J. Periodont.* **24**, 26–31.

[15] SHAPIRO M. (1960) Reattachment operation. *D. Clin. N. Amer.* **15**, 25.

[16] JANSEN M.T., COPPES L. & VERDENIUS H.H.W. (1955) The healing of periodontal wounds in dogs. *J. periodont.* **26**, 292–300.

[17] RAMFJORD S.P. & COSTICH E.R. (1963) Healing after simple gingivectomy. *J. Periodont.* **34**, 401–415.

[18] LINGHORNE W.J. & O'CONNEL D.C. (1957) Studies in reattachment and regeneration of the supporting structures of the teeth i.v. Regeneration in epithelialised pockets following organisation of a blood clot. *J. dent. Res.* **36**, 4–12.

[19] GLICKMAN I. & LAZANSKY J.P. (1950) Reattachment of the marginal gingivae and periodontal membrane in experimental animals. *J. dent. Res.* **29**, 659.

[20] LINGHORNE W.J. & O'CONNEL D.C. (1950) Studies in regeneration and reattachment of the supporting structure of the teeth. I. Soft tissue reattachment. *J. dent. Res.* **29**, 419–428.

[21] MORRIS M.L. (1954) The removal of pocket and attachment epithelium in humans. A histological study. *J. Periodont.* **25**, 7–11.

[22] RAMFJORD S.P., KERR D.A. & ASH M. (eds.) (1966) *World Workshop in Periodontics*, p. 291. Ann Arbor, Michigan.

[23] FRIEDMAN N. (1962) Mucogingival surgery. The apically repositioned flap. *J. Periodont.* **33**, 328–340.

[24] ARIAUDO A.A. (1957) Symposium on the surgical approach to the periodontal problem. Procedure for gingivectomy. *J. Periodont.* **28**, 62.

[25] GLICKMAN I. (1956) The results obtained with an unembellished gingivectomy technique in a clinical study in humans. *J. Periodont.* **27**, 247–255.

[26] RAMFJORD S.P., KERR D.A. & ASH M. (eds.) (1966) *World Workshop in Periodontics*, p. 300. Ann Arbor, Michigan.

[27] McHUGH W.D. & PERSSON P.A. (1958) Fluorescence microscopy of healing gingival epithelium. *Acta. odont. scand.* **16**, 205–218.

[28] PERSSON P.A. (1961) The healing process in the marginal periodontium after gingivectomy with special regard to

the regeneration of epithelium. *Dent. practit. dent. Rec.* **11**, 427–437.

[29] BERNIER J. & KAPLAN H. (1947) The repair of gingival tissue after surgical intervention. *J. Amer. dent. Ass.* **35**, 697.

[30] INNES P.B. (1970) An electron microscopic study of the regeneration of gingival epithelium following gingivectomy in the dog. *J. Periodont. Res.* **5**, 196.

[31] LISTGARTEN M.A. (1967) Electron microscopic features of the newly formed epithelial attachment after gingival surgery. *J. Periodont. Res.* **2**, 46.

[32] LISTGARTEN M.A. (1972) Normal development, structure, physiology and repair of gingival epithelium. *Oral Sciences Reviews*, **1**, 3–68.

[33] STAHL S.S., WITKIN G.J., CANTOR M. & BROWN R. (1968) Gingival healing. 2. Clinical and histologic repair sequences following gingivectomy. *J. Periodont.* **39**, 109–118.

[34] ENGLER W.O., RAMFJORD S.P. & HINIKER J.J. (1966) Healing following simple gingivectomy. A tritiated thymidine radioautographic study. 1. epithelialization. *J. Periodont.* **37**, 298–308.

[35] LEUBKE R.G. & INGLE J.I. (1964) Geometric nomenclature for mucoperiosteal flaps. *Periodontics*, **2**, 301–303.

[36] WRIGHT W. H. (1965) The scalloped reverse bevel incision in mucogingival surgery. *Odont. T.* **73**, 514–526.

[37] KNOWLES J.W., BURGETT F.G., NISSLE R.R., SCHICK R.A., MORRISON E.C. & RAMFJORD S.P. (1979) Results of periodontal treatment related to pocket depth and attachment level. Eight years. *J. Periodont.* **50**, 225–233.

[38] RAMFJORD S.P. & NISSLE R.R. (1974) The modified Widman flap. *J. Periodont.* **45**, 601–607.

[39] RAMFJORD P., KNOWLES J. W., NISSLE R. R., SCHICK R. A. & BURGETT F. G. (1973) Longitudinal study of periodontal therapy. *J. Periodont.* **44**, 66–77.

[40] ROBICSEK (1894) Cited by MERRITT A.H. (1949) *Periodontal Diseases and Soft Tissue Lesions of the Oral Cavity*, p. 110. London, Kimpton.

[41] ZENTLER A. (1918) Suppurative gingivitis with alveolar involvement. A new surgical procedure. *J. Amer. Med. Ass.* **71**, 1530.

[42] ZEMSKY J.L. (1926) Surgical treatment of periodontal disease. *Dent. Cosmos.* **68**, 465.

[43] BLACK G.V. (1915) A work on special dental pathology devoted to the diseases and treatment of the investing tissues of the teeth and dental pulp. Including the sequellae of the death of the pulp. Also systemic effects of mouth infections, in *Oral Prophylaxis and Mouth Hygiene.* Chicago: Medico-Dental Publishing Co.

[44] NEUMANN R. (1921) Die-radikal-chirurgische. Behandlung der Alveolarpyorrhoe. *Vjschr. Zahnheilk*, **37**, 1134. Cited by MADISON W.J. (1939) A review of some surgical methods of treating pyorrohoea. *Amer. J. Orthodont.* **25**, 898–901.

[45] SCHLUGER S. (1949) Osseous resection. A basic principle in periodontal surgery. *Oral surg.* **2**, 316–325.

[46] FRIEDMAN N. (1955) Periodontal osseous surgery, osteoplasty, osteoectomy. *J. Periodont.* **26**, 257–269.

[47] OCHSENBEIN C. (1958) Osseous resection in periodontal surgery. *J. Periodont.* **28**, 15–26.

[48] OCHSENBEIN C. (1960) Newer concepts of mucogingival surgery. *J. Periodont.* **31**, 175–185.

[49] WEINMAN J.P. (1941) Progress of gingival inflammation into the supporting structures of the teeth. *J. Periodont.* **12**, 71–81.

[50] HAM A.W. & LEESON T.S. (1961) *Histology*, 4th Edition. Philadelphia: Lippincott.

[51] WILDERMAN M.N., WENTZ F.M. & ORBAN B.J. (1960) Histogenesis of repair after mucogingival surgery. *J. Periodont.* **31**, 283–299.

[52] PRICHARD J. (1957) Regeneration of bone following periodontal therapy. *Oral Surg.* **10**, 247–252.

[53] NABERS C.L. & O'LEARY T.J. (1965) Autogenous bone transplants in the treatment of osseous defects. *J. Periodont.* **36**, 5–14.

[54] CROSS W.G. (1960) The use of bone implants in the treatment of periodontal pockets. *Dent. Clin. N. Amer.* **March,** 107.

[55] MANN W.V. (1964) Autogenous transplant in the treatment of an infra-bony pocket. Case report. *Periodontics*, **2**, 205–208.

[56] CAFFESSE R.G., RAMFJORD S.P. & NASJLETI C.E. (1968) Reverse bevel periodontal flaps in monkeys. *J. Periodont.* **39**, 219–235.

[57] FRANK R., FIORE-DONNO G., CIMASONI G. & OGILVIE A. (1972) Gingival reattachment after surgery in man: an electron microscopic study. *J. Periodont.* **43**, 597–605.

[58] HIATT W.H. & SCHALLHORN R.G. (1973) Intra oral transplants of cancellous bone and marrow in periodontal lesions. *J. Periodont.* **44**, 194–208.

[59] ARCHER W.H. (1956) *A Manual of Oral Surgery*, p. 183. Philadelphia: Saunders.

[60] BOHANNAN H.N. (1962) Studies in the alteration of vestibular depth I. Complete denudation. *J. Periodont.* **33**, 120–128.

[61] GOLDMAN H.M. (1953) *Periodontia*, 3rd Edition, p. 552. St. Louis: Mosby.

[62] NABERS C.L. (1954) Repositioning the attached gingivae. *J. Periodont.* **25**, 38.

[63] GOLDMAN H.M., SCHLUGER S. & FOX L. (1956) *Periodontal therapy*, p. 301. St. Louis: Mosby.

[64] BOHANNAN H.M. (1962) Studies in alteration of vestibular depth II. Periosteum retention. *J. Periodont.* **33**, 354–359.

[65] CLARK J. (1963) Mucogingival surgical techniques. An appraisal. *J. Periodont.* **34**, 158–165.

[66] FRIEDMAN N. (1963) Mucogingival surgery: The apically repositioned flap. *J. Periodont.* **33**, 328–340.

[67] BOHANNAN H.M. (1963) The fixed long labial mucosal flap in vestibular alteration. *Periodontics*, **1**, 16.

[68] GRUPE H.E. & WARREN R.F. (1956) Repair of gingival defects by a sliding flap operation. *J. Periodont.* **27**, 92–95.

[69] McFALL W.T. (1967) The laterally repositioned flap criteria for success. *Periodontics*, **5**, 82–92.

[70] AURIODO A. & TYRELL H. (1957) Repositioning and increasing the zone of attached gingivae. *J. Periodont.* **28**, 106–110.

[71] ROBINSON R.E. & AGNEW R.G. (1963) Periosteal fenestration at the mucogingival line. *J. Periodont.* **34**, 503–512.

[72] NABERS J.M. (1966) Free gingival grafts. *Periodontics*, **4**, 243–245.

[73] MLINEK A., SMUKLER H. & BUCHNER A. (1973) The use of free gingival grafts for the coverage of denuded roots. *J. Periodont.* **44**, 248–254.

[74] JANSON W.A., RUBIN M.P., KRAMER G.M., BLOOM J.A. & TURNER H. (1969) Development of the blood supply to split thickness free gingival autografts. *J. Periodont. Periodontics*, **40**, 707–716.

CHAPTER 16

Epidemiology of gingivitis and periodontitis

Epidemiology is the study of the distribution and determinants of states of health and disease in human populations. Surveys conducted in many different countries have led the World Health Organization [1] to state: 'periodontal disease is one of the most widespread diseases of mankind. No nation and no area of the world is free from it and in most it has a high prevalence, affecting in some degree approximately half the child population and almost the entire adult population.'

Periodontal disease has been common in every culture, and paleontologic studies indicate that periodontal disease existed in early man [2]. The findings from epidemiological studies can be used for a variety of purposes. The community dentist may be interested in assessing the *prevalence* (number of cases of a disease in existence at a certain time within a community); the *incidence* (number of new cases of a disease occurring during a certain period within a defined community); or the *severity* of disease. The research worker may wish to correlate prevalence or incidence of a particular disease with various aetiological factors, in order to evaluate the importance, if any, of these factors. Such data may enable the clinician or public health planner to direct preventive measures or appropriate treatment against those factors which are found to be of importance. Clinical trials are carried out to determine to what extent a particular type of therapy may prevent or influence the course of a disease.

Although for many diseases it is sufficient to assess their presence or absence, in the case of chronic periodontal disease this is not adequate. Whilst one individual may have mild inflam-mation of a single gingival area, another may have virtually complete loss of supporting alveolar bone. Both would be classed as having periodontal disease; in the first instance the disease is limited and of no consequence, in the second the life of the dentition is threatened. It is essential therefore, to determine not only the presence or absence of periodontal disease but also its distribution within the dentition, and its severity in terms of active tissue destruction.

WHO PLAN OF ASSESSMENT

Types of studies

The World Health Organization in 1978, in a technical report on the epidemiology, aetiology and prevention of periodontal diseases [3], proposed that assessments of gingivitis, pocketing and number of erupted teeth constitute the basic data required for all types of studies of periodontal disease. Because plaque and gingivitis are so closely correlated, it was considered unnecessary to assess plaque in population studies and field trials. However, for clinical testing, the assessment of plaque may be needed, depending on the objective of the study. The assessment of calculus is required for studies of treatment need and for the purpose of evaluation but the WHO considered that as calculus is not of itself a disease it should not be included in disease status measurements.

[The remainder of this section is extracted, with permission, from WHO Technical Report Series, No. 621 (1978) Epidemiology, etiology, and prevention of periodontal diseases, pp. 29–43.]

CLINICAL TESTING

Clinical trials are carefully controlled investigations employing a wide range of procedures to test preventive or curative methods and to define their maximum effectiveness under the best possible conditions, before they are used in a community.

Longitudinal experimental studies in human beings are difficult, time-consuming, and often expensive. The choice of index systems to be used in connexion with clinical testing must be decided on in relation to the objectives of the trial, the size of the population, the period of study, and the type and extent of changes anticipated.

In studies of groups with relatively small amounts of plaque, the criteria of the oral hygiene index [4, 5] have usually proved too crude for demonstration of significant differences between study and control groups. When plaque is evaluated in relation to prevalence and severity of gingivitis, only the amount of plaque in contact with the gingival margins is of critical importance. One of the most accurate clinical methods of scoring bacterial colonization at the gingival margin in short-term trials is the use of the plaque index [6]. Its modification, the visible plaque index, is based on the number of tooth surfaces with clearly visible plaque. In personal oral hygiene education programmes, the progress of the individual patient has been successfully evaluated with charts showing the frequency of surfaces with stained plaque.

In long-term studies, the effects of plaque covering the tooth surfaces may be reliably estimated by determining the health status of gingival tissues. In a classical study on experimental gingivitis, the gingival index [7] was used to show that gingivitis developed after 10–21 days without mechanical oral hygiene measures. Gingivitis may also be assessed by the simpler method of recording only those gingival margins that bleed after gentle probing of the sulcus or pocket area.

If a clinical trial continues for several years, the effect of an agent or procedure may be evaluated by assessing the apical migration of the junctional epithelium, which, in most individuals, seems to be the deleterious end-result of plaque-induced inflammation. In such studies standardized radiographs are often valuable for measuring changes in the height of the alveolar crest.

It is essential to use standard methods of examination in clinical trials. The examiners should be familiar with the criteria and scoring procedure in order to avoid 'drift' during the progress of the study. Close cooperation with a statistician who has a knowledge of biology is desirable in the planning, execution, and evaluation of a research programme.

FIELD TRIALS

Field trials are demonstrations of the feasibility, acceptability, and effectiveness of preventive methods or curative programmes in a defined community. They may involve the training of local personnel in preventive procedures and the essential daily routines in applying them. In the main they test the chosen methods or programmes under real conditions. These trials are usually evaluated by examining random samples of the total population at different points in time rather than by making successive examinations of the same individuals.

A preventive or curative procedure evolved during clinical trials may undergo modifications during a field trial. The feasibility of a regimen, for example, may be shown to be poor because of its complexity, because of a poor cost/effectiveness ratio, or because of the lack of manpower resources to implement it. Acceptability may be low because the public dislike the offered treatment or because religious or cultural factors reduce participation in the programme.

In field trials the preventive or curative programmes are usually conducted by personnel with minimum training and experience who work within the existing system of oral health care. Sound scientific methods of sampling and measurement should be applied in field trials, and they should be applied just as stringently as in clinical testing. The extent of improved health and lowered disease incidence or prevalence determines whether the tested regimen should be incorporated into a routine national health care programme.

POPULATION STUDIES OF PERIODONTAL DISEASE STATUS

Population studies of periodontal disease status are surveys designed to collect descriptive data on the prevalence and distribution of the disease in various populations or subgroups and to evaluate preventive programmes. Such studies reveal only positive or negative associations between the occurrence of the disease and other observed characteristics. To establish causal relationships it is necessary to carry out specific analytical studies and to verify the results by means of experimental clinical and field trials.

DETERMINATION OF TREATMENT NEEDS AND EVALUATION OF EXISTING SERVICES

Surveys for the determination of treatment needs and the evaluation of existing services, which are made for planning purposes, can be based on the assessment of disease status.

For the assessment of disease status, only gingivitis and pocketing are measured, but, for the assessment of treatment needs, calculus is also measured. From these three clearly defined measurements, estimates of preventive and treatment services may be obtained.

The advantages, in terms of savings in cost and time, derived from this simple survey procedure can be enhanced by using the smallest valid sample compatible with the objectives of the study. 'Convenience' samples are often the only type possible in surveys in developing countries, and in such cases the 'pathfinder survey' is an important tool. In this type of survey a sample of 200–300 in a given age-group is often sufficient for the study objectives.

Assessment of periodontal diseases

During the past 20–30 years, many indices have been developed for recording the clinical signs associated with periodontal diseases. The majority were originally designed for a specific research project and were later adopted by other investigators. The multiplicity of indices has tended to inhibit the comparison of results from different studies.

Existing indices have been classified into opposing categories—i.e., reversible as opposed to irreversible indices, combined-feature as opposed to separate-feature indices, and indices based on severity gradings as opposed to indices that record only the presence or absence of a given clinical sign.

Although indices such as the periodontal disease index measure past periodontal disease experience, they do not give information about treatment needs and are therefore unsuitable for public health planning purposes.

In order to obtain comparable data from different parts of the world, it is logical to develop population survey criteria that conform to the scoring procedures used by both the private and the public health dentist. This rules out combined indices such as the periodontal index, which relies largely on visible signs of inflammation on the outer surface of the gingiva and on estimations of deep destruction of tooth attachment.

An alternative to combined indices is the separate scoring of gingival inflammation and pocket depth. In this respect the gingival index has proved valuable in demonstrating the role of plaque in the initiation and progression of gingivitis. However, it has been criticized for its use of severity gradings, because the supporting evidence is insufficient to justify calculation of mathematical means. Also, the more gradings an index system uses, the more difficult it is to achieve reproducibility at an acceptable level.

It would be an advantage if severity gradings could be avoided. Even if pocket depths are measured, one pocket 8 mm deep is certainly not equal in severity to two pockets 4 mm deep. The prevalence or distribution of 8 mm and 4 mm pockets in a population would give a more accurate picture of the situation.

A simple present/absent classification for recording clinical signs associated with periodontal diseases should be adopted only after criteria have been determined that provide valid indications of disease status and estimations of treatment requirements.

DENTAL PLAQUE

Microbial plaque is the primary aetiological

factor in periodontal disease. There is variation among individuals in host resistance; in some persons a small amount of plaque may cause severe disease while in others heavy plaque for decades will produce no major periodontal problem.

The amount of plaque present on tooth surfaces at a given time reflects an equilibrium between the rate of plaque formation and the rate of removal. Plaque scores, and the correlation between plaque and gingivitis, may thus be largely invalidated by an extra cleaning of the teeth before an oral examination. Plaque indices measure the current amounts of plaque resulting from recent oral hygiene activities rather than the usual amounts of microbial deposits. No index yet described includes subgingival plaque scores. This means that, even with a plaque index score of zero, there may be microbial colonization on the root surface in connexion with a periodontal pocket.

There is no reason to believe that the amount of plaque on teeth increases with advancing age. On the contrary, plaque scores have been observed to decrease with age in girls in their early adolescence, probably because of improved oral hygiene practices.

Though plaque scores may be of value in the instruction and motivation of individual patients, the consequences of the presence of plaque (i.e., actual periodontal diseases) are more important in population studies.

GINGIVAL INFLAMMATION

Many studies have shown that the amount of gingival inflammation provides a good estimation of the efficacy of recent oral hygiene measures. No improvement in gingival conditions can be achieved by an extra cleaning of the teeth prior to an examination. Since the amount of gingival inflammation inherently includes the effect of host resistance, the gingival condition may be a more valid criterion of need for improved oral hygiene measures than is the amount of plaque on the tooth surface. Moreover, the gingivae also react to the subgingival plaque, which is not measured by plaque scores and is not easy to assess.

The criteria most often used for gingival

health include pink colour, knife-edge-shaped margins, stippled surface, and firmness of the gingival tissue. These criteria are of great value for an experienced examiner performing longitudinal surveys or clinical trials in which the same individuals are scored and rescored after given periods of time. For the less experienced examiner, these signs may be difficult to observe and record consistently. Moreover, inflammatory reactions on the side of the gingival margin next to the tooth are often undetectable by looking solely at the clinical appearance of the outer gingival surface. Application of the usual criteria poses problems if populations are to be compared. Gingival inflammation cannot be accurately determined if the gingiva is pigmented, and blunt gingival margins lacking stippling may be perfectly healthy in some persons. On the other hand, the gingiva may even look and feel firm in spite of chronic inflammation in a deep pocket on the same tooth surface.

Both clinically and histologically the most appropriate sign of gingival health is absence of bleeding at gentle probing. It has been suggested that gingival bleeding is an earlier sign of gingivitis than is colour change. This seems logical because the inflammation begins on the dental side of the gingiva. Moreover, the use of gingival bleeding as an index is practical, because the pocket should be probed anyway to assess its depth and to record the presence or absence of subgingival calculus.

As with plaque, there is no reason to assume that the amount and severity of gingivitis increase with advancing age. They may even regress. Indeed, an improvement in gingival conditions after puberty and after parturition has been noted in women.

SUPRAGINGIVAL CALCULUS

Light-brown mineralized deposits frequently form on teeth located near the orifices of the major salivary ducts—i.e., lingual to the mandibular incisors and buccal to the maxillary first and second molars. Supragingival calculus normally extends coronally from the gingival margin, and only a small part may be in contact with the soft tissues.

However, because it is easily observed by dentists and patients, its removal often receives priority over that of the more deleterious subgingival calculus, and the latter form is commonly not even diagnosed.

SUBGINGIVAL CALCULUS

Dark-brown subgingival mineralized deposits form on the teeth in the gingival sulci or pockets. The location of subgingival calculus is not influenced by the position of salivary gland duct openings; rather its distribution follows the pattern of periodontal inflammation in individual dentitions.

The surface of subgingival calculus is almost covered with a layer of plaque. The plaque causes more inflammation and an increased flow of gingival fluid, which in turn may contribute to more calculus formation. Subgingival calculus is thus an important link in a causal chain; its diagnosis and removal are essential in the treatment of periodontal disease.

Subgingival calculus can be diagnosed most effectively by means of probing; there are no reliable signs to indicate the presence or absence of these deposits.

PERIODONTAL POCKETS

Pocket formation is a result of long-standing progressive gingival inflammation. Once formed, the periodontal pocket provides a sheltered environment for pathogenic microbial colonies, which may cause further connective-tissue destruction. Pockets 4 mm or more in depth have been regarded as being in need of periodontal treatment.

After surgical eradication of a deep pocket, the exposed root surface and the often bulky gingival margin should be accepted as signs of health as long as no inflammation is present at the gingival margin. Following treatment of periodontal pockets the epithelial attachment may be located more apically than it was formerly and an area of cementum may be exposed. The exposed root surface may be of epidemiological interest because it reflects past periodontal disease experience, but it should not be included in an assessment of further need for treatment. Reliable diagnosis of periodontal pockets can be made only by probing.

Proposed survey methodology

There is dissatisfaction with basic methods for the measurement of periodontal diseases and treatment requirements in populations, and the WHO have therefore proposed a new method of making surveys. The method must be tested against others that have been used to date, and it has been recommended that WHO proceed with this testing as rapidly as possible. If it proves satisfactory the method should be generally adopted.

AGE-GROUPS AND METHODS OF SCORING

It is recommended that results of periodontal assessments should be reported for four separate age-groups: 15–19, 20–29, 30–44, 45–64 years. However, not all these age-groups need necessarily be included in surveys, the choice being dependent on study objectives. Economic considerations may restrict the number of age-groups included in population studies, in which case 15–19 and 30–44 years are probably the groups most useful for planning. The four age-groups recommended are compatible with the WHO standard age-groupings, i.e., single years to 19, then 20–24, 25–29, 30–34, 35–44, 45–54, 55–64, and 65 years and over. However, some of these groups are spanned by the age-groups recommended by the Scientific Group, and data should be collected within the groupings recommended by single years, 5-year groups, or 10-year groups according to the WHO standard. The use of age-groups is recommended because it will provide information on variations with age in the development of periodontal disease.

Subjects younger than 15 years are not included because it is believed that periodontal status should be measured only in subjects with a full complement of fully erupted permanent teeth (excluding third molars). Assessments should not be made in tissues surrounding primary teeth. Fully edentulous persons should be excluded from comparisons of prevalence data, but the percentage of edentulous persons should be reported for each age-group. The mean number of erupted teeth should also be reported.

Various units of measurement for the assessment of periodontal status were considered. It was thought that, from a practical standpoint, findings either for segments or for selected representative teeth would be most suitable, and, in order to restrict probing for periodontal pockets to a minimum, a decision in favour of six teeth was made.

In the maxilla the scorings are made on the facial and mesial aspects of the right first molar, the left central incisor, and the left first premolar. In the mandible the scorings are made on the lingual and mesial aspects of the left first molar, the right central incisor, and the right first premolar. It is important to follow this sequence. The mesial surface is examined from the facial aspect in the maxillary teeth and from the lingual aspect in the mandibular teeth. A positive finding on any part of the designated tooth surfaces is recorded as a positive score for the tooth in question. If any of these teeth

are missing, the distal neighbouring teeth should be substituted.

With this method of partial recording, estimates of disease and treatment may be slightly overestimated or underestimated, but the simplification was considered essential for general population studies. Additional studies should be made to demonstrate the relationship between full and partial recording methods.

In the examination procedure a blunt periodontal probe is inserted gently into the pocket or sulcus of the designated tooth unit. The probe (see fig. 12.16, p. 188) has two principal graduations—one at 3·5 mm and one at 5·5 mm.

The assessments made, in sequence, are the presence or absence of supragingival or subgingival calculus, the depth of the gingival pocket (fig. 16.1a) and the presence or absence of bleeding after probing.

CALCULUS

If calculus is clearly visible and in contact with

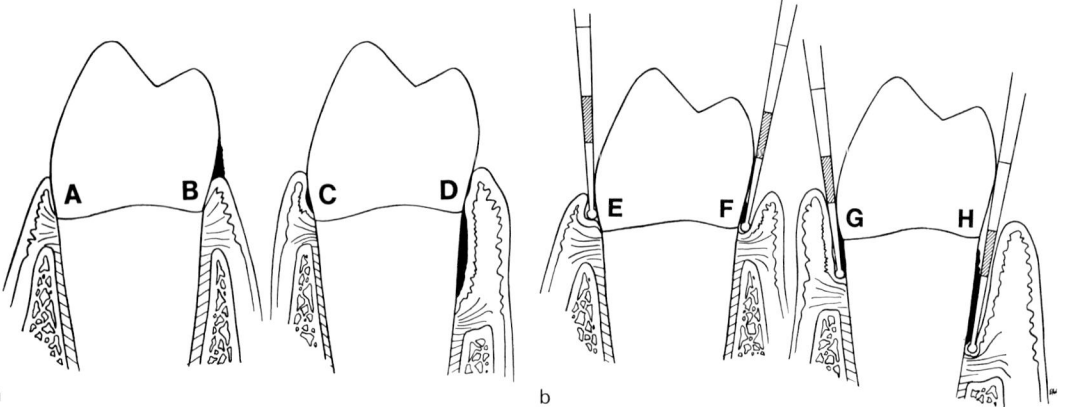

FIG. 16.1. Cross-section of teeth showing (a) supra and subgingival calculus and periodontal pocket: (b) correct probing angles for detecting subgingival calculus and measuring pocket depth.
A. Healthy gingival margin with sulcus depth less than 3·5 mm.
B. Clinically visible supragingival calculus in contact with the gingival margin.
C. Clinically invisible subgingival dental calculus. Pocket less than 3·5 mm.
D. Deepened periodontal pocket with deposition of subgingival calculus.
E. Periodontal probe gently inserted into the healthy gingival sulcus.
F. Periodontal probe gently inserted into shallow pocket with subgingival calculus. Bleeding may occur after probing.
G. Periodontal probe gently inserted into pocket deeper than 3·5 mm. The tooth scores 1 for calculus and pocketing, and probably for gingival bleeding.
H. Periodontal probe gently inserted into a pocket deeper than 5·5 mm. Tooth scores 1 for calculus, 2 for pocketing and, if bleeding follows, 1 for gingivitis.
[Reprinted, with permission, from WHO Technical Report Series No. 261 (1978)]

the gingival margin on any part of the assigned surface, a score of 1 is recorded for the tooth. If calculus is not visible the subgingival tooth surface is probed for calculus. Following the anatomic configuration of the root of the tooth surface (fig. 16.1b), the end of the periodontal probe is gently inserted between the tooth and the gingiva until the resistance of the supra-alveolar fibjes is felt. The force applied should not exceed the weight of the probe, which should be held lightly so that there is no blanching of the thumbnail. 'Gentle probing' should not cause pain when performed on the back of the hand. In the mandibular areas the weight of the probe itself is in many cases sufficient. The form or colour of the gingiva often indicates where subgingival calculus is to be found. Multiple probings may be indicated at a specific surface. As soon as an obvious calculus deposit is felt, a score of 1 is recorded for the tooth. If neither supragingival nor subgingival calculus is found on the surface being examined, the tooth score is 0.

It was not considered necessary to have a measure of the quantity of calculus for each of the six teeth because severity can to some extent be estimated from the number of examined teeth that have calculus.

MEASUREMENT OF POCKET DEPTH

Probing for calculus gives an indication of the presence or absence of a deepened periodontal pocket. An examination of pocket depth is made and recorded according to the following criteria:

    0 = clinical gingival sulcus of 3·5 mm or less
    1 = pockets greater than 3·5 mm and less than or equal to 5·5 mm
    2 = pockets greater than 5·5 mm.

Multiple probings may again be indicated. All pocket depths are to be measured from the gingival margins. The deepest pocket found on the surface determines the score to be assigned to the tooth. According to this classification, gingival sulci with scores of 0 are regarded as free of periodontitis. Pockets with a score of 1 can often be kept free of gingivitis, and loss of additional apical migration of the junctional epithelium can be prevented if plaque and calculus are controlled.

Teeth with a score of 2 usually require more complex treatment.

ASSESSMENT OF GINGIVITIS

When all six teeth have been probed for calculus and pockets, the same teeth are re-examined in the same sequence (starting from the maxillary right molar) to ascertain whether the probing has resulted in obvious bleeding from the gingival pocket or sulcus. Only a mouth mirror is used for this assessment. If evidence of bleeding is detected, the score for the tooth is 1; if no bleeding is detected, the score is 0.

ASSESSMENT OF GINGIVAL RECESSION

In addition to the essential measurements already described, gingival recession may be measured as an indication of past disease or of treatment already provided. However, the value of collecting this information should be assessed after an initial period of use. The following scores are to be recorded:

    0 = root exposure of 3·5 mm or less
    1 = root exposure of more than 3·5 mm but less than or equal to 5·5 mm
    2 = root exposure of more than 5·5 mm.

These intervals were selected largely because they conform to those used for measuring pockets. Recession is to be measured from the cemento-enamel junction to the gingival margin.

TOOTH MOBILITY

No measure of mobility of teeth has been included in the proposed method because it is believed that there are no generally available procedures for stabilizing mobile teeth. Mobile teeth may still function adequately for an indefinite period.

Requirements for prevention and treatment

The measurements of subgingival calculus, gingivitis, and periodontal pocketing can each be related to services required. The requirements vary with age even for similar levels of disease, the need for services to deal with gingivitis in particular being greater for adolescents and young adults owing to the importance of preventing periodontitis at those ages.

Thus, according to the recommended method:

(1) gingivitis scores indicate the need for oral hygiene education,

(2) calculus or shallow pocketing scores indicate the need for scaling in the affected quadrant(s) and oral hygiene education,

(3) deep pocketing scores indicate the need for complex care, which may comprise deep scaling and/or surgery in any age-groups, and for oral hygiene education.

The nature of the dental services available and the estimated time required to deliver them on an individual basis depend on a number of factors. The most important are the attitudes and behaviour of the population, the type of manpower, the type of equipment, the approach to oral hygiene education, and the actual treatment procedures. It is essential to have an estimate of the anticipated success of these treatments and their impact on the overall prevalence of disease in a population. The recommendations must naturally be adapted to local circumstances and possibilities and directed to the groups most in need.

Given these sources of variation, the WHO Expert Committee considered the limited data available and the experience of periodontists and public health dentists to reach preliminary working estimates for the guidance of planners. These estimates are given in Table 16.1. It was not possible to assess such variables as type of dental manpower, available equipment, and the attitude of the population to periodontal diseases and treatment needs. The WHO Expert Group stressed the need to test these estimates and pointed out that each planner should be prepared to adjust them according to local factors.

TABLE 16.1. Estimate of mean time required to provide periodontal services

Age-group (years)	Positive score for	Service	Time required
15–19	Gingivitis	Oral hygiene education (OHE)	60 min
	Calculus or shallow pockets	Scaling + OHE initial follow-up	15 min + 10 min/quadrant + 50 min for OHE 15 min + 5 min/quadrant + 10 min for OHE
	Deep pockets	Deep scaling + OHE initial follow-up	45 min/quadrant + 50 min for OHE 10 min/quadrant + 10 min for OHE
		Surgery	60 min/quadrant + 30 min postoperative care
20–29	Treatment as for age-group 15–19 except that the time required for initial scaling is 15 min/quadrant.		
30–44	Gingivitis	Oral hygiene education (OHE)	10 min
	Calculus or shallow pockets	Scaling + OHE initial follow-up	15 min + 30 min/quadrant + 50 min for OHE 15 min + 5 min/quadrant + 10 min for OHE
	Deep pockets	Deep scaling + OHE initial follow-up	45 min/quadrant + 50 min for OHE 10 min/quadrant + 10 min for OHE
		Surgery	60 min/quadrant + 30 min postoperative care
45 and over	Gingivitis	Oral hygiene education (OHE)	10 min
	Calculus or shallow pockets	Scaling + OHE initial follow-up	15 min + 30 min/quadrant + 50 min for OHE 15 min + 5 min/quadrant + 10 min for OHE
	Deep pockets	Deep scaling + OHE initial follow-up	45 min/quadrant + 50 min for OHE 10 min/quadrant + 10 min for OHE
		Surgery	60 min/quadrant + 30 min postoperative care

All the estimates given in the table are based on quadrants rather than segments because most of the data available have been developed on that basis. It is stressed that, for every population surveyed, an estimate of prevention potential and its effect on reducing the need for follow-up services must be made. The times given in the table allow the administrator to work out the total time to be allowed for initial and follow-up treatments of each subject and to decide on the period necessary between treatment and follow-up. This allows him to estimate the manpower requirements in any one year. As a guideline, follow-up for reinforcement of oral hygiene and removal of retention factors will on average require an estimated 10 minutes for oral hygiene education and 5 minutes per quadrant for scaling per annum.

Planners should decide which age-group and category of disease severity should have the highest priority so that treatment categories can be allocated according to the resources available. For example, it may be considered unnecessary to provide oral hygiene education and scaling for those persons aged 45 years and over who have only gingivitis and shallow pockets, because their chances of maintaining their teeth without treatment are good. Alternatively, it may be decided that a particular age-group will receive treatment only if the mean periodontal score is above a certain (arbitrary) level or that services will be restricted by some other criterion such as risk or demand.

INDICES

Study of the epidemiology of periodontal disease requires precise criteria which can be applied when determining and recording the periodontal status of the individuals being studied. Indices are used to express clinical observations or measurements in terms of numerical values, which can be used for quantitating and evaluating the factors being studied. Many indices have been described and although reproducibility varies to some extent in relation to the precision of the criteria laid down, they have provided valuable data regarding many epidemiologic aspects of periodontal disease.

Gingival index, GI [7]

This index is designed to assess the type, severity and location of gingival disease. The circumference of the gingival margin is divided into four areas (mesial, distal, buccal and lingual). Each of the four areas is scored from zero to three according to the following criteria:

0–Normal gingiva.

1–Mild inflammation, slight change in colour, slight oedema; no bleeding on probing.

2–Moderate inflammation; redness, oedema and glazing; bleeding on probing.

3–Severe inflammation; marked redness and oedema; ulceration; spontaneous bleeding.

The scores for the various areas of each tooth are added and divided by four to determine the GI for the tooth.

By adding all the figures and dividing by the number of teeth in the mouth the GI for the individual can be determined.

PERIODONTAL INDEX, PI [8]

This index has been widely used, and enables quantitative assessment of the more advanced stages of tissue destruction, as well as the presence of gingivitis. In determining the PI, the status of the periodontium of each tooth is scored as follows:

0–Negative. There is neither overt inflammation of the investing tissues nor loss of function due to destruction of supporting tissues.

1–Mild gingivitis. There is an overt area of inflammation in the free gingiva but this area does not circumscribe the tooth.

2–Gingivitis. Inflammation completely circumscribes the tooth but there is no apparent break in the epithelial attachment.

6–Gingivitis with pocket formation. The epithelial attachment has been broken and there is a pocket (not merely a deepened gingival crevice due to swelling in free gingiva). There is no interference with normal masticatory function, the tooth is firm and has not drifted.

8–Advanced destruction with loss of masticatory function. The tooth may be loose; may have drifted; may sound dull on percussion with a metal instrument; may be depressible in its socket.

When there is doubt the lower score is assigned.

The PI for a given mouth is the sum of the scores for individual teeth divided by the number of teeth examined. Most persons with a clinical diagnosis of gingivitis score from 0·1 to 1·0; those with well established periodontitis score from 1·5 to 5·0; and those with terminal periodontitis from about 4·0 to 8·0.

PERIODONTAL DISEASE INDEX, PDI [9]

This index depends on assessment of gingivitis and measurement of the distance by which the bottom of the gingival sulcus extends apically beyond the cemento-enamel junction. It can record, therefore, both reversible changes of gingivitis and irreversible changes of periodontitis.

SIMPLIFIED ORAL HYGIENE INDEX, OHI-S [4]

This index is used as a measure of oral uncleanliness and usually six tooth surfaces are scored: buccal surfaces of upper first molars, the lingual surfaces of lower first molars, and the labial surfaces of the upper right and lower left central incisors. Each surface is scored for soft debris and for calculus respectively.

Criteria for scoring oral debris
(debris index score DI-S)

0–No deris or stain present.
1–Soft debris covering not more than $\frac{1}{3}$ of the tooth surface, or the presence of extrinsic stains without other debris regardless of surface area covered.
2–Soft debris covering more than $\frac{1}{3}$ but not more than $\frac{2}{3}$ of the exposed tooth surface
3–Soft debris covering more than $\frac{2}{3}$ of the exposed tooth surface.

Criteria for scoring calculus
(calculus index score, CI-S)

0–No calculus present.

1–Supragingival calculus covering not more than $\frac{1}{3}$ of the exposed tooth surface.
2–Supragingival calculus covering more than $\frac{1}{3}$ but not more than $\frac{2}{3}$ of the exposed tooth surface or the presence of individual flecks of subgingival calculus around the cervical portion of the tooth, or both.
3–Supragingival calculus covering more than $\frac{2}{3}$ of the exposed tooth surface or a continuous heavy band of subgingival calculus around the cervical portion of tooth, or both.

The mean debris index score plus the mean calculus score gives the OHI-S.

Plaque index, P1I [6]

This index is obtained in the same way as the Gingival Index, except that plaque is scored instead of the condition of the gingiva, using the following criteria:

0–No plaque in the gingival area.
1–A film adhering to the free gingival margin and adjacent area of the tooth. The plaque may only be recognized by running a probe across the tooth surface.
2–Moderate accumulation of soft deposits within the gingival pocket, on the gingival margin and/or adjacent tooth surface which can be seen by the naked eye.
3–Abundance of soft matter within the gingival pocket and/or on the gingival margin and adjacent tooth surface.

CAUSES OF TOOTH LOSS

Study of the literaure reveals that a number of different approaches have been used to obtain information about the loss of teeth in a population. Some investigators have used full mouth radiographs and recorded the number of teeth and the tooth types present in the mouth. Others have used clinical examination at the time of extraction. Another method which has been used is to examine the patient and record teeth that must be extracted, at the same time noting the reason for the extraction. Table 16.2 summarizes the findings of a number of studies on the causes of the tooth loss. The majority of studies were carried out in the

TABLE 16.2. Causes of tooth loss.

No. of teeth	No. of patients	Caries %	Periodontal disease %	Prosthetic reasons %	Other reasons %	Country	Reference No.
13909	2723	51·42	32·2	13·0	3·38	U.S.A.	10
1424	353	48·8	40·7	2·8	7·7	U.S.A.	11
7109	2337	39·7	20·2	20·2	20·1	U.S.A.	12
18030	4278	26·7	66·3	1·7	5·3	India	13
2411	805	38·3	36·0	3·5	22·2	U.S.A.	14
2008 Males	463	30·2	29·2	29·6		U.S.A.	15
1970 Females	567	30·2	17·9	34·9		U.S.A.	
4563	1813	61·0	21·7	8·1	9·2 ·	Canada	16
2816	Not given	86·9	4·9	1·6		Israel	17
5486	2302	50·0	30·0			Denmark	18
34456	17595	47·1	11·1	33·8	7·9	Sweden	19

United States of America, but two were undertaken in Scandinavia and one in India. It can be seen that caries and periodontal disease are the princpal causes for tooth loss, although a considerable difference exists between percentages recorded in the various studies. This is probably due to the fact that few authors have recorded, at the time of removal, the precise cause for extraction of an individual tooth. It is well-known that periodontal disease increases in severity with increasing age (vice infra), thus a direct comparison of the reports on periodontal disease as the cause of tooth extraction is impossible without taking the age groups studied into account. It is clear that if the majority of the patients in one report are of a young age group, periodontal disease would be of minor importance. If comparison is to be made between different groups, it is of the utmost importance that groups having similar age and sex should be compared. Another major problem relates to the defining of criteria for extraction.

Having reviewed the available data, it was the view of Waerhaug [20] that in developed countries extractions due to periodontal disease amount to somewhat less than 40 per cent and dental caries something more than 40 per cent of the total loss. About 10 per cent of the teeth are extracted for prosthetic reasons (periodontal disease is probably indirectly responsible for the loss of some of these teeth). In less well developed countries, the figure for extractions due to

periodontal disease has been calculated to be 66 per cent, and after age 30, the percentage is high as 80 per cent. Within reasonable limits these figures may be taken as indicative of the conditions in the less developed countries. Waerhaug considered that as two-thirds of the world population live in countries comparable to India, on a world wide basis, periodontal disease is the most important cause of tooth loss.

In the event that the marked loss of teeth due to dental caries in the younger age groups in developed countries be reduced significantly by preventive measures, the number of teeth at risk to periodontal disease will increase markedly. Thus, periodontal disease is a public health problem of enormous magnitude both for the individual patient and for the community.

Following a national study into adult dental health in Scotland, Todd and Whitworth [21] drew attention to the fact that teeth are not always extracted for reasons of disease. They suggested that the dentist's attitude, the patient's attitude and technical problems associated with the provision of treatment, carry more weight than is often allowed for in the assessment of reasons for tooth loss.

Localization of periodontal disease within the dentition

Gingivitis and periodontitis are most pronounced in the interdental regions and least obvious on the buccal or labial surfaces [22 & 23]. The same distribution largely holds true for the accumulation of bacterial plaque and calculus, showing the close association between these deposits and clinical signs of disease. The most severe gingivitis and pocket formation occurs around the incisors and first and second molars, with the pre-molars and canines being least affected. The first teeth to be extracted because of periodontal disease are usually the first molars [24].

Prevalence of periodontal disease

If deviation from perfect health is used as a measure, practically all human beings have periodontal disease. Severity varies widely from continent to continent, country to country and from community to community. Within a community there may be variations in severity associated with age, sex, socioeconomic status, presence of systemic disease, use of tobacco, stress and other factors.

Correlation of periodontal disease with age

There is little reliable data on the pre-school child [25] but by the age of fourteen, virtually all children show some gingivitis. In the zero to four year age group it has been shown that approximately 10 per cent of children have some gingivitis [26]. Both the prevalence and severity increase with age, with a sharp rise at 7–8 years associated with the loss of deciduous teeth and the eruption of the permanent dentition [27]. There appears to be an increase in prevalence and severity of gingivitis at the time of puberty and following this, there seems to be a slight decline in prevalence with a greater decline in severity [28]. The prevalence of gingivitis in 13–14 year olds has been reported in several studies to be greater than 99 per cent [29 & 30]. Fourteen per cent of 13 year olds have been shown to have periodontitis in addition to gingivitis. The prevalence of pocketing was reported to increase with increasing age, being 36 per cent at 17 years [30], 48 per cent at 19, 75 per cent at 24 and 97 per cent at 34 years [31]. One study has shown that the average individual aged 19 years had pockets around 6·5 per cent of teeth. This percentage increased to 23 per cent of teeth in 29 year olds, 52 per cent in 39 year olds, 82 per cent at 49 and 88 per cent at 65 years of age [32]. In a further survey, 23 per cent of 29 year olds were found to be in the terminal stages of periodontal disease and about to lose their teeth; 46 per cent of 39, 79 per cent of 49 and 95 per cent of 59 year olds were similarly affected [33]. It may be concluded that in the majority of persons, the break-down of the periodontal tissues progresses in approximately linear fashion from the late teens throughout life [34].

The strong correlation between periodontal destruction and age suggests that age per se might be an important aetiological factor. A close correlation, however, does not necessarily indicate a causal relationship. The effect of age might simply be to afford sufficiently prolonged exposure of the periodontium to pathogenic factors in bacterial deposits. Few studies have thoroughly investigated the direct effect of ageing on the health of the periodontal tissues and further work is clearly necessary in this field. One study has been reported [35] of 60 dentate women aged from 66 to 89 years with the object of determining whether periodontal disease was more highly correlated with chronologic age (reflecting length of exposure to various aetiologic agents plus intrinsic host changes with age). The hypothesis being tested was that individuals showing greater biologic ageing in respect to their chronologic age would also show a greater extent or severity of periodontal disease than those individuals appearing 'biologically younger'. It was found that gingival recession and loss of gingival attachment were significantly more highly correlated with an estimate of biologic age than chronologic age.

Influence of sex

In virtually all surveys carried out in Europe and North America [36], the periodontal condition of females has been found to be significantly better than males. When the oral hygiene status is compared, however, females are found to be considerably better than males [37]. Thus, when comparisons are made between males and females of the same age and oral hygiene status, no difference is found between them.

Influence of oral hygiene

Regardless of whether gingivitis, periodontitis, or bone destruction is measured, there is a strong correlation between the severity of these conditions and oral hygiene. Provided that the sample is sufficiently large, the correlation between PI and OHI is very close to linear and only age shows an equally strong correlation [38 & 39].

In numerous surveys carried out by different investigators in many areas of the world, the correlation of increasing oral uncleanliness and age, with increasing prevalence and severity of periodontal disease has clearly been demonstrated to such an extent that significant contributions by other factors may be masked [40]. When group data have been equalized for oral hygiene and age, in statistical analyses, no correlation has yet been established between periodontal index (PI) and geography, water fluoride levels, race, blood groupings, sex, molar attrition, total serum protein, haemoglobin, socioeconomic factors, or nutritional status with respect of vitamin A, ascorbic acid, thiamine, riboflavin, or nicotinamide. It should be noted, however, that these surveys concerned groups of ambulatory subjects, presumably without gross nutritional deficiencies or obvious systemic diseases predisposing to periodontal disease (see chap. 13). Until now, nearly all surveys have depended on a single examination of each subject. Consequently, they have had to make the assumption, not necessarily valid, that a cross section of present status is an accurate representation of accumulated past and expected future experience of all age groups.

The close relationship between OHI, PI and age has been analyzed for multiple and partial correlations in two different studies of Vietnamese and Lebanese populations. In either statistical array or in the two considered as one, less than 10 per cent of the variance in group PI scores remained to be explained after the combined influence of age and oral uncleanliness had been estimated [41]. In other words, residual factors wholly independent of age and oral hygiene, unless masked, would be expected to have little effect on periodontal disease as scored by these indices in these populations. The fact that the correlations were essentially unchanged when the two arrays were considered as one makes this analysis particularly significant, since each array was a composite of a number of unlike populations, differing ethnologically, culturally, nutritionally and socioeconomically [41]. As previously pointed out, however, it is a truism of statistical analysis that a close correlation is not necessarily a causal relationship. It could be argued that progressive accumulation of bacterial deposits is incidental to the progress of periodontal disease simply because conditions in a periodontal pocket favour microbial growth and mineralization. If this were so, treatment designed to minimize plaque deposition and to remove calculus periodically should not avert the onset of periodontal disease nor should it have an effect on established periodontal disease. A number of studies have shown that this is not the case and have clearly shown the clinical value of prevention or removal of bacterial deposits [22, 42–45].

The very high correlation between age, level of periodontal disease (as assessed by loss of attachment) and oral hygiene was not confirmed, however, in a study of an adult population in the United States [46]. It was found that the combined effects of age, debris, and calculus were sufficient to account statistically for only about 42 per cent of the variability in gingivitis scores. Their coefficient of multiple correlation was 0·65. With attachment loss as the dependent variable and age, debris, calculus and gingivitis scores as independent variables, the coefficient of multiple correlation was 0·57 accounting for about 32 per cent of the variability in attachment loss scored. Comparisons with the data presented by Russell and his co-workers [41] cannot be made precisely because the periodontal status of the American adults was represented by one figure for gingival inflammation and a futher figure for attachment loss, which was not the case in Russell's study. It is clear that further work will be required on this important problem to clarify the role of factors other than age and oral hygiene in the aetiology and severity of periodontal disease.

REFERENCES

[1] WORLD HEALTH ORGANIZATION (1961) Report No. 207, Periodontal Disease. Geneva, W.H.O.

[2] WILKINSON F.C., ADAMSON K.T. & KNIGHT F. (1929) A study of the incidence of dental disease in the Aborigines, from the examination of 65 skulls in the collection found in the Melbourne University. *Aust. J. Dent.* **33**, 109.

[3] WORLD HEALTH ORGANIZATION (1978) Epidemiology, etiology, and prevention of periodontal diseases. *Technical Reprrt Series No. 621.* Geneva, W.H.O.

[4] GREENE J.C. & VERMILLION J.R. (1960) Oral hygiene index: a method of classifying oral hygiene status. *J. Amer. dent. Ass.* **61**, 172.

[5] GREENE J.C. & VERMILLION J.R. (1964) *Journal of the American Dental Association,* **68**, 7–13.

[6] SILNESS J. & LÖE H. (1964) Periodontal disease in pregnancy: II. Correlation between oral hygiene and periodontal condition. *Acta odont. scand.* **22**, 121.

[7] LÖE H. & SILNESS J. (1963) Periodontal disease in prenancy. I. Prevalence and severity. *Acta odont. scand.* **21**, 533.

[8] RUSSELL A.L. (1956) A system of classification and scoring for prevalence surveys of periodontal disease. *J. dent. Res.* **35**, 350.

[9] RAMFJORD S. P. (1959) Indices for the prevalence and incidence of periodontal disease. *J. Periodont.* **30**, 51.

[10] BREKHUS P. J. (1929) Dental disease and its relation to the loss of human teeth. *J. Amer. dent. Ass.* **16**, 2237.

[11] ALLEN E.F. (1944) Statistical study of primary causes of extractions. *J. dent. Res.* **23**, 453.

[12] KROGH H.W. (1958) Permanent tooth mortality: A clinical study of causes of loss. *J. Amer. dent. Ass.* **57**, 670.

[13] MEHTA F.S., SANJANA M.K., SHROFF B.C. & DOCTOR R.H. (1958) Relative importance of the various causes of tooth loss. *J. All India dent. Ass.* **30**, 211.

[14] ANDREWS G. & KROGH H.W. (1961) Permanent tooth mortality. *Dent. Progr.* **1**, 130.

[15] GREWE J.M., GORLIN R.J. & MESKIN L.H. (1966) Human tooth mortality: a clinical-statistical study. *J. Amer. dent. Ass.* **72**, 106.

[16] TROTT J.R. & CROSS H.G. (1966) Analysis of the principle reasons for tooth extractions in 1,813 patients in Manitoba. *Dent. Pract. (Bristol),* **17**, 20.

[17] ABRAMOWSKY Z.L. & BUCHNER A. (1967) Causes of tooth extraction. II. A statistical study. *New York J. Dent.* **37**, 16.

[18] BAY I. & GAD T. (1967) Causes of tooth mortality in Denmark. *J. periodont. Res.* **2**, 246.

[19] LUNDQVIST C. (1967) Tooth mortality in Sweden. A statistical survey of tooth loss in the Swedish population. *Acta odont. scand.* **25**, 298.

[20] WAERHAUG J. (1966) *World Workshop in Periodontics,* p. 192.

[21] TODD J.E. & WHITWORTH A. (1974) *Adult Dental Health in Scotland 1972.* London: HMSO.

[22] LÖE H., THEILADE E. & JENSEN B.S. (1965) Experimental gingivitis in man. *J. Periodont.* **36**, 177.

[23] LOVDAL A., ARNO A. & WAERHAUG J. (1958) Incidence of clinical manifestations of periodontal disease in light of oral hygiene and calculus formation. *J. Amer. dent. Ass.* **56**, 21.

[24] SCHEI O., WAERHAUG J., LOVDAL A. & ARNO A. (1959) Alveolar bone loss as related to oral hygiene and age. *J. Periodont.* **30**, 7.

[25] MACKLER S.B. & CRAWFORD J.J. (1973) Plaque development and gingivitis in the primary dentition. *J. Periodont.* **44**, 18.

[26] BARROS L. & WITKOP C.J. JR. (1963) Oral and genetic study of Chileans 1960. III. Periodontal disease and nutritional factors. *Arch. oral Biol.* **8**, 195.

[27] MASSLER M., SCHOUR I. & CHOPRA B. (1950) Occurrence of gingivitis in suburban Chicago school children. *J. Periodont.* **21**, 146.

[28] PARFITT G.J. (1957) A five year longitudinal study of the gingival condition of a group of children in England. *J. Periodont.* **28**, 26.

[29] MCHUGH W.D., MCEWAN J.D. & HITCHIN A.D. (1964) Dental disease and related factors in thirteen year old children in Dundee. *Brit. dent. J.* **117**, 246.

[30] SHEIHAM A. (1969) The prevalence and severity of periodontal disease in Surrey school children. *Dent. Pract. (Bristol),* **19**, 232.

[31] SHEIHAM A. (1969) The prevalence and severity of periodontal disease in British populations. Dental surveys of employed populations in Great Britain. *Brit. Dent. J.* **126**, 115.

[32] SHEIHAM A. (1971) Dental epidemiological survey of a Northern Ireland population. Dental caries and periodontal disease findings. *J. Irish. dent. Ass.* **17**, 150.

[33] SHEIHAM A. (1971) Prevention and control of periodontal disease. *Dental Health,* **10**, 1.

[34] WAERHAUG J. (1971) Epidemiology of periodontal disease, in *The Prevention of Periodontal Disease.* Eds. Eastoe J.E., Picton D.C.A. & Alexander A.G. p. 5. London: Henry Kimpton.

[35] HANSEN G.C. (1973) An epidemiologic investigation of the effect of biologic ageing on the break-down of periodontal tissue. *J. Periodont.* **44**, 269.

[36] KELLY J.E. & VAN KIRK L.E. (1965) Periodontal disease in adults. *Vital Health Statistics,* **12**, 1.

[37] KELLY J.E., VAN KIRK L.E. & GARST C.C. (1966) Oral hygiene in adults. *Vital Health Statistics,* **11**, 1.

[38] WAERHAUG J. (1967) Prevalence of periodontal disease in Ceylon. *Acta odont. scand.* **25**, 205.

[39] SHEIHAM A. (1970) Dental cleanliness and chronic periodontal disease. Studies on populations in Britain. *Brit. dent. J.* **129**, 413.

[40] BURNETT G.W. & SCHERP H.W. (1969) *Oral Microbiology and Infectious Disease.* 3rd Edn. p. 414. Baltimore: Williams and Wilkins.

[41] RUSSELL A.L. (1963) International nutrition surveys: a summary of preliminary dental findings. *J. dent. Res.* **42**, 233.

[42] LOVDAL A., ARNO A., SCHEI O. & WAERHAUG J. (1961) Combined oral hygiene on the incidence of gingivitis. *Acta. odont. scand.* **19,** 537.

[43] SUOMI J.D., GREENE J.C., VERMILLION J.R., DOYLE J., CHANG J.J. & LEATHERWOOD E.C. (1971) The effect of controlled oral hygiene procedures on the progression of periodontal disease in adults; results after third and final year. *J. Periodont.* **42,** 152.

[44] SUOMI J.D., LEATHERWOOD E.C. & CHANG J.C. (1973) A follow up study of former participants in a controlled and hygiene study. *J. Periodont.* **44,** 662–666.

[45] LIGHTNER L.M., O'LEARY T.J., DRAKE R.B., CRUMP P.P. & ALLEN M.F. (1971) Preventive periodontitis treatment procedures: results over 46 months. *J. Periodont.* **42,** 555.

[46] SUOMI J.D. & DOYLE J. (1972) Oral hygiene and periodontal disease in an adult population in the United States. *J. Periodont.* **43,** 677.

Index